CRC SERIES IN NUTRITION AND FOOD

Editor-in-Chief

Miloslav Rechcigl, Jr.

Handbook of Nutritive Value of
Processed Food
Volume I: Food For Human Use
Volume II: Animal Feedstuffs

Handbook of Nutritional Requirements
in a Functional Context
Volume I: Development and Conditions
of Physiologic Stress
Volume II: Hematopoiesis, Metabolic
Function, and Resistance to
Physical Stress

Handbook of Agricultural Productivity
Volume I: Plant Productivity
Volume II: Animal Productivity

Handbook of Naturally Occurring
Food Toxicants

Handbook of Foodborne Diseases
of Biological Origin

Handbook of Nutritional Supplements
Volume I: Human Use
Volume II: Agricultural Use

HANDBOOK SERIES

Nutritional Requirements
Volume I: Comparative and
Qualitative Requirements

Nutritional Disorders
Volume I: Effect of Nutrient
Excesses and Toxicities in Animal
and Man
Volume II: Effect of Nutrient
Deficiencies in Animals
Volume III: Effect of Nutrient
Deficiencies in Man

Diets, Culture Media, Food
Supplements
Volume I: Diets for Mammals
Volume II: Food Habits of, and
Diets for Invertebrates and
Vertebrates — Zoo Diets
Volume III: Culture Media for
Microorganisms and Plants
Volume IV: Culture Media for
Cells, Organs and Embryos

CRC Handbook of Naturally Occurring Food Toxicants

Editor

Miloslav Rechcigl, Jr.
Nutrition Advisor and Chief
Research and Methodology Division
Agency for International Development
U.S. International Development Cooperation Agency
Washington, D.C.

CRC Series in Nutrition and Food
Editor-in-Chief
Miloslav Rechcigl, Jr.

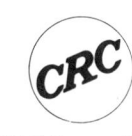

CRC Press, Inc.
Boca Raton, Florida

Library of Congress Cataloging in Publication Data

Main entry under title:

Handbook of Naturally occurring food toxicants.

  (CRC series in nutrition and food)
  Bibliography: p.
  Includes index.
  1. Food—Analysis. 2. Food poisoning.
I. Rechcigl, Miloslav. II. Title. C.R.C. handbook
of naturally occurring food toxicants. III. Series.
TX531.H286   1983   615.9′54   82-9551
ISBN 0-8493-3965-0

This book represents information obtained from authentic and highly regarded sources. Reprinted material is quoted with permission, and sources are indicated. A wide variety of references are listed. Every reasonable effort has been made to give reliable data and information, but the author and the publisher cannot assume responsibility for the validity of all materials or for the consequences of their use.

All rights reserved. This book, or any parts thereof, may not be reproduced in any form without written consent from the publisher.

Direct all inquiries to CRC Press, Inc., 2000 Corporate Blvd., N.W., Boca Raton, Florida, 33431.

© 1983 by CRC Press, Inc.

International Standard Book Number 0-8493-3965-0

Library of Congress Card Number 82-9551
Printed in the United States

PREFACE
CRC SERIES IN NUTRITION AND FOOD

Nutrition means different things to different people, and no other field of endeavor crosses the boundaries of so many different disciplines and abounds with such diverse dimensions. The growth of the field of nutrition, particularly in the last 2 decades, has been phenomenal, the nutritional data being scattered literally in thousands and thousands of not always accessible periodicals and monographs, many of which, furthermore, are not normally identified with nutrition.

To remedy this situation, we have undertaken an ambitious and monumental task of assembling in one publication all the critical data relevant in the field of nutrition.

The *CRC Series in Nutrition and Food* is intended to serve as a ready reference source of current information on experimental and applied human, animal, microbial, and plant nutrition presented in concise tabular, graphical, or narrative form and indexed for ease of use. It is hoped that this projected open-ended multivolume compendium will become for the nutritionist what the *CRC Handbook of Chemistry and Physics* has become for the chemist and physicist.

Apart from supplying specific data, the comprehensive, interdisciplinary, and comparative nature of the *CRC Series in Nutrition and Food* will provide the user with an easy overview of the state of the art, pinpointing the gaps in nutritional knowledge and providing a basis for further research. In addition, the series will enable the researcher to analyze the data in various living systems for commonality or basic differences. On the other hand, an applied scientist or technician will be afforded the opportunity of evaluating a given problem and its solutions from the broadest possible point of view, including the aspects of agronomy, crop science, animal husbandry, aquaculture and fisheries, veterinary medicine, clinical medicine, pathology, parasitology, toxicology, pharmacology, therapeutics, dietetics, food science and technology, physiology, zoology, botany, biochemistry, developmental and cell biology, microbiology, sanitation, pest control, economics, marketing, sociology, anthropology, natural resources, ecology, environmental science, population, law politics, nutritional and food methodology, and others.

To make more facile use of the series, the publication has been organized into separate handbooks of one or more volumes each. In this manner the particular sections of the series can be continuously updated by publishing additional volumes of new data as they become available.

The Editor wishes to thank the numerous contributors many of whom have undertaken their assignment in pioneering spirit, and the Advisory Board members for their continuous counsel and cooperation. Last but not least, he wishes to express his sincere appreciation to the members of the CRC editorial and production staffs, particularly President Bernard J. Starkoff, Earl Starkoff, Sandy Pearlman, Amy G. Skallerup, and Melanie Mortellaro for their encouragement and support.

We invite comments and criticism regarding format and selection of subject matter, as well as specific suggestions for new data which might be included in subsequent editions. We should also appreciate it if the readers would bring to the attention of the Editor any errors or omissions that might appear in the publication.

Miloslav Rechcigl, Jr.
Editor-in-Chief

PREFACE

HANDBOOK OF NATURALLY OCCURRING FOOD TOXICANTS

In the last decade an increased concern has been voiced against various environmental hazards, particularly chemicals that may cause harm to humans or animals. Numerous studies which have dealt with this subject invariably have focused on chemical contaminants of some component of a food chain. In contrast, much less attention has been paid to the potentially harmful substances that may occur in foodstuffs naturally.

Naturally occurring toxicants are often associated with legumes and oil-bearing plants which constitute one of the most important sources of protein, particularly in the countries of the Third World. A prolonged consumption of food containing natural toxicants may bring about chronic toxicity exhibited by reduced growth, digestive disturbances, or aggravation of malnutrition. In the absence of acute toxic symptoms the condition is often undetected. Apart from the obvious health effects, a continuous ingestion of such toxicants can also markedly affect the person's productivity and as a consequence further endanger the existence of those populations that subsist on such foodstuffs.

The purpose of this Handbook is to sensitize the reader to this problem and to provide a systematic overview of the most important naturally occurring food toxicants.

The Handbook should be of interest to anybody who is concerned with nutritive and health aspects of food. Inasmuch as many of the discussed toxicants can be removed or destroyed by a suitable method of food processing it should be of special value to food technologists.

THE EDITOR

Miloslav Rechcigl, Jr. is a Nutrition Advisor and Chief of Research and Methodology Division in the Agency for International Development.

He has a B.S. in Biochemistry (1954), a Master of Nutritional Science degree (1955), and a Ph.D. in nutrition, biochemistry, and physiology (1958), all from Cornell University. He was formerly a Research Biochemist in the National Cancer Institute, National Institutes of Health and subsequently served as Special Assistant for Nutrition and Health in the Health Services and Mental Health Administration, U.S. Department of Health, Education and Welfare.

Dr. Rechcigl is a member of some 30 scientific and professional societies, including being a Fellow of the American Association for the Advancement of Science, Fellow of the Washington Academy of Sciences, Fellow of the American Institute of Chemists, and Fellow of the International College of Applied Nutrition. He holds membership in the Cosmos Club, the Honorary Society of Phi Kappa Pi, and the Society of Sigma Xi, and is recipient of numerous honors, including an honorary membership certificate from the International Social Science Honor Society Delta Tau Kappa. In 1969, he was a delegate to the White House Conference on Food, Nutrition, and Health and in 1975 a delegate to the ARPAC Conference on Research to Meet U.S. and World Food Needs. He served as President of the District of Columbia Institute of Chemists and Councillor of the American Institute of Chemists, and currently is a delegate to the Washington Academy of Sciences and a member of the Program Committee of the American Institute of Nutrition.

His bibliography extends over 100 publications including contributions to books, articles in periodicals, and monographs in the fields of nutrition, biochemistry, physiology, pathology, enzymology, molecular biology, agriculture, and international development. Most recently he authored and edited *Nutrition and the World Food Problem* (S. Karger, Basel, 1979), *World Food Problem: a Selective Bibliography of Reviews* (CRC Press, 1975), and *Man, Food and Nutrition: Strategies and Technological Measures for Alleviating the World Food Problem* (CRC Press, 1973) following his earlier pioneering treatise on *Enzyme Synthesis and Degradation in Mammalian Systems* (S. Karger, Basel, 1971), and that on *Microbodies and Related Particles, Morphology, Biochemistry and Physiology* (Academic Press, New York, 1969). Dr. Rechcigl also has initiated a new series on *Comparative Animal Nutrition* and was Associated Editor of *Nutrition Reports International*.

ADVISORY BOARD MEMBERS

E. J. W. Barrington
Cornerways
Alderton, Tewkesbury
Glascow, Scotland

Charles A. Black
Department of Agronomy
Iowa State University of Science and
 Technology
Ames, Iowa

Ricardo Bressani
Division of Agricultural and Food
 Science
Institute of Nutrition of Central
 America and Panama (INCAP)
Guatemala City, Guatemala

Sir David Cuthbertson
Department of Pathology and
 Chemistry
University of Glasgow
Glasgow, Scotland

William J. Darby
The Nutrition Foundation, Inc.
New York, New York

Emanuel Epstein
Department of Soils and Plant
 Nutrition
University of California, Davis
Davis, California

Leon Golberg
Chemical Industry Institute of
 Toxicology
Research Triangle Park, North
 Carolina

Earl O. Heady
Center for Agricultural and Rural
 Development
Iowa State University of Science and
 Technology
Ames, Iowa

Dorothy Hollingsworth
The British Nutrition Foundation
Alembic House
London, England

B. Connor Johnson
Department of Biochemistry and
 Molecular Biology
The University of Oklahoma Health
 Science Center
Oklahoma City, Oklahoma

O. L. Kline
American Institute of Nutrition
Bethesda, Maryland

Gilbert A. Leveille
General Foods Corporation
Tarrytown, New York

Margaret Mead (deceased)
The American Museum of Natural
 History
New York, New York

Emil M. Mrak
Department of Food Science
University of California, Davis
Davis, California

Anthony H. Rose
School of Biological Sciences
University of Bath
Claverton Down
Bath, England

Howerde E. Sauberlich
Department of Nutrition
Letterman Army Institute of Research
San Francisco, California

Nevin S. Scrimshaw
Department of Nutrition and Food
 Science
Massachusetts Institute of Technology
Cambridge, Massachusetts

ADVISORY BOARD MEMBERS (Continued)

Charity Waymouth
The Jackson Laboratory
Bar Harbor, Maine

E. M. Widdowson
Dunn Nutritional Laboratories
Cambridge, England

Dr. S. H. Wittwer
Agricultural Experiment Station
Michigan State University
East Lansing, Michigan

CONTRIBUTORS

Robert C. Buckner, Ph.D.
Research Agronomist
USDA-Agricultural Research Service
 and University of Kentucky
Lexington, Kentucky

Mordechai Chevion, Ph.D.
Senior Lecturer
Department of Cellular Biochemistry
Hebrew University of Jerusalem
Jerusalem, Israel

G. Cooper-Driver, Ph.D.
Assistant Professor of Plant
 Biochemistry
Boston University
Boston, Massachusetts

N. T. Crosby, Ph.D.
Department of Industry
Laboratory of the Government Chemist
London, England

Christine S. Evans, Ph.D.
Research Fellow
Department of Biology
Imperial College
University of London
London, England

Thomas Fazio, Ph.D.
Division of Chemistry and Physics
Bureau of Foods
Food and Drug Administration
Washington, DC

Frederick A. Fuhrman, Ph.D.
Professor of Physiology Emeritus
Stanford University
Stanford, California

Gad Glaser, M.D., Ph.D.
Senior Lecturer
Department of Cellular Biochemistry
Hebrew University of Jerusalem
Jerusalem, Israel

Bernd Hoffmann, Ph.D., D.V.M.
Director and Professor
Institut für Veterinärmedizin
Bundesgesundheitsamt
Berlin, West Germany

A. W. Hovin, Ph.D.
Professor
Department of Plant and Soil Sciences
Montana State University
Bozeman, Montana

John W. Howard, Ph.D.
Director
Division of Chemistry and Physics
Food and Drug Administration
Washington, DC

Werner Jaffé, Ph.D.
Professor of Biochemistry and
 Nutrition
Universidad Central, Facultad de
 Ciencias
Caracas, Venezuela

Kenneth F. Lampe, Ph.D.
Senior Scientist
American Medical Association
Chicago, Illinois

Pavel Langer, M.D.
Institute of Experimental
 Endocrinology
Center of Physiological Sciences, SAV
Bratislava, Czechoslovakia

Jacob Mager, M.D., Ph.D.*
Professor and Chairman
Department of Cellular Biochemistry
Hebrew University of Jerusalem
Jerusalem, Israel

Hiromu Matsumoto, Ph.D.
Professor of Agricultural Biochemistry
University of Hawaii
Honolulu, Hawaii

* Deceased May 3, 1980.

Theodore Ouzounellis, M.D.
Consultant
Vostanion Hospital
Mytilini, Greece

Russell Pressey, Ph.D.
Research Chemist
Richard B. Russell Agricultural
  Research Center
Athens, Georgia

Irtaza H. Siddique, D.V.M., Ph.D.
Professor of Microbiology and Public
  Health
School of Veterinary Medicine
Tuskegee Institute
Tuskegee, Alabama

Martin Stob, Ph.D.
Professor
Department of Animal Sciences
Purdue University
W. Lafayette, Indiana

Harvey L. Tookey, Ph.D.
Research Leader
Northern Regional Research Center,
  U.S.D.A.
Peoria, Illinois

H. Allen Tucker, M.D.
Professor
Department of Animal Science
Michigan State University
East Lansing, Michigan

Cecil H. Van Etten
Retired Research Chemist
Northern Regional Research Center,
  U.S.D.A.
Peoria, Illinois

Shelly G. Yates
Research Chemist
Northern Regional Research Center,
  U.S.D.A.
Peoria, Illinois

DEDICATION

To my inspiring teachers at Cornell University—Harold H. Williams, John K. Loosli, the late Richard H. Barnes, the late Clive M. McCay, and the late Leonard A. Maynard. And to my supportive and beloved family—Eva, Jack, and Karen.

TABLE OF CONTENTS

TOXIC CHEMICAL CONSTITUENTS
Naturally Occurring Food Toxicants: Toxic Amino Acids......................3
Glucosinolates 15
Nutritional Significance of Lectins 31
Naturally Occurring Inhibitors: Carbohydrase Inhibitors 39
Cycasin 43
Naturally Occurring Food Toxicants: Favism-Producing Agents 63
Naturally Occurring Food Toxicants: Estrogens 81
Naturally Occurring Food Toxicants: Goitrogens..........................101
Nitrosamines: A Review of Their Chemistry, Biological Properties, and
  Occurrence in the Environment..131
Polycyclic Aromatic Hydrocarbons in Foods 161

TOXIC PLANTS
Mushroom Poisoning...193
Chemical Substances in Plants Toxic to Animals 213
Alkaloids in Tall Fescue and Reed Canarygrass: A Review 241
Tall Fescue Toxins..249

TOXIC ANIMAL CONSTITUENTS
Food Contaminants: Animal Growth Promotors (Antibiotic Residues) 277
Naturally Occurring Hormones in Animal Foods: Testosterone...............287
Naturally Occurring Hormones in Animal Foods: Glucocorticoids 295
Toxic Constituents of Animal Foodstuffs: Eggs of Fishes and Amphibians 301
Quail Poisoning (Coturnism)...313

INDEX 323

Toxic Chemical Constituents

NATURALLY OCCURRING FOOD TOXICANTS: TOXIC AMINO ACIDS

Christine S. Evans

INTRODUCTION

More than 200 amino acids have been isolated from living organisms, of these only 25 to 30 are of universal occurrence being incorporated into proteins (for example aspartic acid and glycine) or occurring as metabolic intermediates (for example ornithine or citrulline). The distribution of the nonprotein amino acids is very variable, a few have been isolated from animals such as the N-methylated lysines and arginines from mammalian cells, and some are known to be incorporated into bacterial cell walls and others occur in the free state or as simple peptides or condensation compounds such as γ-glutamyl or acetyl derivatives.

The qualitative and quantitative distribution of amino acids can vary greatly between species of a family or genus, and even between different organs of a single plant. Many of these "uncommon" amino acids occur in extremely high concentrations. For example the West African legume *Griffonia simplicifolia* accumulates 5-hydroxy-L-tryptophan up to 14% of its seed weight[1] and seeds of *Mucuna* species accumulate L-3,4-dihydroxyphenylalanine (L-dopa) up to 10% of their seed weight.[2] Many of these seed amino acids disappear rapidly when the seeds germinate, but not always. Albizzine, for example, occurs in seeds of *Albizzia julibrissin* and remains as the major free amino acid in the growing seedlings, whereas azetidine-2-carboxylic acid is accumulated in the seedlings, of *Delonix regia* but not in its seeds.[3]

Some of these uncommon amino acids are close, structural analogues of the protein amino acids and can act as antimetabolites when introduced into animals, plants, and microorganisms to which they are normally foreign. Different organisms react variously to similar concentrations of the same compound and while low concentrations of one compound can produce a high level of toxicity in a specific organism, other organisms remain unaffected by much greater concentrations of the same compound.

Several reviews[4-6] in recent years have described the possible toxic effects of uncommon amino acids on microorganisms, insects, birds, and mammals. This account will describe the toxic properties of those "nonprotein" amino acids that occur in plants which are likely to be eaten by man and his domestic animals.

TOXIC AMINO ACIDS

The Lathrogens

Seeds of various species of the legume genus *Lathyrus* are eaten by man, cattle, and horses, particularly in the Indian subcontinent. A disease known as lathyrism, which is largely confined to that subcontinent, is characterized in man by muscular weakness and paralysis of the lower limbs. In extreme cases it may be fatal. It occurs when seeds of certain species (*L. sativus* and less frequently *L. cicera* and *L. clymenum*) form a major proportion of the diet. This occurs in poorer areas or during times of famine when other food supplies are scarce (reviewed by Selye,[7] Sharma,[8] and Bell).[9]

3-N-(4-L-Glutamyl)aminopropionitrile

$$NCCH_2CH_2NHOCCH_2CH_2CH(NH_2)CO_2H$$

The first toxic compound to be isolated from a species of *Lathyrus* (*L. odoratus* was identified as 3-*N*-(4-L-glutamyl)aminopropionitrile by Schilling and Strong.[10] The physiologically active part of the molecule is the 3-amino-propionitrile moiety,[11] which causes severe skeletal abnormalities in young rats. The disease lathyrism should be separated into two syndromes, neurolathyrism or classical lathyrism, and osteolathyrism, the syndrome caused by 3-aminopropionitrile. This compound interferes with the formation of cross linkages in polypeptide chains in collagen and elastin and so causes a weakening of blood-vessel walls and bones. It must be emphasized that seeds of *L. odoratus* are not consumed by man and osteolathyrism is not a medical or veterinary problem.

L-2,4-Diaminobutyric Acid

$$H_2NCH_2CH_2CH(NH_2)CO_2H$$

The first compound from *Lathyrus* seeds to be shown to produce neurological effects was L-2,4-diaminobutyric acid. It was isolated by Ressler and co-workers[12] from seeds of *L. latifolius* and later shown to occur in many species of the Leguminosae and Cruciferae.[13] Its toxicity results from its action as an inhibitor of the ornithine transcarbamylase of mammalian liver, which disrupts the urea cycle and induces ammonia toxicity.[14] The neurological symptoms caused by L-2,4-diaminobutyric acid, however, are distinct from those characteristic of classical human neurolathyrism. As previously noted, the species of *Lathyrus* directly implicated in human lathyrism are *L. sativus*, *L. cicera*, and *L. clymenum*, and none of these contain L-2,4-diaminobutyric acid nor 3-*N*-(4-L-glutamyl)aminopropionitrile.

3-*N*-Oxalyl-L-2,3-diaminopropionic Acid

$$HO_2CCONHCH_2CH(NH_2)CO_2H$$

Rao et al.[15] and Murti et al.[16] independently isolated a strongly acidic amino acid from seeds of *L. sativus* identified as 3-*N*-oxalyl-L-2,3-diaminopropionic acid (ODAP). This compound has been shown to produce neurological symptoms in young birds,[17] young mice,[18] young rats, guinea pigs, and dogs[19] which are indistinguishable from those produced by feeding animals with *L. sativus* seed. Rao and co-workers[20] showed that, on intrathecal administration to adult monkeys, paralysis of the hind limbs occurred. The neurological effects that are produced in young birds or mammals cannot be produced to the same extent in the adults. This may be due to the exclusion of the amino acid by a blood-brain barrier in the adult animal that is not fully developed in the young.[21] However, during times of physical stress and malnutrition the permeability of a blood-brain barrier may be altered and the adult animal rendered susceptible to the toxic effects of the compound. Cheema and co-workers[22] have shown that neurological effects in adult animals can be induced by the oxalyl amino acid if the animals are first made acidotic with calcium chloride.

This neurotoxic amino acid has since been found in other legume species, notably in 13 species of *Crotalaria*[23] and 17 species of *Acacia*[24] in addition to seeds of *Lathyrus*. In *L. sativus* it is formed as the 3-isomer by the transfer of the oxalyl group from oxalyl-coenzyme A to the 3-nitrogen of 2,3-diaminopropionic acid,[25] however in the plant it is accompanied by lower concentrations of 2-*N*-oxalyl-L-2,3-diaminopropionic acid formed by a chemical rearrangement of the 3-oxalyl isomer.[26] The toxicity of several species of *Crotalaria* to domestic animals and birds may well be explained in part by the accumulation of this oxalyl amino acid in its seed. It is of economic interest that some ODAP-containing *Acacia* species have been reported to have promise as forage plants in arid areas of the world.[27]

Table 1
DISTRIBUTION OF THE LATHYROGENS IN SPECIES OF *LATHYRUS*[29]

Lathyrus species containing 2,3-diaminobutyric acid, *N*-4-oxalyl-2,4-diaminobutyric acid and *N*-3-oxalyl-2,3-diaminopropionic acid

    L. sylvestris
    L. latifolius
    L. heterophyllus
    L. gorgoni
    L. grandiflorus
    L. arrhosus
    L. rotundifolius
    L. tuberosus
    L. multiflora
    L. undulatus

Additional *Lathyrus* species containing *N*-3-oxalyl-2,3-diaminopropionic acid

    L. setifolius
    L. alatus
    L. articulatus
    L. arvense
    L. pannonicus
    L. ochrus
    L. clymenum
    L. sativus
    L. megallanicus

Seeds of *L. latifolius* in addition contain the higher homologue, 4-*N*-oxalyl-L-2,4-diaminobutyric acid

$$HO_2CCONHCH_2CH_2CH(NH_2)CO_2H$$

which is also neurotoxic to young chicks.[28] The neurological effects of each of the oxalyl amino acids and diaminobutyric acid itself will be superimposed and compounded in animals eating *Lathyrus* seeds.

The distribution of known toxic compounds in *Lathyrus* species is shown in Table 1, as given by Bell.[29]

3-Cyanoalanine and 4-Glutamylcyanoalanine

$$NCCH_2CH(NH_2)CO_2H$$

Vicia sativa is frequently found growing in areas where *L. sativus* is grown, and its seeds are found as contaminants in wheat supplies. Ressler and co-workers[30-32] identified a neurotoxic amino acid in seeds of *Vicia sativa* as 3-cyanoalanine, in association with its 4-glutamyl derivative. The symptoms of *V. sativa* toxicity are convulsions, rigidity, prostration, and death. These symptoms can be reproduced in young or mature rats and chickens with subcutaneous (s.c.) injection of 3-cyanoalanine. The toxicity can be delayed and reduced by pyridoxal. When 3-cyanoalanine is fed to rats, large amounts of cystathionine are excreted. The toxic action of this amino acid is to inhibit the rat liver cystathionase, a vitamin B_6-requiring enzyme which converts cystathionine to cystine.[33] The enzyme inhibition causes the accumulation of cystathionine.

It seems unlikely that 3-cyanoalanine is the neurotoxin responsible for lathyrism despite the frequent contamination of *Lathyrus* seed supplies with seeds of *Vicia sativa*, but the combination of this toxin with ODAP from *Lathyrus* seeds would accentuate the neurological symptoms ascribed to the disease lathyrism.

It is possible to remove the toxins from *L. sativus* seeds by soaking them in hot water and draining off the water, though many essential nutrients such as water-soluble vitamins are also lost in this process. Human lathyrism could be avoided by the replacement of the toxic species of *Lathyrus* by species with little or no toxic amino acids. Perhaps a more readily achievable aim is the selection of toxic-low strains of *L. sativus* and this objective is presently being pursued in India.

Selenoamino Acids

Selenium poisoning occurs in several parts of the world where selenium-rich soils are found, notably in the U.S., Australia, Ireland, and Israel.[34,35] Food plants which grow in these areas may become selenium rich and have toxic effects on man and animals. The selenium is incorporated into amino acids which are analogues of the sulfur amino acids[36] and these in turn may be incorporated into proteins,[37] Two syndromes of chronic selenium toxicity have been ascribed to organic selenium compounds. One is chronic selenosis or "blind-staggers" which occurs in animals grazing on the native weeds in the genera *Astragalus* and *Machaerantha*. Some of these species are accumulator plants and will grow only on selenium-rich soils, accumulating up to 15,000 ppm of selenium in their tissues,[35] whereas other species, while absorbing large amounts of selenium from selenium-rich soils, will grow satisfactorily on normal soils. These species are known as secondary selenium absorbers and contain only a few hundred ppm of selenium in their tissues. The nonprotein amino acids methylselenocysteine and selenocystathionine which occur free in the plants

$$CH_3SeCH_2CH(NH_2)CO_2H$$

$$HO_2CCH(NH_2)CH_2SeCH_2CH_2CH(NH_2)CO_2H$$

are thought to be the cause of toxicity. Peterson and Butler[38] have suggested that the synthesis of these compounds is a detoxification mechanism whereby the selenium analogues of cysteine and methionine are not incorporated into plant proteins. These selenium-rich species do not present a health hazard to man, but have accounted for serious losses of grazing livestock.

The second syndrome of selenium toxicity in livestock is similar to "alkali disease" caused by excess alkaline salts in soil and water. The symptoms include loss of hair, and deformation and sloughing of hooves. They occur after livestock have grazed for some weeks on cereals and forage plants which grow on seleniferous soils. These crop plants are nonaccumulator species, but if growing in the same areas as accumulator species tend to absorb more selenium from the soil in the form of organic compounds originating in accumulator species, because the accumulator species convert the inorganic selenium absorbed from the soil into soluble organic compounds, which are eventually returned to the soil. Crop plants growing in these areas are therefore likely to contain higher concentrations of selenium than crops which have no contact with accumulator species.[39]

The symptoms of selenium poisoning in man include dermatitis, fatigue, dizziness, and loss of hair and nails. Rosenfeld and Beath[35] report that chronic human selenosis in Columbia is probably caused by eating corn grown in seleniferous soil. Similarly, Lemley and co-workers[40,41] have related cases of selenosis in the U.S. to the high concentrations of selenium in foods. Symptoms of toxicity disappear however when the affected persons change to a selenium-free diet. People living in seleniferous areas of the U.S. have been reported to have a higher incidence of dental caries,[42] discoloration of the skin,[43] diseased nails on fingers and toes, and gastrointestinal problems than occur in a normal population. The daily urinary excretion of selenium at 0.2 ppm selenium or more was significantly higher among affected persons than healthy individuals.[43]

In man, selenium toxicity is caused by selenomethionine and selenocystine, selenium analogues

$$CH_3SeCH_2CH_2CH(NH_2)CO_2H$$

$$\begin{array}{l} SeCH_2CH(NH_2)CO_2H \\ | \\ SeCH_2CH(NH_2)CO_2H \end{array}$$

of the sulfur amino acids methionine and cystine found in the proteins of crop plants grown on seleniferous soils.[44-46]

Acute selenium poisoning in man by selenium-accumulating plants has only been reported for one species, *Lecythis ollaria,* which is placed in the order Myrtales. This is a large deciduous tree widely distributed in Central and South America where it is known as the "coco-de-mono" or "monkey nut" tree. The nuts can produce toxic symptoms which include abdominal discomfort, nausea, vomiting, diarrhea, and loss of scalp and body hair. Kerdel-Vegas[47] refers to 9 cases of poisoning by this plant in Venezuela, the most serious of which was fatal to a 2-year-old child. The toxic symptoms occur after very small quantities of nuts are eaten. A boy aged 12 years who ate only 7 nuts suffered nausea and vomiting whereas diarrhea, dizziness, and complete loss of hair occurred when quantities up to 80 nuts were eaten. The toxic compound accumulated in the nuts is a selenium-containing amino acid, selenocystathionine.[48]

$$HOOC.CH(NH_2)CH_2SeCH_2CH_2CH(NH_2)COOH$$

This compound will cause loss of hair in man and experimental animals; Aronow and Kerdel-Vegas[49] suggested that it might be cytotoxic to the hair-follicle cell. It has been shown to inhibit growth in cultures of mouse fibroblasts, this toxicity being reversed by various sulfur compounds of which L-cystine was the most effective.[49]

3-Methylenecyclopropylpropionic Acid (Hypoglycin A)

$$CH_2 = \!\!\bigtriangleup\!\!- CH_2CH(NH_2)CO_2H$$

The fruit of the tropical tree *Blighia sapida* (in the family Sapindaceae) is a common food in the Caribbean and in Nigeria, but the toxicity caused by eating its unripe fruits is well known. The symptoms of toxicity include severe vomiting, coma, and acute hypoglycemia and these sometimes result in death, especially among individuals suffering from malnutrition.

The toxic factor, hypoglycin A, was isolated from both ripe and unripe fruits by Hassall and co-workers[50] who found it to be present in larger concentrations in the unripe fruit. When injected into rats, guinea pigs, and kittens, hypoglycin A caused striking reductions in blood sugar concentration.[51] It is thought to interfere with the oxidation of fatty acids, so that glycogen stores have to be metabolized for energy, with the depletion of carbohydrates resulting in hypoglycemia. Von Holt and Benedict[52] have suggested that it is not the amino acid itself which blocks fatty acid metabolism, but an unsaturated carboxylic acid formed from it in the mammalian system.

Experiments with pregnant rats have shown that hypoglycin A has teratogenic activity.[53] From 125 pregnant rats injected with hypoglycin A there were only 8 normal fetuses compared with 98 normal fetuses produced by the control group of 105 pregnant rats.

The lower homologue of hypoglycin A, 2-methylenecyclopropylglycine, has been isolated by Gray and Fowden[54] from the seeds of *Litchi chinensis*

$$CH_2 = \text{(cyclopropyl)} - CH(NH_2)CO_2H$$

(lychee), also in the family Sapindaceae. The seeds of this plant are not normally eaten, so the toxic effects of this compound are not a problem. It was not found in the fleshy part of the fruit. However Gray and Fowden[54] demonstrated in the laboratory that this amino acid was toxic to mice causing hypoglycemia.

L-3,4-Dihydroxyphenylalanine (L-Dopa)

$$HO-\text{(phenyl)}(OH)-CH_2CH(NH_2)CO_2H$$

The pods of *Vicia faba* (the broad bean) contain up to 0.25% of L-3,4-dihydroxyphenylalanine (L-dopa) either as the free amino acid or in the form of a β-glycoside.[55-56] In individuals deficient in glucose-6-phosphate dehydrogenase (G-6PD), the ingestion of the beans can precipitate a hemolytic anemia known as favism. Kosower and Kosower[57] showed that erythrocytes deficient in G-6PD would lose reduced glutathione on incubation in a medium containing L-dopa, although subsequent in vivo experiments did not produce any hemolytic effects on G-6PD-deficient erythrocytes exposed to high concentrations of L-dopa.[58]

L-Dopa has been used in the treatment of Parkinson's disease,[59] a chronic neurological disorder characterized by tremor, rigidity of the limbs, and poverty of movement. However oral ingestion of high concentrations of L-dopa is known to cause toxic side effects such as nausea, vomiting, and involuntary chewing movements.[60]

Further studies on the distribution of L-dopa within species of the Leguminosae have shown that seeds of several *Mucuna* species may contain up to 10% of free L-dopa.[61,62] The extraction of L-dopa from *Mucuna* seeds will greatly increase the availability of the compound, and its toxicity may become a more serious problem. These large concentrations in the seeds may form a chemical barrier which protects the seeds from insect attack. Rehr and co-workers[63] have shown that even low concentrations of L-dopa can significantly affect the tyrosinase activity in the larvae of *Prodenia eridania* (the southern armyworm).

5-Hydroxy-L-tryptophan (5-HTP)

$$HO-\text{(indole)}-CH_2CH(NH_2)CO_2H$$

Another amino acid which has been used for the medical treatment of neurological disorders is 5-hydroxy-L-tryptophan (5-HTP). It is the precursor of 5-hydroxytryptamine (5-HT, serotonin) which is a physiologically active amine in mammalian brain. It has been shown that 5-HTP readily crosses the blood-brain barrier (unlike 5-HT)[64,65] and experiments with dogs and rats have shown that injection of 5-HTP can produce an increase in the level of 5-HT in the brain. The toxic symptoms so caused consist of "tremors, pupillary dilation, loss of light reflex, apparent blindness, salivation, marked hyperpnea, and tachycardia".

Administration of 5-HTP to infants suffering from Down's syndrome (mongolism) produced an increase in muscle tone, although large doses of 5-HTP had pronounced side effects of motor restlessness, vomiting, diarrhea, and hypertension.[66] Wyatt[67] reports an increase in the rapid eye movement sleep in normal subjects after administration of 5-HTP.

Seeds of the West African legume *Griffonia simplicifolia* contain up to 10% of free 5-HTP.[68,69] The high concentration of this amino acid in the seeds may account for their use in native medicine in parts of West Africa. However this potentially toxic amino acid does not commonly occur in foods eaten by man.

2-Amino-3-methylaminopropionic Acid

$$(H_3C)HNCH_2CH(NH_2)CO_2H$$

In tropical and subtropical areas, species of the Cycadaceae are used as food for man and animals. The roots, stems, and seeds are eaten by man and the leaves eaten by domestic animals. Six of the nine genera of this family have been reported as causing toxic symptoms either in man or animals and some carcinogenic glycosides have been isolated from the seeds and roots of several species.[70] However the acute poisoning by these glycosides does not account for the symptoms of paralysis of the hind limbs occurring in cattle after eating the leaves of *Zamia*[71] nor explain the high occurrence of amyotrophic lateral sclerosis found in Guam among the people who obtain food starch from seeds of *Cycas circinalis*.[72,73]

The seeds of *Cycas circinalis*, however, contain the amino acid 2-amino-3-methylaminopropionic acid[74] which acts as a neurotoxin in rats, mice, and chicks.[75,76] It occurs both as the free amino acid and in a bound form in all *Cycas* species,[77] though the total concentration in the seeds is probably too low to cause any permanent paralysis. However this amino acid may contribute to the toxicity of the Cycads in addition to the effect of the carcinogens also present in these plants.

3-N-(3-Hydroxypyridone-4)-2-aminopropionic Acid (Mimosine)

Mimosine has been found in many species of the Mimosoideae (one of the subfamilies of the Leguminosae), the most important of which is *Leucaena leucocephala* which has been grown extensively as a cover crop in tropical and subtropical areas. Its foliage is toxic to grazing animals. The symptoms of poisoning include decreased weight gain, cataracts in young animals, infertility, and the most striking feature, loss of hair.[78,79] This depilatory effect can be produced by injection or oral administration of the purified amino acid,[80] though the toxic side effects caused by mimosine have been a major obstacle in the development of this compound as a chemical shearing agent.

The mechanism of the toxicity is not fully understood, mimosine is an inhibitor of enzymes which require pyridoxal phosphate, especially the cysteine synthesizing system in rat liver. Hylin[78] has shown that mimosine is a potent inhibitor of both cystathionine synthetase and cystathionase from rat liver. This may partly explain the depilatory effect as hair protein contains an exceptionally large amount of cysteine some of which is probably formed from methionine. Less cysteine available for hair protein synthesis would stop or reduce hair growth resulting in a loss of hair. In ruminants, enlargement of the thyroid also occurs. Hegarty et al.[81] have shown that the goitrogen is not mimosine itself but 3-hydroxy-4(1H)-pyridone which is formed from mimosine by microorganisms of the rumen.

L-2-Amino-6-amidinohexanoic Acid (Indospicine)

$$H_2NC(:NH)CH_2CH_2CH_2CH_2CH(NH_2)CO_2H$$

Animals grazing on the leaves and seeds of the tropical legume *Indigofera spicata* develop liver lesions, initially described by Hutton and co-workers[82,83] in rabbits and mice. An uncommon amino acid, indospicine was isolated from the seeds and leaves of this species by Hegarty and Pound[84] and was subsequently shown to be hepatotoxic in chickens, mice, rabbits, guinea pigs, sheep, pigs, and cows.[85] It also has a teratogenic effect in fetal rats, exposure to the amino acid on day 13 of gestation caused cleft palates.[86]

Indospicine, a close structural analogue of arginine, exerts a toxic effect by competitively inhibiting arginine metabolism.[87] Its major action is to cause a primary blockage of arginine incorporation into protein, resulting in a secondary depression of incorporation of other amino acids.[88-90]

(2-Amino-4-(guanidinooxy)butyric Acid) (Canavanine)

$$H_2NC(:NH)NHOCH_2CH_2CH(NH_2)CO_2H$$

Many species of the Papilionoideae (a subfamily of the Leguminosae) contain canavanine in their seeds,[91] often forming up to 5% of the dry seed weight. Canavanine, first isolated from seeds of *Canavalia ensiformis,* is another close structural analogue of arginine. It is toxic to microorganisms,[92] locusts,[93] and bruchid larvae,[94,95] though less is known of its toxicity to mammals. Tschiersch[96] showed that feeding both the seed of *Canavalia ensiformis* and purified canavanine to mice caused toxicity. The mechanism of action is not fully understood, but in vitro studies on mammalian cells have shown that canavanine is incorporated into nuclear proteins, so interfering with DNA synthesis.[97] Miller and Consigli[98] have shown that canavanine reduces cellular proliferation in embryonic mice cells.

Roasted seeds of some species of *Canavalia* and *Dioclea*, another canavanine-containing legume, are eaten by natives of Costa Rica. Some but not all of the canavanine is destroyed by heating,[29] so this amino acid could produce toxic effects in man if seeds containing it formed a major part of the diet.

SUMMARY

Several food plants contain, in addition to the protein amino acids, many uncommon, nonprotein amino acids. The functions of these secondary compounds in the plant are not fully understood, though much evidence has accumulated over recent years to suggest that they form a part of a chemical defense mechanism of the plant against predators. Some of these compounds are toxic to specific microorganisms, insects, birds, or mammals. Most of the amino acids which are toxic to man give rise to chronic rather than acute symptoms of poisoning, which suggests that low concentrations of a particular toxin can have a cumulative harmful effect if supplied as part of the diet over a long period of time. In many cases, the symptoms of toxicity induced by a compound in laboratory animals are comparable with those observed in an animal suffering from toxicity in the field, though the concentration and toxicity of the toxin in the plant may not always be sufficient to explain the full symptoms.

Some of the uncommon amino acids described are neurotoxins, such as 3-oxalyl-2,3-diaminopropionic acid, which is responsible for the disease classical lathyrism in man. Other toxic amino acids are close structural analogues of protein amino acids and exert their toxicity by disrupting enzyme systems, for example the seleno-amino acids are incorporated into enzymes in place of the normal sulfur amino acids and canavanine replaces arginine in nuclear proteins. Mimosine is a potent inhibitor of cystathionine synthetase enzymes in the liver, but its depilatory effect in animals has encouraged investigation into its use as a defleecing agent in sheep despite its toxicity.

Some uncommon amino acids are precursors of normal metabolites, for example 5-hydroxytryptophan gives rise to 5-hydroxytryptamine, a physiologically active amine in the mammalian brain, and has been used medicinally to improve the condition of mongolism in which the blood level of 5-HT is low. Similarly L-dopa has been used for the treatment of Parkinson's disease. Both these compounds are potentially toxic to man.

It is likely that the nonprotein amino acids in plants may give rise to increased problems of toxicity in the future, as attempts are made to increase the food supply of the world by growing plants not traditionally used for food and fodder.

REFERENCES

1. Bell, E. A., Fellows, L. E., and Qureshi, M. Y., 5-Hydroxy-L-tryptophan; taxonomic character and chemical defence in *Griffonia*, *Phytochemistry*, 15, 823, 1976.
2. Bell, E. A. and Janzen, D. H., Medical and ecological considerations of L-dopa and 5-HTP in seeds, *Nature (London)*, 229, 136—137, 1971.
3. Watson, R. and Fowden, L., Amino acids of *Caesalpinia tinctoria* and some allied species, *Phytochemistry*, 12, 617—622, 1973.
4. Bell, E. A., Uncommon amino acids in plants, *FEBS Lett.*, 64, 29—35, 1976.
5. Hylin, J. W., Toxic peptides and amino acids in foods and feeds, *J. Agric. Food Chem.*, 17, 492—496, 1969.
6. Fowden, L., Non-protein amino acids from plants: distribution, biosynthesis and analog functions, *Recent Adv. Phytochem.*, 8, 95—122, 1974.
7. Selye, H., Lathyrism, *Rev. Can. Biol.*, 16, 1—82, 1957.
8. Sharma, D. N., Lathyrism. The old and new concepts, *J. Indian Med. Assoc.*, 36, 299—304, 1961.
9. Bell, E. A., The structure and biosynthesis of lathyrogens and related compounds, *Food Chem.*, 6, 213—222, 1981.
10. Schilling, E. D. and Strong, F. M., Isolation, structure and synthesis of a lathyrus factor from *L. odoratus*, *J. Am. Chem. Soc.*, 76, 2848, 1954.

11. Dasler, W., Isolation of toxic crystals from sweet peas *(Lathyrus odoratus), Science,* 120, 307—308, 1954.
12. Ressler, C., Redstone, P. A., and Erenberg, R. H., Isolation and identification of a neuroactive factor from *Lathyrus latifolius, Science,* 134, 188—190, 1961.
13. Van Etten, C. H. and Miller, R. W., The neuroactive factor αγ-diamino-butyric acid in angiosperm seeds, *Econ. Bot.,* 17, 107—109, 1963.
14. O'Neal, R. M., Chen, C. H., Reynolds, C. S., Meghal, S. K., and Koeppe, R. E., The neurotoxicity of L-2,4-diaminobutyric acid, *Biochem. J.,* 106, 699—706, 1968.
15. Rao, S.L. N., Adiga, P. R., and Sarma, P. S., The isolation and characterisation of β-N-oxalyl-L-αβ-diaminopropionic acid: a neurotoxin from seeds of *Lathyrus sativus, Biochemistry,* 3, 432—436, 1964.
16. Murti, V. V. S., Seshadri, T. R., and Venkitasubramanian, T. A., Neurotoxic compounds of the seeds of *Lathyrus sativus, Phytochemistry,* 3, 73—78, 1964.
17. Adiga, P. R., Rao, S. L. N., and Sarma, P. S., Some structural features and neurotoxic action of a compound from *Lathyrus sativus* seeds, *Curr. Sci.,* 32, 153—155, 1963.
18. Olney, J. W., Misra, C. H., and Rhee, V., Brain and retinal damage from lathyrus excitotoxin, β-N-oxalyl-L-α,β-diaminopropionic acid, *Nature (London),* 264, 659—661, 1976.
19. Rao, S. L. N. and Sarma, P. S., Neurotoxic action of β-N-oxalyl-L-α,β-diaminopropionic acid, *Biochem. Pharmacol.,* 16, 218—219, 1967.
20. Rao, S. L., Sarma, P. S., Mani, K. S., Raghunatha Rao, T. R., and Sriramachari, S., Experimental neurolathyrism in monkeys, *Nature (London),* 214, 610—611, 1967.
21. Curtis, D. R. and Watkins, J. C., The pharmacology of amino acids related to γ-aminobutyric acid, *Pharmacol. Rev.,* 17, 347—391, 1965.
22. Cheema, P. S., Padmanaban, G., and Sarma, P. S., Neurotoxic action of β-N-oxalyl-L-α,β-diaminopropionic acid in acidotic adult rats, *Indian J. Biochem.,* 6, 146—147, 1969.
23. Qureshi, M. Y., Pilbeam, D. J., Evans, C. S., and Bell, E. A., The neurolathyrogen, α-amino-β-oxalylaminopropionic acid in legume seeds, *Phytochemistry,* 16, 477—479, 1977.
24. Evans, C. S., Qureshi, M. Y., and Bell, E. A., Free amino acids in the seeds of *Acacia* species, *Phytochemistry,* 16, 565—570, 1977.
25. Malathi, K., Padmanaban, G., and Sarma, P. S., Biosynthesis of β-N-oxalyl-L-α,β-diaminopropionic acid, the *Lathyrus sativus* neurotoxin, *Phytochemistry,* 9, 1603—1610, 1970.
26. Bell, E. A. and O'Donovan, J. P., The isolation of α and γ-oxalyl derivatives of α,γ-diaminobutyric acid from seeds of *Lathyrus latifolius* and the detection of the α-oxalyl isomer of the neurotoxin α-amino-β-oxalyl aminopropionic acid which occurs together with the neurotoxin in this and other species, *Phytochemistry,* 5, 1211—1219, 1966.
27. Underexploited Tropical Plants with Promising Economic Value, Report, National Academy of Sciences, Washington, D.C., 1975, 111.
28. Rao, S. L. N. and Sharma, P. S., Neurotoxic properties of N-substituted oxamic Acids, *Indian J. Biochem.,* 3, 57—58, 1966.
29. Bell, E. A., Aminonitriles and amino acids not derived from proteins, in *Toxicants Occurring Naturally in Foods,* National Academy of Sciences, Washington, D.C., 1973, 153—169.
30. Ressler, C., Isolation and identification from common vetch of the neurotoxin β-cyano-L-alanine, a possible factor in neurolathyrism, *J. Biol. Chem.,* 237, 733—735, 1962.
31. Ressler, C., Nigam, S. N., Giza, Y-H., and Nelson, J., Isolation and identification from common vetch of γ-L-glutamyl-β-cyano-L-alanine, a bound form of the neurotoxin β-cyano-L-alanine, *J. Am. Chem. Soc.,* 85, 3311—3312, 1963.
32. Ressler, C., Nigam, S. N., and Giza, Y.-H., Toxic principle in vetch. Isolation and identification of γ-L-glutamyl-L-β-cyanoalanine from common vetch seeds. Distribution in some legumes, *J. Am. Chem. Soc.,* 91, 2758—2765, 1969.
33. Pfeffer, M. and Ressler, C., β-Cyanoalanine, an inhibitor of rat liver cystathionase, *Biochem. Pharmacol.,* 16, 2299—2308, 1967.
34. Kingsbury, J. M., *Poisonous Plants of the United States and Canada,* Prentice-Hall, Englewood Cliffs, N. J., 1964.
35. Rosenfeld. I. and Beath, O. A., *Selenium,* Academic Press, New York, 1964.
36. Shrift, A. and Virupaksha, T. K., Biosynthesis of se-methyl-seleno-cysteine from selenite in selenium accumulating plants, *Biochim. Biophys. Acta,* 71, 483—485, 1963.
37. Shrift, A. and Virupaksha, T. K., Seleno-amino acids in selenium accumulating plants, *Biochim. Biophys. Acta,* 100, 65—75, 1965.
38. Peterson, P. J. and Butler, G. W., Significance of selenocystathionine in an Australian selenium-accumulating plant, *Neptunia amplexicaulis, Nature (London),* 213, 599—600, 1967.
39. Peterson, P. J., Sulphur and selenium containing amino acids, *Phytochemistry,* 9, 916, 1970.
40. Lemley, R. E., Selenium poisoning in the human. A preliminary case report, *J. Lancet,* 60, 528—531, 1940.

41. Lemley, R. E. and Merryman, M. P., Selenium poisoning in the human, *J. Lancet,* 61, 435—438, 1941.
42. Hadjimarkos, D. M., Effect of selenium on dental caries, *Arch. Environ. Health,* 10, 893—899, 1965.
43. Smith, M. I. and Westfall, B. B., Further field studies on the selenium problem in relation to public health, *Public Health Rep.,* 52, 1375, 1937.
44. Olson, O. E., Novacek, E. J., Whitehead, E. I., and Palmer, I. S., Investigations on selenium in wheat, *Phytochemistry,* 9, 1181—1188, 1970.
45. Shrift, A., Aspects of selenium metabolism in higher plants, *Annu. Rev. Plant Physiol.,* 20, 475—494, 1969.
46. Shrift, A., Selenium toxicity, in *Phytochemical Ecology: Proceedings,* Harbourne, J. B., Ed., Academic Press, New York, 1972, 145—161.
47. Kerdel-Vegas, F., Generalised hair loss due to the ingestion of "coco de mono" *(Lecythis ollaria), J. Invest. Dermatol.,* 42, 91—94, 1964.
48. Kerdel-Vegas, F., Wagner, F., Russell, P. B., Grant, N. H., Alburn, H. E., Clark, D. E., and Miller, J. A., Structure of the pharmacologically active factor in the seeds of *Lecythis ollaria, Nature (London),* 205, 1186—1187, 1965.
49. Aronow, L. and Kerdel-Vegas, F., Cytotoxic and depilatory effects of extracts of *Lecythis ollaria, Nature (London),* 205, 1185—1186, 1965.
50. Hassall, C. H., Reyle, K., and Feng, P., Hypoglycin, A. B., biologically active polypeptides from *Blighia sapida, Nature (London),* 173, 356—357, 1954.
51. Hassall, C.H. and Reyle, K., Hypoglycin A and B, two biologically active polypeptides from *Blighia sapida, Biochem. J.,* 60, 334—339, 1955.
52. Von Holt, C. and Benedict, I., Biochemie des Hypoglycin A. II. Der Einflues des Hypoglycins auf Oxidation von Glucose und Fettsauren, *Biochem. Z.,* 331, 430—435, 1959.
53. Persaud, T. V. N., Teratogenic effects of hypoglycin A, *Nature (London),* 217, 471, 1968.
54. Gray, D. O. and Fowden, L., α-Methylenecyclopropyl glycine from *Litchi* seeds, *Biochem. J.,* 82, 385—389, 1962.
55. Guggenheim, M., Dioxyphenylalanine, eine neue Aminosäure aus *Vicia faba, Z. Physiol. Chem.,* 88, 276—277, 1913.
56. Andrews, R. S. and Pridham, J. B., Structure of a dopa glucoside from *Vicia faba, Nature (London),* 205, 1213—1214, 1965.
57. Kosower, N. S. and Kosower, E. M., Does 3,4-dihydroxyphenylalanine play a part in favism?, *Nature (London),* 215, 285—286, 1967.
58. Gaetani, G., Salvidio, E., Pannacciulli, I., Ajmar, F., and Paravidino, G., Absence of haemolytic effects of L-dopa on transfused G-6PD-deficient erythrocytes, *Experimentia,* 26, 785, 1970.
59. Calne, D. B. and Sandler, M., L-dopa and Parkinsonism, *Nature (London),* 226, 21—24, 1970.
60. Van Woert, M. H. and Bowers, M. B., The effect of L-dopa on monoamine metabolites in Parkinson's disease, *Experimentia,* 26, 161—163, 1970.
61. Bell, E. A. and Janzen, D. H., Medical and ecological considerations of L-dopa and 5-HTP in seeds, *Nature (London),* 229, 136—137, 1971.
62. Daxenbichler, M. E., Van Etten, C. H., Hallinan, E. A., and Earle, F. R., Seeds as sources of L-dopa, *J. Med. Chem.,* 14, 463—465, 1971.
63. Rehr, S. S., Janzen, D. H., and Feeny, P. P., L-dopa in legume seeds; a chemical barrier to insect attack, *Science,* 181, 81—82, 1973.
64. Udenfriend, S., Titus, E., Weissbach, H., and Peterson, R. E., Biogenesis and metabolism of 5 hydroxyindole compounds, *J. Biol. Chem.,* 219, 335—344, 1956.
65. Udenfriend, S., Weissbach, H., and Bogdanski, D. F., Increase in tissue serotonin following administration of its precursor 5-hydroxytryptophan, *J. Biol. Chem.,* 224, 803—810, 1957.
66. Bazelon, M., Paine, R. S., Cowie, V. A., Hunt, P., Houck, J. C., and Mahanand, D., Reversal of hypotonia in infants with Down's syndrome by administration of 5-hydroxytryptophan, *Lancet,* i, 1130—1133, 1967.
67. Wyatt, R. J., Serotonin now: clinical implications of inhibiting its synthesis with p-chlorophenylalanine, *Ann. Intern. Med.,* 73, 607—629, 1970.
68. Bell, E. A. and Fellows, L. E., Occurrence of 5-hydroxytryptophan as a free plant amino acid, *Nature (London),* 210, 529, 1966.
69. Fellows, L. E. and Bell, E. A., 5-Hydroxytryptophan, 5-hydroxytryptamine and L-tryptophan-5-hydroxylase in *Griffonia simplicifolia, Phytochemistry,* 9, 2389—2396, 1970.
70. Nishida, K., Kobayashi, A., and Nagahama, T., Studies on cycasin, a new toxic glycoside of *Cycas revoluta* Thunb. *Bull. Agric. Chem. Soc. Jpn.,* 19, 77-84, 1955.
71. Mason, M. M. and Whiting, M. G., Demyelination in the bovine spinal cord caused by *Zamia* neurotoxicity, *Fed. Proc. Fed. Am. Soc. Exp. Biol.,* 25, 533, 1966.

72. Whiting, M. G., Toxicity of cycads, *Econ. Bot.*, 17, 271—302, 1963.
73. Yang, M. C. and Mickelsen, O., Cycads, in *Toxic Consituents of Foodstuffs*, Liener, I. E., Ed., Academic Press, New York, 1969, 159—167.
74. Vega, A. and Bell, E. A., α-amino-β-methylaminopropionic acid, a new amino acid from seeds of *Cycas circinalis*, *Phytochemistry*, 6, 759—762, 1967.
75. Vega, A., Bell, E. A., and Nunn, P. B., The preparation of L- and D-α-amino-β-methylaminopropionic acids and the identification of the compound isolated from *Cycas circinalis* as the L-isomer, *Phytochemistry*, 7, 1885—1887, 1968.
76. Polsky, F. I., Nunn, P. B., and Bell, E. A., Distribution and toxicity of α-amino-β-methylaminopropionic acid, *Fed. Proc. Fed. Am. Soc. Exp. Biol.*, 31, 1473—1475, 1972.
77. Dossaji, S. F. and Bell, E. A., Distribution of α-amino-β-methylamino-propionic acid in *Cycas*, *Phytochemistry*, 12, 143—144, 1973.
78. Hylin, J. W., Toxic peptides and amino acids in foods and feeds, *J. Agric. Food Chem.*, 17, 492—496, 1969.
79. Hegarty, M. P., Schinckel, P. G. and Court, R. D., Reaction of sheep to the consumption of *Leucaena glauca* Benth and to its toxic principle mimosine, *Aust. J. Agric. Res.*, 15, 153—167, 1964.
80. Reis, P. J., Tunks, D. A., and Hegarty, M. P., Fate of mimosine administered orally to sheep and its effectiveness as a defleecing agent, *Aust. J. Biol. Sci.*, 28, 495—501, 1975.
81. Hegarty, M. P., Lee, C. P., Christie, G. S., Court, R. D., and Haydock, K. P., The goitrogen 3-hydroxy-4(1H)-pyridone, a ruminal metabolite from *Leucaena leucocephala*: effects in mice and rats, *Aust. J. Biol. Sci.*, 32, 27—40, 1979.
82. Hutton, E. M., Windrum, G. M., and Kratzing, C. C., Studies on the toxicity of *Indigofera endecaphylla*. I. Toxicity for rabbits, *J. Nutr.*, 64, 321—333, 1958.
83. Hutton, E. M., Windrum, G. M., and Kratzing, C. C., Studies on the toxicity of *Indigofera endecaphylla*. II. Toxicity for mice, *J. Nutr.*, 65, 429—440, 1958.
84. Hegarty, M. P. and Pound, A. W., Indospicine, a new hepatotoxic amino acid from *Indigofera spicata*, *Nature (London)*, 217, 354—355, 1968.
85. Hegarty, M. P. and Pound, A. W., Indospicine, a hepatotoxic amino acid from *Indigofera spicata*: isolation, structure and biological studies, *Aust. J. Biol. Sci.*, 23, 831—842, 1970.
86. Pearn, J. H. and Hegarty, M. P., Indospicine — the teratogenic factor from *Indigofera spicata* extract causing cleft palate, *Br. J. Exp. Pathol.*, 51, 34—36, 1970.
87. Christie, G. S., Wilson, M., and Hegarty, M. P., Effects on the liver in the rat of ingestion of *Indigofera spicata*, a legume containing an inhibitor of arginine metabolism, *J. Pathol.*, 117, 195—205, 1975.
88. De Munk, F. G., Christie, G. S., and Hegarty, M. P., The effects of indospicine on bone marrow cells in liquid culture, *Pathology*, 4, 133—137, 1972.
89. Madsen, N. P., Christie, G. S., and Hegarty, M. P., Effect of indospicine on incorporation of L-arginine-^{14}C into protein and transfer ribonucleic acid by cell-free systems from rat liver, *Biochem. Pharmacol.*, 19, 853—857, 1970.
90. Madsen, N. P. and Hegarty, M. P., Inhibition of rat liver homogenate arginase activity *in vitro* by the hepatoxic amino acid indospicine, *Biochem. Pharmacol.*, 19, 2391—2393, 1970.
91. Bell, E. A., Lackey, J. A., and Polhill, R. M., Systematic significance of canavanine in the Papilionoideae, *Biochem. Syst. Ecol.*, 6, 201—212, 1978.
92. Schachtele, C. F. and Rogers, P., Canavanine death in *Escherichia coli*, *J. Mol. Biol.*, 14, 474—489, 1965.
93. Navon, A. and Bernays, E. A., Inhibition of feeding in acridids by non-protein amino acids, *Comp. Biochem. Physiol.*, 59A, 161—164, 1978.
94. Rosenthal, G. A., Janzen, D. H., and Dahlman, D. L., Degradation and detoxification of canavanine by a specialised seed predator, *Science*, 196, 658—660, 1977.
95. Dahlman, D. L. and Rosenthal, G. A., Non-protein amino acid-insect interactions. I. Growth effects and symptomology of L-canavanine consumption by tobacco hornworm, *Manduca sexta* (L.), *Comp. Biochem. Physiol.*, 51A, 33—36, 1975.
96. Tschiersch, B., Zur toxischen Wirkung der Jackbohne, *Pharmazie*, 17, 621—623, 1962.
97. Hare, J. D., Nuclear alterations in mammalian cells induced by L-canavanine, *J. Cell. Physiol.*, 75, 129—131, 1970.
98. Miller, G. C. and Consigli, R. A., The effect of canavanine on cultured mouse cells, *Proc. Soc. Exp. Biol. Med.*, 146, 549—553, 1974.

GLUCOSINOLATES*

Cecil H. VanEtten and Harvey L. Tookey

INTRODUCTION

The natural glucosinolates, formerly called thioglucosides, are found in all crucifer plants including horticultural crops such as cabbage, oilseed crops such as rapeseed, condiments such as mustard seed, and herbage such as *Brassica* kale. Many of the species in families closely related to Cruciferae, such as Capparaceae, Limnanthaceae, and Resedaceae, also contain glucosinolates.[1] One species, *Carica papaya*, from the unrelated family Caricaceae is the source of papain. This species contains large amounts of benzylglucosinolate (benzyl-GS).[2] Nearly 80 naturally occurring glucosinolates have been discovered.[3]

Glucosinolates are the source of organic nitriles, isothiocyanates, and SCN ion. Some of these compounds have been shown to be harmful if consumed in sufficient amounts by humans and by animals. They contribute to the flavor of the food or condiment that contains them. The compounds are most commonly formed by hydrolysis of the glucosinolates by an enzyme system that accompanies them but that does not become active until the wet raw plant material is crushed. (In the early literature the name myrosinase was given to the enzyme. Thioglucosidase glucohydrolase EC 3.2.3.1 or thioglucosidase is recommended by the International Union of Biochemistry.)[4] Less frequently, the aglucon products from the glucosinolates may be formed by chemical hydrolysis or by the action of enzymes from nonplant sources such as microorganisms of the digestive tract.[5,6]

Reviews which may be consulted include those concerning biological effects from ingestion of crucifers,[7-12] chemistry of the glucosinolates,[1,10,11,13] problems in the use of rapeseed meals in animal feeds,[14-16] and transfer of deleterious substances into milk from animals fed crucifers.[17,18] A book on the biology and chemistry of the Cruciferae is recommended.[19]

HYDROLYTIC PRODUCTS FROM GLUCOSINOLATES

Upon enzymatic hydrolysis, most of the glucosinolates form stable isothiocyanates or nitriles as well as glucose and HSO_4 ion (Scheme 1). The formation of organic thiocyanates in significant amounts has rarely been observed.[20] Whether isothiocyanates or nitriles are formed depends on the glucosinolates present, the kind and part of the plant, treatment of plant material prior to hydrolysis of glucosinolates, and conditions during the hydrolysis.[11,21] Nitriles are more apt to be formed in fresh tissue that is crushed than in plant tissue that has been heated. If a hydroxyl group is in the aglucon as shown in Scheme 2, the isothiocyanate is unstable and cyclizes to give an oxazolidinethione.[22] If a glucosinolate containing terminal unsaturation is hydrolyzed under conditions favoring nitrile formation, the sulfur may be retained as an episulfide group.[23-25] Episulfide formation depends on the presence of a labile protein during the thioglucosidase hydrolysis.[26,27]

The indolylmethyl-GSs (Scheme 3) form unstable isothiocyanates which decompose quantitatively to give inorganic SCN ion along with other products.[28-30] Of the domestic crops, only white mustard seed, *Brassica hirta* or *Sinapis alba*, contains large amounts of *p*-hydroxybenzyl-GS (sinalbin). The isothiocyanate from this glucosinolate

---

* This chapter was prepared on official government time by members of the U. S. Department of Agriculture and reports research paid for by the American taxpayer.

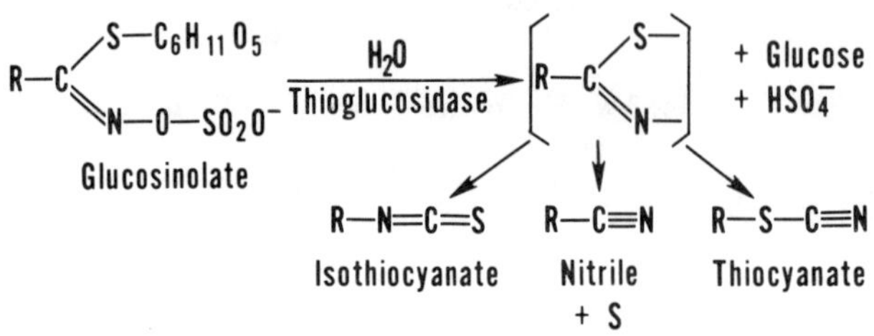

SCHEME 1.

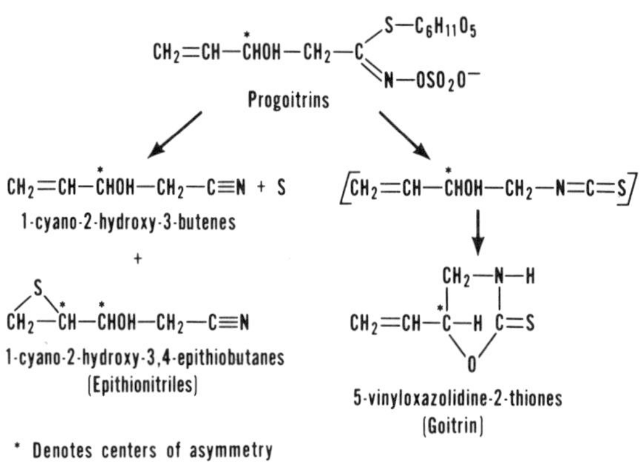

SCHEME 2.

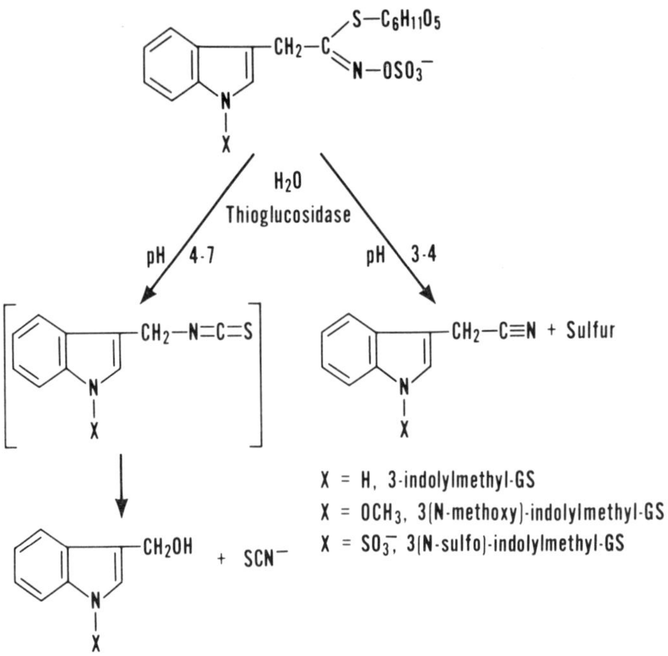

SCHEME 3.

readily decomposes at high pH to give SCN ion.[13] It appears that SCN ion is found in at least small amounts in all glucosinolate-containing plants after thioglucosidase hydrolysis under conditions favorable for isothiocyanate formation.

GLUCOSINOLATE COMPOSITION OF COMMERCIAL CROPS

Glucosinolates that are found in crucifer crops are listed in Table 1. The composition of common cabbage *(Brassica oleracea* var. *capitata)* and of Chinese cabbage *(B. campestris* ssp. *pekinensis)* are given in Table 2. The data on common cabbage do not include the core and cambial cortex which have a significantly different composition from the leaves.[37] Glucosinolate products in roots of turnips *(B. campestris* ssp. *rapifera)* and rutabagas *(B. napus* ssp. *rapifera)* are shown in Table 3. The data of Tables 2 and 3 were obtained by enzymatic hydrolysis of glucosinolates under analytical conditions that yield only isothiocyanates, oxazolidinethione (goitrin), or SCN ion.[39] Estimation of the isothiocyanates and oxazolidinethione was accomplished by gas-liquid chromatography[39] and ultraviolet (UV) absorption.[40] The SCN ion, determined by colorimetry of its reaction product with ferric iron,[41] was used as a measure of indolymethyl-GSs (Scheme 3). Total glucosinolates were determined by measurement of the glucose released during enzymatic hydrolysis of the glucosinolates.[42]

Table 4 shows the composition of oilseed meals from rapeseeds of commerce by methods given in the table. Tower and Candle are among the recent Canadian cultivars of low-glucosinolate rape. Table 5 gives the amounts of glucosinolates in less widely grown crops. For many of these, quantitative data are not available. Data presented are the best available, but represent diverse methods of analysis. Brussels sprouts were analyzed by a recent method[47] that allows a separate, direct measurement of each indolylmethyl-GS (Nos. 23, 24 of Table 1). A new method involving high-performance liquid chromatography of intact glucosinolates[63] appears promising, but few applications have yet appeared.

Reports of flavor volatiles from crucifer vegetables include many compounds derived from glucosinolates found in radish,[64] cooked cabbage,[65] horseradish,[66] Brussels sprout,[67] and others. These studies are not quantitative, but show trace amounts of products presumably from glucosinolates that have not appeared in compositional studies.

KNOWN BIOLOGICAL EFFECTS OF SPECIFIC GLUCOSINOLATES AND THEIR HYDROLYTIC PRODUCTS

Allyl isothiocyanate (from sinigrin) — In common with other volatile isothiocyanates, this compound has poor water solubility and acts as a lacrimator and vesicant. Daily doses of 2 to 4 mg fed to rats by stomach tube for 60 days inhibit radioactive iodine uptake of the thyroid and increase the SCN ion content of the blood plasma 3- to 6-fold. At autopsy the rat thyroids show histological changes indicative of goiter.[68] Presumably the allyl isothiocyanate was detoxified by conversion to products including SCN ion, which is a known goitrogen. Allyl isothiocyanate is mutagenic in the Ames test.[69] It is not teratogenic in the rat, but does cause embryonal death and lowered fetal weights.[70]

1-Cyano-3,4-*epi*-thiobutane (from butenyl-GS) — This compound has an LD_{50} of 109 mg/kg in the rat (s.c.). It is not teratogenic, but causes embryonal death and decreased fetal weights.[70]

1-Cyano-2-*(S)*-hydroxy-3-butene (from *epi*-progoitrin) — The stable, water-soluble oil has an LD_{50} of 170 mg/kg in mice (oral)[9] and 200 mg/kg in rats (s.c.).[70] In pregnant rats treated with 175 mg/kg, the adrenals are enlarged and the liver partially necrotic.[70]

Table 1
GLUCOSINOLATES IDENTIFIED IN COMMERCIAL CROPS

No.	R-Group	Glucosinolate Trivial name	Structure	Ref.[a]
1.	Methyl-	Glucocapparin	CH_3-	13
2.	Allyl-	Sinigrin	$CH_2=CH-CH_2-$	13
3.	1-Methylpropyl-	Glucocochlearin	$CH_3-CH_2-CH(CH_3)-$	13
4.	2-Methyl-2-hydroxypropyl-	Glucoconringiin	$(CH_3)_2COH-CH_2-$[b]	13
5.	3-Methylthiopropyl-	Glucoibervirin	$CH_3-S-(CH_2)_3-$	13
6.	3-Methylsulfinylpropyl-	Glucoiberin	$CH_3-SO-(CH_2)_3-$	13
7.	3-Butenyl-	Gluconapin	$CH_2=CH-(CH_2)_2-$	13
8.	2(R)-Hydroxy-3-butenyl-	Progoitrin	$CH_2=CH-*CHOHCH_2-$[b]	13
9.	2(S)-Hydroxy-3-butenyl-	epi-Progoitrin	$CH_2=CH-*CHOHCH_2-$[b]	31
10.	2-Methyl-2-hydroxybutyl-	Glucocleomin	$CH_3-CH_2-\underset{CH_3}{\overset{}{C}}OH-CH_2-$[b]	32
11.	4-Methylthiobutyl-	Glucoerucin	$CH_3-S-(CH_2)_4-$	13
12.	4-Methylthio-3-butenyl-		$CH_3S-CH=CH-(CH_2)_2-$	33
13.	4-Methylsulfinylbutyl-	Glucoraphanin	$CH_3SO(CH_2)_4-$	13
14.	4-Methylsulfonylbutyl-	Glucoerysolin	$CH_3SO_2(CH_2)_4-$	13
15.	4-Pentenyl-	Glucobrassicanapin	$CH_2=CH-(CH_2)_3-$	13
16.	2-Hydroxy-4-pentenyl-		$CH_2=CH-CH_2-CHOH-CH_2-$[b]	34
17.	5-Methylthiopentyl-	Glucoberteroin	$CH_3-S-(CH_2)_5-$	13
18.	5-Methylsulfinylpentyl-	Glucoalyssin	$CH_3-SO-(CH_2)_5-$	13
19.	Benzyl-	Glucotropaeolin	$C_6H_5-CH_2-$	13
20.	2-Phenylethyl-	Gluconasturtiin	$C_6H_5CH_2CH_2-$	13
21.	p-Hydroxybenzyl-	Sinalbin	$p\text{-}HOC_6H_4-CH_2-$[c]	13
22.	m-Methoxybenzyl-	Glucolimnanthin	$m\text{-}CH_3OC_6H_4-CH_2-$	13
23.	3-Indolylmethyl-	Glucobrassicin	(indole-3-CH₂-)[c]	28
24.	3(N-Methoxy)indolylmethyl-	Neoglucobrassicin	(1-methoxyindole-3-CH₂-)[c]	29

Note: *Denotes centers of asymmetry.

[a] Those known prior to 1960 were taken from a review by Kjaer.
[b] These unstable isothiocyanates cyclize to form oxazolidinethiones.
[c] Decomposition products from these unstable isothiocyanates include SCN ion.

1-Cyano-2(S)-hydroxy-3(R)(S)-epi-thiobutanes (from epi-progoitrin) — These water-soluble oils tend to polymerize with rise in temperature.[23] The isomers tested orally in mice have LD_{50}s ranging from 178 to 240 mg/kg.[9] Poor growth and dose-dependent kidney and liver lesions develop in rats fed the mixed isomers at 75 to 300 ppm for 90 days.[71]

Table 2
COMPOSITION OF CABBAGE HEADS:[a] GLUCOSINOLATES AND AGLUCON PRODUCTS

	Brassica oleracea L.[b,c]			B. campestris L.,
	var. capitata		var.	ssp. pekinensis[d]
Component	f. alba (white)	f. rubra (red)	sabauda (Savoy)	(Chinese cabbage)
Allyl-NCS (2)[e]				
Mean, ppm	26	10	14	0
Range, ppm	5—146	2—26	0.1—39	—
3-Methylsulfinylpropyl-NCS (6)				
Mean, ppm	46	24	76	0
Range, ppm	5—92	8—49	23—144	—
3-Butenyl-NCS (7)				
Mean, ppm	2	11	0.3	15
Range, ppm	0—14	5—18	0—0.9	1—69
5 (S)-Vinyloxazolidinethione (8)				
Mean, ppm	4	11	0.6	11
Range, ppm	0—22	6—20	0—1.7	1—59
4-Methylsulfinylbutyl-NCS (13)				
Mean, ppm	9	93	9	0
Range, ppm	0—54	56—146	0.5—15	—
4-Methylsulfonylbutyl-NCS (14)				
Mean, ppm	4	5	11	0
Range, ppm	0—15	1—10	8—13	—
4-Pentenyl-NCS (15)				
Mean, ppm	0	0	0	26
Range, ppm	—	—	—	4—82
5-Allyloxazolidinethione (16)				
Mean, ppm	0	0	0	4
Range, ppm	—	—	—	0—19
5-Methylthiopentyl-NCS (17)				
Mean, ppm	0	0	0	11
Range, ppm	—	—	—	0.4—64
5-Methylsulfinylpentyl-NCS (18)				
Mean, ppm	0	0	0	25
Range, ppm	—	—	—	2—59
2-Phenylethyl-NCS (20)				
Mean, ppm	2	1	2	21
Range, ppm	0—6	0.5—2	0.2—4	6—91
Thiocyanate ion (23, 24)				
Mean, ppm	18	—	47	24
Range, ppm	8—59	—	35—61	11—50
Total glucosinolates[f]				
Mean, ppm	510	766	770	541
Range, ppm	264—1016	565—1088	413—1239	174—1357
Number of cultivars	67	8	4	14

[a] Calculated on a fresh (as-is) basis.
[b] Sampling did not include the cambial cortex and pith. Data from VanEtten et al.[35]
[c] 3-Methylthiopropyl-NCS (4),[e] 4-methylthiobutyl-NCS (10), and benzyl-NCS (18) were also found in small amounts in B. oleracea.
[d] Data from Daxenbichler et al.[36]
[e] Numbers in parentheses refer to parent glucosinolate in Table 1.
[f] Calculated from glucose measurement on the average molecular weight of glucosinolates present.

Table 3
COMPOSITION OF TURNIP AND RUTABAGA ROOTS:[a]
GLUCOSINOLATES AND AGLUCON PRODUCTS

Component	Brassica campestris L. ssp. rapifera (turnip)		Brassica napus L. ssp. rapifera (rutabaga)	
	Mean (ppm)	Range (ppm)	Mean (ppm)	Range (ppm)
1-Methylpropyl-NCS (3)[b]	20	0—46	29	0—64
3-Butenyl-NCS (7)	32	1—138	11	tr—73
5(S)-Vinyloxazolidinethione (8)	69	0—135	108	66—188
4-Methylthiobutyl-NCS (11)	14	5—23	52	24—132
4-Pentenyl-NCS (15)	35	1—74	5	tr—15
5-Allyloxazolidinethione (16)	20	0—122	4	0—17
5-Methylthiopentyl-NCS (17)	32	9—80	43	2—100
5-Methylsulfinylpentyl-NCS (18)	7	0—13	13	0—34
2-Phenylethyl-NCS (20)	83	10—166	64	16—166
Thiocyanate ion (23, 24)	34	7—65	25	8—66
Total glucosinolates[c]	1350	593—2307	1544	868—2641

[a] Calculated on fresh weight of peeled roots.[38]
[b] Numbers in parentheses refer to parent glucosinolate in Table 1.
[c] Calculated from glucose measurement using mol wt = 457.

5,5-Dimethyloxazolidinethione (from 2-methyl-2-hydroxypropyl-GS) — Isolated from hare's ear mustard *(Conringia orientalis)*,[72] this compound has about the same antithyroid activity as *R* and *S* goitrin.[73]

p-Hydroxybenzyl-GS (sinalbin) — Isolated sinalbin causes marked growth depression in mice when fed at a level that would be expected if white mustard seed was used as a sole source of protein.[74] Our calculations indicate this level to be about 2% sinalbin in the ration.

(R)- and (S)-2-Hydroxy-3-butenyl-GSs (progoitrin and *epi*-progoitrin) — Following oral administration of crystalline progoitrin to humans and to rats, the compound slowly hydrolyzes to give goitrin as one of the products.[8] Increased goitrin content of the blood serum and urine and suppression of radioiodine uptake of the thyroid followed ingestion of 1 to 4 g of progoitrin by humans. The goitrin content of the blood serum reached a maximum in 35 hr. In contrast, serum goitrin peaked at 30 min after ingestion of an equivalent amount of goitrin. In vitro experiments with *Paracolobactrum,* commonly found in the intestinal tract of man,[5] and *Enterobacter cloacae*[6] demonstrated that these organisms hydrolyze progoitrin to give goitrin. Isolated *epi*-progoitrin fed to rats for 90 days as 0.5, 0.85, 1.5, and 2.6% of the ration caused decreased growth proportional to the amount fed.[75] At 2.6% of the ration, all the animals died within 56 days. Pathological lesions were observed in enlarged kidneys, liver and thyroids. Similar but more severe lesions and poorer growth were observed in animals fed crambe meal with its active thioglucosidase and *epi*-progoitrin present. Those animals fed such crambe meal died if the *epi*-progoitrin level reached 0.5 to 1.0% of the total ration.[75]

3-Methylsulfinylpropyl isothiocyanate (from glucoiberin) — The LD_{50} in rats (s.c.) is 90 mg/kg. It is not teratogenic, but does cause embryonal death and lowered fetal weights.[70]

3-Methylsulfonylpropyl isothiocyanate (cheirolin from methyl sulfonylpropyl-GS) — This compound is a nonvolatile liquid (bp 200°C, 3 mm) and has some solubility

Table 4
COMPOSITION OF CRUCIFER SEED MEALS:[a] GLUCOSINOLATES AND AGLUCON PRODUCTS

Plant name	Number of cultivars	3-Butenyl-NCS(6)[b]		(S)-Goitrin (7)		4-Pentenyl-NCS (14)		Total glucosinolates[c]		Ref.
		Mean (%)	Range (%)	Mean (%)	Range (%)	Mean (%)	Range (%)	Mean (%)	Range (%)	
Rapeseed, European										
Brassica napus L.										
Winter type	17	0.47	0.30—0.63	1.19	0.75—1.55			6.0	3.9—6.9	43
Summer type	5	0.41	0.35—0.49	1.00	0.86—1.12			5.0	4.3—5.6	43
Bronowski	5	0.12	0.02—0.35	0.16	0.03—0.8			1.5	0.18—3.7	43
B. campestris L.										
Winter type	4	0.89	0.81—1.05	0.13	0.06—0.17			3.7	3.3—4.3	43
Summer type	2	0.56	0.49—0.59	0.34	0.32—0.35			3.3	3.3—3.3	43
Rapeseed, Canadian										
B. napus L.										
Common cultivars	3	0.20	0.19—0.25	1.2	0.80—1.38	0.05	0.03—0.07	4.6	3.4—5.7	44, 45
Bronowski	1	0.03		0.03				0.21		44, 45
Tower	1	0.10		0.19		tr.				46
B. campestris L.										
Common cultivars	2	0.2		0.17		0.15		1.8		44
Candle	1	0.05		0.07		0.05				46

[a] Calculated on basis of air-dry, fat-free meal. May also contain other glucosinolates in small amounts.
[b] Numbers in parentheses refer to parent glucosinolate in Table 1.
[c] Calculated from glucose measurement and the average molecular weight of glucosinolates present.

Table 5
GLUCOSINOLATES IN MINOR CROPS

Plant name	Part of plant	Aglucon[a] and parent glucosinolate[b]	Ref.
For Food			
Broccoli, cauliflower, collards, kale *Brassica oleracea* L.	Leaf, flower, stem	Similar to cabbage	48
Brussels sprout *B. oleracea* L., var. *gemmifera* D.C.	Button (bud)	165 ppm (2), 51 ppm (7) 115 ppm (8), 85 ppm (23, 24)	47
Garden cress *Lepidium sativum* L.	Leaf	L (19), S (7) S (15), S (20)	49
Kohlrabi *B. oleracea* L. var. *gongylodes*	Stem	32 ppm (3), 34 ppm (6), 14 ppm (7), 17 ppm (23, 24)	50
Papaya *Carica papaya* L.	Fruit pulp (immature)	0.02% (19)	51
	Latex, dry	2.6—4.1% (19)	2
Radish *Raphanus sativus* L.	Root	L (12) S (23, 24)	33
Rocket mustard *Eruca sativa* Mill.	Whole plant	L (11)	52
Turnips *B. campestris* L.	Leaf	127 ppm (7), 109 ppm (15), 38 ppm (23, 24)	38
Water cress, *Nasturtium officinale* R. Br.	Leaf	L (20)	53
For Condiment			
Black mustard *B. nigra* L. Koch	Seed meal	1.0—1.2% (2)	54
Brown or Indian mustard *B. juncea* L. Coss	Seed meal	2.8% (2), S (7)	46, 55
White mustard *B. hirta* (*Sinapis alba* L.)	Seed meal	3.3% (21)	56
Capers *Capparis spinosa* L.	Bud	L (1), S (2), S (6), S (10)	57
Charlock *B. kaber* (D.C.) L.C. Wheeler or *Sinapis arvensis*	Seed	L (21)	54
Ethiopian rapeseed *B. carinata* Braun.	Seed	L (2)	54
Horseradish *Armoracia rusticana*	Root	0.2—0.4% (2), 0.08—0.4% (20)	58
For Feed			
Crambe *Crambe abyssinica* Hochst. ex. R. E. Fries	Defatted dehulled seed meal	2.4—2.9% (9), S (2), S (7), S (20)	31, 59
Limnanthes alba Benth	Defatted seed meal	1.2—2.0% (22), 0.0—0.2% (4)	60—62

[a] L = large amount, S = small amount; numerical values are for isothiocyanate, oxazolidinethione, or SCN ion.
[b] Numbers in parentheses refer to parent glucosinolates of Table 1.

in water. It is a glucosinolate hydrolysis product from mature fruit and leaves of a pasture weed (turnip weed, *Rapistrum rugosum*). The isolated compound fed to rats causes a depression of radioiodine uptake by the thyroid.[76]

2-Phenylethyl isothiocyanate (from 2-phenylethyl-GS) — This is a volatile liquid, bp 102 to 103° (1.4 to 1.5 mm). The LD_{50} in male mice is approximately 700 mg/kg orally, 150 mg/kg s.c. or 50 mg/kg i.v. A 0.5% solution of the compound gave 96 to 100% knock-down of house flies and pea aphids. The compound is less active against Mexican bean beetles, German cockroaches, and mites.[77]

5-Phenyloxazolidinethione (from 2-hydroxy-2-phenylethyl-GS) — Isolated from species of *Barbarea* and *Reseda luteola*,[78] this compound has about half the antithyroid activity of *R* and *S* goitrin.[79]

Thiocyanate ion — Thyroid enlargement caused by SCN was observed in some of the patients that were treated for hypertension with potassium thiocyanate.[80] With the feeding of 0.5g KSCN per day, the SCN ion content of the blood was increased 5 to 10 mg/100 mℓ.[81] At this dosage level, iodine uptake of the thyroid was inhibited. Thyroid enlargement in animals is prevented by increasing the iodine content of the ration unless the SCN ion is fed at high level.[83] The feeding of SCN ion to milk cows at 1.5 to 3 g/day (the amount found in a daily feeding of 15 to 30 kilo of *Brassica* fodder) gave an increase in SCN ion in the milk from 1.7 to 3.5 mg/ℓ to 6.2 to 9.3 mg/ℓ, but this was considered not to be harmful for those drinking the milk.[84] However, as the SCN ion increased, the iodine content of the milk decreased markedly, but then increased to normal levels after the feeding of the SCN ion was stopped. Apparently the SCN ion prevents iodine absorption by both the thyroid and the mammary gland. From this observation, which has been confirmed by others, it is concluded an iodine deficiency might develop in those consuming large amounts of milk from cows that have high levels of SCN ion in their ration.

(S)- or *(R)*-5-Vinyloxazolidinethione (goitrin, from progoitrin or *epi*-progoitrin) — When *(S)*-goitrin is taken by man in a single dose ranging from 50 to 200 mg, marked to complete inhibition of iodine uptake by the thyroid occurs for up to 24 hr.[85] This effect is not overcome by larger amounts of iodine in the diet.[86] *(S)*-Goitrin from progoitrin in rapeseed and *(R)*-goitrin from *epi*-progoitrin in crambe seed have equal antithyroid activity. They possess 2% of the potency of propylthiouracil when tested in the rat, but 133% of the potency of propylthiouracil when tested in man.[8] *(R)*-Goitrin fed to rats for 90 days as 0.23% of the ration caused a mild hyperplasia of the thyroid and reduced the body weight to 85% of that of the controls.[75] *(R)*- and *(S)*-goitrin fed to broilers for 30 days as 0.05% of the ration depressed weight gains and enlarged the thyroids. After about 3 to 4 weeks of feeding, the radioiodine uptake of the thyroid increased and the secretion rate from the gland became normal. It appears the chicks fed the goitrogen eventually reach physiological equilibrium at an increased thyroid-to-body weight ratio.[87] Similar results with chicks were reported by others.[88] The oral LD_{50} in mice for *(R)*-goitrin is 1260 to 1415 mg/kg.[9] *(R)*- and *(S)*-goitrin are not teratogenic to the rat.[70,89] The feeding of goitrin at levels up to 2.0 μg per rat per day on a diet marginal in iodine content caused enlargement of the thyroids as the dosage was increased.[90] These results were not confirmed by others, who found that a dose of 50 μg/day was required to cause enlargement of the thyroid.[91]

PROBLEM AREAS

Crucifer Oilseed Meals

In the use of crucifer plants for food or feed, the most obvious problems have been those arising from attempts to use seed meal for animal feed. Most harmful effects are caused by the glucosinolates or products derived from them that are found in processed seed meal. The older standard varieties of rape contain 3 to 7% glucosinolates in fat-free meal.[16] In contrast, the known glucosinolate content of the horticultural crucifer crops ranges from 175 to 3900 ppm based on fresh weight.[36,47,92] In the early development of the rape and mustard oilseed industry, the byproduct meal was used for fertilizer either because livestock refused to eat the meal or because growth response was poor, with development of enlarged thyroids and pathologic changes in other body organs. Problems with breeding animals occurred even when the meal was fed at low levels. Ruminants were the most tolerant to the meal; consequently, some of the meal was utilized in feeding beef cattle.[14] Controlling heat and moisture content of the seed during processing made it possible to inactivate the thioglucosidase without hydrolysis of the glucosinolates. Meals processed this way gave a better growth response and could be fed to monogastric animals as 10% of the ration.[14,16]

Insight into the problems encountered in the use of crucifer crops for food or feed has improved in the last decade because of research on the nature of the natural glucosinolates and recognition of organic nitriles as products from thioglucosidase hydrolysis[23,25] as well as isothiocyanates and goitrin.[85] Development of faster and more accurate methods of testing for antithyroid activity was also essential.[8] From this background it was apparent that improvement in crucifer oilseed meals for feed uses depends on extraction or inactivation of the glucosinolates in existing varieties or the development of new varieties low in total glucosinolates.[93] Crucial to progress in either of these areas was the development of better quantitative analytical methods.

Outstanding progress has been made in the development of new rapeseed varieties that are low in total glucosinolates. A variety named Bronowski, developed in Northern Europe through selection over many years, contains as low as 0.2% total glucosinolates in the defatted seed meal. Pigs fed processed seed meal from a Bronowski variety did as well as those fed soybean meal and better than those fed processed seed meal from a standard *Brassica napus* rape.[94] However, the feeding to mice of Bronowski seed meal that has not been heated to inactivate the thioglucosidase still shows the presence of growth-inhibiting substances; they are found in a glucosinolate-containing fraction from the meal.[95] Bronowski seed was crossed with other varieties to improve the agronomic characteristics of the plant and to lower the erucic acid content of the seed oil. At the present time, several new varieties, of both *Brassica napus* and *B. campestris*, that are very low in erucic acid and glucosinolates have been introduced in Canada. These varieties, collectively named Canola,[96] may be fed to broiler chicks as 20% of the ration, to growing pigs at 12%, or to calves at 20%.[97]

In the recent literature, at least 25 publications describe procedures with water as an essential part of the solvent for extraction of glucoinsolates from crucifer seeds. Most of the glucosinolates are removed, but cost of the additional steps prohibit processing meal for use in animal feeds. The best of the procedures is a preparation of protein isolate that is satisfactory in dogs and rats as a source of 40% of their protein.[98] A critical appraisal of the problems encountered in establishing such isolates as safe for food use has been reported.[99] In making protein isolates, consideration should be given to the reaction of isothiocyanates with proteins at pH 6 and above.[100]

Condiments

Those crucifers consumed as condiments, although high in total glucosinolates, appear in practice not to be hazardous because their pungency limits their use in large amounts. For example, rats fed defatted *Brassica carinata* seed containing thioglucosidase and unhydrolyzed allyl-GS, as 20% of their ration, grew very slowly and at autopsy showed no pathology except abscesses in their throats. The abscesses were attributed to the vesicant action of allyl isothiocyanate liberated during mastication and swallowing of the seed meal.[101]

Crucifer Vegetable Crops

Brassica oleracea var. *capitata* (cabbage) and related cole crops are the major horticultural crops that contain glucosinolates. From the extensive literature on the goitrogenic properties of cabbage, no firm conclusions can be drawn because of the diverse results from feeding vegetables to experimental animals.[7] The wide range of the glucosinolates in these vegetables and the variability of glucosinolate hydrolytic products account in part for the many different biological effects reported from the feeding of these crops to experimental animals. When rats on a ration marginal in iodine content are fed cabbage *ad libitum,* abnormal function and enlargement of the thyroid has consistently been obtained.[68] When the rats are fed SCN ion, allyl isothiocyanate, or goitrin at the levels they would be expected to ingest if fed cabbage, depression of iodine uptake and enlargement of the thyroid occurs.[102] In contrast, by a test in which depression of radioactive iodine uptake of the thyroid was measured in man after eating a large serving of cabbage, no significant goitrogenic activity could be detected. (Tests utilizing rutabaga and turnip roots consistently gave positive results.)[103] What appears to be contradictory results by different groups of investigators may be explained in the following way. Thyroid inhibition is not a problem when cabbage or other crucifer vegetables are consumed at intervals even in large amounts, if the diet is adequate in iodine content; however, if these foods are consumed over long periods of time as a major component of a relatively low iodine diet, thyroid malfunction may develop. Most of the work on goitrogenicity of cabbage was carried out before the major glucosinolates in cabbage, 3-methylsulfinylpropyl-GS and 3-indolymethyl-GS, were recognized. The compositions of the cabbage in the diets as consumed were not known with respect to the presence of isothiocyanates, goitrin, nitriles, or intact glucosinolates.

There has been concern that new plant varieties may contain larger amounts of natural toxicants.[104] Since current varieties of cabbage differ fourfold in total glucosinolate,[92] the development of new varieties of low glucosinolate content should be possible. Although total glucosinolate content may vary with growing conditions,[47,105] the relative proportions of individual glucosinolates (pattern) in *Brassica* cultivars usually follow genetic lines.[35,36,106,107] For example, red cabbages are rich in 4-carbon glucosinolates (Nos. 7, 8, 11, 13 of Table 1) compared to most white cabbages.[35] Glucosinolate patterns of seed differ significantly from the corresponding heads, but have predictive value for glucosinolate pattern in the heads.[108]

The biological effects of the aglucons that may be formed from the glucosinolates and the conditions under which the aglucons form should be more thoroughly explored. Fresh, crushed roots of turnip and rutabaga yield 0.01 to 0.1% goitrin, yet little goitrin was found in the leaf tissue of other *Brassica* vegetables.[85] Leaf tissue autolyzes to form predominantly organic nitriles.[25,52,109] Commercial sauerkraut contained from 16 to 25 ppm 1-cyano-3-methylsulfinylpropane, but no isothiocyanates or goitrin.[110]

Toxicants From Milk and Body Parts of Farm Animals Fed Crucifer Crops

Crucifers are grown for forage in Australia and parts of Europe as a major part of the ration for ruminants. In 1956, a hypothesis was advanced that a significant amount of endemic goiter in Tasmania and in Australia was due to the action of a goitrogen in milk from cows fed *Brassica* forage.[111] Evidence to support the hypothesis included the failure of potassium iodide to correct the development of goiter in school children who drank the milk and the development of hyperplasia of the thyroid in calves of the cows fed the forage. The hypothesis has been refuted by others[112] who presented convincing evidence that goitrin, in sufficient amounts to show inhibition of radioiodine uptake by the thyroid, cannot be transferred to the milk of cows by feeding high levels of *Brassica* forage. Concentration of goitrin in the milk ranged from 30 to 80 µg/ℓ. Rat feeding for a year on this milk at the maximum *ad libitum* level of 20 mℓ per rat per day caused no enlargement of the thyroids or other evidence of their malfunction. However, a third group did show enlargement of thyroids of rats fed milk from cows in an endemic goiter region of Finland.[90] Also according to these workers, increasing enlargement of the thyroids occurred in rats fed daily doses of goitrin ranging from 0 to 2 µg/day. This concentration was in the range that they received from the milk. These results demonstrate the difficulties in establishing the subchronic to chronic levels at which the goitrogen shows an effect.

Kale anemia, a disease of cattle feeding on *Brassica* kale, is not caused by the glucosinolates, but by free *S*-methylcysteine sulfoxide in the plant tissue or compounds formed from the sulfoxide by microorganisms in the digestive tract.[113]

There is no evidence for the transfer of *(R)*-goitrin, organic nitriles, or unhydrolyzed *epi*-progoitrin to the body parts of beef cattle fed optimum levels of processed crambe seed meal that contained these compounds.[114]

Glucobrassicins

These 3-indolylmethyl-GSs (Scheme 3) are of special interest because 3-indolylmethyl-GS and 3-(*N*-methoxy)indolylmethyl-GS are found in large amounts in rapidly growing leaf tissue, such as in edible cabbage. The third member of the group, 3-(*N*-sulfonate)indolylmethyl-GS, isolated from *Isatis tinctoria* L. seed, is also probably present in edible crucifers.[115]

Metabolism of Glucosinolate Hydrolysis Products

Recent review includes the metabolism of SCN-, organic isothiocyanates, thiocyanates, and nitriles,[116] but the pharmacology of many of the glucosinolate products remains unknown.

REFERENCES

1. **Ettlinger, M. G. and Kjaer, A.**, Sulfur compounds in plants, in *Recent Advances in Phytochemistry*, Vol. 1, Mabry, T. J., Ed., Appleton-Century-Crofts, New York, 1968, 59—144.
2. **Tang, C. S.**, Localization of benzyl glucosinolate and thioglucosidase in *Carica papaya* fruit, *Phytochemistry*, 12, 769—773, 1973.
3. **Kjaer, A.**, Glucosinolates in the Cruciferae, in *The Biology and Chemistry of the Cruciferae*, Vaughn, J. G., MacLeod, A. J., and Jones, B. M. G., Eds., Academic Press, New York, 1976, 207—219.
4. **Florkin, M. and Stotz, E. H.**, in *Comprehensive Biochemistry*, Vol. 13, Florkin, M. and Stotz, E. H., Eds., Elsevier, New York, 1965, 142.
5. **Oginsky, E. L., Stein, A. E., and Greer, M. A.**, Myrosinase activity in bacteria as demonstrated by the conversion of progoitrin to goitrin, *Proc. Soc. Exp. Biol. Med.*, 119, 360—364, 1965.
6. **Tani, N., Ohtsuru, M., and Hata, T.**, Purification and general characteristics of bacterial myrosinase produced by *Enterobacter cloacae*, *Agric. Biol. Chem.*, 38, 1623—1630, 1974.
7. **Greer, M. A.**, Nutrition and goiter, *Physiol. Rev.*, 30, 513—548, 1950.
8. **Greer, M. A.**, The natural occurrence of goitrogenic agents, *Recent Prog. Horm. Res.*, 18, 187—219, 1962.
9. **VanEtten, C. H., Daxenbichler, M. E., and Wolff, I. A.**, Natural glucosinolates (thioglucosides) in foods and feeds, *J. Agric. Food Chem.*, 17, 483—491, 1969.
10. **VanEtten, C. H. and Tookey, H. L.**, Chemistry and biological effects of glucosinolates, in *Herbivores Their Interaction with Secondary Plant Metabolites*, Rosenthal, G. A. and Janzen, D. H., Eds., Academic Press, New York, 1979, 471—500.
11. **Tookey, H. L., VanEtten, C. H., and Daxenbichler, M. E.**, Glucosinolates, in *Toxic Constituents of Plant Foodstuffs*, 2nd ed., Liener, I. E., Ed., Academic Press, New York, 1980, 103—142.

12. Tapper, B. A. and Reay, P. F., Cyanogenic glucosides and glucosinolates, in *Chemistry and Biochemistry of Herbage,* Vol. 1, Butler, G. W. and Bailey, R. W., Eds., Academic Press, New York, 1973, 447—476.
13. Kjaer, A., Naturally derived isothiocyanates (mustard oils) and their parent glucosides, in *Progress in the Chemistry of Organic Natural Products,* Zechmeister, L., Ed., Springer-Verlag, Basel, 1960, 122—175.
14. Bowland, J. P., Clandinin, D. R., and Wetter, L. R., Eds., Rapeseed meal for livestock and poultry — a review. Publ. 1257, The Canada Department of Agriculture, Ottawa, 1965, 1—96.
15. Rutkowski, A., The feed value of rapeseed meal, *J. Am. Oil Chem. Soc.,* 48, 863—868, 1971.
16. Appelqvist, L. A. and Ohlson, R., *Rapeseed,* Elsevier, New York, 1972, 1—391.
17. Virtanen, A. I., On the chemistry of the *Brassica* factor: its effect on the function of the thyroid gland and its transfer to milk, *Experientia,* 17, 241—252, 1961.
18. Walker, N. J. and Gray, I. K., The glucosinolate of land cress *(Coronopus didymus)* and its enzymic degradation products as precursors of off-flavor in milk — a review, *J. Agric. Food Chem.,* 18, 346—352, 1970.
19. Vaughan, J. G., MacLeod, A. J., and Jones, B. M. G., Eds., *The Biology and Chemistry of the Cruciferae,* Academic Press, New York, 1976, 1—355.
20. Gmelin, R. and Virtanen, A. I., A new type of enzymatic cleavage of mustard oil glucosides. Formation of allyl thiocyanate in *Thlaspi arvense* L. and benzyl thiocyanate in *Lepidium ruderale* L. and *L. sativum* L., *Acta Chem. Scand.,* 13, 1474—1475, 1959.
21. Cole, R. A., Volatile components produced during ontogeny of some cultivated crucifers, *J. Sci. Food Agric.,* 31, 549—557, 1980.
22. Greer, M. A., The isolation and identification of progoitrin from *Brassica* seed, *Arch. Biochem. Biophys.,* 99, 369—371, 1962.
23. Daxenbichler, M. E., VanEtten, C. H., and Wolff, I. A., Diastereomeric episulfides from *epi*-progoitrin upon autolysis of crambe seed meal, *Phytochemistry,* 7, 989—996, 1968.
24. Kirk, J. T. O. and Macdonald, C. G., 1-Cyano-3,4-epithiobutane: a major product of glucosinolate hydrolysis in seeds from certain varieties of *Brassica campestris, Phytochemistry,* 13, 2611—2615, 1974.
25. Daxenbichler, M. E., VanEtten, C. H., and Spencer, G. F., Glucosinolates and derived products in cruciferous vegetables. Identification of organic nitriles from cabbage, *J. Agric. Food Chem.,* 25, 121—124, 1977.
26. Tookey, H. L., Crambe thioglucosidase glucohydrolase (EC 3.2.3.1): separation of a protein required for epithiobutane formation, *Can. J. Biochem.,* 51, 1654—1660, 1973.
27. Cole, R. A., Epithiospecifier protein in turnip and changes in products of autolysis during ontogeny, *Phytochemistry,* 17, 1563—1565, 1978.
28. Gmelin, R. and Virtanen, A. I., Glucobrassicin, the precursor of 3-indolylacetonitrile, ascorbigen, and SCN⁻ in *Brassica oleracea* species, *S. Kemistilehti,* B34, 15—18, 1961.
29. Gmelin, R. and Virtanen, A. I., Neoglucobrassicin, ein zweiter SCN-precursor vom indoltyp in *Brassica*-arten, *Acta Chem. Scand.,* 16, 1378—1386, 1962.
30. Elliott, M. C. and Stowe, B. B., Indole compounds related to auxins and goitrogens of woad *(Isatis tinctoria* L.), *Plant Physiol.,* 47, 366—372, 1971.
31. Daxenbichler, M. E., VanEtten, C. H., and Wolff, I. A., A new thioglucoside, (R)-2-hydroxy-3-butenylglucosinolate (sic) from *Crambe abyssinica* seed, *Biochemistry,* 4, 318—323, 1965.
32. Kjaer, A. and Thomsen, H., Glucocleomin, a new natural glucoside, furnishing (-)-5-ethyl-5-methyl-2-oxazolidinethione on enzymic hydrolysis, *Acta Chem. Scand.,* 16, 591—598, 1962.
33. Friis, P. and Kjaer, A., 4-Methylthio-3-butenyl isothiocyanate, the pungent principle of radish root, *Acta Chem. Scand.,* 20, 698—705, 1966.
34. Tapper, B. A. and MacGibbon, D. B., Isolation of (-)-5-allyl-2-thiooxazolidone from *Brassica napus* L., *Phytochemistry,* 6, 749—753, 1967.
35. VanEtten, C. H., Daxenbichler, M. E., Tookey, H. L., Kwolek, W. F., Williams, P. H., and Yoder, O. C., Glucosinolates: potential toxicants in cabbage cultivars, *J. Am. Soc. Hort. Sci.,* 105, 710—714, 1980.
36. Daxenbichler, M. E., VanEtten, C. H., and Williams, P. H., Glucosinolates and derived products in Cruciferous vegetables: analysis of 14 varieties of Chinese cabbage, *J. Agric. Food Chem.,* 27, 34—37, 1979
37. VanEtten, C. H., Daxenbichler, M. E., Kwolek, W. F., and Williams, P. H., Distribution of glucosinolates in the pith, cambial-cortex, and leaves of the head in cabbage, *Brassica oleracea* L., *J. Agric. Food Chem.,* 27, 648—650, 1979.
38. Carlson, D. G., Daxenbichler, M. E., VanEtten, C. H., Tookey, H. L., and Williams, P. H., Glucosinolates in crucifer vegetables: turnips and rutabagas, *J. Agric. Food Chem.,* 29, 1235—1239, 1982.

39. Daxenbichler, M. E. and VanEtten, C. H., Glucosinolate and derived products in cruciferous vegetables: gas-liquid chromatographic determination of the aglucon derivatives from cabbage. *J. Assoc. Off. Anal. Chem.*, 60, 950—953, 1977.
40. Appelqvist, L. A. and Josefsson, E., Method for quantitative determination of isothiocyanates and oxazolidinethiones in digests of seed meals of rape and turnip rape, *J. Sci. Food Agric.*, 18, 510—519, 1967.
41. Josefsson, E., Method for quantitative determination of *p*-hydroxybenzyl isothiocyanate in digests of seed meal of *Sinapis alba* L., *J. Sci. Food Agric.*, 19, 192—194, 1968.
42. VanEtten, C. H. and Daxenbichler, M. E., Glucosinolates and derived products in cruciferous vegetables: total glucosinolates by retention on anion exchange resin and enzymatic hydrolysis to measure released glucose, *J. Assoc. Off. Anal. Chem.*, 60, 946—949, 1977.
43. Josefsson, E. and Appelqvist, L. A., Glucosinolates in seed of rape and turnip rape as affected by variety and environment, *J. Sci. Food Agric.*, 19, 564—570, 1968.
44. Downey, R. K., Craig, B. M., and Youngs, C. G., Breeding rapeseed for oil and meal quality, *J. Am. Oil Chem. Soc.*, 46, 121—123, 1969.
45. Finlayson, A. J., Krzymanski, J., and Downey, R. K., Comparison of chemical and agronomic characteristics of two *Brassica napus* L. cultivars, Bronowski and Target, *J. Am. Oil Chem. Soc.*, 50, 407—410, 1973.
46. Maheshwari, P. N., Stanley, D. W., Gray, J. I., and Van de Voort, F. R., An HPLC method for simultaneous quantitation of individual isothiocyanates and oxazolidinethione in myrosinase digests of rapeseed meal, *J. Am. Oil Chem. Soc.*, 56, 837—841, 1979.
47. Heaney, R. K. and Fenwick, G. R., Glucosinolates in *Brassica* vegetables. Analysis of 22 varieties of Brussels sprout (*Brassica oleracea* var. *gemmifera*), *J. Sci. Food Agric.*, 31, 785—793, 1980.
48. Josefsson, E., Distribution of thioglucosides in different parts of *Brassica* plants, *Phytochemistry*, 6, 1617—1627, 1967.
49. MacLeod, A. J. and Islam, R., Volatile flavour components of garden cress, *J. Sci. Food Agric.*, 27, 909—912, 1976.
50. Michajlovskij, N., Sedlak, J., and Kostekova, O., Effect of thermal treatment on the content of goitrogenic substances in plant food, *Rev. Czech. Med.*, 15, 132—144, 1969.
51. Tang, C. S., Benzyl isothiocyanate of papaya fruit, *Phytochemistry*, 10, 117—121, 1971.
52. Cole, R. A., Isothiocyanates, nitriles, and thiocyanates as products of autolysis of glucosinolates in Cruciferae, *Phytochemistry*, 15, 759—762, 1976.
53. Schultz, O. E. and Gmelin, R., Paper chromatography of mustard oil drugs, *Z. Naturforsch.*, 7b, 500—508, 1952.
54. Ettlinger, M. G. and Thompson, C. P., in Studies of Mustard Oil Glucosides II. Contract No. DA19-129 QM-1689 Project No. 7-99-01-001, Simplified food logistics. Final Report, Department of Chemistry, Rice Institute, Houston, Texas, 1962, 1—106.
55. Jensen, K. A., Conti, J., and Kjaer, A., Isothiocyanates. II. Volatile isothiocyanates in seeds and roots of various *Brassica* plants, *Acta Chem. Scand.*, 7, 1267—1270, 1953.
56. Josefsson, E., Content of *p*-hydroxybenzyl glucosinolate in seed meals of *Sinapis alba* as affected by heredity, environment and seed part, *J. Sci. Food Agric.*, 21, 94—97, 1970.
57. Ahmed, Z. F., Rizk, A. M., Harnonouda, F. M., and Seif El-Nasr, M. M., Glucosinolates of Egyptian *Capparis* species, *Phytochemistry*, 11, 251—256, 1972.
58. Daxenbichler, M. E. and Rhodes, A. M., unpublished data, 1981.
59. Daxenbichler, M. E., VanEtten, C. H., Brown, F. S., and Jones, Q., Oxazolidinethiones and volatile isothiocyanates in enzyme-treated seed meals from 65 species of Cruciferae, *J. Agric. Food Chem.*, 12, 127—130, 1965.
60. Ettlinger, M. G. and Lundeen, A. J., The mustard oil of *Limnanthes douglasii* seed, *m*-methoxybenzyl isothiocyanate, *J. Am. Chem. Soc.*, 78, 1952—1956, 1956.
61. Miller, R. W., Daxenbichler, M. E., Earle, F. R., and Gentry, H. S., Search for new industrial oils. VIII. The genus *Limnanthes*, *J. Am. Oil Chem. Soc.*, 41, 167—169, 1964.
62. Daxenbichler, M. E. and VanEtten, C. H., 5,5-Dimethyl oxazolidine-2-thione formation from glucosinolate in *Limnanthes alba* Benth. seed, *J. Am. Oil Chem. Soc.*, 51, 449—450, 1974.
63. Helboe, P., Olsen, O., and Sorensen, H., Separation of glucosinolates by high performance liquid chromatography, *J. Chromatrogr.*, 197, 199—205, 1980.
64. Kjaer, A., Madsen, J. O., Maeda, Y., Ozawa, Y., and Uda, Y., Volatiles in distillates of fresh radish of Japanese and Kenyan origin, *Agric. Biol. Chem.*, 42, 1715—1721, 1978.
65. Buttery, R. G., Griadagni, B. G., Ling, L. C., Seifert, R. M., and Lipton, W., Additional volatile components of cabbage, broccoli and cauliflower, *J. Agric. Food Chem.*, 24, 829—832, 1976.
66. Grob, K. and Matile, P., Capillary GC of glucoinsolate-derived horseradish constituents, *Phytochemistry*, 19, 1789—1793, 1980.

67. MacLeod, A. J. and Pikk, H. E., A comparision of the chemical flavour composition of some Brussels sprouts cultivars grown at different crop spacings, *Phytochemistry*, 17, 1029—1032, 1978.
68. Langer, P. and Stolc, V., Goitrogenic activity of allylisothiocyanate a wide spread natural mustard oil, *Endocrinology*, 76, 151—155, 1965.
69. Yamaguchi, T., Mutagenicity of isothiocyanates, isocyanates, and thioureas on *Salmonella typhimurium*, *Agric. Biol. Chem.*, 44, 3017—3018, 1980.
70. Nishie, K. and Daxenbichler, M. E., Toxicology of glucosinolates, related compounds (nitriles, R-goitrin, isothiocyanates) and vitamin U found in Cruciferae, *Food Cosmet. Toxicol.*, 18, 159—172, 1980.
71. Gould, D. H., Gumbmann, M. R., and Daxenbichler, M. E., Pathological changes in rats fed the crambe meal-glucosinolate hydrolytic products, 2S-l-cyano-2-hydroxy-3,4-epithiobutanes *(erythro* and *threo)* for 90 days, *Food Cosmet Toxicol.*, 18, 619—625, 1980.
72. Hopkins, C. Y., A sulfur containing substance from the seed of *Conringia orientalis*, *Can. J. Res.*, 16B, 341—344, 1938.
73. Astwood, E. B., Bissell, A., and Hughes, A. M., Further studies on the nature of compounds which inhibit the function of the thyroid gland, *Endocrinology*, 37, 456—481, 1945.
74. Josefsson, E. and Uppström, B., Influence of sinapine and *p*-hydroxybenzyl glucosinolate on the nutritional value of rapeseed and white mustard meals, *J. Sci. Food Agric.*, 27, 438—442, 1976.
75. VanEtten, C. H., Gagne, W. E., Robbins, D. J., Booth, A. N., Daxenbichler, M. E., and Wolff, I. A., Biological evaluation of crambe seed meals and derived products by rat feeding, *Cereal Chem.*, 46, 145—155, 1969.
76. Bachelard, H. S. and Trikojus, V. M., Plant thioglycosides and the problem of endemic goitre in Australia, *Nature (London)*, 185, 80—82, 1960.
77. Lichtenstein, E. P., Strong, F. M., and Morgan, D. G., Naturally occurring insecticides, identification of 2-phenylethyl isothiocyanate as an insecticide occurring naturally in the edible part of turnips, *J. Agric. Food Chem.*, 10, 30—33, 1962.
78. Kjaer, A. and Gmelin, R., A new isothiocyanate glucoside (glucobarbarin) furnishing (-)-phenyl-2-oxazolidinethione upon enzymic hydrolysis, *Acta Chem. Scand.*, 11, 906—907, 1957.
79. Greer, M. A. and Whallon, J., Antithyroid effect of barbarin (phenyl-thiooxazolidone) a natural occurring compound from *Barbarea*, *Proc. Soc. Exp. Biol. Med.*, 107, 802—804, 1961.
80. Barker, M. H., The blood cyanates in the treatment of hypertension, *JAMA*, 106, 762—767, 1936.
81. Atwood, E. B., The chemical nature of compounds which inhibit the function of the thyroid gland, *J. Pharmacol. Exp. Ther.*, 78, 79—89, 1943.
82. Stanley, M. M. and Astwood, E. B., Determination of the relative activities of antithyroid compounds in man using radioactive iodine, *Endocrinology*, 41, 66—85, 1947.
83. Greer, M. A., Stott, A. K., and Milne, K. A., Effect of thiocyanate, perchlorate and other ions on thyroidal iodine metabolism, *Endocrinology*, 79, 237—247, 1966.
84. Piironen, E. and Virtanen, A. I., The effect of thiocyanate in nutrition on the iodine content of cow's milk, *Z. Ernaehrungswiss.*, 3, 140—147, 1963.
85. Astwood, E. B., Greer, M. A., and Ettlinger, M. G., L-5-Vinyl-2-thiooxazolidone, an antithyroid compound from yellow turnip and from *Brassica* seeds, *J. Biol. Chem.*, 181, 121—130, 1949.
86. Greer, M. A., Kendall, J. W., and Smith, M., Antithyroid compounds, in *The Thyroid Gland*, Pitt-Rivers, R. and Trotter, W. R., Eds., Butterworths, Washington, D.C., 1964, 357—389.
87. Clandin, D. R., Bayly, L., and Caballero, A., Effects of (-)-5-vinyl-2-oxazolidinethione, a goitrogen in rapeseed meal, on the rate of growth and thyroid function of chicks, *Poultry Sci.*, 45, 833—837, 1966.
88. Matsumoto, T., Itoh, H., and Akiba, Y., Goitrogen effects of (-)-5-vinyl-2-oxazolidinethione, a goitrogen in rapeseed, in growing chicks, *Poultry Sci.*, 47, 1323—1330, 1968.
89. Khera, K. S., Non-teratogenicity of D- and L-goitrin in the rat, *Food Cosmet. Toxicol.*, 15, 61—62, 1977.
90. Peltola, P., The role of L-5-vinyl-2-thiooxazolidone in the genesis of endemic goiter in Finland, in *Current Topics in Thyroid Research*, Cassano, C. and Andreoli, M., Eds., Academic Press, New York, 1965, 872—876.
91. Langer, P. and Michajlovskij, N., Studies on the antithyroid activity of naturally occurring L-5-vinyl-2-thiooxazolidone and its urinary metabolite in rats, *Acta Endocrinol.*, 62, 21—30, 1969.
92. VanEtten, C. H., Daxenbichler, M. E., Williams, P. H., and Kwolek, W. F., Glucosinolates and derived products in cruciferous vegetables. Analysis of the edible part from twenty-two varieties of cabbage, *J. Agric. Food Chem.*, 24, 452—455, 1976.
93. Tallent, W. H., Improving high-erucic oilseeds: chemically or genetically, *J. Am. Oil Chem. Soc.*, 49, 15—19, 1972.
94. Bell, J. M., Nutritional value of low glucosinolate rapeseed meal for swine, *Can. J. Anim. Sci.*, 55, 61—70, 1975.

95. Josefsson, E. and Uppström, B., Influence of glucosinolates and native enzymes on the nutritional value of low glucosinolate meal, *J. Sci. Food Agric.*, 27, 433—437, 1976.
96. Rapeseed Assoc. of Canada, 1017-837 W. Hastings, St., Vancouver, B. C., Canada, *Rapeseed Digest*, 13(4), 2, April 1979.
97. Canola Council of Canada, *Canola Meal for Livestock and Poultry*, Publ. No. 59, Winnipeg, Manitoba, Canada, June 1981, 1—25.
98. Loew, F. M., Doige, C. E., Manns, J. G., Searey, G. P., Bell, J. M., and Jones, J. D., Evaluation of dietary rapeseed protein concentrate flours in rats and dogs, *Toxicol. Appl. Pharmacol.*, 35, 257—267, 1976.
99. Jones, J. D., Problems associated with substitution of plant proteins in human nutrition. Preparation and tests on rapeseed proteins, Can. Fed. Biol. Soc., 18th Annu. Meeting, University of Manitoba, Winnipeg, 1975.
100. Björkman, R., Interaction between proteins and glucosinolate isothiocyanates and oxazolidinethiones from *Brassica napus* seed, *Phytochemistry*, 12, 1585—1590, 1973.
101. VanEtten, C. H., Wolff, I. A., Kirk, L. D., and Booth, A. W., Unpublished results, Northern Regional Research Center, Peoria, Illinois, 1965.
102. Langer, P., Antithyroid action in rats of small doses of some naturally occurring compounds, *Endocrinology*, 79, 1117—1122, 1966.
103. Greer, M. A. and Astwood, E. B., The antithyroid effect of certain foods in man as determined with radioactive iodine, *Endocrinology*, 43, 105—119, 1948.
104. Hanson, C. H., Ed., The Effect of FDA Regulation (GRAS) on Plant Breeding and Processing, CSSA special publication number 5, Crop Science Society of America, Madison, Wisc., 1974, 1—63.
105. Bible, B. B., Ju, H-Y., and Chong, C., Influence of cultivar, season, irrigation, and date of planting on SCN ion content in cabbages, *J. Am. Soc. Hort. Sci.*, 105, 88—91, 1980.
106. Heaney, R. K. and Fenwick, G. R., The glucosinolate content of *Brassica* vegetables, a chemotaxonomic approach to cultivar identification, *J. Sci. Food Agric.*, 31, 794—801, 1980.
107. Cole, R. A. and Phelps, K., Use of canonical variate analysis in the differentiation of swede cultivars by gas-liquid chromatography of volatile hydrolysis products, *J. Sci. Food Agric.*, 30, 669—676, 1979.
108. Tookey, H. L., Daxenbichler, M. E., VanEtten, C. H., Kwolek, W. F., and Williams, P. H., Cabbage glucosinolates: correspondence of patterns in seeds and leafy heads, *J. Am. Soc. Hort. Sci.*, 105, 714—717, 1980.
109. VanEtten, C. H. and Daxenbichler, M. E., Formation of organic nitriles from progoitrins in leaves of *Crambe abyssinica* and *Brassica napus*, *J. Agric. Food Chem.*, 19, 194—195, 1971.
110. Daxenbichler, M. E., VanEtten, C. H., and Williams, P. H., Glucosinolate products in commercial sauerkraut, *J. Agric. Food Chem.*, 28, 809—811, 1980.
111. Clements, F. W. and Wishart, J. W., A thyroid-blocking agent in the etiology of endemic goiter, *Metab. Clin. Exp.*, 5, 623—639, 1956.
112. Virtanen, A. I., Kreula, M., and Kiesvaara, M., Investigation on the alleged goitrogenic properties of cow's milk, *Z. Ernaehrungswiss. Suppl.*, 3, 23—37, 1963.
113. Smith, R. H., Kale poisoning, *Rep. Rowett Inst.*, 30, 112—131, 1974.
114. VanEtten, C. H., Daxenbichler, M. E., Schroeder, W., Princen, L. H., and Perry, T. W., Tests for *epi*-progoitrin derived nitriles, and goitrin in body tissues from cattle fed crambe meal, *Can. J. Anim. Sci.*, 57, 75—80, 1977.
115. Elliott, M. C. and Stowe, B. B., Distribution and variation of indole glucosinolates in woad (*Isatis tinctoria* L.), *Plant Physiol.*, 48, 498—503, 1971.
116. Wood, J. L., Biochemistry, in *Chemistry and Biochemistry of Thiocyanic Acid and Derivatives*, Newman, A. A., Ed., Academic Press, New York, 1975, 156—221.

NUTRITIONAL SIGNIFICANCE OF LECTINS

Werner G. Jaffé

Lectins or hemagglutinins are proteins which can interact in a very specific way with certain carbohydrates. In its specificity this interaction is comparable to that of an antibody with its antigen or even to the binding of an enzyme to its substrate. The lectins can bind to free sugars or to sugar residues existing in polysaccharides, glycoproteins, or glycolipids, which may be free or may exist in bound form, for example in cell membranes.

The term "hemagglutinin" derives from the visible interaction of lectin-containing material with red blood cells. This agglutination reaction was known since the last century when it was observed that an extract from castor beans would agglutinate a suspension of washed red blood cells of different animal species. This activity was related at this time to the high toxicity of the castor beans. Since these first observations, lectins or lectin-like proteins have been detected in many plant species including fungus and lichens, and also in animals, both invertebrates and vertebrates. The term "lectin" points to the specifity of the reaction (legere = to choose).

In order to produce clumping of erythrocytes and other cells, a lectin must bear at least two receptor sites. The capacity to aggregate red blood cells, which have many surface carbohydrate residues, is a common criterion used to identify lectins. Agglutination is inhibited if the lectin-specific sugar is present in the solution in which the cells are suspended. This is similar to the inhibition a hapten exerts on the reaction between an antibody and its specific antigen and allows study of the specificity of the lectins.

Some lectins will stimulate human and animal lymphocytes to undergo mitosis in vitro, a fact which has been very useful for the study of lymphocyte dynamics and function. Carbohydrate-containing molecules are found in the membranes of many cells and may undergo characteristic changes during embryonic development and malign transformation which may be followed by the use of lectins.

The chemical structure of only a few lectins has been studied in some detail. Many, but not all, are glycoproteins and contain bivalent metal ions (Mn^{++}, Ca^{++}, Zn^{++}). Some can be split in subunits which may be of one or two different types. Several different lectins exist frequently in plant sources and are called "isolectins".

The chemical,[1,2] taxonomic,[3] botanical,[4] immunological,[5] and regulatory[6] aspects of lectins have been reviewed. Compared with this extensive literature, the number of review papers dealing with the antinutritional properties of lectins is rather small.[7,8]

Lectins bound to insoluble support material are useful for affinity chromatography of complex sugar-bearing compounds. At the same time, the lectins can be obtained by affinity chromatography on their specific sugars, immobilized by binding to support material or directly on insoluble polysaccharides like sephardex, sepharose, quitine, etc. Several lectins and immobilized lectins are now commercially available.

FUNCTION OF LECTINS

Very little is known about the function the lectins perform in the organisms in which they occur. There is growing evidence that lectins participate in the recognition processes between cells or between cells and various carbohydrate-containing molecules. Thus they may participate in regulating a variety of normal physiological functions.[6] They also may be involved in defense mechanisms of plants against invasion of harmful microorganisms and insect attack.[9] The possible role played by lectins in the process of recognizing the nitrogen-fixing bacteria of the genus *Rhizobium* by their legume host has received particular attention. The bacterial cells have sugar-containing substances on their surfaces. There is growing evidence that they may be bound by lectins existing in the roots of legumes, thus establishing the relationship between plants and bacteria.[10]

DETECTION

For screening, the hemagglutinating test is still preferred. Activation of the red blood cells by treatment with trypsin or pronase enhances the sensibility of this test which has been critically evaluated by Burger.[11] Not all blood samples of a given animal species may react in an identical fashion due to the existence of different blood groups.

LECTINS IN FOODS

Lectins have been detected in a great number of edible plants: many legume seeds, potatoes, wheat germ, etc. (Table 1) (see also Reference 74). It is likely that there are still more undiscovered lectins for which the right detection method has not yet been devised. The first lectin to be discovered was the highly toxic ricin from castor beans.[12] It has since been found that a hemagglutinin of low toxicity exists in these seeds together with a toxin. The latter has only one receptor group for sugar residues and therefore will attach itself to the surface of susceptible cells but will not clump them, while the hemagglutinin has two receptor sites.[13] The toxicity of the castor beans stimulated the search for other toxic lectins and led to the discovery of the hemagglutinating activity of the extract of many of the edible legume seeds.[14]

SOYBEAN LECTIN

As early as 1917 it was found that diets prepared with raw soybeans would not support normal growth of experimental animals as do the diets containing heated soybeans, indicating the probable presence of heat-labile, antinutritional compounds in these seeds.[15] Lectins, enzyme inhibitors, and undefined compounds have been implicated.

Liener[16] was the first to isolate a soybean lectin which was toxic when injected into rats. Several isolectins have been detected later in soybeans.[17] The role of the lectin in the oral toxicity of raw soybeans is still a matter of dispute. When the soybean lectin was incorporated into the diet at a level equivalent to the activity found in raw soybean meal, a significant depression of the growth of rats was obtained.[18] On the other hand, Liener et al.[19] could not detect any correlation between the level of hemagglutinating activity in the extracts from different soybean cultivars and the growth-depressing action of the raw beans when added to an experimental rat ration. No such relation was either found between trypsin inhibitor activity and growth-promoting action. The soybean lectin can be removed from a raw seed extract by affinity chromatography. Added to a casein diet, this extract did not cause a significantly different growth depression than did the crude extract.[20] These results seem to indicate that the growth-depressing activity of raw soybeans is due to the interaction of various factors, one of which may well be the lectin. There exist considerable differences between different animal species in their growth response to diets containing raw soybeans, but it is unknown whether this fact is related to the lectin content of the rations.

LECTINS IN BEANS: *(PHASEOLUS VULGARIS)*

Rats fed a diet prepared with raw ground garden beans and supplemented with all essential nutrients will lose weight and die within 1 to 2 weeks. Poor acceptibility and

Table 1
LECTINS FOUND IN EDIBLE PLANTS

Source	Isolation	Molecular weights	Metal requirement	Carbohydrate (%)	Erythrocytes agglutinated	Toxicity
Soy bean *Glycine Max*	17, 18, 19, 31, 32, 33	110.000	+	5.0	Rabbit	+ 16
Garden bean *Phaseolus vulgaris*	21, 23, 25, 27, 34, 35, 36	91.000—130.000	+	4.10	All[a]	+ Type A and C − Type B and D 28, 38, 43
Broad bean[39,40] *Vicia faba*	38, 39	50.000	—	3	All	— 41
Lima bean *Phaseolus limensis*	42	124.000 247.000	+	4.0	Human blood group A	— 41, 43
Lentil *Lens esculenta*	44, 45, 46	52.000	+	0 (?)	Rabbit	—
Garden pea *Pisum sativum*	47, 48, 49	54.000	+	0—0.3	Rabbit	— 50
Field bean *Dolichos lablab*	51, 52	?	—	2	Rabbit	+ 43, 53, 54
Runner bean *Phaseolus cocineus (multifloris)*	55	120.000	+	40	All	+ 41
Horse gram *Dolichos biflorus*	56, 57	109.000 122.000	+	2	Human blood group A	— 43

Table 1 (continued)
LECTINS FOUND IN EDIBLE PLANTS

Source	Isolation	Molecular weights	Metal requirement	Carbohydrate (%)	Erythrocytes agglutinated	Toxicity
Potato *Solanum tuberosum*	58, 59	80.000 100.000	?	5, 2	All	?
Wheat germ *Triticum vulgaris*	60, 61, 62	17.000—35.000	?	0	Tumor cells	(?) 63
Jack bean *Canavalia ensiformis*	64, 65, 66	112.000	+	0	Rabbit	+ 41, 67

^a Only type A beans agglutinate all blood types.[27]

digestibility, enzyme inhibitors, and lectins could be responsible, but there is good evidence that the latter are at least one of the major causes. Experiments by Hanover et al.[21] and by Jaffé[22] clearly established that the lectins are most likely responsible for the toxicity. Since then several authors purified toxic bean lectins.[23-25]

Five heterogeneous proteins can be separated from bean lectin. Each consists of isomeric, noncovalently bound tetramers made of two different subunits.[26] The toxicity of different bean cultivars may be quite different. Four groups of cultivars can be distinguished according to their toxicity and the type of lectins they contain.[27] The latter can be distinguished by their specificity toward red blood cells of various animal species.[28]

A possible explanation for the toxic action of some legumes is that they combine with cells lining the intestinal wall, thus causing localized lesions and a nonspecific interference with the absorption of nutrients.[22] Only lectins resistant to gastric and intestinal digestion can be expected to exhibit such an action.

Etzler and Branstrator demonstrated the binding of several fluorescence-labeled lectins to cells of intestinal vellies of rat intestine.[68] King et al.,[69] and Sotello et al.[70] produced evidence that bean lectins can damage and kill intestinal cells both in vitro and in vivo. Intestinal invertase is strongly inhibited by bean lectin[71] and so is the uptake of vitamin B.[72]

Jayne-Williams and Burgess observed that raw navy beans are toxic for Japanese quail but not for germ-free birds.[24] When the intestines of the latter were infected with several coliform strains, death occurred, which was attributed to impairment of body defense mechanisms by the lectin. Dramatic overgrowth of *Escherichia coli* may occur in the small intestine of rats fed bean lectin and may contribute to the toxic action.[73]

Several cases of human intoxication through the ingestion of raw or partially cooked bean products have been reported.[29,30] Lectins are quite common in foods generally consumed in the U.S. as Nachbar and Oppenheimer[74] have recently pointed out. They observed hemagglutinating activity in about one third of the different food samples tested. Nothing is known about the possible consequences on human health of such widespread exposure.

The data presented in Table 1 summarize some of the published information on lectins in plant food products. The details described by different authors frequently differ from each other in some aspects. One of the reasons is that the lectins from different varieties or cultivars of one plant species may vary considerably in chemical, physical, and biological aspects. Moreover, different isolectins may exist, and subunit aggregation or dissociation depends on the special experimental conditions used. The information on sugar content is also often inconsistent.

The published data on the toxicity of plant lectins are very scarce. Therefore, in the column on toxicity, information on growth-depressing activity of the raw plant material is included, although in most cases it has not been proven that the lectin is the only responsible factor, or even that it is involved as a causative agent of the toxic effect.

Hemagglutination specifity is not well known in many cases. Therefore, only the most frequently used kind of cell is registered.

REFERENCES

1. Sharon, N. and Lis, H., Lectins: cell-agglutinating and sugar-specific proteins, *Science*, 177, 949, 1972.
2. Lis, H. and Sharon, N., The biochemistry of plant lectins (phytohemagglutinins), *Ann. Rev. Biochem.*, 42, 541, 1973.

3. Liener, I. E., Phytohemagglutinins (phytolectins), *Ann. Rev. Plant Physiol.*, 27, 291, 1976.
4. Toms, G. L. and Western, A., Haemagglutinins, in *Chemotaxonomy of the Legumes*, Harborne, J. B., Boulter, D., and Turner, B. L., Eds., Academic Press, London, 1971, 367.
5. Jaffé, W. G., Immunology of plant lectins, in *Immunological Aspects of Foods*, Catsimpooles, N., Ed., John Wiley & Sons, New York, 1977, 170.
6. Oppenheimer, S. B., Interaction of lectins with embrionic cell surface, *Curr. Top. Dev. Biol.*, 11, 3, 1977.
7. Liener, I. E., Phytohemagglutinins. Their nutritional significance, *J. Agric. Chem.*, 22, 17, 1974.
8. Jaffé, W. G., Phytohemagglutinins, in *Toxic Constitutents of Plant Foodstuffs*, 2nd ed., Liener, I. E., Ed., Academic Press, New York, 1980, 73.
9. Janzen, D. H., Juster, H. B., and Liener, I. E., Insecticidal action of the phytohemagglutinin in black beans on a bruchid beetle, *Science*, 192, 795, 1976.
10. Bohlool, B. B. and Schmidt, E. L., Lectins: a possible basis for specificity in the *Rizobium*-legume root nodule symbiosis, *Science*, 185, 269, 1974.
11. Burger, M. M., Assays for agglutination with lectins. *Meth. Enzymol.*, 32, 615, 1974.
12. Stillmark, H., Über Ricin, *Arch. Pharmakol. Inst. Dorpat*, 3, 59, 1889.
13. Olsnes, S., Abrin and ricin: structure and mechanism of two toxic lectins, *Bull. Inst. Pasteur*, 74, 85, 1975.
14. Landsteiner, K. and Raubitschek, H., Beobachtungen über Hämolyse und Hämagglutination, *Zentralbl. Bakteriol. Parasitenkd. Infektionskr. Hyg. Abt. 2*, 45, 660, 1908.
15. Osborne, T. B. and Mendel, L. B., The use of soybeans as food, *J. Biol. Chem.*, 32, 369, 1917.
16. Liener, I. E., Soyin, a toxic protein from the soybean. I. Inhibition of rat growth, *J. Nutr.*, 49, 527, 1953.
17. Lotan, R., Lis, H., and Sharon, N., Aggregation and fragmentation of soybean agglutinin, *Biochem. Biophys. Res. Commun.*, 63, 144, 1975.
18. Liener, I. E. and Pallansch, M. J., Purification of a toxic substance from defatted soybean flour, *J. Biol. Chem.*, 197, 29, 1962.
19. Kakade, M. L., Simons, N. R., Liener, I. E., and Lambert, I. W., Biochemical and nutritional assessment of different varieties of soybeans, *J. Agric. Food Chem.*, 20, 87, 1972.
20. Turner, R. H. and Liener, I. E., The effect of the selective removal of hemagglutinin on the nutritive value of soybean, *J. Agric. Food Chem.*, 23, 484, 1975.
21. Hanovar, P. M., Shih, C. V., and Liener, E. E., The inhibition of growth of rats by purified hemagglutinin fraction isolated from *Phaseolus vulgaris*, *J. Nutr.*, 77, 109, 1962.
22. Jaffé, W. G., Über Phytotoxine aus Bohnen, *Arzneim. Forsch.*, 10, 1012, 1960.
23. Pusztai, A. and Palmer, R., Nutritional evaluation of kidney beans *(Phaseolus vulgaris)*: the toxic principle, *J. Sci. Food Agric.*, 28, 620, 1977.
24. Jayne-Williams, D. J. and Burgess, C. D., Further observations on the toxicity of navy bean *(Phaseolus vulgaris)* for Japanese quail *(Coturnix coturnix japonica)*, *J. Appl. Bacteriol.*, 37, 149, 1974.
25. Andrew, A. T., Navy (haricot) bean *(Phaseolus vulgaris)* lectin. Isolation and characterization of two components from a toxic agglutinating extract, *Biochem. J.*, 13, 421, 1974.
26. Yachnin, S. and Svenson, R. H., The immunological and physicochemical properties of mitogenic proteins derived from *Phaseolus vulgaris*, *Immunology*, 22, 871, 1972.
27. Jaffé, W. G., Levy, A., and Gonzalez, I. D., Isolation and partial characterization of bean phytohemagglutinins, *Phytochemistry*, 13, 2685, 1974.
28. Jaffé, W. G. and Gomez, M. J., Beans of high or low toxicity, *Qual. Plant Foods Hum. Nutr.*, 24, 359, 1975.
29. Griebel, C., Erkrankungen durch Bohnenflocken *(Phaseolus vulgaris)* und Platterbsen *(Lathyrus tingitanus)* *Z. Lebensm. Unter. Forsch.*, 90, 1991, 1950.
30. Anon., An unusual outbreak of food poisoning, *Br. J. Nutr.*, 6046, 1268, 1976.
31. Catsimpoolas, N. and Meyer, E. W., Isolation of soybean hemagglutinin and demonstration of multiple forms by isoelectric focusing, *Arch. Biochem. Biophys.*, 132, 279, 1969.
32. Lotan, R., Lis, H., and Sharon, N., Aggregation and fragmentation of soybean agglutinin, *Biochim. Biophys. Res. Commun.*, 62, 144, 1975.
33. Allen, A. K. and Neuberger, A., A simple method for the preparation of an affinity absorbent for soybean agglutinin using galactosamine on CH-Sepharose, *FEBS Lett.*, 50, 362, 1975.
34. Jaffé, W. G. and Hannig, K., Fractionation of proteins from kidney beans, *(Phaseolus vulgaris)*, *Arch. Biochem. Biophys.*, 109, 80, 1965.
35. Dahlgren, K., Porath, J., and Lindahl-Kiessling, K., On the purification of phytohemagglutinins from *Phaseolus vulgaris* seeds, *Arch. Biochem. Biophys.*, 137, 306, 1970.
36. Felsted, R. L., Leavitt, R. D., and Bahcur, N. R., Purification of the phytohemagglutinin family of proteins from red bean *(Phaseolus vulgaris)*, by affinity chromatography, *Biochim. Biophys. Acta*, 405, 72, 1975.

37. Miller, J. B., Hsu, R., Heinnikson, R., and Yachnin, S., Extensive homology between the subunits of the phytohemagglutinin mitogenic proteins derived from *Phaseolus vulgaris, Proc. Natl. Acad. Sci. U.S.A.,* 72, 1388, 1975.
38. Evans, R. J., Pusztai, A., Watt, W. B., and Baner, D. H., Isolation and properties of protein fraction from navy beans *(Phaseolus vulgaris)* which inhibit growth of rats, *Biochim. Biophys. Acta,* 303, 175, 1973.
39. Allen, H. J. and Johnson, E. A., Isolation and partial characterization of a lectin from *Vicia faba, Biochim. Biophys. Acta,* 444, 374, 1976.
40. Allen, A. K., Deasi, N. N., and Neuberger, A., The purification of the glycoprotein lectin from the broad bean *(Vicia faba)* and a comparision with lectins of a similar specifity, *Biochem. J.,* 155, 127, 1976.
41. De Muelenaere, H. J. H., Toxicity and haemagglutinating activity of legumes, *Nature (London),* 206, 827, 1965.
42. Galbraith, W. and Goldstein, I. J., Phytohemagglutinin of the Lima bean *(Phaseolus lunatus).* Isolation, characterisation, and interaction with a type A blood-group substance, *Biochemistry,* 11, 3976, 1972.
43. Manage, L., Joshi, A., and Sohonie, K., Toxicity to rats and mice of purified, phytohemagglutinins from four Indian legumes, *Toxicon,* 10, 89, 1972.
44. Howard, I. K. and Sage, H. J., Isolation and characterisation of a phytohemagglutinin from the lentil, *Biochemistry,* 8, 2436, 1969.
45. Tichá, M., Entlicher, G., Kostir, J. V., and Kocourek, J., Studies on phytohemagglutinins. IV. Isolation and characterization of hemagglutinin from the lentil, *Biochim. Biophys. Acta,* 221, 282, 1970.
46. Strosberg, A. D., Foriers, A., Van Driessche, F., Mole, L. E., and Kanarek, L., Studies on the structure of lectins. II. Lentin lectin, *Arch. Int. Physiol. Biochem.,* 84, 660, 1976.
47. Entlicher, G., Kostir, J. V., and Kocourek, J., Studies on hemagglutinins. III. Isolation and characterisation of hemagglutinins from the pea *(Pisum sativum* L.), *Biochim. Biophys. Acta,* 221, 272, 1970.
48. Trowbridge, I. S., Isolation and chemical characterization of a mitogenic lectin from *Pisum sativum, J. Biol. Chem.,* 249, 6004, 1974.
49. Van Driessche, E., Strosberg, A. D., and Kanarek, L., Studies on the structure of lectins. I. Pea *(Pisum sativum)* lectin, *Arch. Int. Physiol. Biochem.,* 84, 677, 1976.
50. Huprikar, S. V. and Sohonie, K., Haemagglutinins from Indian pulses. II. Purification and properties of haemagglutinin from white pea *(Pisum* sp.), *Enzymology,* 28, 333, 1965.
51. Salgarkar, S. and Sohonie, K., Haemagglutinins of field bean *(Dolichos lablab).* I. Isolation, purification and properties of haemagglutinins, *Indian J. Biochem.,* 2, 193, 1965.
52. Rao, D. N., Hariharan, K., and Rajagopal, R. D., Purification and properties of a phytohemagglutinin from *Dolichos lablab* (field bean), *Lebensm. Wiss. Technol.,* 9, 246, 1976.
53. Jaffé, W. G., Estudio sobre la inhibición del crecimiento de ratas causada por algunas semillas de leguminosas, *Acta Cient. Venez.,* 1, 62, 1950.
54. Salgarkar, S. and Sohonie, K., Haemagglutinins of the field bean *(Dolichos lablab).* II. Effect of feeding field bean haemagglutinin A on rat growth, *Indian J. Biochem.,* 2, 197, 1965.
55. Nowaková, N. and Kocourek, J., Studies on phytohemagglutinins. XX. Isolation and characterisation of hemagglutinins from scarlet runner seeds *(Phaseolus coccineus* L.), *Biochim. Biophys. Acta,* 359, 320, 1974.
56. Carter, W. G. and Etzler, M. E., Isolation, characterization and subunit structures of multiple forms of *Dolichos biflorus* lectin, *J. Biol. Chem.,* 250, 2756, 1975.
57. Kocourek, J., Jamieson, G. A., Votruba, T., and Horeji, V., Studies on phytohemagglutinins. I. Some properties of the lectins of horse gram seeds, (*Dolichos biflorus* L.), *Biochim. Biophys. Acta,* 500, 344, 1977.
58. Delmotte, F., Keida, D., and Monsigny, M., Protein-sugar interaction: purification by affinity chromatography of *Solanum tuberosum* agglutinin (STA lectin), *FEBS Lett.,* 53, 324, 1975.
59. Allen, A. K. and Neuberger, A., The purification and properties of the lectin from the potatoe tuber, a hydroxyproline-containing glycoprotein, *Biochem. J.,* 135, 307, 1973.
60. Nagata, Y. and Burger, M. M., Wheat germ agglutinin, molecular characteristics and specificity for sugar binding, *J. Biol. Chem.,* 249, 3116, 1974.
61. Levine, D. I., Kaplan, M. J., and Greenway, P. I., The purification and characterisation of wheatgerm agglutinin, *Biochem. J.,* 129, 847, 1972.
62. Thomas, M. W., Walborg, E. E., Jr., and Jirgensons, B., Circular dichroiism and sacchride-induced conformational transitions of wheat germ agglutinin, *Arch. Biochem. Biophys.,* 178, 625, 1977.
63. Attia, F. and Creek, R. D., Studies on raw and heated wheat germ for young chicks, *Cereal Chem.,* 42, 492, 1965.

64. Agrawal, B. B. L. and Goldstein, I. J., Physical and chemical characterization of concanavalin A, the hemagglutinin from jack bean *(Canavalia ensiformis), Biochim. Biophys. Acta,* 133, 376, 1967.
65. Olson, M. O. J. and Liener, I. E., Some physical and chemical properties of concanavalia A, the phytohemagglutinin of the jack bean, *Biochemistry,* 6, 105, 1967.
66. Wang, J. L., Cunningham, B. A., Waxdal, M. I., and Edelman, G. M., *J. Biol. Chem.,* 250, 1490, 1975.
67. Jayne-Williams, D. J., Influence of dietary jack beans *(Canavalia ensiformis)* and of Concanavalin A on the growth of conventional and gnotobiotic Japanese quail, *(Coturnix coturnix japonica), Nature (London), New Biol.,* 243, 150, 1973.
68. Etzler, M. and Branstrator, M. L., Differential localization of cell surface and secretory components in rat intestinal epithelium by use of lectins, *J. Cell Biol.,* 62, 452, 1974.
69. King, T. P., Pusztai, A., and Clarke, E. M. W., Kidney bean *(Phaseolus vulgaris)* Lectin-induced lesions in rat small intestine. I. Light microscope studies, *J. Comp. Pathol.,* 90, 585, 1980.
70. Sotello, A., Arteaga, M. E., Frias, M. I., and Gonzáles Garze, M. T., Cytotoxic effect of two legumes in epithelial cells of the small intestine, *Qual. Plant Plant Food, Hum. Nutr.,* 30, 79, 1980.
71. Rovanet, J. M. and Besancon, P., Effects d' un extrait de phytohemagglutinines sur la croissance, la digestibilité de l' azote et l' activite' de l' invertase et de le (Na + -K +) - ATPase de la muqueuse intestinale chez le rat, *Ann. Nutr. Aliment.,* 33, 405, 1979.
72. Bawell, I., Miller, B., and Balder, D., Inhibition of vitamin B12 absorption by a dietary lectin: effect of phytohemagglutinin in the rat, *Am. J. Clin. Nutr.,* 33, 930, 1980.
73. Wilson, A. B., King, T. P., Clarke, E. M. W., and Pusztai, A., Kidney bean *(Phaseolus vulgaris)* lectin induced lesions in rat small intestine. II. Microbiological studies, *J. Comp. Pathol.,* 90, 597, 1980.
74. Nachbar, M. S. and Oppenheim, J. D., Lectins in the United States diet: a survey of lectins in consumed foods and a review of the literature, *Am. J. Clin. Nutr.,* 33, 2338, 1980.

NATURALLY OCCURRING INHIBITORS: CARBOHYDRASE INHIBITORS

Russell Pressey

The list of natural inhibitors of carbohydrases in Table 1 includes only those that have been proven to be proteinaceous[2,3,11,21,24] or are believed to be so on the basis of such properties as thermolability and molecular weight. An inhibitor that had been assumed to be a protein, the amylase inhibitor from sorghum,[6] has been shown to be a series of oligomeric condensed tannins of the leucocyanide group.[27] Similarly, the pectinase inhibitor from Sericea[28] has been shown to be a polymer of proanthocyanidin.[29] Both of the sorghum and Sericea inhibitors appear to be general protein denaturants. Most of the inhibitors listed, however, are highly specific with respect to the carbohydrase and its source(s). Some are reactive with endogenous enzymes, notably the invertase inhibitors, and may thus have a regulatory function. Others are reactive with enzymes from unrelated sources but not with the endogenous enzymes; these proteins may function as protective agents against microbial and insect damage. The possibility also exists that the ability of certain proteins to inhibit enzymes is fortuitous.

Table 1
PROTEINACEOUS NATURAL INHIBITORS OF CARBOHYDRASES

Inhibitor source	Mol wt of inhibitor	Carbohydrase inhibited	Source of enzyme inhibited	Source of enzyme not inhibited	Ref.
1. Navy bean	—	α-Amylase	Human pancreas	—	1
2. Kidney bean	49,000	α-Amylase	Human pancreas and saliva, hog pancreas, *Helix pomatia*	Barley malt, rye, *Bacillus amyloliquefaciens*, *Bacillus subtilis*, *Bacillus licheniformis*, *Aspergillus oryza*	2
3. Wheat	18,215	α-Amylase	*Tenebrio molitor*, *Blatella germanica*, *Tribolium confusm*	Wheat, human saliva, hog pancreas, fungal, microbial	3—5
4. Wheat	26,200	α-Amylase	Human saliva and pancreas, *Tenebrio molitor*, *Blatella germanica*, *Tribolium confusum*, chick pancreas	Wheat, fungal, microbial, hog pancreas	3—8
5. Wheat	21,000	α-Amylase	Chick pancreas	—	7
6. Wheat	60,000	α-Amylase	*Tenebrio molitor*	Human saliva and pancreas, hog pancreas	5
7. Mango	—	α-Amylase	Mango, banana	—	9
8. Potato	17,000	Invertase	Potato tuber, foliage of many plants including potato, tomato, and tobacco	Yeast, *Neurospora*, foliage of some plants	10, 11
9. Sweet potato	22,900	Invertase	Potato tuber, sweet potato leaf	Yeast, *Neurospora*	13
10. Sweet potato	19,500	Invertase	Sweet potato root	Yeast	14
11. Sugar beet	18,100	Invertase	Potato tuber, sugar beet root, sugar beet foliage	Yeast, *Neurospora*	13, 15
12. Corn	<75,000	Invertase	Corn endosperm	—	16
13. Morning glory	—	Invertase	Morning glory petals	—	17
14. Pear	—	Polygalacturonase	Fungal	—	18
15. Avocado	—	Polygalacturonase	Avocado	—	19
16. Cucumber	—	Polygalacturonase	Fungal	Cucumber, Tomato	20
17. Red kidney bean hypocotyls	50,000	Polygalacturonase	*Aspergillus niger*, *Colletotrichum lindemuthianum*, *Fusarium oxysporum*, *Sclerotium rolfsii*	—	21, 22

Table 1
PROTEINACEOUS NATURAL INHIBITORS OF CARBOHYDRASES

Inhibitor source	Mol wt of inhibitor	Carbohydrase inhibited	Source of enzyme inhibited	Source of enzyme not inhibited	Ref.
18. Tomato stems and suspension—cultured sycamore cells	—	Polygalacturonase	*Colletotrichum lindemuthianum, Fusarium oxysporum,* and *Sclerotium rolfsii*	—	21
19. Cucumber, bean, pepper, onion, cabbage	—	Pectin lyase	*Aspergillus* sp.,	—	23
20. Cucumber, bean, pepper, onion, cabbage	—	Pectate lyase	*Bacillus polymyxa*	—	23
21. Human saliva	380,000	β-Glucuronidase		—	25
22. Porcine sublingual gland	340,000	β-Glucuronidase		—	24
23. Porcine submaxillary glands	340,000	β-Glucuronidase		—	26

REFERENCES

1. Bowman, D. E., Amylase inhibitor of navy beans, *Science*, 102, 358—359, 1945.
2. Marshall, J. J. and Lauda, C. M., Purification and properties of phaseolamin, an inhibitor of α-amylase, from the kidney bean, *Phaseolus vulgaris*, *J. Biol. Chem.*, 250, 8030—8037, 1975.
3. Shainkin, R. and Birk, Y., α-Amylase inhibitors from wheat — Isolation and characterization, *Biochim. Biophys. Acta*, 221, 502—513, 1970.
4. Silano, V., Pocchiari, F., and Kasarda, D. D., Physical characterization of α-amylase inhibitors from wheat, *Biochim. Biophys. Acta*, 317, 139—148, 1973.
5. Petrucci, T., Tomasi, M., Cantagalli, P., and Silano, V., Comparison of wheat albumin inhibitors of α-amylase and trypsin, *Phytochemistry*, 13, 2487—2495, 1974.
6. Kneen, E. and Sandstedt, R. M., Distribution and general properties of an amylase inhibitor in cereals, *Arch. Biochem.*, 9, 235—249, 1946.
7. Saunders, R. M. and Lang, J. A., α-Amylase inhibitors in Triticum aestivum: purification and physical-chemical properties, *Phytochemistry*, 12, 1237—1241, 1973.
8. Sodini, G., Silano, V., DeAgazio, M., Pocchiari, F., Tenori, L., and Vivaldi, G., Purification and properties of a Triticum aestivum specific albumin, *Phytochemistry*, 9, 1167—1172, 1970.
9. Mattoo, A. K. and Modi, V. V., Partial purification and properties of enzyme inhibitors from unripe mangoes, *Enzymologia*, 39, 237—247, 1970.
10. Schwimmer, S., Makower, R. U., and Rorem, E. S., Invertase and invertase inhibitor in potato, *Plant Physiol.*, 36, 313—316, 1961.
11. Pressey, R., Separation and properties of potato invertase and invertase inhibitor, *Arch. Biochem. Biophys.*, 113, 667—674, 1966.
12. Pressey, R., Invertase inhibitor from potatoes: purification, characterization, and reactivity with plant invertases, *Plant Physiol.*, 42, 1780—1786, 1967.
13. Pressey, R., Invertase inhibitors from red beet, sugar beet, and sweet potato roots, *Plant Physiol.*, 43, 1430—1430, 1968.
14. Matsushita, K. and Uritani, I., Isolation and characterization of acid invertase inhibitor from sweet potato, *J. Biochem.*, 79, 633—639, 1976.
15. Kursanov, A. L., Dubinina, I. M., and Burakhanova, E. A., A natural inhibitor of invertase from sugar beet roots, *Fiziol. Rast.*, 18, 568—574, 1971.
16. Jaynes, T. A. and Nelson, O. E., An invertase inactivator in maize endosperm and factors affecting inactivation, *Plant Physiol.*, 47, 629—634, 1971.
17. Winkenback, F. and Matile, P., Evidence for *de novo* synthesis of an invertase inhibitor protein in senescing petals of *Ipomoea*, *Z. Pflanzenphysiol.*, 63, 292—295, 1970.
18. Weurman, C., Pectinase inhibitors in pears, *Acta Botan. Neerl.*, 2, 107—121, 1953.
19. Reymond, D. and Phaff, H. J., Purification and certain properties of avocado polygalacturonase, *J. Food Sci.*, 30, 266—273, 1965.
20. Bock, W., Krause, M., and Dongowski, G., Differences in efficacy between vegetable polygalacturonase inhibitors, *Nahrung*, 14, 375—381, 1970.
21. Albersheim, P. and Anderson, A. J., Proteins from plant cell walls inhibit polygalacturonases secreted by plant pathogens, *Proc. Natl. Acad. Sci.*, 68, 1815—1819, 1971.
22. Fisher, M. L., Anderson, A. J., and Alberskeim, P., Host-pathogen interactions. VI. A single plant protein efficiently inhibits endopolygalacturonases secreted by *Colletotrichum lindemuthianum* and *Aspergillus niger*, *Plant Physiol.*, 51, 489—491, 1973.
23. Bock, W., Dongowski, G., Goebel, H., and Krause, M., Detection of the inhibition of microbial pectin and pectate lyases using inhibitors of vegetable origin, *Nahrung*, 19, 411—416, 1975.
24. Sakamoto, W., Nishikaze, O., and Sugimura, T., Isolation of β-glucuronidase inhibitor from human saliva, *Arch. Oral Biol.*, 19, 703—708, 1974.
25. Sakamoto, W., Nishikaze, O., and Sakakibara, E., Isolation of an inhibitor of β-glucuronidase from porcine sublingual gland, *Biochim. Biophys. Acta*, 329, 72—80, 1973.
26. Sakamoto, W., Nishikaze, O., and Sakakibara, E., Comparison of two inhibitors of β-glucuronidase from porcine sublingual and submaxillary glands, *Biochim. Biophys. Acta*, 343, 409—415, 1974.
27. Strumeyer, D. H. and Malin, M. J., Identification of the amylase inhibitor from seeds of *Leoti sorghum*, *Biochim. Biophys. Acta*, 184, 643—645, 1969.
28. Bell, T. A., Etchells, J. L., and Smart, W. W. G., Pectinase and cellulase enzyme inhibitor from Sericea and certain other plants, *Botan. Gaz.*, 126, 40—45, 1965.
29. Cook, C. E., Buhrman, J. A., Tallent, C. R., and Wall, M. E., The pectinase inhibitor from Sericea (*Lespedeza cuneata*), *Lloydia*, 33, 255—260, 1970.

CYCASIN

Hiromu Matsumoto

INTRODUCTION

Cycads, which contain cycasin, provide a food starch for small groups of people in some tropical and subtropical areas of the world. Chemical investigations on the toxic constituents of cycads had been carried out in Australia and Japan over a period of 4 decades, but they attracted little notice.[1] During the 1950s, attention was focused on the clinical observations that unusually high rates of morbidity and mortality from amyotrophic lateral sclerosis (ALS) occurred among the native Chamorro on the island of Guam.[2-4] The natives suggested that *Cycas circinalis* may be a causative agent for the paralytic disease, ALS. Published observations that cattle grazing on cycads frequently developed gait disturbances, which progressed through states of motor weakness to paralysis of the hindquarters, gave some support to the suggestion that eating cycad could be a cause of ALS.

No evidence of neurotoxicity resembling ALS developed in laboratory animals fed cycad material. However, those that survived for a long period developed tumors. This observation provided an impetus for experimentation in carcinogenesis with a naturally occurring toxicant. Later, it was demonstrated that derivatives of cycasin administered to animals at a specific period during fetal development induced malformation or structural disorganization of the brain. These observations stimulated the use of compounds related to cycasin for studies on experimental brain malformations.

CYCADS

Distribution of Cycads

Cycads are slow-growing plants with a cylindrical trunk or a swollen underground tuber-like stem and a crown of very large, coarse, stiff palm-like evergreen leaves. Modern cycads are among the most primitive of living seed plants and are the surviving remnants of an ancient cycad flora, which were common in the Mesozoic Era and may have been the ancestors to flowering plants.

Cycads belong to nine genera and are confined mainly to the tropics and subtropics but extend to some warm temperate regions in Australia, South Africa, Japan, and Florida. The most widely distributed genus is *Cycas,* which ranges from East Africa, across the Indian Ocean, southeast Asia, Oceania, and to northeastern Australia. *Cycas circinalis* L. and *C. revoluta* Thunb., two important species of this genus, are widely cultivated as ornamentals and the glossy foliage is often cut for decorative greens or wreaths. The genus *Zamia* is distributed from Florida, West Indies, Mexico, and south to Brazil and Chile. Three other genera are found in the western hemisphere, *Microcycas* in Cuba, and *Dioon* and *Ceratozamia* in Mexico. *Macrozamia* grows in the eastern, central, and southwestern parts of Australia while *Bowenia* is located in northeastern Queensland. *Encephalartos,* one of two genera found in Africa, ranges from South Africa, Mozambique, Rhodesia, northward to Kenya, Sudan, and Ghana. The ninth genus *Stangeria* is limited to the eastern coastal region of South Africa.[5,6]

Cycads as Food

The reader is referred to review articles on cycads as economic plants by Thieret[6] and Whiting[1] for detailed information on the use of cycads as food. Cycads are well adapted for adverse climatic conditions and can survive when other plants are destroyed by typhoon, flood, or drought. They have been a source of sustenance during emergencies and seasonal shortages, and even a staple in areas where the food supply is limited. The references cited by Thieret and Whiting are old and it is difficult to determine whether or not the use of cycads as food, by small groups of people who live in relatively isolated areas, continues to be a general practice. A few recent articles on cycads indicate that they are still occasionally used as food by native Chamorros of Guam,[1] the Wasanga tribe of Kenya,[7] and the natives of Amami Oshima,[8] and Miyako Island (Ryukyus)[9] in southern Japan.

Cycads are used mainly as a source of starch from either the seeds or the stem, although all parts of the plants of one or another species are used as food. It is known to people who use cycads as food that they contain poisonous substances which must be removed before the plants can be safely consumed. Detoxification procedures developed for the preparation of flour, in widely scattered geographic areas, are remarkably similar. The starchy endosperm is removed from the cycad seed and cut into small pieces and soaked in frequent changes of water over several days, or the pieces are placed in a sack or basket and kept in running water. They are then dried in the sun and ground into flour for immediate use or stored for later use. The effectiveness in leaching toxicants from the seed kernel pieces depends on the size of the pieces, and the frequency of change of fresh water. Thus, the possibility of incomplete extraction of the toxicants exists. Cases of human poisoning reported in the literature could be due to inadequate preparation of cycad flour (Figure 1A and B).[6,7]

Toxicity of the Cycads

Recent investigations on the naturally occurring toxicants in cycads were started as a search for neurotoxins, which possibly could be etiological factors in the high incidence of ALS in Guam. A crude meal prepared from *Cycas circinalis* seeds collected in Guam was fed to rats as part of their feed by Laquer and co-workers.[10] Acute toxic manifestations were recognizable by light microscopy within 24 hr and consisted of loss of cytoplasmic basophilia and glycogen from isolated liver cells around the central vein. Focal cellular necrosis, pyknosis of nuclei, and cytoplasmic eosinophilia were well established within 48 hr. Rats which died within a few days were found at autopsy to have accumulations of free, slightly yellowish fluid in the serosal cavities, occasionally a mild degree of subcutaneous edema, and often a marked edema of the perilobular pancreatic connective tissue. Small punctate hemorrhages were seen beneath the serosal surfaces, sometimes at many sites. The mortality was high among rats fed 2% or more of the cycad flour, the majority dying within 2 weeks. Those surviving developed benign and malignant tumors in the liver and kidneys, with one case in the lung and one in the small intestine.[10] This was the first demonstration of carcinogenicity of cycads.

A systematic separation of the constituents of cycad seed, coupled with a bioassay for toxicity, was carried out in another study conducted during the same period by Matsumoto and Strong.[11] *C. circinalis* seeds collected on Guam were chemically separated into nine fractions. Three of these fractions were acutely toxic to rats and the biological effects were similar to those described above. A compound isolated from one of the fractions was identified as cycasin, an azoxyglucoside. The chemical structure of this compound was already established from earlier work on cycads. The chemical and physical properties of cycasin and related compounds are described in the next section. The aglycone of cycasin, methylazoxymethanol (MAM), was present in another fraction and evidence was obtained that the compound was reasonably stable and could be isolated. This aglycone fraction, when fed to rats at a high level, produced acute liver damage, causing death. Smaller doses over a long period of time produced hepatomas. This work presented the first experimental proof that the active carcinogen is the aglycone of cycasin, MAM.[11]

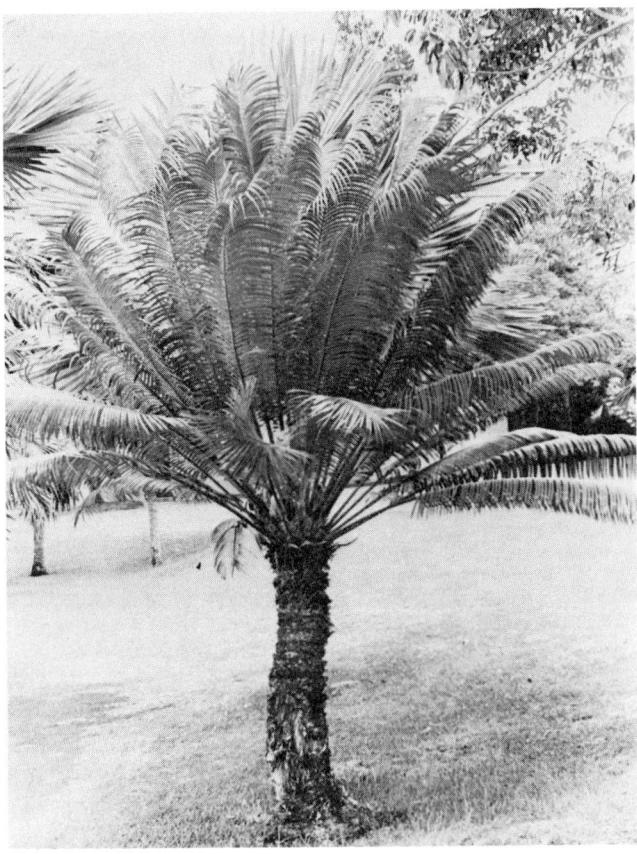

FIGURE 1A. Small *Cycas circinalis* tree with cylindrical trunk and palm-like evergreen leaves.

Earlier, when cycasin was first isolated, Nishida et al.[12] had concluded that cycasin itself is not toxic but it is cleaved, probably by microbial enzymes of the intestinal tract, to yield the aglycone, MAM, which is responsible for the toxic action. Recent experiments proved that Nishida's conclusion was correct. Cycasin injected into rats was excreted almost quantitatively in the urine, but when the compound was given orally the quantity excreted in the urine varied from 30 to 63%. No cycasin was detected in the feces. The animals which excreted the least amount of cycasin showed the most severe signs of toxicity. The results suggested that intestinal microorganisms play an important role in the activation of cycasin.

The importance of the intestinal microorganisms was demonstrated conclusively by the lack of toxicity of cycasin orally administered to germ-free rats. Sprague-Dawley germ-free rats fed large amounts of cycasin (200 mg/100 g feed) gained weight and were alive and well after 20 days, whereas conventional rats fed the same ration had died or were moribund. Moreover, the livers of germ-free rats were normal in contrast to the conventional rat liver, which showed evidence of severe diffuse, centrilobular liver cell necrosis often accompanied by hemorrhage.[13] Ninety-seven per cent of orally administered cycasin was excreted in the urine and feces of germ-free rats, while only 20 per cent was excreted by conventional rats. Substantial amounts of cycasin were excreted in the feces of germ-free but not in conventional rats.[14] The results suggest that intestinal mucosal enzymes apparently do not play a part in the hydrolysis of cycasin. Monocontamination of germ-free rats with microorganisms known to produce the enzyme β-glucosidase produced toxicity, whereas microorganisms which did not have β-glucosidase activity caused no toxicity.[15]

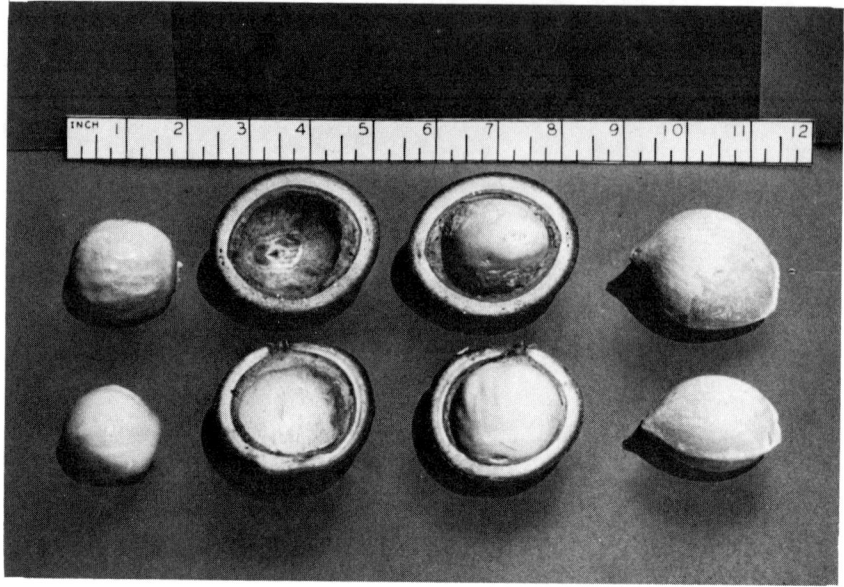

FIGURE 1B. *Cycas. circinalis* seeds (from left): 1. kernel (endosperm). 2. Cross section of fleshy outer shell (pericarp) without and with kernel. 3. Cross section of outer shell and whole kernel in place. 4. Seed with seed coat.

The aglycone of cycasin, MAM, however, proved to be toxic by injection. Graded doses of MAM were injected intraperitoneally into 11 female rats. All animals were visibly affected in about 5 hr. Of the animals given high doses, 6 died in 1 to 3 days.[16] Thus, it was proved that toxicity of cycasin administered orally is dependent upon the intestinal bacterial β-glucosidase, which is needed to free MAM from the glucose of cycasin.

CHEMISTRY OF CYCASIN

Cycasin and Other Azoxyglycosides

Cooper,[17] in 1941, isolated a toxic crystalline compound from *Macrozamia spiralis* and named it macrozamin. The aglycone part of this compound, although not isolated, was shown 10 years later to be an aliphatic azoxy-compound, hydroxyazoxymethane or methylazoxymethanol, MAM. The aglycone was believed to be incapable of independent existence.[18] The sugar moiety of macrozamin was identified 2 years earlier as primeverose, 6-[β-D-xylopyranosyl]-D-glucopyranose.[19]

Nishida,[20] in 1955, surmised that the toxic compound in *Cycas revoluta* was related to the azoxyglycoside isolated from *Macrozamia*, which proved to be correct. The compound had an azoxy moiety attached to glucose instead of to primeverose. The compound was named cycasin. Riggs showed that the same compound was present in *C. circinalis*.[21] Evidence was obtained from proton resonance spectroscopy that the unsubstituted methyl group of cycasin was attached to the quarternary nitrogen atom and the chemical structure was established to be the one shown in Figure 2.[22] Cycasin is soluble in water and in aqueous ethanol, but sparingly soluble in ethanol. It is insoluble in most organic solvents. It gives a positive Molish reaction, produces a greenish-blue color with anthrone, it has an optical rotation of $[\alpha]^{28}_D = -41.3$, and melts at 144 to 145°C with decomposition.[21]

The glycosides, cycasin and macrozamin, are readily hydrolyzed with 0.1 N acid at

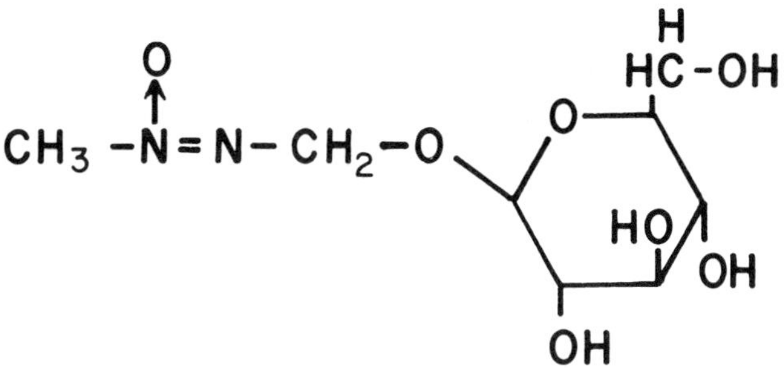

$$CH_3-\overset{\overset{O}{\uparrow}}{N}=N-CH_2-O-\text{[sugar ring]}$$

Cycasin

FIGURE 2. The chemical structure of cycasin: β-D-glycosyl-oxy-azoxymethane, or methylazoxymethyl-β-D-glucopyranoside.

100°C. The rate of hydrolysis is that expected for O- or N- glycopyranosides. The liberation of the aglycone from the glycoside by acid hydrolysis causes it to rapidly decompose stoichiometrically as follows:

$$CH_3-\overset{\overset{O}{\uparrow}}{N}=N-CH_2O-\text{sugar} \xrightarrow{H^+} HCHO + CH_3OH + N_2 + \text{sugar}$$

The reaction of basic hydrolysis is complex and among the products identified are cyanide ion (about 0.5 mol), formic acid (0.5 mol), and traces of methylamine and ammonia.[18]

The aglycone moiety has two linked nitrogen atoms, a feature not previously known in a natural product. There is a characteristic ultraviolet absorption maximum at 217 nm and an inflection around 275 nm. A strong infrared band appears near 1530 cm^{-1}, which can be attributed to the azoxy nature of the aglycone.[18]

Nishida and co-workers have shown that there is in *C. revoluta* a series of seven other azoxyglycosides, which occur in minute quantities.[23,24] These compounds are thought to be products of transglucosylation and could be considered as β-glucosyl-cycasins. Thus, they have been named neocycasins. The aglycone of these glycosides was considered too unstable to isolate so the azoxy structure was deduced from the degradation products of acid hydrolysis and from spectral information.

C. revoluta has been the most thoroughly examined of the cycads. All parts of the plant, the seed, leaf, stem, and male strobil have been analyzed for the presence of azoxyglycosides.[24] The azoxyglycosides probably exist in all the cycad genera. They have been identified thus far in five of the nine genera. Cycasin and macrozamin appear to be the major azoxyglycosides. Cycasin is present in *Cycas*[20,21] and *Zamia*,[25] while macrozamin is found in *Macrozamia*,[18,26] *Encephalartos*,[26] *Bowenia*,[26] *Cycas*,[27] and *Zamia*.[25] The distribution of azoxyglycosides in the underground stem of *Zamia* and *Cycas* seed husk is interesting in that cycasin and macrozamin are present in large and about equal amounts (about 1% each, dry weight basis).[25,27]

Isolation of Cycasin

Nishida et al.[20] developed a separation procedure which can be used for the isolation of small to large amounts of cycasin. Kernels of *Cycas revoluta,* which have a high concentration of cycasin, were used. The hulled kernels were immediately boiled to inactivate the enzymes. The kernels were minced, dried, and ground. The powdered material was extracted four times with cold water. The combined extract was filtered and concentrated under reduced pressure to a small volume. Three volumes of ethanol were added to the concentrate and the precipitated material consisting of proteins, starch, and other polysaccharides was removed. The filtrate was concentrated to a small volume of syrup. The syrupy liquid was passed through a cation exchanger and an anion exchanger to remove organic acids, bases, and inorganic salts. The eluate was concentrated to a syrupy consistency. The syrup, which now consisted primarily of glycosides and simple sugars was chromatographed on a Darco G-60-celite column. The simple sugars were washed off the carbon column with water. The cycasin adsorbed on the column was eluted with 10% ethanol. The eluate was concentrated to a syrup, three volumes of ethanol were added, and the mixture was stored in a refrigerator. Colorless needles were obtained after several days. The compound was recrystallized from ethanol-water.

The procedure was subsequently modified and simplified for large-scale preparation of cycasin. The enzymes were inactivated by autoclaving the whole seed prior to removal of kernel, and the extraction was made with 0.1 N HCl instead of water. The acid had no apparent effect on cycasin, but it inverted sucrose which, if present, interfered with the crystallization of cycasin. The yield of cycasin was improved, and as much as 285 g of cycasin was isolated from a 170 kg batch of kernel.[28]

Methylazoxymethanol, MAM

The aglycone of macrozamin and cycasin was considered an entity incapable of independent existence. Thus, the structural elucidation of the aglycone of macrozamin and cycasin was accomplished by comparing its infrared and ultraviolet spectra with model aliphatic compounds and by chemical degradation studies.[19,20] Enzymatic hydrolysis of cycasin by crude cycad β-glucosidase resulted in the decomposition of the aglycone.[20] Kobayashi and Murozono[29] hydrolyzed cycasin with purified cycad β-glucosidase and obtained evidence that as long as heat is not applied to the reaction mixture the free aglycone can exist, but they did not attempt its isolation. Matsumoto and Strong first obtained the aglycone in the free state and showed that it is reasonably stable.[11] The aglycone was found in the ether-soluble lipid fraction when *Cycas circinalis* seeds were chemically fractionated and bioassayed for toxicity. The aglycone was separated from the lipid material and purified. The ultraviolet spectrum of the purified material indicated that it was an azoxy compound and it was demonstrated that the material was the aglycone and not cycasin. Kobayashi and Matsumoto used a commercially available β-glucosidase, almond emulsin, to hydrolyze cycasin and extracted the free aglycone with ether in a continuous liquid-liquid extractor. A system in which 5% cycasin dissolved in 0.3 M phosphate buffer at pH 5.2 and incubated at 35° for 5 hr with 0.2% emulsin was established to be satisfactory for large-scale hydrolysis of cycasin. The aglycone was purified by repeated vacuum fractional distillation. The compound is a colorless liquid with the following physical properties: bp 51° C (0.6 mm), mp 1—3°C. It is completely miscible in water or alcohol, soluble in chloroform, less soluble in and decomposes at room temperature in aqueous solution. The ultraviolet spectrum is the same and infrared spectrum is similar to that of cycasin.[30]

It became apparent, as the interest in cycasin and its aglycone increased, that isolation of cycasin is too time-consuming and difficult and that a synthetic compound was needed to meet research needs. The ideal compound would have been MAM, but because of its relative instability, the acetate ester of the compound was synthesized. The symmetrical 1,2-dimethylhydrazine was oxidized to azomethane, then to azoxymethane. The azoxymethane was brominated in the allylic position by the Wohl-Ziegler reaction and subsequently, in a two-phase reaction, converted to MAM-acetate (MAM-Ac) with silver acetate.[31] This compound is now commercially available. The starting compound, 1,2-dimethylhydrazine, and the oxidation product, azoxymethane, have since become well-established carcinogens for colon and rectum in experimental animals.[32-34] This synthesis also made possible the preparation of a radioisotope-labeled MAM-Ac. The preparation of the starting compound was modified and a tritium-labeled methyl group was incorporated into 1,2-dimethylhydrazine.[35]

The MAM-Ac has been shown to be deacetylated by serum esterase, probably choline esterase.[36] Thus, free MAM is generated in experimental animals parenterally administered the acetate.

Analytical Methods

The unusual chemical and physical properties of cycasin have been utilized for the qualitative detection and quantitative determination of cycasin. A convenient and rapid qualitative test for the presence of cycasin is to detect the cyanide ion formed when the compound is treated with alkali. A sample solution in test tube is made alkaline with a few drops of 2 N NaOH and heated to boiling. The solution is acidified with sulfuric acid and the evolution of hydrocyanic acid is detected by a blue coloration of copper-benzidine test paper placed at the mouth of the test tube. The tube is gently heated, if necessary.[21] This test is useful in testing for the completeness of extraction of cycasin from cycad nut.

Separation of the glycoside from other compounds can be carried out with either paper or thin-layer chromatography. The developing solvent is *n*-butanol/acetic acid/water (4/1/1), and visualization is with a 1% resorcinol solution in ethanol-2 N HCl (1:9), or with aniline hydrogen phthalate in butanol. The sprays detect the glucose of cycasin.[21] A specific reaction for the azoxy group of cycasin is obtained by spraying 0.2% chromotropic acid in 2 M sulfuric acid and heating a thin layer plate at 100 to 110°C for 5 to 10 min.[11] These two qualitative tests have been adapted for quantitative determination. The separated cycasin can be quantitated by eluting the compound from the paper chromatogram and the glucose determined by a micro method.[21]

Cycasin can also be determined quantitatively by generating formaldehyde in an acidic solution and by developing a color by heating the solution with chromotropic acid in 12 M sulfuric acid. The intensity of the color developed is determined colorimetrically at 570 nm and the quantity of cycasin is read off a standard curve. The standard curve can be calibrated with a standardized formaldehyde solution and chromotropic acid, if pure cycasin is not available.[11]

Direct polarographic reduction of the aliphatic azoxy group has been utilized for quantitative analysis of cycasin in the cycad seed. An aqueous alcoholic extract is cleared of interfering substances by treating it with lead acetate followed by the addition of hydrogen sulfide or potassium oxalate. The clarified extract is determined at pH 1 or at pH 7 by polarography.[37]

Both the chromotropic acid and polarographic methods determine all the azoxy glycosides and do not distinguish cycasin from macrozamin and neocycasins. A gas chromatographic method has been used for the determination of cycasin. The cycad nut or prepared flour is extracted with 70% ethanol and the residue from the dried extract is directly trimethylsilyated.[38] This method can separate cycasin from macrozamin, but macrozamin is barely detectable. A more satisfactory method for the estimation of a mixture of cycasin and macrozamin is to dissolve the residue in 1% ethanol and determine the azoxyglycosides by liquid chromatography using a reverse-phase mode. The method separates cycasin and macrozamin and for equimolar amounts of the two compounds the peak heights are essentially equal.[39]

All of these procedures were developed for the determination of cycasin in the cycad nut or prepared crude meal. The determination of cycasin and macrozamin in urine and animal tissue is more difficult. It is necessary to remove the interfering materials and concentrate the glycosides. The method of Kobayashi and Matsumoto of adsorbing the glycosides on Darco-celite column and eluting them with 20% ethanol, after thoroughly washing the column with water to remove the interfering impurities, works well in these cases.[30] The eluate is dried and the azoxyglycosides in the residue are quantitated either by gas or liquid chromatography.

BIOLOGICAL EFFECTS OF CYCASIN

Carcinogenicity of Cycasin

The development of neoplastic lesions was first observed in rats which were fed crude cycad meal to test for the presence of neurotoxins in cycad nuts,[10,11] as described in a preceding section. The experiment in which *Cycas circinalis* was chemically separated and each fraction tested on rats indicated that both cycasin and its aglycone, MAM, fractions were carcinogenic.[11] Pure cycasin fed to Osborne-Mendel strain of rats proved to be carcinogenic. Cycasin-containing diets were fed for 13 days to groups of weanling rats and 21 days to young adult rats, after which animals were raised on a standard ration. Neoplasms of the kidneys were found in 32 of 34 rats autopsied 8 months later.[14] Germ-free rats, in contrast, fed for 20 consecutive days a diet containing 200 mg cycasin per 100 g feed showed no evidence of neoplastic disease 1 year after exposure to the large amount of cycasin.[14]

Intraperitoneal injection of the free MAM into conventional Fischer rats resulted in a variety of neoplasms principally of the liver, kidney, and intestinal tract.[16] MAM, when administered intraperitoneally to germ-free rats, was also hepatotoxic and carcinogenic, manifestations which can be produced by cycasin only when fed to conventional rats. These experiments confirmed the hypothesis that the ingested cycasin is hydrolyzed by bacterial β-glucosidase and that the released aglycone, MAM, is the proximate carcinogen.

Primary cancer of the liver (Figure 3) generally resulted from long-term feeding of cycasin while tumors of the kidneys were most frequently observed after short-term or single exposure to cycasin. Colonic tumors which ranked third in frequency developed in the proximal colon when cycasin was fed, but a wider distribution of carcinomas of the colon, rectum, and small intestine were more frequent when MAM was parenterally administered.[40] The interval between the 1st feeding of cycasin to rats and the appearance of neoplasms was about 6 months.

Fresh or dried husks of *C. circinalis* added to rat ration at 5 or 10% levels induced malignant tumors of liver and kidneys. Similar observations of benign and malignant tumors of liver and kidneys in rats fed low concentrations (0.5 and 1.0%) of cycad husks have been reported.[41] Tubers of *Zamia floridana* also have been found to be carcinogenic. At a 3% level, 60% of the rats developed liver and kidney tumors.[40]

Although most of the studies have been carried out on rats, other species have been shown to be sensitive to cycasin carcinogenesis. Liver and kidney tumors in C56BL/6 mice were induced with topical application of an aqueous extract of *C. circinalis* seeds on artificially induced skin ulcers.[42] Hepatomas, kidney, and pulmonary adenomas have been produced in adult mice with intragastrically administered cycasin.[43,44] Hamsters given cycasin developed hepatocellular and bile duct carcinomas.[45] Liver tumors were found in 9 of 27 guinea pigs fed crude cycad meal.[46] MAM injected intraperitoneally into guinea pigs also produced hepatocellular carcinomas, which confirmed the susceptibility of this species to cycasin carcinogenesis.[47] Aquarium fishes *(Bracydanio reris* and *Lebistes reticulatus)* developed acute degenerative changes in the liver and pancreas after feeding in water to which cycad meal or cycasin was added. Hepatic cells of various structure developed in the residual hepatic tissue and many of these foci had all the characteristics of malignant neoplasms.[48] Cycad was toxic and microscopic lesions were found in the liver and kidneys in chickens when 0.5 or 1% cycad kernels or cycad husks were added to their rations for as long as 68 weeks. However, no tumors developed.[49]

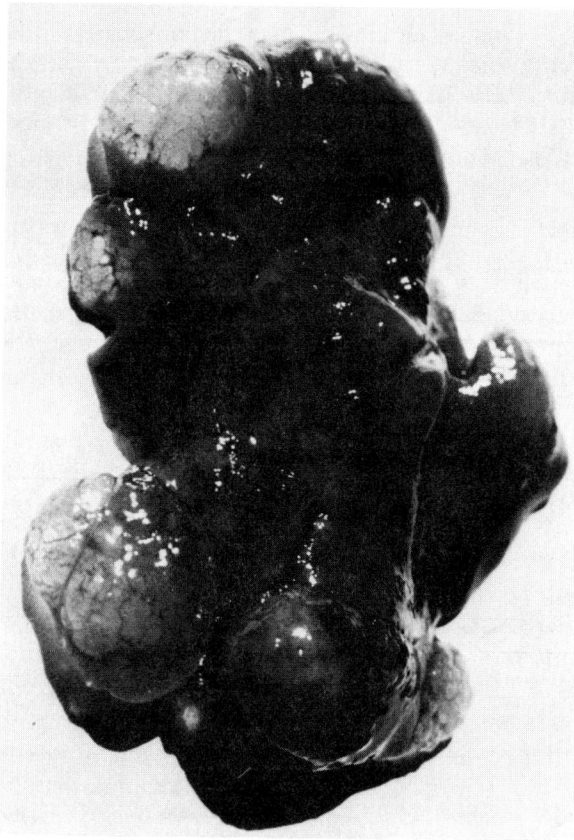

FIGURE 3. Liver of cycasin-fed rat showing nodular hepatoma and multiple small cysts.

The incidence and localization of tumors varied with the species of the test animals. Rats treated with a single administration of cycasin developed high incidence of kidney and intestinal tumors. Hepatocellular carcinomas, lung adenomas or lung carcinomas were frequent in mice, especially when treated with cycasin as newborns. A high incidence of proliferative changes and carcinomas of the intrahepatic bile ducts were observed in hamsters. Young adult rabbits and guinea pigs which received a single oral administration of cycasin near its LD_{50} failed to develop tumors.[50]

The organ specificity of tumor induction in the rat also varied with the quantity of cycasin orally administered. Sprague-Dawley female rats given a low quantity of 4 mg cycasin per kilogram bodyweight per day over a period of 24 months developed a considerable number of mammary tumors, while ACI males developed interstitial tumors in the testis. A high level of cycasin of 500 mg/kg bodyweight per week for 12 weeks produced liver cirrhosis and a high incidence of intestinal and renal tumors. A single dose of 25 mg/kg bodyweight also induced intestinal and renal tumors.[51]

The importance of oral administration and the role of intestinal bacterial β-glucosidase in cycasin carcinogenesis has been described above. However, the induction of kidney tumors in rats, which were subcutaneously injected with cycasin as newborns, indicated that a different mechanism was involved in rats younger than 1 month.[52] One mechanism suggested was that the cycasin injected into newborns was excreted in the urine and the dams, in the process of cleaning their young, swallowed the cycasin-containing urine. The cycasin was hydrolyzed by the bacterial enzymes in the intestine of the dams and the free MAM was transferred back to the young through the milk.[53]

Evidence that MAM can pass into the milk was demonstrated earlier.[54] Germ-free newborns subcutaneously injected with cycasin and nursed by germ-free mothers developed kidney tumors.[47] Similarly, intraperitoneally injected 16, 17, 18, 19, and 20 day old rats immediately weaned also developed kidney tumors.[55] These results suggested that the tissue of the young had an enzyme capable of hydrolyzing cycasin. It was shown that the enzyme β-glucosidase is present in the subcutaneous tissue.[56] Subsequently, it was demonstrated that the enzyme activity of the small intestine of the rat increased gradually to a maximum at about the 16th postnatal day and decreased rapidly to a minimum shortly after weaning at 21 days. There was excellent correlation between the β-glucosidase activity in the small intestine and the incidence of tumors induced in rats injected subcutaneously or intraperitoneally with cycasin at different ages ranging from day 1 to day 25. The authors suggest that the induction of tumors is related to the enzyme activity of the small intestine.[55]

The active component of cycasin, MAM, can cross the placenta and induce neoplasms in the progeny. First evidence of transplacental tumor induction was obtained in Sprague-Dawley rat offsprings of mothers fed various concentrations of cycad meal added to their rations. Of offspring which survived for 6 months, 15 developed tumors at various sites.[57] Experiments with single dose of MAM injected intraperitoneally or intraveneously into Fischer rats at different days during gestation indicated that the last day of intrauterine life was the most sensitive day for later pulmonary and cerebral tumor development in the offsprings. The incidence of tumors was not high, but unusual aggregation of certain neoplasms occurred.[47] Chemical evidence that MAM crossed the placenta was obtained by thin-layer chromatography of fetal extract.[58] Later studies confirmed the transplacental passage of MAM into the fetuses and demonstrated that MAM had reacted with fetal nucleic acids and proteins.[59]

The reader who is interested in more detailed pathology is referred to the review by Laqueur.[41]

Neurotoxicity of Cycasin

Indication that MAM could affect the development of the brain was first noted in experiments designed to answer the question of whether or not it was possible to induce tumors by the transplacental route in rat offspring exposed to cycasin during fetal development. Brain tumors were found in both male and female offspring, the earliest at 11 months.[57] Further indication of brain involvement was obtained when MAM was tested for teratogenic effect on hamsters. Malformations of the fetuses were observed in pregnant golden hamsters injected with MAM on the 8th day of gestation. Among the malformations were microencephalus, hydrocephalus, exencephalus, and spina bifida.[60] Subsequent experiments with rats and mice have demonstrated that malformations can be induced in either the cerebrum or cerebellum depending on the time of MAM administration.

Various degrees of microencephaly were noticed in 4 litters of Fischer rats 14 months old. There was a reduction in brain weight and this was mainly due to the uniform reduction in the cerebral hemispheres (Figure 4). The remainder of the brain was essentially normal and there was no evidence of a deformed skull. A single injection of MAM (20 mg/kg bodyweight) on days 14 or 15 of gestation produced identical malformation in the litter.[61] Microencephaly has been induced by administration of the synthetic MAM-Ac on day 14 or 15 of gestation in the Long-Evans strain of rats. Unlike those animals treated with the free aglycone, these animals suffered a general weight reduction. At 35 days of age, body, brain, kidney, liver, spleen, and testis were significantly reduced, whereas at 14 days of age only the brain weights were significantly less than the controls. The brain was the only organ that showed macroscopic malformation, characterized by greatly reduced cerebral hemispheres and defects in the cortical mantle.[62]

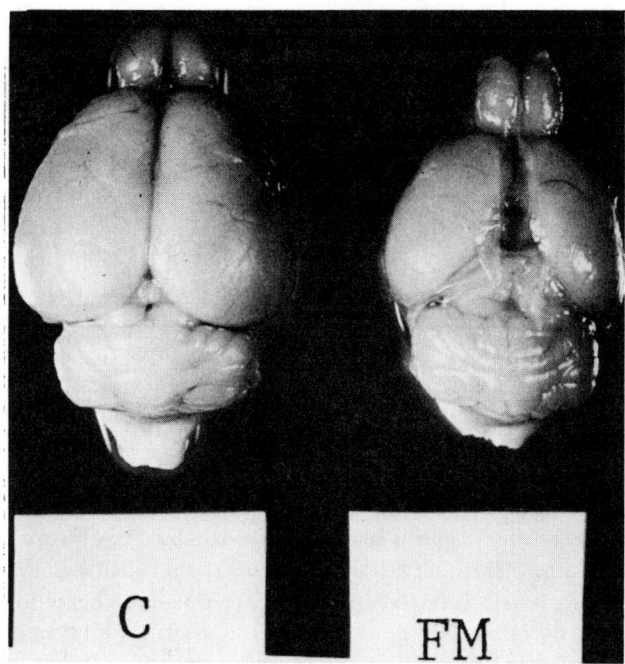

FIGURE 4. Dorsal view of rat brains: Control brain (C) and methylazoxymethyl-acetate treated microencephalic brain (FM), with reduced size of cerebral hemispheres and broad exposure of the copora quadrigemina. (Courtesy of Maria Spatz, National Institute of Neurological, Communicative Disorders and Stroke.)

Microencephaly has been induced in a number of different species. The cerebral mass of the hamster and ferret was reduced by prenatal treatment with MAM-Ac while the structure of the cerebellum of hamster, rabbit, ferret, cat, and dog was readily modified by postnatal treatment.[63]

The quantitative cellular loss in the hemispheres was correlated with morphological changes which occurred in the developing microencephalic brain. The cellular loss was indicated by the loss of DNA. The loss of DNA in the fetal brain apparently occurred during the first 3 days after the injection of MAM into the mother rat. Thereafter, the MAM-treated brain grew almost at a normal rate, but the loss in DNA persisted through maturity of the animal. There was approximately a 25% difference in the quantity of DNA between control and MAM-treated whole brain at birth. This deficiency in DNA was restricted to the cerebral hemispheres.[64] Microencephalic rats of the Fischer strain tested in a Hebb-Williams maze performed substantially and significantly below the control rats.[65]

The first experimental induction by cycasin of a neurological disorder, which resulted in locomotor difficulty, was produced in mice. It was observed in C57B1/6 strain of mice which had received a single subcutaneous injection of 0.5 mg of cycasin per gram bodyweight at birth. The animals developed varying degrees of locomotor difficulty from slight posterior weakness with excessive swaying of the hindquarters and a slow gait to complete paralysis of the hindquarters, with movement by dragging the paralyzed hindquarters.[66] These symptoms were irreversible and closely resembled those described in the literature for cattle.[1] Similar results were produced in the dd strain of mice. Histopathologic findings were limited to the cerebellum. Nuclear debris were found in the external cellular layer 24 hr after the administration of cycasin; 72

hr later the external granular layer had nearly disappeared. As late as 260 days after the injection of cycasin the molecular and internal granular layer had failed to form, the Purkinje cells were scattered irregularly among the granule cells, and there was a greatly reduced number of granular cells within the brain substance beneath the cortical surface.[67] Similar cerebellar changes were produced in Swiss albino mice with both cycasin and MAM-Ac. The deficiency of brain weight was due mainly to the markedly decreased mass of the cerebellum. The changes tended to be more severe with MAM treatment and more variable with cycasin.[68] These microanatomic changes also were observed in the newborn hamster,[69] and in the dog.[70] Cerebellar malformation has been induced in the rat, but without any apparent abnormality of motor function. Hamsters, in contrast, showed gross motor dysfunction. They had consistent difficulty in properly executing coordinated movements in walking or running, but there seemed to be no impairment of the vestibular function or of other righting reflexes. A malformed cerebellum was produced in both the cat and ferret, but only the ferret showed a lasting motor deficit.[63]

Mutagenicity of Cycasin

Radiomimetic effects of cycasin were demonstrated by Teas, et al.[71] by measuring the induction of chromosome aberrations in the root-tip cells of onion, *Allium cepa*. A 0.05% solution of cycasin induced as many chromosome aberrations in the onion root-tip as produced by about 200 R of gamma radiation. Similar chromosome aberrations have been noted in the root-tips of *Zamia intergrifolia* when treated with cycasin and β-glucosidase.[72] The common bean (*Phaseolus vulgaris* L.) seed was treated with cycasin to test its mutagenicity. The seeds were grown and chlorophyll mutations (which change leaf color) and morphological mutations (which change the shape, size, and growth patterns or growth habits of an organ or the whole plant) were observed.[73] Cycasin, its aglycone, MAM, and MAM-Ac were tested for the induction of sex-linked recessive lethal mutations in *Drosophila melongaster* males. Cycasin was not mutagenic, but MAM and MAM-Ac were potent mutagens.[74]

MAM was found by Smith[75] to be a good mutagen in *Salmonella typhimurium*. The mutagenic activity was tested by measuring the frequency of reversion to histidine independence of several histidine-requiring mutants of *Salmonella*. Cycasin neither inhibited nor caused reversion in any of the mutants. A host-mediated assay, which incorporates a microbial indicator in the murine host, was used to demonstrate the mutagenicity of cycasin. Histidine auxotrophs of *S. typhimurium* G-46 were injected intraperitoneally and cycasin was administered orally to the mice. A 2% cycasin or a 1% MAM administration resulted in increased mutation frequency. The mutation was increased 30-fold by cycasin and 100-fold by MAM, when the compounds were given 2 hr before the test organisms were introduced into the mouse peritoneum. Cycasin given parenterally did not cause an increase over the spontaneous-mutation frequency.[76] This agrees with the earlier reports mentioned above that cycasin if given by injection to adult animals is inactive. The Ames assay utilizes a rat liver microsomal enzyme mixture, commonly called the S-9 Mix, for the activation of some compounds to their mutagenic form.[77] However, this system is incapable of activating glucosides such as cycasin. A system of preincubation of glucosides with β-glucosidase before testing with the Ames *Salmonella* test was successful in demonstrating the mutagenicity of cycasin in vitro.[78]

Biochemical Actions of Cycasin

Numerous biochemical studies on the reaction of cycasin and MAM on cellular constituents and the effect of these compounds on certain enzyme activities have been carried out in order to understand the nature of the carcinogenic action of the compounds. The primary reaction is methylation and the effects reported range from what apparently appears to be cell membrane destruction to inhibition or inactivation of enzyme systems responsible for the synthesis of nucleic acids and proteins.

Cycasin or cycad meal fed at increasing levels for 48 hr produced a progressive loss, up to approximately 30% of the total rat liver RNA. The change in liver phospholipids following cycasin and cycad meal feeding almost duplicated the results of RNA.[79,80] The almost identical loss of RNA and phospholipids correlated closely with the disintegration of cytoplasmic basophilia, as observed with the light microscope,[10] and with the disaggregation of polysomes and depletion of rough endoplasmic reticulum, observed with the electron microscope.[81] These changes in concentration of RNA and phospholipoproteins suggested that the primary effect of cycasin toxicity could be on the lipoprotein-rich membrane of the endoplasmic reticulum.

A single nonlethal dose of MAM inhibited the incorporation of thymidine into DNA of rat liver, small intestine, and kidneys. The rat liver showed marked inhibition of RNA and protein synthesis.[82] Inhibition of RNA synthesis in vitro also has been demonstrated. Uridine triphosphate (UTP) incorporation was inhibited in hepatic nuclei isolated from rats that had been treated with MAM. Orotic acid incorporation into nucleolar RNA was unaffected, but cytidine incorporation was significantly decreased.[83] The failure of the MAM-treated isolated nuclei to incorporate UTP into RNA could have been that the precursors necessary for RNA synthesis could not penetrate the nucleus because of permeability changes in the nuclear membrane. However, an "aggregate" enzyme system containing chromatin and RNA polymerase, which basically is a nuclear preparation devoid of membrane, showed that there was marked inhibition of UTP incorporation into RNA.[84]

The distribution patterns of liver ribosomes indicated that while monomer-plus-dimer represented approximately 35% for control rat liver, the monomer-dimer in the cycasin-treated rats increased to 52% and 67% in MAM-Ac treated animals. MAM, which methylates liver RNA, deaggregates polyribosomes, but cycasin was not as effective as MAM-Ac. The lower capacity of cycasin was ascribed to the inefficiency of the hydrolysis of cycasin by the intestinal microflora.[85]

MAM-induced single-strand breaks in liver DNA in vivo, which could be monitored by centrifugation in alkaline sucrose gradient. The damage to DNA was apparently maximal within a few hours after administration of MAM, but the repair process was not completely ended at 14 days.[86]

The inhibition of protein synthesis by cycasin in the rat liver has been observed. This inhibition was not evident for about 5 hr after cycasin administration, but once established it persisted for the next 20 hr. Cycasin inhibited protein synthesis in the liver but not in the kidney, spleen, or ileum.[87] Similar inhibition of liver protein synthesis, but no effect in kidney and small intestine, was observed after MAM-Ac administration to rats.[82] Protein synthesis also was inhibited in the liver of rats treated with an aqueous extract of *Macrozamia communis*.[88] The azoxyglycoside in this species is macrozamin, but the inhibition of microsomal protein was similar. Synthesis of microsomal proteins was inhibited in rat livers of animals treated with MAM-Ac. Protein synthesis was 50% below control levels in 1 hr after a single MAM injection and maximum inhibition of 70% was observed in 2 hr and synthesis returned to control levels in 24 hr.[89] Circular dichroism analysis of the "aggregate" enzyme preparation from MAM-treated rat liver indicated a change in conformation of the nuclear proteins component. The results suggested that MAM interacted with nuclear proteins and produced conformational changes which resulted in decreased RNA synthesis.[84]

Methylation of nucleic acids was detected in some organs of rats administered cycasin. The methylated compound was identified as 7-methyl-guanine. Liver RNA was methylated to a greater extent than was either kidney or small intestine RNA.[87] Meth-

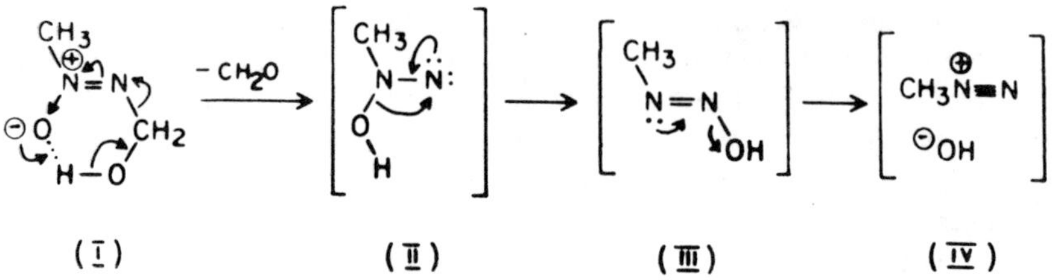

FIGURE 5. The formation of the transient methyl donor, methyldiazonium hydroxide (IV), by way of the azene (II) and diazo hydroxide (III) from methylazoxymethanol, MAM, (I).

ylation of nucleic acids of fetuses of rats which were injected with MAM during pregnancy has been shown. Guanine, methylated in the seven position, was found in both DNA and RNA.[59] It also has been demonstrated that MAM can methylate RNA and DNA in vitro. RNA or DNA mixed with MAM in 1 mℓ of 0.2 M phosphate buffer at pH 7.0 was kept at 37° for 16 hr. A single methylated derivative, identified as 7-methylguanine was found in both the hydrolyzate of the treated RNA and DNA.[90]

Other biochemical effects of cycasin toxicity have been reported. Liver catalase activity has attracted much attention since the observation was made that its activity is decreased in cancer patients and tumor-bearing animals. The level of catalase activity was lowered in liver of rats fed 0.2% of cycasin with their feed. A 3% cycad meal diet, in place of cycasin, caused a 50% reduction in catalase activity. The kidney catalase activity was not significantly affected by cycasin or cycad nut meal.[93] The synthesis of catalase decreased from 5 to 1.2 units/hr in the liver of rats fed a ration of 0.2% cycasin. The degradation of liver catalase decreased from 2.9 to 1.4%/hr. Although the total catalase activity did not change, catalase synthesis as well as degradation decreased in the rat kidney. Apparently, cycasin can alter both the rates of synthesis and degradation of catalase.[94] Histochemically, it was demonstrated that glucose 6-phosphatase activity decreased, even in the absence of microscopic evidence of injury, in the liver of guinea pigs fed cycad meal for 5 days. Adenosine triphosphatase activity was decreased while the alkaline phosphatase was increased. In the rat liver, glucose 6-phosphatase and 5-nucleotidase activities decreased but the adenosine triphosphatase decreased in centrilobular areas and increased in the periportal zones. The activity changes were dose dependent. The hepatocellular distribution of esterase activities was altered to some degree.[95] The level of activity of rat blood plasma choline cholinesterase was consistently elevated by the feeding of a diet containing cycasin. The elevation in plasma cholinesterase activity level appeared within 24 hr after the initial feeding of cycasin. The elevation persisted for at least 5 days after discontinuing feeding of cycasin diet. Continuous feeding of cycasin for 10 days elevated the cholinesterase activity level significantly above the 5-day level. Cycasin did not inhibit or activate the action of rat plasma cholinesterase in vitro.[96]

There have been speculations on the mode of action of MAM in the methylation process (Figure 5). Miller[91] first suggested that MAM might act biologically in a manner similar to N-nitrosodimethylamine and form diazomethane as an intermediate. He also suggested that if azoxymethane is oxidized in vivo it would yield the aglycone of cycasin, MAM, and would be highly toxic. Subsequently, azoxymethane was shown to be carcinogenic and Druckrey and Lange[33] suggested that the mechanism of action of this compound is through its conversion to MAM by enzymatic hydroxylation. The resulting MAM spontaneously breaks down by concerted reaction and yields methyl diazonium hydroxide, the active intermediate. Nagasawa, et al.[92] obtained spectroscopic evidence that diazomethane is not an intermediate in the decomposition of MAM in aqueous solutions. Proton magnetic resonance spectra of the MAM decomposition in D₂O was obtained. Diazomethane has a reactive CH₂- group and it would be expected that from solvolysis of the compound a C-D bond would be present in the new methyl group (CH_2D-), if formed it was not detected. It was concluded that the transient methyl donor is most likely methyldiazonium hydroxide as proposed by Druckrey and Lange.[33]

Effect of Cycasin on Humans

The discovery of the carcinogenic effects of cycasin caused concern for the well-being of those people who consume cycads. Cycad flour prepared for human consumption was examined for presence of cycasin. Experimental animals, including nonhuman primates, were fed cycad flour or cycasin to determine the long-term effects of cycasin.

Kobayashi examined the flour as well as a number of food products which contained from one quarter to one third of flour prepared from *C. revoluta* seeds, but was not able to detect any cycasin.[8]

Flour prepared from *C. circinalis* by native Guamanians for human consumption was tested on rats. The animals were fed diets containing as much as 10% of processed *C. circinalis* seeds for a period of 23 months to determine whether or not the flour was carcinogenic. No neoplastic lesions were observed similar to those induced in rats after long-term ingestion of unprocessed cycad flour.[100]

Hirono, et al.[9] surveyed the people of Miyako Islands, Okinawa, to determine whether or not they suffered long-term detrimental effects from having subsisted on cycads as an emergency food when their Islands were devastated by a series of typhoons in 1959. Cases of acute toxicity were noted, but there was no indication that the incidence of neoplasms had increased in that population 10 years after the disaster. However, the death rate for liver cirrhosis was found to be higher than in Japan proper. The authors concluded that the high death rate for liver cirrhosis may be related to the practice of consuming cycads by the natives of Miyako Islands.

Cycasin administered orally for a long period to nonhuman primates was hepatotoxic and hepatocarcinogenic. One Old World monkey out of nine animals necropsied had a well-differentiated hepatocellular carcinoma and a second one had multiple tumors, including hepatocellular carcinoma, intrahepatic bile duct adenocarcinoma, renal carcinoma and adenomas, and adenomatous polyps of the colon. Hepatotoxic effects were found in monkeys fed as little as 133 mg of cycasin. All but one monkey in the experiment had hepatic lesions.[101] The liver lesions included toxic hepatitis, centrilobular liver necrosis, hyperplastic nodules and cirrhosis which were simlar to those lesions described by Dastur and Palekar in rhesus monkeys fed a diet containing cycad seeds.[102] It is uncertain whether the hepatic lesions noted in the necropsied monkeys would have progressed to tumors had the monkeys survived longer.[101] However, liver cirrhosis is thought to precede hepatocellular carcinomas in some instances in humans.[103]

The results of the administration of cycasin in the nonhuman primates experiment strongly suggest that the high rate of death from liver cirrhosis in the population of Miyako Islands could well be related to the ingestion of cycads as concluded by Hirono, et al.[9] Generally, those who use cycad seeds as food process them well to remove the toxins when there is ample time, as indicated by the absence of cycasin in cycad flour prepared for human consumption. However, under adverse conditions, such as after a typhoon, when there is urgent need to prepare some food for survival, there is the possibility that the removal of cycasin from the seeds may be incomplete. The fact that cases of acute liver toxicity and even death were noted in the Miyako Island survey indicates that accidental ingestion of improperly prepared cycad material does occur. As in the case of nonhuman primates, it is not certain whether those people who died of cirrhosis of the liver would eventually have developed neoplasms had they survived, but it is evident that there is need to prepare cycad materials with great care.

Concluding Comments

The emphasis in the early cycad toxicity studies was on acute signs and the need for chronic toxicity experiments probably was not fully appreciated even after the toxic components, the azoxyglycosides, were isolated from the cycads. The search for neurotoxins, which would be expected to produce their paralytic effects after a long period, undoubtedly influenced the experimental plan to maintain the cycad-fed rats for as long a time as possible. The rats developed tumors long before any neurologic effects were observed, but this would have been missed if only acute toxicity signs had been followed.

The discovery of microencephaly was a reverse case of that for carcinogenicity. The objective was to observe the induction of brain tumors by transplacental transport of MAM to the fetus. Tumors were produced in a few cases, but the anatomical changes noted in the brain were a chance observation. An interest in brain tumors and transplacental induction of tumors had resulted in an interesting brain malformation observation.

There is only suggestive evidence at this time that ingestion of cycads produces cancer in humans. The major contribution of these carcinogenesis studies is that it pointed to the possible role intestinal microflora could play in carcinogenesis, and it provided a stimulus to explore the role of intestinal microorganisms in the metabolism of other compounds that could be converted to carcinogens.[97]

A considerable amount of work on MAM-induced cerebral and cerebellar malformations has been carried out and a review on neurotoxicity of cycasin and MAM has been written.[98] However, there is no evidence that the cycads are responsible for ALS. It was recently reported that the retentrate of an aqueous extract of seeds of *Encephalartos altensteinii* passed through an Amicon UM-2 ultrafiltration membrane was neurotoxic to guinea pigs.[99] Thus, the search for neurotoxins in cycads continues.

REFERENCES

1. Whiting, M. G., Toxicity of cycads, *Econ. Bot.* 17, 270, 1963.
2. Kurland, L. T. and Mulder, D. W., Epidemiologic investigations of amyotrophic lateral sclerosis. I. Preliminary Report on geographic distribution, with special reference to the Mariana Islands, including clinical and pathologic observations, *Neurology*, 4, 355, 1954.
3. Kurland, L. T., Introductory remarks — Third Conference on the Toxicity of Cycads, *Fed. Proc. Fed. Am. Soc. Exp. Biol.*, 23, 1337, 1964.
4. Hirano, A., Malamud, N., Elizan, T. S., and Kurland, L. T., Amyotrophic lateral sclerosis and parkinsonism-dementia complex on Guam, *Arch. Neurol.*, 15, 35, 1966.
5. Fosberg, F. R., Resume of the Cycadaceae, *Fed. Proc. Fed. Am. Soc. Exp. Biol.* 23, 1340, 1964.
6. Theiret, J. W., Economic botany of the cycads, *Econ. Bot.*, 12, 3, 1958.
7. Mugera, G. M. and Nderito, P., Toxic properties of *Encephalartos hildebrandtii*, *East Afr. Med. J.*, 45, 732, 1968.
8. Kobayashi, A. Cycasin in cycad materials used in Japan, *Fed. Proc. Fed. Am. Soc. Exp. Biol.*, 31, 1476, 1972.
9. Hirono, I., Kachi, H., and Kato, T., A survey of acute toxicity of cycads and mortality rate from cancer in the Miyako Islands, Okinawa, *Acta Pathol.*, 20, 327, 1970.
10. Laquer, G. L., Mickelsen, O., Whiting, M. G., and Kurland, L. T., Carcinogenic properties of nuts from *Cycas circinalis* L. indigenous to Guam, *J. Natl. Cancer Inst.*, 31, 919, 1963.
11. Matsumoto, H. and Strong, F. M., The occurrence of methylazoxymethanol in *Cycas circinalis* L., *Arch. Biochem. Biophys.*, 101, 299, 1963.
12. Nishida, K., Kobayashi, A., Nagahama, T., Kojima, K., and Yamane, M., Studies on cycasin, a new toxic glycoside from *Cycas revoluta* Thunb. IV. Pharmacological study of cycasin, *Seikagaku*, 28, 218, 1956.

13. Laquer, G. L., Carcinogenic effects of cycad meal and cycasin methylazoxymethanol glycoside in rats and effects of cycasin in germfree rats, *Fed. Proc. Fed. Am. Soc. Exp. Biol.*, 23, 1386, 1964.
14. Spatz, M., McDaniel, E. G., and Laquer, G. L., Cycasin excretion in conventional and germ-free rats, *Proc. Soc. Exp. Biol. Med.*, 121, 417, 1966.
15. Spatz, M., Smith, D. W. E., McDaniel, E. G., and Laqueur, G. L., Role of intestinal microorganisms in determining cycasin toxicity, *Proc. Soc. Exp. Biol. Med.* 124, 691, 1967.
16. Laquer, G. L. and Matsumoto, H., Neoplasms in female Fischer rats following intraperitoneal injection of methylazoxymethanol, *J. Natl. Cancer Inst.*, 37, 217, 1966.
17. Cooper, J. M., Isolation of a toxic principle from the seeds of *Macrozamia spiralis*, *J. Proc. R. Soc. N. S. Wales*, LXXIV, 450, 1941.
18. Langley, B. W., Lythgoe, B., and Riggs, N. V., Macrozamin. II. The aliphatic azoxy structure of the aglycone part, *J. Chem. Soc.*, 1951, 2309, 1951.
19. Lythgoe, B. and Riggs, N. V., Macrozamin. I. The identity of the carbohydrate component, *J. Chem. Soc.*, 1949, 2716, 1949.
20. Nishida, K., Kobayashi, A., and Nagahama, T., Studies on cycasin, a new toxic glycoside of *Cycas revoluta* Thunb., *Bull. Agric. Chem. Soc. (Jpn)*, 19, 77, 1955.
21. Riggs, N. V. Glycosyloxyazoxymethane, a constituent of the seeds of *Cycas circinalis* L., *Chem. Ind.*, 926, 1956.
22. Korsch, B. H. and Riggs, N. V., Proton magnetic resonance spectra of aliphatic azoxy compounds and the structure of cycasin, *Tetrahedron Lett.*, 10, 523, 1964.
23. Nishida, K., Kobayashi, A., Nagahama, T., and Numata, T., Studies on some new azoxy glycosides of *Cycas revoluta* Thunb. I. On neocycasin A, β-laminaribosyloxyazoxymethane, *Bull. Agric. Soc. (Jpn)*, 23, 460, 1959.
24. Nagahama, T., Studies on neocycasins, new glycosides of cycads, *Bull. Fac. Agric. Kagoshima Univ.*, 14, 1, 1964.
25. Matsumoto, H. and Nagahama, T., Unpublished data.
26. Riggs, N. V., The occurrence of macrozamin in the seeds of cycads, *Aust. J. Chem.*, 7, 123, 1954.
27. Nagahama, T., Ijuin, I., and Watabe, T., Azoxyglycosides occurring in the outer shells of *Cycas circinalis* L. nuts, *Agric. Biol. Chem. (Jpn).*, 28, 573, 1964.
28. Kobayashi, A. and Murozono, T., A trial for large-scale preparation of cycasin, *Bull. Fac. Agric. Kagoshima Univ.*, 21, 129, 1971.
29. Kobayashi, A., Biochemical studies on cycasin. II. Existence of free aglycone of cycasin in its enzymatic hydrolysis. *Agric. Biol. Chem. (Jpn)*, 26, 208, 1962.
30. Kobayashi, A. and Matsumoto, H., Studies on methylazoxymethanol, the aglycone of cycasin: isolation, biological and chemical properties, *Arch. Biochem. Biophys.*, 110, 373, 1965.
31. Matsumoto, H., Nagahama, T., and Larson, H. O., Studies on methylazoxymethanol, the aglycone of cycasin: a synthesis of methylazoxymethyl acetate, *Biochem. J.*, 95, 13C, 1965.
32. Druckrey, H., Preussman, R., Matzkies, F., and Ivankovic, S., Selective erzeugnung von darmkrebs bei ratten durch, 1,2-dimethylhydrazin, *Naturwissenschaften*, 54, 285, 1967.
33. Druckrey, H. and Lang, A., Carcinogenicity of azoxymethane dependent on age in BD rats, *Fed. Proc. Fed. Am. Soc. Exp. Biol.*, 31, 1482, 1972.
34. Druckrey, H., Specific carcinogenic and teratogenic effects of indirect alkylating methyl and ethyl compounds and their dependency on stages of ontogenic developments, *Xenobiotica*, 3, 271, 1973.
35. Horisberger, M. and Matsumoto, H., Studies on methylazoxymethanol, Synthesis of ^{14}C and ^{3}H labelled methylazoxymethyl-acetate, *J. Labelled Comp.*, 4, 164, 1968.
36. Poynter, R. W., Ball, C. R., Goodban, J., and Thackrah, T., The influence of physostigmine on the activation of methylazoxymethanol acetate, a potent carcinogen, by a serum factor in vitro. *Chem. Biol. Interact.*, 4, 139, 1972.
37. Nishida, K., Kobayashi, A., and Nagahama, T., Studies on cycasin, a new toxic glycoside, of *Cycas revoluta*, Thunb. VI. Polarography of cycasin, *Bull. Agric. Chem. Soc. (Jpn)*, 20, 122, 1956.
38. Wells, W. W., Yang, M. G., Bolzer, W., and Mickelsen, O., Gas-liquid chromatographic analysis of cycasin in cycad flour, *Anal. Biochem.*, 25, 325, 1968.
39. Matsumoto, H., unpublished data.
40. Laqueur, G. L., Oncogenicity of cycads and its implications, in *Advances in Modern Toxicology*, Vol. 3, Kraybill, H. F. and Mehlman, M. A., Eds., John Wiley & Sons, New York, 1977, 231.
41. Hoch-Ligeti, C., Stutzman, E., and Arvin, J. M., Cellular composition during tumor induction in rats by cycad husks, *J. Natl. Cancer Inst.*, 41, 605, 1968.
42. O'Gara, R. W., Brown, J. M., and Whiting, M. G., Induction of hepatic and renal tumors by topical application of aqueous extract of cycad nut to artificial skin ulcer in mice, *Fed. Proc. Fed. Am. Soc. Exp. Biol.*, 23, 1383, 1964.
43. Hirono, I., Shibuya, C., and Fushimi, K., Tumor induction in C57BL/6 mice by a single administration of cycasin, *Cancer Res.*, 29, 1658, 1969.

44. Hirono, I. and Shibuya, C., High incidence of pulmonary tumors in dd mice by a single injection of cycasin, *Gann,* 61, 403, 1970.
45. Hirono, I., Hayashi, K., Mori, H., and Miwa, T., Carcinogenic effects of cycasin in Syrian golden hamsters and the transplantibility of induced tumors, *Cancer Res.,* 31, 283, 1971.
46. Spatz, M., Carcinogenic effect of cycad meal in guinea pigs, *Fed. Proc. Fed. Am. Soc. Exp. Biol.,* 23, 1384, 1964.
47. Laqueur, G. L. and Spatz, M., Oncogenicity of cycasin and methylazoxymethanol, *Gann (Monogr.,)* 17, 189, 1975.
48. Stanton, M. F., Hepatic neoplasms of aquarium fish exposed to *Cycas circinalis, Fed. Proc. Fed. Am. Soc. Exp. Biol.,* 25, 661, 1966.
49. Sanger, V. L., Yang, M. G., and Mickelsen, O., Cycad toxicosis in chicken, *J. Natl. Cancer Inst.,* 43, 391, 1969.
50. Hirono, I., Carcinogenicity and neurotoxicity of cycasin with special reference to species differences, *Fed. Proc. Fed. Am. Soc. Exp. Biol.,* 31, 1493, 1972.
51. Fukunishi, R., Watanabe, K., Terashi, S., and Kawaji, K., Shift of target organs in cycasin carcinogenesis, *Gann,* 62, 353, 1971.
52. Hirono, I., Laquer, G. L., and Spatz, M., Tumor induction in Fischer and Osborne-Mendel rats by a single administration of cycasin, *J. Natl. Cancer Inst.,* 40, 1003, 1968.
53. Yang, M. G., Mickelsen, O., and Sanger, V. L., Cycling of cycasin from newborn rats to their mother and back to the newborn, *Proc. Soc. Exp. Biol. Med.* 131, 135, 1969.
54. Mickelsen, O., Campbell, E., Yang, M., Mugera, G., and Whitehair, C. B., Studies with cycad, *Fed. Proc. Fed. Am. Soc. Exp. Biol.,* 23, 1363, 1964.
55. Matsumoto, H., Nagata, Y., Nishimura, E. T., Bristol, R., and Haber, M., β-glucosidase modulation in preweanling rats and its association with tumor induction by cycasin, *J. Natl. Cancer Inst.,* 49, 423, 1972.
56. Spatz, M., Hydrolysis of cycasin by β-D-glucosidase in skin of newborn rats, *Proc. Soc. Exp. Biol. Med.,* 128, 1005, 1968.
57. Spatz, M. and Laqueur, G. L., Transplacental induction of tumors in Sprague-Dawley rats with crude cycad material, *J. Natl. Cancer Inst.,* 38, 233, 1967.
58. Spatz, M. and Laqueur, G. L., Evidence for transplacental passage of the natural carcinogen cycasin and its aglycone, *Proc. Soc. Exp. Biol. Med.,* 127, 281, 1968.
59. Nagata, Y. and Matsumoto, H., Studies on methylazoxymethanol: methylation of nucleic acids in the fetal rat brain, *Proc. Soc. Exp. Biol. Med.,* 132, 383, 1969.
60. Spatz, M., Dougherty, W. J., and Smith, D. W. E., Teratogenic effects of methylazoxymethanol, *Proc. Soc. Exp. Biol. Med.,* 124, 476, 1967.
61. Spatz, M. and Laqueur, G. L., Transplacental chemical induction of microencephaly in two strains of rats, *Proc. Soc. Exp. Biol. Med.,* 129, 705, 1968.
62. Fischer, M. H., Welker, C., and Waisman, H. A., Generalized growth retardation in rats induced by prenatal exposure to methylazoxymethyl acetate, *Teratology,* 5, 223, 1972.
63. Haddad, R. K., Rabe, A., and Dumas, R., Comparison of effects of methylazoxymethanol acetate on development in different species, *Fed. Proc. Fed. Am. Soc. Exp. Biol.,* 31, 1520, 1972.
64. Matsumoto, H., Spatz, M., and Laqueur, G. L,. Quantitative changes with age in the DNA content of methylazoxymethanol induced microencephalic rat brain, *J. Neurochem.,* 19, 297, 1972.
65. Haddad, R. K., Rabe, A., Laqueur, G. L., Spatz, M., and Valsamis, M. P., Intellectual deficit associated with transplacentally induced microcephaly in the rat, *Science,* 163, 88, 1969.
66. Hirono, I. and Shibuya, C., Induction of neurological disorder by cycasin in mice, *Nature (London),* 216, 1311, 1967.
67. Hirono, I., Shibuya, C., and Hayashi, K., Induction of a cerebellar disorder with cycasin in newborn mice and hamsters, *Proc. Soc. Exp. Biol. Med.,* 131, 593, 1969.
68. Jones, M., Yang, M., and Mickelsen, O., Effects of methylazoxymethanol glucoside on the cerebellum of the postnatal Swiss albino mouse, *Fed. Proc. Fed. Am. Soc. Exp. Biol.,* 31, 1508, 1972.
69. Shimada, M. and Langman, J., Repair of the external granular layer of the hamster cerebellum after prenatal and postnatal administration of methylazoxymethanol, *Teratology,* 3, 119, 1979.
70. Sanger, V. L., Yang, M., and Mickelsen, O., Cycasin-induced central nervous system lesions in postnatal mice, *Fed. Proc. Fed. Am. Soc. Exp. Biol.,* 31, 1524, 1972.
71. Teas, H. J., Sax, H. J., and Sax, K., Cycasin: radiomimetic effect, *Science,* 149, 541, 1965.
72. Porter, E. D. and Teas, H. J., Comparative radiomimetic effect of emulsin, cycasin, methylazoxymethanol and X-rays in *Zamia integrifolia, Rad. Bot.,* 11, 21, 1971.
73. Moh, C. C., Mutagenic effect of cycasin in beans (*Phaseolus vulgaris* L.), *Mutation Res.,* 10, 251, 1970.
74. Teas, H. J. and Dyson, J. G., Mutation in *Drosophila* by methylazoxymethanol, the aglycone of cycasin, *Proc. Soc. Exp. Biol. Med.,* 125, 988, 1967.

75. Smith, D. W. E., Mutagenicity of cycasin aglycone (methylazoxymethanol), a naturally occurring carcinogen, *Science,* 152, 1273, 1966.
76. Gabridge, M. G. and Legator, M. S., Cycasin: detection of associated mutagenic activity, *in vivo, Science,* 163, 689, 1969.
77. Ames, B. N., McCann, J., and Yamasaki, E., Methods for detecting carcinogens and mutagens with the *Salmonella*/mammalian-microsome mutagenicity test, *Mutation Res.,* 31, 347, 1975.
78. Matsushima, T., Matsumoto, H., Shirai, A., Sawamura, M., and Sugimura, T., Mutagenicity of the naturally occurring carcinogen cycasin and synthetic MAM-conjugates on *Salmonella typhimurium, Cancer Res.,* 39, 3780, 1979.
79. Williams, J. N., Effect of cycad and cycasin feeding on liver RNA, DNA, succinic oxidase, and lipids in the rat, *Fed. Proc. Fed. Am. Soc. Exp. Biol.,* 23, 1374, 1964.
80. Williams, J. N. and Laqueur, G. L., Response of liver nucleic acids and lipids in rats fed *Cycas circinalis* L. endosperm or cycasin, *Proc. Soc. Exp. Biol. Med.,* 118, 1, 1965.
81. Ganote, C. E. and Rosenthal, A. S., Characteristic lesions of methylazoxymethanol-induced liver damage, a comparative ultrastructural study with dimethylnitrosamine, hydrazine sulfate, and carbon tetrachloride, *Lab. Invest.,* 19, 382, 1968.
82. Zedeck, M. S., Sternberg, S. S., Poynter, R. W., and McGowan, J., Biochemical and pathological effects of methylazoxymethanol acetate, a potent carcinogen, *Cancer Res.,* 30, 801, 1970.
83. Zedeck, M. S., Sternberg, S. S., McGowan, J., and Poynter, R. W., Methylazoxymethanol acetate: induction of tumors and early effects on RNA synthesis, *Fed. Proc. Fed. Am. Soc. Exp. Biol.,* 31, 1485, 1972.
84. Grab, D. J., Zedeck, M. S., Swislocki, N. I., and Sonnenberg, M., In vitro synthesis of RNA with "aggregate" enzyme, chromatin, and DNA from liver of methylazoxymethanol acetate-treated rats, *Chem. Biol. Interact.,* 6, 259, 1973.
85. Shank, R. C., Effect of cycasin on protein synthesis, *Biochem. Biophys. Acta,* 166, 578, 1968.
86. Damjanov, I., Cox, R., Sarma, D. S. R., and Farber, E., Patterns of damage and repair of liver DNA induced by carcinogenic methylating agents, *in vivo, Cancer Res.,* 33, 2122, 1973.
87. Shank, R. C. and Magree, P. N., Similarities between the biochemical actions of cycasin and dimethylnitrosamine, *Biochem. J.,* 105, 521, 1967.
88. Healy, P. J., Studies on poisoning by Macrozamia communis. I. Biochemical disturbances in the liver, *Biochem. Pharmacol.,* 18, 85, 1969.
89. Lundeen, P. B., Banks, G. S., and Ruddon, R. W., Effects of the carcinogen methylazoxymethanol acetate on protein synthesis and drug metabolism, *Biochem. Pharmacol.,* 20, 2522, 1971.
90. Matsumoto, H. and Higa, H. H., Studies on methylazoxymethanol, the aglycone of cycasin: methylation of nucleic acids, *in vitro, Biochem. J.,* 98, 20C, 1966.
91. Miller, J. A., Comments on chemistry of cycads, *Fed. Proc. Fed. Am. Soc. Exp. Biol.,* 23, 1361, 1964.
92. Nagasawa, H. T., Shirota, F. N., and Matsumoto, H., Decomposition of methylazoxymethanol, the aglycone of cycasin, in D_2O, *Nature (London),* 236, 234, 1972.
93. Rechcigl, M., Jr., Rates and kinetics of catalase synthesis and destruction in rats fed cycad and cycasin *in vivo, Fed. Proc. Fed. Am. Soc. Exp. Biol.,* 23, 1376, 1964.
94. Rechcigl, M., Jr. and Laqueur, G. L., Carcinogen-mediated alteration of rates of enzyme synthesis and degradation, *Enzymol. Biol. Clin.,* 9, 276, 1968.
95. Spatz, M,. Effects of cycad meal and cycasin on histochemical demonstrable liver phosphatase and nonspecific esterases, *Fed. Proc. Fed. Am. Soc. Exp. Biol.,* 23, 1381, 1964.
96. Orgell, W. H. and Laqueur, G. L., Effect of ingested cycasin on blood plasma cholinesterase, *Fed. Proc. Fed. Am. Soc. Exp. Biol.,* 23, 1378, 1964.
97. Weisburger, J. H., Colonic carcinogens: their metabolism and mode of action, *Cancer,* 28, 60, 1971.
98. Jones, M., Mickelsen, O., and Yang, M., Methylazoxymethanol neurotoxicity, in *Progress in Neuropathology,* Vol. 2, Zimmerman, H. M., Ed., Grune & Stratton, New York, 1973, 91—114.
99. Louw, W. K. A. and Oelofsen, W., Carcinogenic and neurotoxic components in the cycad *Encephalartos alternsteinii* Lehm. (family Zamiaceae), *Toxicon,* 13, 447, 1975.
100. Yang, M. G., Mickelsen, O., Campbell, M. E., Laqueur, G. L., and Keresztesy, J. C., Cycad flour used by Guamanians: effects produced in rats by long-term feeding, *J. Nutrit.,* 90, 153, 1966.
101. Sieber, S. M., Correa, P., Dalgard, D. W., McIntire, K. R., and Adamson, R. H., Carcinogenicity and hepatotoxicity of cycasin and its aglycone methylazoxymethanol acetate in nonhuman primates, *J. Natl. Cancer Inst.,* 65, 177, 1980.
102. Dastur, D. K. and Palekar, R. S., The experimental pathology of cycad with special reference to oncogenic effects, *Indian J. Cancer,* 11, 33, 1976.
103. Anthony, P. P., Precursor lesions for liver cancer in humans, *Cancer Res.,* 36, 2579, 1976.

NATURALLY OCCURRING FOOD TOXICANTS: FAVISM-PRODUCING AGENTS

M. Chevion, J. Mager, and G. Glaser

ETIOLOGY OF FAVISM: EPIDEMIOLOGICAL, GENETIC, AND BIOCHEMICAL ASPECTS

Brief Description of the Clinical Manifestations of Favism

The occurrence of sproradic cases of an acute hemolysis following ingestion of broad beans (seeds of the *Vicia faba* plant, fava beans) was first recorded in the medical literature around the mid 1850s.[4] Since then a vast number of clinical reports as well as epidemiological, genetic, and biochemical studies have jointly contributed to the characterization of this disorder, termed "favism", and to the elucidation of its etiology and pathogenesis.[83,119]

The fava bean-induced hemolysis varies in intensity in different cases and in its more severe form may be accompanied by jaundice and hemoglobinuria.[10] The other clinical manifestations of the disease, such as pallor, fatigue, nausea, dyspnea, fever and chills, abdominal or dorsal pain are all attributable to the underlying hemolytic event. In the majority of cases the onset of the hemolytic crisis occurs 5 to 24 hr following the consumption of the broad beans, while in rare instances it may be delayed for 2 to 3 days.[56,80] The course of the disease is essentially benign, the acute stage which usually lasts 1 to 2 days being followed by prompt recovery.

Epidemiological Aspects of Favism

Epidemiological studies revealed a number of characteristic and rather puzzling features of the disease.

Favism shows a striking prevalence in the islands and coastal regions of the Mediterranean Sea and in the Middle East (Rhodes, Sardinia, Sicily, Cyprus, Balearic Islands, Southern Italy, Greece, Turkey, Lebanon, Israel, Spain, Algeria, Egypt, Sudan, and Iraq).[2,5,55,56,80] This selective geographic distribution is of particular significance in view of the fact that fava beans are being grown and consumed almost all over the world as a cheap staple food, distinguished by its relatively high content (in percentage of dry weight) of carbohydrates (58%) and proteins (25 to 33%) with a biological value close to that of soybean proteins (50 and 62%, respectively).[53,129]

The seasonal incidence, as reported in various areas, seems to coincide with the period of harvesting of the fava beans.[42]

Genetic and Biochemical Aspects of Favism: Role of Glucose-6-Phosphate Dehydrogenase Deficiency

The early concepts on the infectious,[80] toxic,[49] or immunological[27,37,62,84,90,99] origin of favism appear today completely obsolete, as they fail to account for some of the most characteristic features of the disease, i.e., its selective geographic and ethnic distribution and its striking familial tendency.

A major clue for the understanding of the pathogenesis of favism was provided by the discovery of an inborn error of metabolism as the underlying cause of "drug sensitivity", i.e., a tendency of certain individuals to develop acute hemolysis in response to administration of primaquine and a large variety of other drugs. Beutler et al.[11,12] observed that the red blood cells of the drug-sensitive subjects exhibited a relatively low content of reduced glutathione (GSH), as well as an accelerated rate of GSH oxidation to glutathione disulfide (GSSG) on incubation with 1-acetyl-2-phenylhydrazine in the presence of glucose.[7,13] Carson et al.[29] revealed that this "GSH instability" of the susceptible red blood cells was attributable to a deficiency of the NADP-linked glucose-6-phosphate dehydrogenase (G6PD) and the resultant inability of these cells to maintain an adequate supply of NADPH required for the continuous reduction of GSSG through the action of GSSG reductase.

Prompted by these discoveries, Sansone and Segni[115-118] in Italy and Szeinberg and his collaborators[124-127] in Israel independently observed that the GSH level in red blood cells from persons with a past history of favism tended to be significantly below the average range of normal values. Furthermore, the red-cell GSH content exhibited a sharp decline during the acute phase of favism.[70,124] Moreover, the GSH in erythrocytes from persons with a history of favism proved to be unstable in Beutler's acetylphenylhydrazine test and this property was invariably associated with a pronounced G6PD-deficiency of the red blood cells.[70,116,118,126,127,142]

G6PD-deficiency is of wide-spread occurrence in humans, affecting about 100 million people of all races throughout the world.[28] The incidence of this genetic defect, however, is widely dissimilar in different ethnic groups, with the highest figures of frequency observed, in decreasing order, in some of the oriental Jewish communities of Israel, Sardinians, Cypriot Greeks, American Negroes, and certain African tribes. On the other hand, the deficient trait is virutally absent in Northern European populations, Jews of European descent (Ashkenazic Jews), North American Indians, and Eskimos.[89]

The incidence of favism does not parallel the occurrence of G6PD-deficiency in the different ethnic groups, most conspicuous in this respect being the complete absence of favism in North American Negroes.[9]

G6PD-deficiency is a sex-linked trait, i.e., it is transmitted by a gene located in the X chromosome.[32,71,128] Accordingly, the enzyme deficiency is fully expressed in the hemizygous ($\overline{X}Y$) male, since the mutant gene ($\overline{X}$) is not counterbalanced by the normal allelic X gene. In contrast, full expression of G6PD-deficiency is rare in females, as it depends on a homozygous mutant genotype ($\overline{X}\overline{X}$) with a statistically low probability of occurrence. In the majority of afflicted females, the G6PD-deficiency is therefore of partial or intermediate nature.[71] The rarity of the homozygous constellation of the deficient gene ($\overline{X}\overline{X}$) seems to account also for the striking preponderance of favism in the male sex.[5,56]

Enzymological studies revealed that the normal G6PD enzyme exists in several oligomeric forms (consisting of 2,4, or 6 identical subunits), the catalytically active species being predominantly the dimeric form. The latter species is stabilized by the tight association of the enzyme molecule with NADP or NADPH, while in the absence of the coenzymes, the apoenzyme tends to dissociate into the inactive monomeric subunits.[137-140] By applying starch gel electrophoresis to normal red-cell hemolysates, two major molecular variants of G6PD were differentiated as a fast migrating band A and a slow band B.[24] The more common type B form is found both in Caucasian subjects and in North American Negroes, whereas type A occurs in Negroes only.[24,63] Subsequently, about 80 additional molecular and genetic variants were identified by a combination of various enzymological criteria, such as electrophoretic mobility, Km values, and other kinetic constants.[9,64,141]

About 40 variants exhibit a severely reduced G6PD activity of the red blood cells associated with a tendency to develop hemolytic anemia when challenged with certain drugs or fava beans.[9,139]

While G6PD-deficiency has been unequivocally shown to be an essential prerequisite for the individual susceptibility to favism, some epidemiological features of this disease cannot be accounted for solely by the enzyme deficiency.

The relatively low incidence of favism in G6PD-deficient individuals, its total absence in American Negroes, the bizarre and rather unpredictable mode of its occurrence which shows no correlation with the severity of the enzyme deficiency, and the frequency of exposure to fava beans, suggest that some additional factor(s) may be operative in determining the hemolytic response to the noxious agent present in the fava beans. In fact, a study conducted by Stamatoyannopoulos et al.[122] seems to bear out the conclusion that some genetically determined "extracorpuscular factor" is instrumental in rendering G6PD-deficient subjects susceptible to favism. While the biochemical function of this hypothetical genetic determinant remains as yet to be defined, it appears reasonable to surmise that the extracorpuscular factor may act by governing the absorption, enzymic release, detoxication, or excretion of the causative agent of favism present in the broad beans.

STUDIES ON THE CAUSATIVE AGENT OF FAVISM IN THE BROAD BEANS

Studies In Vivo

Attempts to identify the toxic principle in the fava beans capable of affecting selectively G6PD-deficient individuals are greatly hampered by the lack of a suitable experimental animal (see Hutton, 1971).[59] Some investigators tried to overcome this difficulty by applying the procedure of Dern et al.,[41] which consists of transfusing ^{51}Cr-tagged G6PD-deficient red blood cells into normal compatible recipients and following their survival after administration of fava beans or fava bean extracts.

Using this experimental stratagem, Panizon and Vullo[95] were able to demonstrate a definite shortening of the life span of the transfused G6PD-deficient erythrocytes, following administration of fresh fava beans or juice prepared from them to normal recipients. However, the hemolytic effect of the broad beans was much more pronounced when susceptible individuals in the early stage of recovery from a favic crisis, rather than normal volunteers, were used as recipients. The latter results seemed, therefore, to support the previously referred to conclusion regarding the adjuvant role of an intrinsic factor other than G6PD-deficiency in the pathogenesis of favism. It should be mentioned, however, that other investigators[39,51] failed to obtain any significant effect on the survival of transfused G6PD-deficient erythrocytes, when healthy recipients were challenged with a dose of fava beans.

Studies In Vitro

Experiments designed to demonstrate the presence in the fava beans of a noxious agent with a specific action on G6PD-deficient erythrocytes have thus far been only partially successful.

Thus, Mela and Perona[86] observed a decline of GSH in G6PD-deficient red blood cells following their incubation with a broad bean extract obtained by crushing the seeds with a hydraulic press. Walker and Bowman[130] reported that aqueous extracts of fava beans induced a rapid fall of the GSH level in G6PD-deficient red blood cells, but had no significant effect on normal erythrocytes. The activity of the extracts was abolished by boiling for 90 min. Extracts prepared from peas or other leguminous seeds were without effect.[23] Panizon and Zacchello[96] found that homogenates or juice prepared from fresh fava beans produced a decrease of GSH in vitro and a shortening of the survival of ^{51}-Cr-labeled G6PD-deficient erythrocytes transfused into healthy recipients, but failed to affect normal red blood cells. Panizon[94] also isolated from fava beans a material soluble in lipid solvents which induced a marked oxidation of GSH both in red blood cells and in pure solution. More recently, Bottini and his co-workers[21,22] described the separation of crude fava bean extracts into two fractions, both capable of oxidizing GSH in pure solution and in G6PD-deficient erythrocytes. However, the criteria of separation employed by these authors are of questionable validity.

Fractionation of Fava Bean Extracts

In our laboratory, the search for the toxic agent in broad beans was guided by its presumed selective capacity for oxidizing GSH in G6PD-deficient, but not in normal erythrocytes, when incubated in the presence of glucose. Using aqueous extracts of broad beans as starting material, fractions conforming to this criterion could be isolated by ion exchange chromatography. Some of these fractions were sparingly soluble in water and in neutral solution exhibited a rapid loss of their GSH-oxidizing property concomitant with a profound change in their ultraviolet (UV) spectra. The structural instability of the purified material appeared to be inherent in its tendency to undergo rapid autooxidation on exposure to air, since the decomposition could be prevented by storage under nitrogen.[16] The spectral characteristics and other properties of these substances resembled those described in the literature for some pyrimidine derivatives occurring in fava beans as the aglycone moieties of β-glycosides termed vicine *(1)* and convicine *(2)*. Our subsequent efforts, therefore, concentrated primarily on exploring the possible causative role of these aglycones in producing favism.

Chemical Structure and Properties of Vicine, Convicine and Their Respective Aglycones

Vicine was discovered by Ritthausen and Kreusler[112] in vetch seeds *(Vicia sativa)* using an isolation procedure which involved extraction with dilute H_2SO_4 or 80% ethanol and precipitation with $HgSO_4$; following removal of Hg^{2+} with H_2S and crystallization from dilute ethanol the yield of the pure material was about 0.35%.[107] Vicine was subsequently found to occur also in other species of *Vicia* including *Vicia faba*.[107,136] The glycosidic characteristics of the compound were recognized already by Ritthausen,[109] who also described the isolation of the aglycone and determined its empirical formula.[109,111]

The pyrimidine nature of the aglycone moiety was revealed by Johnson.[61] However, the different structures assigned to vicine by Johnson[61] and Levene[73] were disproved by Bendich and Clements,[6] who finally established the correct formula of vicine as 2,6 diamino-4,5-dihydroxypyrimidine 5-(β-D-glucopyranoside). *(1)*.

Convicine too was discovered by Ritthausen[108] in the seeds of *Vicia faba* and *Vicia sativa*. It was characterized by Johnson[61] as a monoglucoside of 6-iminodialuric acid (isouramil), while the 5-position of the glycosidic bond was suggested by Bendich and Clements.[6] The formulation of convicine as 2,4,5-trihydroxy-6-aminopyrimidine 5-(β-D-glucopyranoside) *(2)* was unambiguously established by Bien et al.[14]

The aglycones, divicine *(3)* and isouramil *(4)*, can be obtained from the corresponding glycosides (vicine and convicine) by mild acid hydrolysis or by enzymic splitting with β-glucosidase.[57,82]

Divicine and isouramil, as well as the corresponding glycosides, react with the Folin-Ciocalteu phenol reagent yielding a blue color similar to that elicited by tyrosine and tryptophan. This reaction has been employed by Higazi and Read[58] for developing a quantitative assay of vicine in plant material and blood. In our hands, however, the method failed to bear out the authors' claim for specificity and, therefore, did not lend itself to direct determination of the pyrimidine glycosides in natural materials.[143] Both divicine and isouramil reduce vigorously alkaline solutions of 2,6-dichlorophenolindophenol (Tillman's reagent), phosphomolybdate, or phosphotungstate. They also elicit an intense blue color reaction with ammoniacal ferric chloridine solution, indicative of the presence of an enolic hydroxyl group[6] (Table 1).

Neutral solutions of isouramil and divicine when tested under nitrogen exhibit single absorption peaks at 280 and 285 nm, respectively. Following exposure of the solutions to oxygen, these peaks show a rapid decline with concomitant appearance of new absorption bands at 255 nm (isouramil) and 245 nm (divicine). This hypsochromic shift, which is readily reversible by addition of reducing agents, such as sodium borohydride, cysteine, or dithiothreitol, is attributable to formation of the oxidized species of the respective pyrimidine molecules.[105] However, more prolonged exposure to oxygen results in total obliteration of the characteristic peaks with attendant increase of end absorption (Figure 1). The latter change, which is no longer reversible by reduction, is suggestive of the rupture of the pyrimidine ring structure. It is interesting to note that closely similar spectral transitions are observed when dialuric acid *(5)* is oxidized to alloxan *(6)*. Based on this analogy, the above interrelationships can be represented as follows:

R	COMPOUND
−OH	ISOURAMIL
−NH$_2$	DIVICINE

The rate of the oxidative breakdown of the aglycones, as measured by following the spectral changes, is strongly pH-dependent,[6] exhibiting a sigmoidal curve with inflection points at pH 7.7 and 7.3 for isouramil and divicine, respectively.[31] The halflives

Table 1
CHARACTERISTIC COLOR TESTS OF FAVA BEAN PYRIMIDINES AND THEIR CONGENERS; STRUCTURE-ACTIVITY CORRELATIONS[6,40]

Compound No.	Positions of the pyrimidine ring[a] substituents				Tests[b]		
	2	4	5	6	A	B	C
1	H	OH	OH	OH	+	+	+
2	OH	OH	OH	OH	+	+	+
3	OH	OH	OH	NH$_2$	+	+	+
4	NH$_2$	OH	OH	NH$_2$	+	+	+
5	NH$_2$	OH	OH	OH	+	+	+
6	NH$_2$	H	OH	OH	+	+	+
7	OH	OH	NH$_2$	NH$_2$	+	+	—
8	NH$_2$	OH	NH$_2$	OH	+	+	—
9	OH	OH	OH	H	+	—	+
10	CH$_3$	H	OH	OH	+	—	+
11	OH	H	OH	H	—	—	+
12	H	OH	H	OH	—	—	—

[a] Numbering system according to IUPAC (see Formula 1).
[b] Tests:
  A. Phosphomolybdic acid. One drop of 10 N NaOH added, followed by a few drops of 2% phosphomolybdic acid; + denotes formation of a deep-blue color.
  B. 2,6-Dichlorophenolindophenol. One drop of 10 N NaOH added, followed by a few drops of 0.1% 2,6-dichlorophenolindophenol; + denotes rapid bleaching of the dye.
  C. Ferric chloride. One drop of 1% FeCl$_3$ added, followed by a few drops of concentrated ammonia; + denotes formation of a deep-blue or violet-blue color.

Information compiled from References 6 and 40.

of divicine and isouramil in neutral solution and at room temperature are about 10 and 15 min, respectively. From the temperature dependence of the rate constants of the breakdown of isouramil, an activation energy of about 14 kcal/mol was calculated.[31] The oxidative decomposition of the two aglycones is markedly enhanced in the presence of traces of transition metal ions (Cu^{2+}, Fe^{3+}).

Bendich and Clements[6] pointed out in their comprehensive study that some of the salient features of divicine and its congeners, viz., their powerful reducing activity, spectral characteristics, and molecular instability show a striking resemblance to those of triose reductone (7), reductic acid (8), and ascorbic acid (9). Furthermore, these authors inferred from a comparison of different substitutions that the common structural denominator underlying these properties is a carbonyl-conjugated enediol (A) or aminoenol (B) system (see Tables 1 and 2).

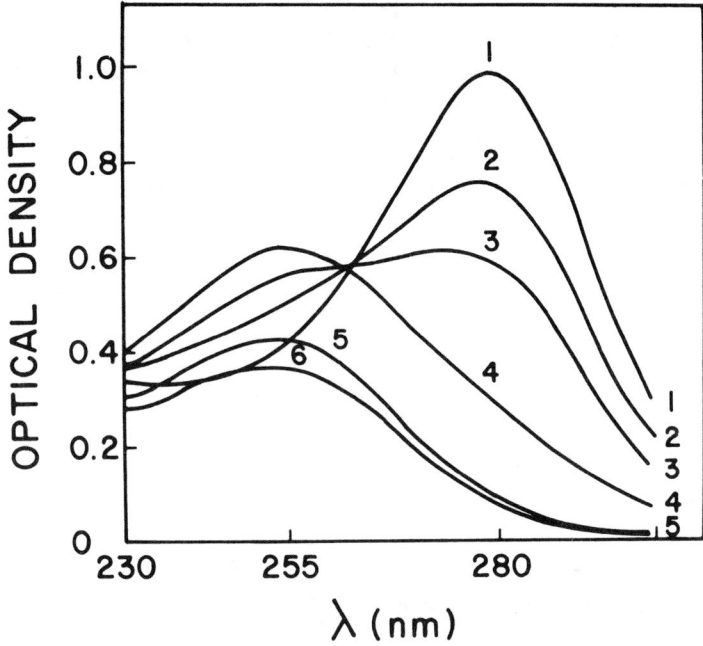

FIGURE 1. Ultraviolet absorption spectra of an isouramil solution incubated under nitrogen or in air. A 0.07 mM solution of isouramil in 0.05 M phosphate buffer (pH 7) was incubated at room temperature under nitrogen or in air. Curve 1, under nitrogen (no change throughout a 60 min period); curves 2, in air for 1, 2, 5, 25, and 30 min, respectively.

It may be mentioned in this connection that these structural arrangements serve to characterize a broad class of compounds designated by the general name of reductones.[120]

Consequently, all the characteristic properties of the pyrimidine aglycones concerned are abolished by substitution of the highly reactive hydroxyl group at C-5, such as that represented by the glycosidic linkage in vicine and convicine. Thus, unlike the free aglycones, the glycosides show no reducing ability, do not undergo oxidation in the presence of oxygen, resist boiling in aqueous solution, and their UV spectra differ significantly from those of their constituent pyrimidines[6,14,31] (see Table 2).

Of particular relevance to the problem of favism appears to be the ability of the pyrimidine aglycones to oxidize reduced GSH as well as a variety of other thiol compounds, such as cysteine or cysteamine (β-mercaptoethylamine). The oxidation of GSH by the pyrimidines proceeds to completion even at a 40-fold or higher molar excess of GSH; it is markedly enhanced by shaking in air and completely suppressed in an atmosphere of nitrogen.[105] The oxygen dependence as well as the nonstoichiometric nature of this phenomenon suggest that the reaction between the pyrimidine and GSH is mediated by a catalytic oxidoreduction mechanism similar to that observed by Borsook et al.[20] with the GSH-ascorbic acid system. This mechanism, involving a cyclic sequence of oxidation of the pyrimidine (isouramil, divicine, or dialuric acid) by the atmospheric oxygen and its renewed reduction by GSH, can be represented as follows:

$$\text{Pyrimidine (red)}^* + O_2 \longrightarrow \text{Pyrimidine (ox)}^{**} + H_2O_2$$
$$\text{Pyrmidine (ox)} + 2\text{GSH} \longrightarrow \text{Pyrimidine (red)} + \text{GSSG}$$

* Reduced form.
** Oxidized form.

Table 2
UV ABSORPTION SPECTRA OF THE FAVA BEAN GLYCOSIDES, THEIR AGLYCONES AND RELATED PYRIMIDINES

Compound	Oxidation state	pH	λ^{max}(nm), [ε(M^{-1} cm^{-1})]	Ref.
Vicine		1	274,[16,400]	6
		6.8	275,[13,200]; 236,[4,400]	6
		13	269,[9,500]; 235,[5,200]	6
Convicine		1	271,[17,400]; 220,[6,000]	14
		7	271,[14,450]	14
		13	273,[14,450]	14
Divicine	Reduced	1	281,[12,900]	40
	Reduced	1	281,[15,850]	30
	Reduced	7	285,[11,280]	31
	Oxidized	7	245	31
Isouramil	Reduced	1	280,[13,600]	40
	Reduced	7	280,[14,400]	31
	Oxidized	7	255	31
Dialuric Acid	Reduced	1% HCl	270,[3,200]	72,98
	Reduced	10% H$_2$SO$_4$	270,[2,900]	98
	Reduced	6.8	275,[16,500]	40
	Reduced	7.4	275,[16,600]	72,98
Alloxan	Oxidized	7.4	245,[4,800]	72,98
	Oxidized	7.8	245,[4,800]	98

A more quantitative study[31] revealed that the oxidation of the pyrimidines takes place with formation of stoichiometric amounts of H_2O_2. Thus, in addition to the direct oxidation of two molecules of GSH by the oxidized form of the pyrimidine, the concomitantly generated H_2O_2 can serve to oxidize another pair of GSH molecules.

Divicine and isouramil, apart from their oxidant effect on thiol compounds, are also capable of forming with GSH additional products with characteristic absorption at 305 nm,[74,105] similar to that produced by the structurally related pyrimidine, alloxan, with GSH.[98] This reaction appears to be specific with respect to GSH, since it does not occur with other sulfhydryl derivatives, such as cysteine or cysteamine, nor can GSSG substitute for GSH. When the pyrimidines are allowed to interact with GSH in air, the appearance of the 305 nm peak exhibits a time lag which coincides with the incipient accumulation of the oxidized form, as indicated by the concurrent hypsochromic shift (vide supra). On the other hand, the formation of the 305-nm absorbing material fails to take place in the absence of oxygen (under nitrogen) and can be completely suppressed or reversed by addition of reducing substances, such as cysteine, dithiothreitol, or borohydride. These data, therefore, seem to concur in favoring the conclusion that the oxidized form of the pyrimidine is the reactive molecular species which takes part in the adduct formation with GSH.[31,105]

Chemical Synthesis of Isouramil, Divicine, and Convicine

The synthesis of isouramil was first accomplished by Davidson and Bogert.[38] These authors used as starting material isobarbituric acid (10) which was either subjected to nitrosation or coupled with p-chlorophenyl diazonium salt and the reaction products (11) and (12) were reduced with (NH$_4$)$_2$S to yield isouramil (4). This synthesis was subsequently modified by McOmie and Chesterfield,[85] who replaced ammonium sulfide with sodium dithionite as the reducing agent and thereby greatly increased the yield, as well as the purity of the final product. This synthetic route was further facilitated by the relatively simple synthesis of isobarbituric acid from 5-bromouracil devised by Wang[134,135] (Scheme 2).

An elegant, though rather tedious synthetic approach was adopted by Davoll and Laney.[40] In this method, ethyl tetrahydropyran-2-yloxycyanoacetate *(13)* was condensed with urea in the presence of sodium ethoxide and the product, tetrahydropyranyl ether of isouramil (6-amino-2,4-dihydroxy-5-tetrahydropyran-2′-yloxypyrimidine) *(14)*, was converted to isouramil by acid hydrolysis (Scheme 3).

An essentially similar method in which urea was replaced by guanidine afforded divicine.[40]

More recently, Bien et al.[15] succeeded in preparing convicine by a procedure consisting of condensation of 6-acetamido-5-hydroxyuracil with tetra-*O*-acetyl-β-D-glucopyranosyl bormide and hydrolytic deacetylation of the resultant convicine pentaacetate derivative to the free glycoside.

PATHOGENESIS OF FAVISM

Biochemical Alterations Induced by Isouramil and Divicine in Red Blood Cells and Their Possible Role in the Pathogenesis of Favism

Red blood cells incubated in the presence of 0.2 to 1 m*M* amounts of isouramil for divicine (to be referred to as aglycones) exhibit a rapid decline of their GSH level, followed by a slower decrease of their ATP content.[82] Addition of glucose to the incubation medium obviates the noxious effect of the aglycones on normal erythrocytes, but fails to protect the G6PD-deficient cells. Convicine and vicine, in which the autooxidizable hydroxyl group at C-5 of the pyrimidine moiety is blocked by the β-glycosidic bond, proved to be inert.

The oxidant effect of the aglycones on the red-cell GSH is on a molar basis, about one order of magnitude higher than that of acetylphenylhydrazine (APH), a compound employed by Beutler[7] for determining "glutathione stability" as a measure of the drug sensitivity of red blood cells. Furthermore, the aglycones are capable of oxidizing GSH in pure solution (see section on the chemical structure of vicine and convicine), thus differing essentially from APH and primaquine which require the presence of hemoglobin for mediating GSH oxidation.

As pointed out previously, the catalytic nature of the oxidant action of the aglycones on GSH is reminiscent of the mechanism involved in the GSH-ascorbic acid oxidoreduction system described by Borsook et al.[20] This analogy is further borne out by the observation that sodium ascorbate at relatively high concentrations (10 m*M*) is capable of producing a marked decrease in the GSH level in G6PD-deficient erythrocytes.[102,131]

Moreover, combined addition of small amounts of isouramil and ascorbic acid results in a pronounced synergistic potentiation of their oxidizing effect on GSH.[105]

In a more recent study,[50] rabbit erythrocytes labeled in vitro with ^{51}Cr were incubated at 37°C with isouramil in the absence of glucose. The cells were then reinfused into the donor rabbit and their halflife was determined. It was found that incubation of the erythrocytes with 2 mM isouramil for 75 min resulted in a shortening of their ^{51}Cr-halflife to less than 5% of the average normal value (9 hr and 9 days, respectively). Lower concentrations of isouramil or shorter exposure times impaired the red-cell survival to a correspondingly lesser extent. In addition, here again, isouramil and ascorbic acid exhibited a synergistic type of interaction in reducing the life span of the red blood cells.

Lin and Ling,[75-77] who have been first in suggesting a possible relation of vicine to favism, described a transient hemoglobinuria occurring in puppies 3 hr after oral administration of vicine (0.2 g/kg body weight). These authors also reported some minor inhibitory effects of vicine on the catalytic rates of glucose-6-phosphate and 6-phosphogluconate-dehydrogenases in red-cell hemolysates.[77] However, the relevance of these phenomena to the pathogenesis of favism is rather questionable.

In conclusion, the potent GSH-oxidizing capacity of the aglycones of vicine and convicine, as well as their deleterious effect on red-cell survival, are strongly suggestive of a causative role of these substances in the induction of favism. The free aglycones may arise from the parent glycosides through the hydrolytic action of β-glucosidase either in the fava beans or, more likely, in the digestive tract.

It is conceivable that individual differences in the ability of the intestinal mucosa to absorb the glycosides and/or to release the aglycones by splitting of the β-glycosidic bond, as well as possible variations in the pyrimidine glycoside content of different crops of fava beans, may account for the "capricious" and rather unpredictable mode of occurrence of favic crises in susceptible individuals, irrespective of the frequency of their exposure to the noxious agent (see Luisada).[80] It may be pertinent to mention in this context that *Vicia faba* L. is distinguished by its remarkable intraspecific variability. The species comprises 3 well-defined toxonomic groups, *major, equina,* and *minor* which differ from each other by the shape and size of their pods and seeds. These subspecies are further differentiated into a large number (over 150) of distinct varieties and land races.[54,69]

Does 3,4-Dihydroxyphenylalanine Play a Role in the Etiology of Favism?

Kosower and Kosower[65] argue that 3,4-L-dihydroxyphenylalanine (dopa) may be one of the toxic principles in the fava beans capable of inducing a hemolysis in G6PD-deficient subjects. This substance is present in broad beans in appreciable amounts (0.25% of the fava pods),[52] mainly in the free state and partly in the form of the β-glycoside of dopa.[3,101] The above authors observed that G6PD-deficient red blood cells incubated for 3 hr in the presence of glucose and millimolar amounts of dopa exhibited a significant loss of GSH. However, a reexamination of their data reveals that the rather inconspicuous dopa-induced oxidation of GSH was of noncatalytic nature. Futhermore, our own experiments showed that dopa at a concentration as high as 10 mM failed to affect the GSH level in normal human erythrocytes incubated for 3 hr in the absence of glucose, while under the same conditions 1 mM isouramil caused almost complete disappearance of the intracellular GSH.

On the other hand, joint addition of subminimal amounts of isouramil and dopa resulted in a striking supra-additive enhancement of GSH oxidation.[105] Similar synergistic effects of dopa and isouramil on GSH oxidation were obtained with glucose-deprived rabbit erythrocytes. However, dopa failed to influence the effect of isouramil on the survival of ^{51}Cr-tagged erythrocytes, treated in vitro and then reinfused into the donor rabbit.[50]

The hypothesis of Kosower and Kosower[65] was modified by Beutler,[8] who suggested that dopaquinone arising in vivo by oxidation of dopa, rather than dopa itself, might be the causative agent of favism. However, the claim for an etiological role of dopa in favism seems to be refuted by the outcome of a direct experiment in vivo which showed that the survival of ^{51}Cr-labeled G6PD-deficient erythrocytes transfused into a normal volunteer was not affected by repeated intravenous (i.v.) injections of dopa into the recipient.[48] In addition, as indicated by Beutler,[8] since L-dopa is being used in large doses for treating Parkinson's disease, G6PD-deficient Parkinsonian patients in favism-prone areas would be at risk of developing hemolysis in the course of the prolonged therapy. To our knowledge, however, not a single case report has been forthcoming in the medical literature to bear out this expectation.

The Biochemical Lesion Underlying the Hemolytic Effect of the Fava Bean Pyrimidine Aglycones

The fava bean pyrimidine aglycones share with acetylphenylhydrazine and the other noxious drugs the ability to bring about irreversible oxidation of GSH in G6PD-deficient erythrocytes. In normal erythrocytes, the oxidant effect of these substances is offset by the powerful capacity of these cells for GSH regeneration mediated by the NADPH-linked GSSG reductase. The activity of the latter system is critically dependent upon the normal functioning of G6PD, as part of the oxidative pentose phosphate cycle which constitutes the only route available in red blood cells for NADPH supply. In G6PD-deficient erythrocytes, the residual activity of this enzyme is barely sufficient to maintain an adequate level of GSH under physiological conditions, but unable to cope with the inordinate demand for NADPH created by the oxidative stress.

The loss of GSH appears to be the primary metabolic disturbance leading to the ultimate destruction of the G6PD-deficient erythrocyte, both in favism and in drug-induced hemolysis. The validity of this concept, implying a crucial role of GSH in preserving the functional and structural integrity of the red blood cells, is attested to by the finding that red blood cells affected with an inborn defect in the biosynthesis of GSH are susceptible to drug-induced hemolysis and favism, much like G6PD-deficient erythrocytes.[17,87,93,103,132] Likewise, the genetically determined GSSG reductase deficiency of the red blood cells manifests itself by drug sensitivity.[79,133]

The oxidant action of the aglycones on the G6PD-deficient red blood cells resembles that of acetylphenylhydrazine or primaquine in inducing the formation of methemoglobin with concomitant appearance of basophilic inclusions, called Heinz-Ehrlich bodies. These inclusion bodies, usually adhering to the cell membrane, appear to be aggregates of denatured hemoglobin, resulting from oxidation of its sulfhydryl groups with attendant formation of mixed glutathione disulfides and loss of the heme groups.[1,11,26,60,104]

It has been suggested that the membrane-attached Heinz bodies and possibly some other less drastic biochemical alterations of the red-cell surface are instrumental in rendering the cells liable to sequestration and thereby vulnerable to destruction by the reticuloendothelial system.[9,106] Such a mechanism may account for the hemolytic action of the offensive drugs on sensitive red blood cells in vivo, contrasting with their failure to induce appreciable red-cell lysis in vitro.[10,82,97]

Cohen and Hochstein[4-36] concluded from their experiments that the noxious drugs interact with oxyhemoglobin, producing methemoglobin and hydrogen peroxide. The relatively small, but nevertheless harmful, amounts of H_2O_2 cannot be efficiently destroyed by catalase and are normally disposed of through the action of GSH peroxidase which catalyzes the oxidation of GSH by H_2O_2 with formation of GSSG and water. The resultant GSSG is promptly reduced by GSSG reductase, thus ensuring continuous regeneration of GSH. Consequently, the overall pathway comprising the oxidative pentose phosphate shunt, GSSG reductase and GSH peroxidase, serves to eliminate the metabolically produced hydrogen peroxide, so as to forestall its injurious effects on hemoglobin and the red cell membrane (see also Cohen[33] and Flohé and Brand[44]).

The notion that GSH peroxidase plays a vital role in preventing the hemolytic action of the peroxide-forming drugs has gained further support from the discovery of a hereditary deficiency of this enzyme as the underlying cause of certain cases of spontaneous or drug-induced hemolysis.[18,19,91,92,123] Furthermore, the recent elucidation of the role of selenium as an essential component of the GSH peroxidase molecule[46,114] has led to the understanding of the biochemical mechanism inherent in the protective effect of dietary selenium against the hydrogen peroxide-induced hemolysis.[113]

The above interrelationships can be summarized as follows (Scheme 4):

1. Isouramil (Divicine) (red)* $\xrightarrow{O_2}$ Isouramil (Divicine) (ox)** + H_2O_2

2. Isouramil (Divicine) (ox) + 2GSH $\longrightarrow$ Isouramil (Divicine) (red) + GSSG

3. 2GSH + H_2O_2 $\xrightarrow{\text{peroxidase}}$ GSSG + $2H_2O$

4. 2GSSG + 2NADPH + $2H^+$ $\xrightarrow{\text{reductase}}$ 4GSH + $2NADP^+$

5. Glucose-6-phosphate + $NADP^+$ $\xrightarrow{\text{dehydrogenase}}$ 6-Phosphogluconic acid + NADPH + H^+

6. 6-Phosphogluconic acid + $NADP^+$ $\xrightarrow{\text{dehydrogenase}}$ Ribulose-5-phosphate + CO_2 + NADPH + H^+

* — Reduced form.
** — Oxidized form.

Some authors indicated that in the course of the oxidative metabolism of the noxious drugs or divicine, free radicals are produced, the latter interacting either with GSH and protein sulfhydryl groups to form GSSG and protein disulfides,[66,68] or with the unsaturated fatty acids of the cell membrane to bring about lipid peroxidation.[45]

In other studies, a derangement of the energy metabolism was observed and its possible role in the shortening of red-cell survival was explored. Several investigators reported that incubation of erythrocytes in the presence of primaquine, phenylhydrazine, or acetylphenylhydrazine causes a marked inhibition of the red-cell glycolysis[67,78] and a progressive decline of the intracellular ATP level.[78,81,88] Similar effects were noted when red blood cells were incubated with isouramil or divicine.[82] Addition of glucose prevented the deleterious action of the drugs on the energy-yielding metabolism in normal but not in G6PD-deficient erythrocytes. The primary site of the inhibitory effect was located at the stage of hexokinase[67] and was shown to be attributable to GSSG formation,[81] thus representing a particular case of the so called "disulfide poisoning", previously described by Eldjarn and Bremer.[43]

While the role of impaired glycolysis and ATP depletion in reducing the red-cell life span is well established,[25,47,100,121] its actual significance in the mechanism of the acute hemolytic syndrome remains as yet to be evaluated.

In concluding this chapter, it appears appropriate to emphasize once again that further study will be needed to provide unequivocal evidence for the as yet presumptive causative role of the fava bean aglycones in the induction of favism. Considerable effort may be also required to fill in the gaps in our current understanding of the pathogenesis of favism and to elucidate the still elusive nature of the factors governing the puzzling epidemiological features of this disease.

ACKNOWLEDGMENTS

Part of the original work of the authors referred to in the text and the preparation of the manuscript of this review were supported by a grant (No. P15/181/16) from the World Health Organization and an award from the Chief Scientist's Office of the Ministry of Health, Israel.

Prof. J. Mager, whose vision and encouragement have extensively contributed to the development of the scientific knowledge and biochemical understanding in this field, died on May 3, 1980, after the completion of this manuscript.

The excellent and devoted secretarial help of Miss Malca Gelb is hereby gratefully acknowledged.

REFERENCES

1. Allen, D. W. and Jandl, J. H., Oxidative hemolysis and precipitation of hemoglobin. II. Role of thiols in oxidant drug action, *J. Clin. Invest.*, 40, 454, 1961.
2. Amin-Zaki, L., El-Din, S., and Kubba, K., Glucose-6-phosphate dehydrogenase deficiency among ethnic groups in Iraq, *Bull WHO*, 47, 1, 1972.
3. Andrews, R. S. and Pridham, J. R., Structure of a Dopa glucoside from *Vicia faba, Nature (London)*, 205, 1213, 1965.
4. Aurichio, L., Sul facismo, *Rass. Clin. Sci. 1st. Biochim. Ital.*, 13, 20, 1935.
5. Belsey, M. A., The epidemiology of favism, *Bull. WHO*, 48, 1, 1973.
6. Bendich, A. and Clements, G. C., A revision of the structural formulation of vicine and its pyrimidine aglycone, divicine, *Biochim. Biophys. Acta*, 12, 462, 1953.
7. Beutler, E., The glutathione instability of drug sensitive red cells, *J. Lab. Clin. Med.*, 49, 84, 1957.
8. Beutler, E., L-Dopa and favism, *Blood*, 36, 523, 1970.
9. Beutler, E., Abnormalities of the hexose monophosphate shunt, *Semin. Hematol.*, 8, 311, 1971.
10. Beutler, E., Glucose-6-phosphate dehydrogenase deficiency, in *The Metabolic Basis of Inherited Disease*, Stanbury, J. B., Wyngaarden, J. B., and Frederickson, D. B., Eds., McGraw-Hill, New York, 1972, 1358.
11. Beutler, E., Dern, R. J., and Alving, A. S., The hemolytic effect of primaquine. VI. An *in vitro* test for sensitivity of erythrocytes to primaquine, *J. Lab. Clin. Med.*, 45, 40, 1955.
12. Beutler, E., Dern, R. J., Flanagan, C. L., and Alving, A. S., The hemolytic effect of primaquine. VII. Biochemical studies of drug-sensitive erythrocytes, *J. Lab. Clin. Med.*, 45, 286, 1955.
13. Beutler, E., Robson, M., and Buttenwieser, E., The mechanism of glutathione destruction and protection in drug-sensitive and non-sensitive erythrocytes. *In vitro* studies, *J. Clin. Invest.*, 36, 617, 1957.
14. Bien, S., Salemnik, G., and Zamir, L., The structure of convicine, *J. Chem. Soc. C (London)*, p. 496, 1968.
15. Bien, S., Amith, D., and Ber, M., Synthesis of convicine (6-amino-5-β-glucopyranosyloxyuracil), *J. Chem. Soc. Perkin Trans.*, I, 1089, 1973.
16. Bien, S., Noam, M., Glaser, G., Razin, A., and Mager, J., unpublished results.
17. Boivin, P. and Galand, C., La synthese du glutathion au cours de l'anemie hemolytique congenitale avec deficit en glutathion reduit, *Nouv. Rev. Fr. Hematol.*, 5, 707, 1965.
18. Boivin, P., Roge, G., and Gueroult, N., Anemie hemolytique avec deficit en glutathion-peroxydase chez un adulte, *Enzymol. Biol. Clin. (Basel)*, 10, 68, 1969.
19. Boivin, P., Hakim, J., and Blery, M., Déficit en glutathion-peroxydase erythrocytaire et anemie hémolytique medicamenteus, *Presse Med.*, 78, 171, 1970.
20. Borsook, H., Davenport, H. W., Jeffreys, C. E. P., and Warner, R. C., The oxidation of ascorbic acid and its reduction *in vitro* and *in vivo*, *J. Biol. Chem.*, 117, 237, 1937.
21. Bottini, E., Favism. Current problems and investigations, *J. Med. Genet.*, 10, 154, 1973.
22. Bottini, E., Lucarelli, P., Spennati, G. F., Businov, L., and Palmarino, R., Presence in *Vicia faba* of different substances with activity *in vitro* on Gd(−) Med. red blood cell reduced glutathione, *Clin. Chim. Acta*, 30, 831, 1970.
23. Bowman, J. E. and Walker, D. G., Action of *Vicia faba* on erythrocytes: possible relationship to favism, *Nature (London)*, 189, 555, 1961.

24. Boyer, S. H., Porter, I. H., and Weilbacher, R. G., Electrophoretic heterogeneity of glucose 6-phosphate dehydrogenase and its relationship to enzyme deficiency in man, *Proc. Natl. Acad. Sci. U.S.A.*, 48, 1868, 1962.
25. Brewer, G. J., Powell, R. D., Swanson, S. H., and Alving, A. S., Hemolytic effect of primaquine. XVII. Hexokinase activity of glucose-6-phosphate dehydrogenase deficient and normal erythrocytes, *J. Lab. Clin. Med.*, 64, 601, 1964.
26. Bunn, H. F. and Jandl, J. H., Exchange of heme among hemoglobin molecules, *Proc. Nat. Acad. Sci. U.S.A.*, 56, 974, 1966.
27. Carcassi, U., Eritroenzimpoatie e anemie emolitiche, *Omnia Med. Pisa*, 1958.
28. Carson, P. E., Glucose-6-phosphate dehydrogenase deficiency in hemolytic anemia, *Fed. Proc. Fed. Am. Soc. Exp. Biol.*, 19, 995, 1960.
29. Carson, P. E., Flanagan, C. L., Ickes, C. E., and Alving, A. S., Enzymatic deficiency in primaquine-sensitive erythrocytes, *Science*, 124, 484, 1956.
30. Chesterfield, J. H., Hurst, D. T., McOmie, J. F. W., and Tute, M. S., Pyrimidines. XIII. Electrophilic substitution at position 6 and a synthesis of divicine (2,4-diamino-5,6-dihydroxy pyrimidine), *J. Chem. Soc.*, 1001, 1964.
31. Chevion, M., Navok, T., Glaser, G., and Mager, J., The chemistry of favism-inducing compounds: the properties of isouramil and divicine and their reaction with glutathione, *Eur. J. Biochem*, 1982, in press.
32. Childs, B., Zinkham, W., Browne, E. A., Kimbro, E. L, and Torbert, J. V., A genetic study of a defect in glutathione metabolism of the erythrocyte, *Bull. Johns Hopkins Hosp.*, 102, 21, 1958.
33. Cohen, G., On the generation of hydrogen peroxide in erythrocytes by acetylphenylhydrazine, *Biochem. Pharmacol.*, 15, 1775, 1966.
34. Cohen, G. and Hochstein, P., Glucose-6-phosphate dehydrogenase and detoxification of hydrogen peroxide in human erythrocytes, *Science*, 134, 1756, 1961.
35. Cohen, G. and Hochstein, P., Glutathione peroxidase: the primary agent for the elimination of hydrogen peroxide in erythrocytes, *Biochemistry*, 2, 1420, 1963.
36. Cohen, G. and Hochstein, P., Generation of hydrogen peroxide in erythrocytes by hemolytic agents, *Biochemistry*, 3, 895, 1964.
37. Dacie, J. V., *The Hemolytic anemias*, Churchill Livingstone, London, 1954, 354.
38. Davidson, D. and Bogert, M. T., Isovioluric Acid (Alloxan 6-Oxime), *Proc. Nat. Acad. Sci. U.S.A.*, 18, 490, 1932.
39. Davies, P., Favism: a family study, *Q. J. Med.*, 31, 157, 1962.
40. Davoll, J. and Laney, D. H., Synthesis of Divicine (2:4-Diamino-5:6 dihydroxypyrimidine) and other derivatives of 4:5 (5:6)-Dihydroxypyrimidine, *J. Chem. Soc. (London)*, p. 2124, 1956.
41. Dern, R. J., Weinstein, I. M., Leroy, G. V., Talmage, D. W., and Alving, A. S., The hemolytic effect of primaquine. I. The localization of the drug-induced hemolytic defect in primaquine sensitive individuals, *J. Lab. Clin. Med.*, 43, 303, 1954.
42. Donoso, G., Hedayat, H., and Khayatyan, H., Favism with special reference to Iran, *Bull. WHO*, 40, 513, 1969.
43. Eldjarn, L. and Bremer, J., The inhibitory effect at the hexokinase level of disulphides on glucose metabolism in human erythrocytes, *Biochem. J.*, 84, 286, 1962.
44. Flohé, L. and Brand, J., Kinetics of glutathione peroxidase, *Biochim. Biophys. Acta*, 191, 541, 1969.
45. Flohé, L., Niebch, G., and Reiber, H., Zur Wirkung von Divicin in menschlichen Erythrocyten, *Z. Klin. Chem. Klin. Biochem.*, 9, 431, 1971.
46. Flohé, L., Günzler, W. A., and Schocke, H. H., Glutathione peroxidase: a selenoenzyme, *FEBS Lett.*, 32, 132, 1973.
47. Gabrio, B.W., Stevens, A. R., Jr., and Finch, C. A., Erythrocyte preservation. III. The reversibility of the storage lesion, *J. Clin. Invest.*, 33, 252, 1954.
48. Gaetani, G., Salvidio, E., Panaciulli, I., Ajmar, F., and Paravidino, G., Absence of hemolytic effects of L-dopa on transfused G6PD-deficiency erythrocytes, *Experientia*, 26, 785, 1970.
49. Gasbarrini, A., II, Favismo, *Policlinico Sez. Prat.*, 22, 1505, 1915.
50. Glaser, G., Weissberg, J., Chevion, M., and Mager, J., To be published.
51. Greenberg, M. S. and Wong, H., The influence of fava beans and primaquine on GSH-unstable red blood cells, *in vivo, J. Lab. Clin. Med.*, 57, 733, 1961.
52. Guggenheim, M., Dioxyphenylalanine, eine neue Amónosaüre aus *Vicia faba, Z. Phys. Chem.*, 88, 276, 1913.
53. Hagberg, A. and Sjödin, J., Broad bean, in *International Biological Programme 4: Food Protein Sources*, Pirie, N. W., Ed., Cambridge University Press, London, 1975, 117.
54. Hanelt, P., Die intraspezifische Variabilitaet von Vicia faba L. und ihre Gliederung, *Kulturpflanze*, 20, 75, 1972.
55. Hassan, M. M., Glucose-6-phosphate dehydrogenase deficiency in the Sudan, *J. Trop. Med. Hyg.*, 74, 187, 1971.

56. Hedayat, Sh., Rahbar, S., Mahbooli, E., Ghaffarpour, M., and Sobhi, N., Favism in the Caspian littoral area of Iran, *Trop. Geogr. Med.*, 23, 149, 1971.
57. Hérissey, H. and Cheymol, J., Sur le Vicioside, *Bull. Soc. Chim. Biol.*, 13, 29, 1931.
58. Higazi, M. L. and Read, W. W. C., Method for determination of vicine in plant material and blood, *J. Agric. Food. Chem.*, 22, 570, 1974.
59. Hutton, J. H., Genetic regulation of glucose-6-phosphate dehydrogenase activity in the inbred mouse, *Biochem. Gen.*, 5, 315, 1971.
60. Jacob, H. S., Mechanisms of Heinz body formation and attachment to the red cell membrane, *Semin. Hematol.*, 7, 341, 1970.
61. Johnson, T. B., The origin of purines in plants, *J. Am. Chem. Soc.*, 36, 337, 1914.
62. Kantor, S. Z., Pinkhas, J., and Djaletti, M., Immunologic studies in a case of favism, *J. Allergy*, 33, 390, 1962.
63. Kirkman, H. N. and Hendrickson, E. M., Sex-linked electrophoretic difference in glucose-6-phosphate dehydrogenase, *Am. J. Human Genet.*, 15, 241, 1963.
64. Kirkman, H. N., McGurdy, P. R., and Naiman, I. L., Functionally abnormal glucose-6-phosphate dehydrogenase, *Cold Spring Harbor Symp. Quant. Biol.*, 29, 361, 1964.
65. Kosower, N. S. and Kosower, E. M., Does 3,4-dihydroxyphenylalanine play a part in favism? *Nature (London)*, 215, 286, 1967.
66. Kosower, N. S. and Kosower, E. M., The glutathione-glutathione disulfide system, in *Free Radicals in Biology*, Vol. 2, Pryor, W. A., Ed., Academic Press, New York, 1976, 5.
67. Kosower, N. S., Vanderhoff, G. A., and London, I. M., Hexokinase activity in normal and glucose-6-phosphate dehydrogenase deficient erythrocytes, *Nature (London)*, 201, 684, 1964.
68. Kosower, N. S., Song, K. R., and Kosower, E. M., Glutathione. III. Biological apsects of the azoester procedure for oxidation within the normal human erythrocyte, *Biochim. Biophys. Acta*, 192, 15, 1969.
69. Ladizinsky, G., Seed protein electrophoresis of the wild and cultivated species of section Faba of Vicia, *Euphytica*, 24, 785, 1975.
70. Larizza, P., Brunetti, P., Grignani, F., and Ventura, S., L'individualita bioenzymatica dell' eritrocito "fabico", *Hameatologica (Pavia)*, 43, 205, 1958.
71. Larizza, P., Brunetti, P., and Grignani, F., Anemie emolitiche enzymopenische *Haematologica (Pavia)*, 45, 1, 1960.
72. Lazarow, A., Patterson, T. W., and Levey, S. The mechanism of cysteine and glutathione protection against alloxan diabetes, *Science*, 108, 308, 1948.
73. Levene, P. A., On vicine, *J. Biol. Chem.*, 18, 305, 1914.
74. Lin, J. Y., Favism. IV. Reactions of vicine and divicine with sulfhydryl group of glutathione and cysteine, *J. Formosan Med. Assoc.*, 62, 777, 1963.
75. Lin, J. Y. and Ling, K. H., Favism. I. Isolation of an active principle from fava beans, *J. Formosan Med. Assoc.*, 61, 484, 1962; cited after *Chem. Abstr.*, 65, 4143, 1966.
76. Lin, J. Y. and Ling, K. H., Favism. II. The physiological activities of vicine *in vivo*, *J. Formosan Med. Assoc.*, 61, 490, 1962; cited after *Chem. Abstr.*, 65, 4144, 1966.
77. Lin, J. Y. and Ling, K. H,. Favism. III. The physiological activities of vicine, *in vitro*, *J. Formosan Med. Assoc.*, 61, 579, 1962.
78. Loehr, G. W. and Waller, H. D., Biochemie und Pathogenese der enzymopenischen haemolytischen Anaemien, *Dtsch. Med. Wochenschr.*, 86, 27, 1961.
79. Loehr, G. W. and Waller, H. D., Eine neue enzymophenische haemolytische Anaemie mit Glutathionreduktasemangel, *Med. Klin. (Munich)*, 36, 1521, 1962.
80. Luisada, A., Favism: a singular disease chiefly affecting the red blood cells, *Medicine*, 20, 229, 1941.
81. Mager, J., Razin, A., Hershko, A., and Izak, G., The mechanism of red-cell hexokinase inhibition induced by oxidation of intracellular glutathione and its relation to drug-sensitivity, *Biochem. Biophys. Res. Commun.*, 17, 703, 1964.
82. Mager, J., Glaser, G., Razin, A., Izak, G., Bien, S., and Noam, J., Metabolic effects of pyrimidines derived from fava bean glycosides on human erythrocytes deficient in glucose-6-phosphate dehydrogenase, *Biochem. Biophys. Res. Commun.*, 20, 235, 1965.
83. Mager, J., Razin, A., and Hershko, A., Favism, in *Toxic Constituents of Plant Foodstuffs*, Liener, L. I., Ed., Academic Press, New York, 1969, 293.
84. Manai, A., Il favismo. Edit. Stamp. Libreria Ital. e Stran, Sassari, 1929.
85. McOmie, J. F. W. and Chesterfield, J. H., Synthesis of 5-hydroxypyrimidine and a new synthesis of divicine, *Chem. Ind. (London)*, 2, 1453, 1956.
86. Mela, C. and Perona, G. P., Sulla resistenza *in vitro* del glutatione ridotto eritrocitario al succo di fava fresche, *Boll. Soc. Ital. Biol. Sper.*, 35,.146, 1959.
87. Minnich, V., Smith, M. B., Brauner, M. J., and Majerus, P. W., Glutathione biosynthesis in human erythrocytes. I. Identification of the enzymes of glutathione synthesis in hemolysate, *J. Clin. Invest.*, 50, 507, 1971.

88. Mohler, D. N. and Williams, W. J., The effect of phenylhydrazine on the adenosine triphosphate content of normal and glucose-6-phosphate dehydrogenase-deficient human blood, *J. Clin. Invest.,* 40, 1753, 1961.
89. Motulsky, A. G., Metabolic polymorphism and the role of infectious diseases in human evolution, *Human Biol.,* 32, 28, 1960.
90. Nathan, R. D., Pachtman, E. A., Fiorelli, G., and Frumin, A. M., A serum defect in favism, *Am. J. Clin. Pathol.,* 61, 462, 1974.
91. Necheles, T., Boles, T., and Allen, D., Erythrocyte glutathione-peroxidase deficiency and hemolytic disease of the newborn infant, *J. Pediatr.,* 72, 319, 1968.
92. Necheles, T. F., Steinberg, M. H., and Cameron, D., Erythrocyte glutathione-peroxidase deficiency, *Br. J. Haematol.,* 19, 605, 1970.
93. Oort, M., Loos, J. A., and Prins, H. K,. Hereditary absence of reduced glutathione in the erythrocytes — a new clinical and biochemical entity, *Vox. Sanguinis,* 6, 370, 1961.
94. Panizon, F., La patogenesi del favismo, *Minerva Pediatr.,* 19, 1391, 1967.
95. Panizon, F. and Vullo, C., Effetti della somministrazione di fava e di primachina sull emazie glucoso-6-fosfato-deidrogenasi-peniche marcate con Cr^{51}, *Haematologica (Pavia),* 47, 205, 1962.
96. Panizon, F. and Zacchello, F., The mechanism of hemolysis in favism. Some analogy in the activity of primaquine and fava juice, *Acta Haematol.,* 33, 129, 1965.
97. Panizon, F. and Zacchello, F., Sulla patogensi dell' anemia de primachina. Effetti della incubazione con primachina e menadione sulla sopravvivenza eritrocitaria, *Atti. Soc. Med. Chir. Padova,* 41, 5, 1966.
98. Patterson, J. W., Lazarow, A., and Levey, S., Reactions of alloxan and dialuric acid with the sulfhydryl group, *J. Biol. Chem.,* 177, 187, 1949.
99. Perera, C. B. and Frumin, A. M., Agglutination of human erythrocytes by fava bean extract, *Bibliotheca Haematol.,* 23, 589, 1965.
100. Prankerd, T. A. J., *The Red Cell. An Account of Its Chemical Physiology and Pathology,* Blackwell Scientific, Oxford, 1961.
101. Pridham, J. B. and Saltmarsh, M. J., The biosynthesis of phenolic glucosides in plants, *Biochem. J.,* 87, 218, 1963.
102. Prins, H. K. and Loos, J. A., Glutathione, in *Biochemical Methods in Red Cell Genetics,* Yunis, Y. Y., Ed., Academic Press, New York, 1969, 123.
103. Prins, H. K., Oort, M., Loos, J. A., Zurcher, C., and Beckers, T., Congenital non-spherocytic hemolytic anemia, associated with glutathione deficiency of the erythrocytes, *Blood,* 27, 145, 1966.
104. Rachmilewitz, E. A., Peisach, J., Bradley, T. B., Jr., and Blumberg, W. E., Role of haemichromes in the formation of inclusion bodies in hemoglobin H disease, *Nature (London),* 222, 248, 1969.
105. Razin, A., Hershko, A., Glaser, G., and Mager, J., The oxidant effect of isouramil on red cell glutathione and its synergistic enhancement by ascorbic acid or 3,4-dihydroxyphenylalanine. Possible relation to the pathogenesis of favism, *Israel J. Med. Sci.,* 4, 862, 1968.
106. Rifkind, R. A., Heinz body anemia: an ultrastructural study. II. Red cell sequestration and destruction, *Blood,* 26, 433, 1965.
107. Ritthausen, H., Ueber Vicin, Bestandteil der Samen von *Vicia sativa, Ber. Dtsch. Chem. Ges.,* 9, 301, 1876.
108. Ritthausen, H., Ueber Vicin und eine zweite stickstoffreiche Substanz der Wickensamen, Convicin, *J. Prakt. Chem.,* 24(2), 202, 1881.
109. Ritthausen, H., Vicin ein Glycosid, *Ber. Dtsch. Chem. Ges.,* 29, 2108, 1896.
110. Ritthausen, H., Ueber die Zusammenzetzung des Vicins, *J. Prakt. Chem.,* 59, 480, 1899.
111. Ritthausen, H., Ueber Divicin, *J. Prakt. Chem.,* 59, 482, 1899.
112. Ritthausen, H. and Kreusler, U., Ueber das Vorkommen von Amygdalin und eine neue dem Asparagin aehnliche Substanz in Wickensamen, *J. Prakt. Chem.,* 2(2), 333, 1870.
113. Rotruck, J. T., Pope, A. L., Ganther, H. E., and Hoekstra, W. G., Prevention of oxidative damage to rat erythrocytes by dietary selenium, *J. Nutr.,* 102, 689, 1972.
114. Rotruck, J. T., Pope, A. L., Ganther, H. E., Swanson, A. B., Hafeman, D. G., and Hoekstra, W. G., Selenium: biochemical role as a component of glutathione peroxidase, *Science,* 179, 588, 1973.
115. Sansone, G. and Segni, G., Prime determinazioni del glutatione (GSH) ematico nel favismo, *Boll. Soc. Ital. Biol. Sper.,* 32, 456, 1956.
116. Sansone, G. and Segni, G., Sensitivity to broad beans, *Lancet,* ii, 295, 1957.
117. Sansone, G. and Segni, G., L'instabilitá del glutatione ematico (GSH) nel favismo: utilizzazione di um test selettivo. Introduzione al problema genetico, *Boll. Soc. Ital. Biol. Sper.,* 33, 1057, 1957.
118. Sansone, G. and Sengi, G., Nuovi aspetti dell'alterato biochimismo delgi eritrociti di favici: assenza pressoche completa della glucoso-6-P-deidrogenasi, *Boll. Soc. Ital. Biol. Sper.,* 34, 327, 1958.
119. Sansone, G., Piga, A. M., and Segni, G., Il favismo, *Minerva Med.,* 1958.
120. Schank, K., Reductones, *Synthesis,* 176, 1972.

121. Simon, E. R., Adenine and purine nucleosides in human red cell preservation. A review, *Transfusion,* 7, 395, 1967.
122. Stamatoyannopoulos, G., Fraser, G. R., Motulsky, A. G., Fessas, P., Akrivakis, A., and Papayonnopoulos, T., On the familial predisposition to favism, *Am. J. Human Genet.,* 18, 253, 1966.
123. Steinberg, M., Brewer, M., and Necheles, T., Acute hemolytic anemia associated with erythrocyte glutathione peroxidase deficiency, *Arch. Intern. Med.,* 125, 302, 1970.
124. Szeinberg, A. and Chari-Bitron, A., Blood glutathione concentration in haemolytic anaemia due to *Vicia faba* or sulfonamides, *Acta Haematol.,* 18, 229, 1957.
125. Szeinberg, A., Sheba, C., Hirshorn, N., and Bodonyi, E., Studies on erythrocytes in cases with past history of favism and drug-induced acute hemolytic anemia, *Blood,* 12, 603, 1957.
126. Szeinberg, A., Asher, Y., and Sheba, C., Studies on glutathione stability in erythrocytes of cases with past history of favism or sulfa drug-induced hemolysis, *Blood,* 13, 348, 1958.
127. Szeinberg, A., Sheba, C., and Adam, A., Enzymatic abnormality in erythrocytes of a population sensitive to *Vicia faba* hemolytic anemia induced by drugs, *Nature (London),* 181, 1256, 1958.
128. Szeinberg, A., Sheba, C., and Adam, A., Selective occurrence of glutathione instability in red blood corpuscles of the various Jewish tribes, *Blood,* 13, 1043, 1958.
129. United States Department of Agriculture, Agriculture Handbook No. 8, Washington, D.C., 1963.
130. Walker, D. G. and Bowman, J. E., *In vitro* effect of *Vicia faba* extracts upon reduced glutathione of erythrocytes, *Proc. Soc. Exptl. Biol. Med.,* 103, 476, 1960.
131. Waller, H. D. and Benoehr, H. C., Studies on the reduction of methemoglobin by ascorbic acid, in *Erythrocytes, Thrombocytes, Leukocytes,* Int. Symp. 2nd, Gerlach, E., Ed., Georg Tieme Verlag, Stuttgart, 1973, 200.
132. Waller, H. D. and Gerok, W., Schwere strahleninduzierte Haemolyse bei hereditaerem Mangel an reduziertem Glutathion in Blutzellen, *Klin. Wochenschr.,* 42, 948, 1964.
133. Waller, H. D., Benoehr, H. C., and Waumans, P., Zur Entstehung der medikameteninduzierten Anaemie bei Glutathionreduktase-Mangeltraegern, *Klin. Wochenschr.,* 47, 25, 1969.
134. Wang, S. Y., Pyrimidines. I. Reaction of Bromide with Uracil, *J. Org. Chem.,* 24, 11, 1959.
135. Wang, S. Y., Chemistry of Pyrimidines. II. The conversion of 5-bromo to 5-hydroxyuracils, *J. Am. Chem. Soc.,* 81, 3786, 1959.
136. Winterstein, A. and Somló, F., in *Handbuch der Pflanzenanalyse,* Klein, G., Ed., Springer-Verlag, Basel, 1933, 362.
137. Yoshida, A., Glucose-6-phosphate dehydrogenase of human erythrocytes. I. Purification and characterization of normal (B⁺) enzyme, *J. Biol. Chem.,* 241, 4966, 1966.
138. Yoshida, A., Human glucose-6-phosphate dehydrogenase; purification and characterization of the Negro type Variant (A⁺) and comparison with normal enzyme (B⁺), *Biochem. Genet.,* 1, 81, 1967.
139. Yoshida, A., Hemolytic anemia and G6PD deficiency, *Science,* 179, 532, 1973.
140. Yoshida, A. and Hoagland, V. D., Jr., Active molecular unit and NADP content of human glucose-6-phosphate dehydrogenase, *Biochem. Biophys. Res. Commun.,* 40, 1167, 1970.
141. Yoshida, A., Beutler, E., and Motulsky, A. G., Human glucose-6-phosphate dehydrogenase variants, *Bull. WHO,* 45, 243, 1971.
142. Zinkham, W. H., Lenhard, R. E., Jr., and Childs, B., A deficiency of glucose-6-phosphate dehydrogenase activity in erythrocytes from patients with favism, *Bull. Johns Hopkins Hosp.,* 102, 169, 1958.
143. Chevion, M. and Mager, J., unpublished results.

NATURALLY OCCURRING FOOD TOXICANTS: ESTROGENS

Martin Stob

INTRODUCTION

Estrogens are compounds which produce a number of predictable responses when administered to animals. Probably the two best known of these effects are vaginal cornification and uterine hypertrophy of intact, immature, or castrated, mature female mice or rats. Both of these effects serve as the basis of bioassays[1,2] for the detection of estrogenic activity of feeds or the determination of the biological potency of specific compounds. The increase in uterine weight (uterotropic effect) is a more sensitive response[3,4] than vaginal cornification, but lacks complete specificity for estrogens since androgens and progesterone will also cause uterine hypertrophy, although at much higher doses than estrogens.[5] Based on these two responses, an incredible number and variety of compounds are estrogenic,[5,6-9] including analogues of DDT[10,11] and delta-9-tetrahydrocannabinol.[12]

Because of the large number of compounds which are estrogenic, it is not surprising that some occur in plants or plant products used for human and animal foods.[7,13-18] In the majority of these cases, the specific compounds which cause the estrogenic effect(s) have been identified; the physiological consequences of consuming the estrogenic foods or plants have been described.

THE OCCURRENCE OF ESTROGENS IN FOODS

This discussion will be limited to the estrogens found in plants. The estrogens which are naturally produced by plants are commonly referred to as phytoestrogens and would not include compounds such as estrone or estriol, both of which have been reported in plants, but are normally produced by the ovaries. The estrogens present in meat and milk are discussed elsewhere in this book; the estrogenic activity present in other foods such as honey and egg yolk have been mentioned in the reviews cited previously.

Bradbury and White[7] identified 53 plants with estrogenic activity. The plants which are used for food for man or animals are presented in Table 1. Subsequently, estrogenic activity has been reported in other plants or products including carrots *(Daucus carota* var. *sativa)*,[19] the hormonal activity of which may be due to 3-methyl-6-methoxy-8-hydroxy-3,4-dihydroisocoumarin.[20] Date palm seeds (*Phoenix dactylifera* L.)[21] and seed oil[22] and seeds[23] from the pomegranate fruit (*Punica granatum*) contain estrone. The estrogenic activity of fennel and anise oil may be due to anethole[24] and perhaps estriol in licorice roots.[25] Hops *(Humulus lupulus),* contain the three beta bitter acids, colupulon, lupulon and adlupulon,[26] which may account for its estrogenicity. The tuberous roots of the plant *Pueraria mirifica* contain the miroestrol.[17] The estrogen zearalenone was first discovered in corn infectd with the fungus *Gibberella zeae*[28] but the compound has been isolated from other grains such as barley,[29,30,31] oats,[29,30,31,32] rice,[31] sesame meal,[33] sorghum,[34,35] and wheat.[29,30,36] *Gibberella zeae* may also produce zearalenol in corn and oats.[32] In addition to the isoflavones, soybeans may also contain coumestrol.[37]

PRINCIPAL PHYTOESTROGENS: BIOLOGICAL POTENCY

The compounds which are most likely to be responsible for the estrogenic activity of plants or plant products are the isoflavones, the coumestans, and the resorcyclic

Table 1
PLANTS REPORTED TO HAVE ESTROGENIC ACTIVITY

Scientific name	Common name	Part examined	Activity, rat(R) or mouse (M) units/kg
Allium sativum L.	Garlic	Bulb	4000 M
Avena sativa L.	Oats	Seeds (meal), seeds, sprouts	6.6 R, 50 R 50 R, 5500 R, 16,000 R
Brassica campestris L.	Rape	Seeds	+
Coffea arabica L.	Coffee	Seed (oil)	+
Dactylis glomerata L.	Orchard grass	Leaf, stem, flower	+
Foeniculum vulgare Mill.	Fennel	Oil	+
Glycyrrhiza glabra L.	Licorice	Root	+ +
Hordeum vulgare L.	Barley	Embryo	+
Lolium perenne L.	Ryegrass	Leaves, stems	+
Malus sylvestris Mill.	Apple	Fruits	+
Oryza sativa L.	Rice	Seeds, embryo	+
Pimpinella anisum L.	Anise	Oil	+
Petroselinum crispum Nym.	Parsley	Root	+
Poa pratensis L.	Blue grass	—	+
Prunus avium L.	Cherry	Fruit	+
Saccharomyces sp.	Yeast	—	+ to 250 M
Salvia officinalis L.	Sage	Leaves	6000 M
Solanum tuberosum L.	Potato	Tubers	+
Trifolium sp.	Clovers	Leaves, stems	+ to 1000 M
Triticum aestivum L.	Wheat	Flour, seeds, germ oil	+

Adapted from Bradbury, R. B. and White, D. E., *Vitamins and Hormones,* Vol. XII, Harris, R. S., Marrian, G. F., and Thimann, K. V., Eds., Academic Press, New York, 1954, 207-230.

acid lactones. Although it was reported that B-sitosterol is estrogenic,[38] which could contribute to the hormonal activity of plants, the 1 uterotropic activity of this compound could not be confirmed by Bickoff.[17] The isoflavones, coumestans, and resorcyclic acid found in plants or plant products are listed in Table 2.

The isoflavones most likely to account for the estrogenic activity of plants are genistein, genistin, daidzein, biochanin A, formononetin, and pratensein. In the mouse, and by oral administration, genistein is more uterotropically active than daidzein, biochanin A, or formononetin.[9] Based on uterine hypertrophy in the mouse, genistein and genistin are equally active by either oral or subcutaneous route of administration.[39] In sheep, by intraruminal infusion, genistein, biochanin A, and formononetin appear to be equally active and genistein and biochanin A are more active when administered intramuscularly than by intraruminal infusion.[40] However, formononetin appears to be more active by the intraruminal than intramuscular route of administration.[40] Pratensein may have lower estrogenic activity than any of the aforementioned isoflavones.[41]

The two most important coumestans are coumestrol[42] and 4'-O-methylcoumestrol[43] which is approximately 10 times less active than coumestrol based on the uterine response of mice to oral administration of the compounds.[44] Coumestrol is more uterotropically active in mice than the isoflavones.[9] In sheep, coumestrol is 15 times more active than the isoflavones when administered intraruminally and is less active by that route of administration than by intramuscular injection.[40]

The two resorcyclic acid lactones most apt to occur in plant parts or products are zearalenone and zearalenol. Comparisons of the biological potency of zearalenone

Table 2
THE ESTROGENIC ISOFLAVONES, COUMESTANS, AND RESORCYCLIC ACID LACTONES

Common name	Chemical name	Source	Ref.
Isoflavones			
Biochanin A	5,7-Dihydroxy-4'-methoxy isoflavone	Red clover	13
Daidzein	4',7-Dihydroxyisoflavone	Soybeans	13
Genistein	4',5,7-Trihydroxy isoflavone	Soybeans	13
Genistin	Genistein-7-glycoside	Soybeans	13
Formononetin	7-Hydroxy-4-methoxy isoflavone	Red clover	13
Pratensein	5,7,3'-Trihydroxy-4'-methoxy isoflavone	Red and subterranean clovers	41
Coumestans			
Coumestrol	4',7-Dihydroxy-benzo-furo-coumarin	Ladino clover	42
4'-O-methyl-coumestrol	4'-O-Methyl-7-hydroxy-benzofurocoumarin	Alfalfa	43
Resorcyclic acid lactones			
Zearalenone	3,4,5,6,9,10-Hexahydro-14,16-dihydroxy-3-methyl-1H-2-benzoxacyclotetradecin-1,7(8H)-dione	*Fusarium* sp.	28
Zearalenol	3,4,5,6,7,8,9,10-Octahydro-7,14,16-trihydroxy-3-methyl-1H-2-benzoxacyclotetradecin-1-one	*Fusarium* sp.	32

with some isoflavones and coumestrol have been made using the affinity of these compounds for estrogen receptors. Thus the comparative binding affinity for receptor in rat uterine cytosol is: estradiol-17β > coumestrol > zearalenone > genistein > daidzein > biochanin A > formononetin.[45] Competition for binding sites in steroid-binding globulin is estradiol-17β > genistein > formononetin > coumestrol > zearalenone.[46]

Generally, the phytoestrogens have lower biological potencies than stilbene estrogens such as diethylstilbestrol (DES) or steroidal estrogens such as estradiol-17β, estrone or estriol. However, tissue and species differences in responses must be considered when comparing potencies. In the ewe, two seasons of grazing clover containing phytoestrogens were necessary to produce the same type of cystic uterine hyperplasia caused by daily injections of 0.11 mg DES for 6 months.[47] Affinity for binding to estrogen receptor sites in uterine cytosol of various species: rabbit, estradiol-17β > coumestrol > genistein;[48] sheep, estradiol-17β > coumestrol > daidzein > formononetin;[49] calf, estradiol-17β > coumestrol.[50] Affinity for rat uterine cytosol and steroid-binding globulin have already been presented. In the mouse, by oral administration, both DES and estrone are much more potent stimulators of uterine hypertrophy than coumestrol or the isoflavones,[9] and DES is approximately 1000 times more active than zearalenone.[51] Estrone is 1600 times more active by subcutaneous injection and 12.5 times more active orally than zearalenone.[52] In the rat, by subcutaneous injection, estradiol-17β is 500 times more active than zearalenone in causing uterine hypertrophy.[53] In young chickens zearalenone was only 1.37% as effective as estradiol dipropionate when injected intramuscularly.[54] In rhesus monkeys, by subcutaneous injection, estradiol-17β was 3.5 and DES 28 times more effective than zearalenone in suppressing the release of luteinizing hormone (LH) from the anterior pituitary; with oral administration, estradiol was 80 and DES 160 times more effective in inhibiting LH release.[55] In swine, estradiol-17β-cyclo-pentylpropionate administered intramuscularly was approximately 20 times more active in causing uterine hypertrophy and 50 times more active in causing vulvar tumefaction than zearalenone administered orally.[56] Direct comparisons cannot be made, but by inference, zearalenone may be equal to DES, when administered orally, in causing hypertrophy of the vulva in young female swine.[56,57,58] Swine may be uniquely sensitive to zearalenone in the feed since as little as 1 to 5 ppm in the ration will cause estrogenic effects.[59] In chickens[54] and monkeys,[55] zearalenone is more effective by injection than by oral administration; it seems to have little or no oral activity in cattle or sheep. Zearalenol is more estrogenic than zearalenone.[32,60] Comparisons of the biological potencies of the isoflavones coumestrol and zearalenone are presented in Tables 3 to 6. The compounds which may be responsible for the estrogenic activity of some feeds consumed by man and animals are identified in Table 7.

FACTORS AFFECTING THE OCCURRENCE OF ESTROGENS IN PLANTS

It may be appropriate to consider why compounds capable of producing estrogenic effects in animals should occur in plants. Some intriguing possibilities include an association with the production of flower pigments,[74] or the specific example of anethole acting as an attractant to the larvae of black swallowtail butterflies,[75] a role in the lignification process,[76] or that they are simply excretion products.[77] There doesn't seem to be much evidence that the phytoestrogens are directly associated with the reproductive processes of plants, although zearalenone may stimulate the development of the perithecia (sexual stage) of some isolates of *Fusarium graminearum*[78] and other organisms.[79]

There is genetic variation in the uterotropic activity of alfalfa[80] and subterranean clover.[81] The estrogenic activity of alfalfa will vary with location of growth, cutting, year of harvest, and stage of growth.[82] The uterotropic activity of subterranean clover varies in different parts of the plant.[83]

Estrogenic compounds occurring in plants may be associated with plant diseases. Phloretin and phloridzin, both estrogenic,[6] appear in apple leaves following injury or innoculation with the pathogen *Venturia inaequalis*.[84,85] The coumestrol content of alfalfa is increased when the plant is attacked by the fungi, *Ascochyta imperfecta, Cylindrocladium scoparium, Colletotricum trifolii, Uromyces striatus,*[86] *Leptosphaerulina briosiana,* and *Pseudopeziza medicagnis.*[87] Sherwood et al.[86] observed that the

Table 3
DOSE-RESPONSE DATA AND RELATIVE POTENCY OF FORAGE ESTROGENS VS. DIETHYLSTILBESTROL AND ESTRONE

Compound	Quantity fed per mouse (μg)	Number of mice	Uterine wt. ± S.E. (mg)[a]	Quantity to produce 25 mg (uterus) (μg)	Relative potency
Control	0.000	300	9.6 ± 0.3		
Diethylstilbestrol	0.025	16	11.8 ± 0.2	0.083	100,000
	0.050	50	18.1 ± 0.7		
	0.075	40	23.7 ± 0.8		
	0.100	491	29.2 ± 0.4		
	0.200	31	78.1 ± 6.2		
Estrone	0.50	23	14.7 ± 0.9	1.20	6,900
	0.75	15	16.0 ± 1.3		
	1.00	22	23.8 ± 2.5		
	1.50	40	36.1 ± 2.3		
	2.00	5	45.3 ± 6.7		
Coumestrol	100	20	13.8 ± 0.2	240	35
	200	44			
	300	126	29.2 ± 1.3		
	400	79	40.7 ± 1.9		
	500	36	76.0 ± 6.0		
Genistein	5,000	18	19.4 ± 0.9	8,000	1.00
	7,500	15	28.0 ± 5.0		
	8,000	19	27.0 ± 1.6		
	12,000	25	32.4 ± 1.9		
	15,000	35	36.6 ± 0.6		
	20,000	25	52.7 ± 1.9		
Daidzein	5,000	20	17.3 ± 1.3	11,000	0.75
	7,500	15	18.5 ± 2.6		
	10,000	20	24.8 ± 1.3		
	15,000	33	31.2 ± 1.4		
Biochanin A	10,000	30	20.3 ± 2.5	18,000	0.46
	20,000	59	27.9 ± 2.1		
	30,000	20	27.9 ± 2.6		
	40,000	38	45.5 ± 3.8		
Formononetin	15,000	20	16.8 ± 0.8	32,000	0.26
	20,000	15	17.9 ± 1.4		
	25,000	19	23.2 ± 1.0		
	30,000	20	27.5 ± 2.3		
	40,000	15	26.1 ± 2.0		

[a] SE, standard error mean.

[b] Measured at the dosage required to produce a 25 mg uterus.

Adapted from Bickoff, E. M., Livingston, A. L., Hendrickson, A. P., and Booth, A. N., *Agric. Food Chem.*, 10, 410—412, 1962. With permission.

concentration of coumestrol was related to the degree of infection and hypothesized that the plant contributes enzymes and coumestrol precursors, but the organism(s) may actually produce it. They report concentrations of coumestrol as follows: none in disease-free leaves, 115 ppm in infected leaves, 168 ppm in the pustules caused by the organisms, and 746 ppm in the urediospores. A high concentration of coumestrol in the urediospores was also reported by Loper et al.[88] However, aphid-damaged portions of alfalfa contain elevated coumestrol[89] and alfalfa "free" of foliar pathogens contains coumestrol.[90] Very high concentrations of coumestrol (2000 ppm) were found in heavily spotted barrel medic leaves which were free of bacteria or fungi.[62]

Table 4
RELATIVE UTEROTROPIC ACTIVITY OF ORALLY ADMINISTERED ZEARALENONE VS. DIETHYLSTILBESTROL IN CASTRATED FEMALE MICE[51]

Treatment	Number of mice	Uterine weight, mg ± standard error, mean
Control ration	10	22.3 ± 1.4
Zearalenone[a]	µg	
1	10	21.2 ± 0.7
10	9	32.1 ± 2.5
25	9	41.8 ± 4.6
50	9	73.8 ± 7.8
100	10	59.6 ± 5.7
125	10	93.5 ± 8.9
Diethylstilbestrol[a]	µg	
0.01	10	30.7 ± 1.5
0.025	10	40.4 ± 3.4
0.05	10	73.6 ± 4.4
0.1	10	110.3 ± 6.6
0.25	10	124.2 ± 7.2

[a] Represents micrograms of compound per gram of diet. Animals were fed 3 g of diet per mouse per day for 6 days.

Table 5
"F-2" MOUSE ESTROGEN ASSAY (SUBCUTANEOUS INJECTION)

Material administered	Total dose (µg)	No. of mice	Mean uterine ratio ± SE
Control	0	10	0.75 ± 0.19
Estrone	0.05	10	1.48 ± 0.09
	0.1	10	2.66 ± 0.36
	0.2	10	3.37 ± 0.32
	0.4	10	3.60 ± 0.18
F-2[a]	5	10	0.72 ± 0.05
	20	10	0.88 ± 0.03
	80	9	1.41 ± 0.11

[a] F-2 = zearalenone.

Data of Dr. R. I. Dorfman, taken from Mirocha, C. J., Christensen, C. M., and Nelson, G. H., *Biotech. Bioeng.*, 10, 469—482, 1968. With permission.

Several factors affect the concentration of zearalenone in moldy grains. In the first reports of an association of hyperestrogenism with the consumption of moldy grain, invariably the animals had been fed grain which had been harvested during cold, wet weather, conditions which favored the growth of the *Fusarium* molds and their production of zearalenone.[91-94] Little zearalenone is found when climatic conditions are not favorable to the growth of the fungus.[35,36] Zearalenone is more apt to be present in stored[95] than freshly harvested corn.[96] *Fusarium* species differ in their ability to produce zearalenone[97] and time and temperature also play important roles in zearalenone production.[98]

Table 6
"F-2" MOUSE ESTROGEN ASSAY
(GAVAGE)

Material administered	Total dose (µg)	No. of mice	Mean uterine ratio ± SE
Control	0	10	0.76 ± 0.06
Estrone	0.5	10	1.21 ± 0.12
	1	9	1.19 ± 0.10
	2	9	2.12 ± 0.23
	4	10	2.93 ± 0.21
F-2[a]	12.5	10	1.11 ± 0.04
	25	10	1.48 ± 0.18
	50	10	1.80 ± 0.12
	100	9	2.35 ± 0.17

[a] F-2 = zearalenone.

Data of Dr. R. I. Dorfman, taken from Mirocha, C. J., Christensen, C. M., and Nelson, G. H., *Biotech. Bioeng.*, 10, 469—482, 1968. With permission.

PHYSIOLOGIC VS. "TOXIC" EFFECTS OF PHYTOESTROGENS

Physiologic Effects

It is apparent that the isoflavones, coumestans and zearalenone, are estrogenic because of the effects they produce: hypertrophy of the vulva, vagina, and uterus of female mammals; hypertrophy of the accessory glands of male mammals; hypertrophy of the mammae and inhibition of the hypothalamus, anterior pituitary, and gonads of mammals of both sexes; and enlargement of the vent and oviduct of avian females. All of these effects are typical and predictable estrogenic responses. Degree of effect can and does vary however. The alteration of the chemical configuration of phytoestrogens, as is the case with other types of estrogens, may cause an alteration in physiological activity.[4,9,44,98,99,100] Differences in estrogenic response will vary with the method of administration.[39,54,55] Response will also vary with species, sheep seemingly more sensitive to isoflavones and coumestans than cattle,[15] and swine more sensitive to zearalenone than avians.[54,59] The number of effects seen will vary with the amounts of phytoestrogen to which the animal is exposed, e.g., at low levels, coumestrol causes vagino-uterotropic effects, but higher levels are required for antigonadotropic action.[101] Prolonged exposure of ewes to phytoestrogens results in a persistent desensitization of the hypothalamus to estrogen.[102] Prior reference has been made to binding of phytoestrogens to the same receptor sites as estradiol, but they have a lesser affinity for those sites than estradiol.

The effects observed in animals consuming feeds containing isoflavones or coumestans are presented in Table 8 and those feeds containing zearalenone and zearalenol in Table 9. The effects of administering known amounts of authentic isoflavones and coumestans are presented in Table 10 and zearalenone in Table 11.

"Toxic" Effects

There have been suggestions of beneficial effects of phytoestrogens, e.g., galactopoiesis,[118] but it is doubtful that estrogens occur in pasture plants in quantities sufficient to stimulate milk production.[119] Alfalfa containing large amounts of coumestrol was reported to stimulate growth and improve carcass quality of lambs,[120] but various doses of pure coumestrol did not stimulate growth when fed to cattle.[121]

Table 7
IDENTIFICATION OF COMPOUNDS RESPONSIBLE FOR THE ESTROGENIC ACTIVITY OF SOME ANIMAL AND HUMAN FEEDS

Feed	Compounds	Ref.
Alfalfa (*Medicago sativa* L.)	Biochanin A	61
	Coumestrol	42
	4'-O-Methyl Coumestrol	43
	Daidzein	61
	Formononetin	61
	Genistein	61
Barrel medic (*Medicago littoralis*)	Coumestrol	62
Barley (*Hordeum vulgare*)	Zearaleone	29—31
Birdsfoot trefoil (*Lotus corniculatus* L.)	?	63
Chick peas (*Cicer arietinum* L.)	Biochanin A	64
Chick pea seedlings (*Cicer arietinum* L.)	Daidzein	65
	Pratensein	65
Clovers (*Trifolium* spp.) (more than 100 species and varieties tested)	Biochanin A	61, 66, 67
	Coumestrol	42, 68
	Daidzein	61, 66, 67
	Formononetin	61, 66, 67
	Genistein	61, 66, 67
	Pratesein	41
Corn (*Zea mays*)	Zearalenone	33
	Zearalenol	32
Hay	Zearalenone	69
Oats (*Avena sativa*)	Zearalenone	32
	Zearalenol	32
Rice (*Oryza sativa*)	Zearalenone	31
Rye (*Secale cereale*)	Zearalenone	29,30
Sesame meal (*Sesamum indicum*)	Zearalenone	33
Sorghum (*Sorghum vulgare*)	Zearalenone	34,35
Soybeans (*Soja max*)	Coumestrol	37
	Daidzein	70
	Genistein	71
	Genistin	71
Soybean sprouts	Coumestrol	37
Wheat (*Triticum vulgare*)	Zearalenone	29, 30
Vegetable oils, including corn, coconut, cottonseed, linseed, olive, peanut, rice bran, safflower, soybean, wheat germ	?	72,73

Although most of the effects of phytoestrogens on animal performance have been detrimental, it is doubtful that these compounds should be labeled toxic or as toxicants. Phytoestrogens were not positively incriminated in causing an increase in the incidence of mastitis in cattle.[103] "Clover disease" in sheep, first reported in Australia, due to the ingestion of forages containing large amounts of genistein and other isoflavones and the "hyperestrogen syndrome" reported in cattle consuming alfalfa which due to the ingestion of forages containing large amounts of genistein and other isoflavones and the "hyperestrogen syndrome" reported in cattle consuming alfalfa which presumably contained high levels of coumestans were associated with signs of typical estrogenic responses, i.e., hypertrophy of the vulva, vagina, and uterus of females, the accessory glands of males, and the mammae of both sexes. Seldom, if ever, was the term toxic used in describing these responses. The pathological conditions which were seen, e.g., cystic glandular hyperplasia of the endometrium, were recognized as effects of chronic estrogen administration. If there is any evidence of a toxicity of the isoflavones, it may be in the reports of the effects of genistin on growth depression in

Table 8
ESTROGENIC EFFECTS IN ANIMALS CONSUMING FEEDS CONTAINING ISOFLAVONES OR COUMESTANS

Animal (sex)	Feed	Effects	Ref.
Cattle (F)	Alfalfa, estrogenic pastures, subterranean clover	Infertility, nymphomania	15
Cattle (F)	Alfalfa and brome grass	Mastitis	103
Sheep (F)	Subterranean clover	Infertility, dystocia, postnatal mortality of lambs, uterine prolapse, fetal retention, metritis, sterility, cystic endometrial hyperplasia, delayed conception, vulvar hypertrophy	15
Sheep (M castrated)	Subterranean clover	Hypertrophy of seminal vesicles, bulbo-urethral glands, mammae and death	15
Guinea pig (F)	Subterranean clover	Infertility, cystic hyperplasia of endometrium	15
Guinea pig (M)	Subterranean clover	Hypertrophy of mammae	7
Rabbit (F)	Ladino clover	Reduced conception, litter size	104
Mice (F)	Ladino clover	Inhibition of estrus and ovulation	105
Quail (both sexes)	Forbs	Impaired reproduction	106

Table 9
ESTROGENIC EFFECTS IN ANIMALS CONSUMING FEEDS CONTAINING ZEARALENONE

Animal (sex)	Feed	Effect(s)	Ref.
Cattle (F)	Hay	Infertility	69
Cattle (F)	Sorghum	Abortion	140
Swine (F)	Corn	Hypertrophy of vulva, uterus, mammae, vaginal prolapse, infertility, anal prolapse (sic)[a]	107
Swine (F)	Corn	Abortion	33
Swine (M)	Corn	Hypertrophy of mammae, atrophy of testes, anal prolapse (sic)[a]	107
Turkeys (M)	"Feeds"	Infertility	107
Turkeys (M,F)	Sesame meal	Enlargement of vent	107
Turkeys (M,F)	Corn	Enlargement of vent	79
Chickens (M,F)	Corn	Enlargement of vent	79
Geese (M)	"Feeds"	Infertility	107

[a] Rectal prolapse.

the mouse[111] and the effects of both genistin and genistein on growth depression in rats.[114] The inhibitory effects of estrogens on the growth of rodents, at the doses reported, are well known,[122-124] and are allegedly due to suppression of growth hormone

Table 10
THE EFFECTS OF ADMINISTERING VARIOUS DOSAGES OF AUTHENTIC ISOFLAVONES OR COUMESTANS IN ANIMALS

Compound/dose	Effects	Ref.
Mouse		
Biochanin A, 10,000—40,000 µg/g diet	Uterine hypertrophy	9
Coumestrol, 100-500 µg/g diet	Uterine hypertrophy	9
Coumestrol, 500 µg/g diet	Antigonadotropic	101
Daidzein, 5,000—15,000 µg/g diet	Uterine hypertrophy	9
Formononetin, 15,000—40,000 µg/g diet	Uterine hypertrophy	9
Genistein, 5,000—20,000 µg/g diet	Uterine hypertrophy	9
Genistein, 15 mg/day, diet	Infertility, both sexes	108
Genistein, 10 mg injected	Displace estradiol from uterine receptors	109
Genistin, 5 mg/day, diet	Uterine hypertrophy	39
Genistin, 0.2% of diet	Infertility, females	110
Genistin, 9—72 mg/day, diet	Testes atrophy, depressed growth	111
Rat		
Coumestrol, 1000 µg injected, 5 days neonatally	Persistent estrus syndrome	112
Coumestrol diacetate, 125 µg injected	Increased protein and phospholipid synthesis in uterus	113
Genistein, 0.5% of diet	Testes atrophy, depressed growth	114
Genistein, 400 µg injected	Increased protein and phospholipid synthesis in uterus	113
Genistin, 0.5% of diet	Testes atrophy, depressed growth	114
Sheep		
Biochanin A, 1 g injected	Uterine hypertrophy	40
Coumestrol, 0.012 g injected, 1.4 g intraruminally	Uterine hypertrophy	40
Formononetin, 24 g injected	Uterine hypertrophy	40
Genistein, 1 g injected	Uterine hypertrophy	40

production by the anterior pituitary gland[122] or depression of appetite.[123,124] However, in the mouse[111] and rat[114] studies, the authors indicate the effects "are not the same" as estrogens,[114] or that "the effects of genistin may be primarily non-estrogenic".[111] The depressing effects of genistin on reproduction in the mouse[110] may not be due to an estrogenic effect since feeding as much as 2.2 µg DES per 100 g body weight for 3 days prior to breeding and during gestation and lactation had no effect on conception or gestation in rats.[125] The stimulatory effects of estrogens on growth and improvement in feed efficiency in cattle are also well known,[126,127,128] and these effects may be due to a stimulation of appetite[129] or an increase in the production of growth hormone by

Table 11
EFFECTS OF ADMINISTERING VARIOUS DOSAGES OF AUTHENTIC ZEARALENONE IN ANIMALS

Animal	Dose	Effects	Ref.
Mouse	10 μg/g feed	Uterine hypertrophy	51
	20 μg injected	Uterine hypertrophy	52
Rat	1 mg, oral	Uterine hypertrophy	115
	0.6 mg, topical to skin	Uterine hypertrophy	115
Swine	1—50 mg daily, oral	Hypertrophy vulva, vagina, uterus and mammae; metaplasia of cervical epithelial cells	56
	100 ppm in feed	Infertility	116
	25—100 ppm in feed	Infertility, nymphomania, pseudopregnancy, reduced litter size, smaller pigs, malformations, juvenile hyperestrogenism, probable fetal resorption	117
Chicken	300—800 ppm in feed	Hypertrophy of vent. oviducts and cloacal bursa; eversion of cloaca	79
Turkey	300—800 ppm in feed	Hypertrophy of vent, oviducts and cloacal bursa; eversion of cloaca	79
Monkey	14 or 56 μg/kg injected	Stimulation, LH surge	55
	14 μg/kg injected	Serum LH depression	55
	400 μg daily, orally for 4 days	Serum LH depression	55

the anterior pituitary[130] or both. This difference in growth response to estrogens between rats and cattle may simply be due to species, but may also be due to the dosages employed, those for the rat being much greater relative to body weight and therefore may represent pharmacologic or "toxic" doses and responses.

Zearalenone has frequently been identified as "toxic" or as a mycotoxin.[29,33,35,36,52,56,79,99,107,115,116,131,132] This, in part, may be due to the use of the term "vulvovaginitis" in describing one of the effects resulting from swine eating moldy corn,[91,92,94] but as Kurtz and Mirocha accurately indicate, "vulvovaginitis" is a misnomer since no primary inflammatory changes occur in the vulva or vagina as a result of zearalenone toxicosis.[116] The first use of the term "toxin" as applied to zearalenone[132] may have been due to the common usage of that label to any fungal product or to a misunderstanding of the physiological nature of the compound. The term "fungal estrogen"[69,78] or "estrogenic metabolite"[133] is more descriptive. The first report of the existence of zearalenone was accurate in describing it as a uterotropic, anabolic agent.[28] Much of the confusion also probably stems from the production of substances by *Fusarium* molds which indeed do produce toxic effects: monoacetoxyscirpenol, diacetoxyscirpenol (associated with hemorrhagic bowel syndrome in swine), deoxynivalenol (associated with feed refusal, emesis, and bloody stools in swine), and T-2 toxin (associated with bloody stools in cattle).[33] These four compounds are included in the so-called trichothecene toxins. Therefore, reports of the death of swine eating rations with traces of zearalenone,[134] or its implication in causing abortion,[33] stillbirths, neonatal mortality, and small litters,[135] or feed refusal[136] in swine must be viewed with suspicion, since zearalenone and deoxynivalenol commonly occur in the same feed sample.[33] Toxicity and poor reproductive performance in swine eating corn inoculated with *Fusarium roseum* was said specifically not to be due to an estrogenic factor.[137,138] Detrimental effects in swine such as infertility, weakened offspring, mummified fetuses, reduced litter size, stillbirths, splay legs, and agalactia, have not been satisfactorily proven scientifically to be due to zearalenone contamination of feed.[116] Feeds which are implicated in various types of mycotoxicoses and assayed for zearalenone should also be assayed for the trichothecenes.[33] Deoxynivalenol has been positively identified as the feed refusal and emesis factor and the dosages required to produce these effects in swine have been established.[139] If present in sufficient amounts, zearalenone may cause effects detrimental to reproduction in swine: failure to conceive[56] and nymphomania, pseudopregnancy, reduced litter size, malformations, and possible fetal resorption.[117] It is unlikely that short-term exposure of swine to zearalenone will permanently impair reproduction since a gilt fed 25 mg DES for 64 days showed no ill effects from that treatment.[58]

The reports that feeding hay containing 14 ppm zearalenone caused infertility[69] or eating sorghum with 12 ppm zearalenone caused abortion[140] in cattle are subject to doubt for two reasons: (1) the rations were not assayed for the presence of the trichothecene toxins, and (2) the relatively low physiological activity of orally administered estrogens in cattle. Feeding as much as 20 mg DES per 1000 lb body weight daily to pregnant cows had no effect on pregnancy.[141] Feeding 20 mg DES daily for 148 days had no effect on subsequent fertility of heifers.[142] An intramuscular injection of 100 mg DES is required to cause abortion during the first trimester of pregnancy in cows.[143] An additional point might be considered when implicating zearalenone as a cause for infertility in cattle. A more potent estrogenic derivative of zearalenone, zearalanol (tradename, RALGRO®), is used as an anabolic agent to stimulate the growth of cattle[126] and sheep.[144] This product is administered in pellets implanted subcutaneously because the compound is ineffective by the oral route of administration. It seems unlikely therefore, that the weaker estrogen, zearalenone, would be orally active in cattle. Feeding corn which had been invaded by *Gibberella zeae* (containing 500 ppb zearalenone and which had been refused by swine) to dairy cows had no significant effect on feed consumption or milk or butterfat production.[145]

In rhesus monkeys, the subcutaneous injection of zearalenone caused a surge of the luteinizing hormone (LH) from the anterior pituitary, which is a typical estrogenic response, but was not as effective as estradiol-17β or DES in producing this effect. By subcutaneous injection, estradiol-17β was 3.5 and DES 28 times more effective than zearalenone in suppressing LH release; with oral administration, estradiol-17β was 80 and DES 160 times more effective than zearalenone in inhibiting LH release.[55]

Chickens are quite resistant to the effects of zearalenone. In birds up to 21 days of age, the only effect was hypertrophy of the oviduct in some of the females fed 800 ppm.[146] In finishing broilers and young turkeys, addition of 800 ppm zearalenone in the diet had minimal effects.[147] In mature chickens, feeding 800 ppm zearalenone to hens for 8 weeks had no effect on egg production, egg size, or fertility; feeding the same level to males had no effect on their fertility.[148]

The actual toxicity of zearalenone is very low. The LD_{50} (mg/kg) in female mice is more than 20,000; more than 10,000 in female rats; more than 5,000 in female guinea pigs.[98] It seems hardly appropriate to use the term "mycotoxin" for zearalenone. "Mycoestrogen" would be more accurate.

If phytoestrogens are present in physiologic amounts, they will cause their effects by typical estrogenic mechanisms, i.e., attached to receptors in tissues such as the vagina,[140] uterus,[48,49,53,109] and mammary glands[131] which result in the expected response. Inhibition of the hypothalamus[55,102] and the anterior pituitary[55,101] probably also results from a phytoestrogen-receptor affinity.

CARCINOGENICITY OF PHYTOESTROGENS

Since some of the plants or plant products identified in Table 7 eventually become part of the human diet, a very brief discussion of carcinogenicity of phytoestrogens is appropriate. Since estrogens are implicated in a number of malignancies, it is not surprising to find some studies conducted to determine the possible role of phytoestrogens in the induction of cancer. A possible role of *Fusarium* mycotoxins, i.e., the tricothecenes and zearalenone, in the etiology of tumors of the digestive tract and the gonads and related organs has been suggested.[150] However, using the *Salmonella*/mammalian microsome assay, coumestrol, zearalenone, daidzein, genistein, formononetin, and biochanin A were not mutagenic.[151] The oral administration of coumestrol did not appear to support the growth of chemically induced rat mammary tumors, but subcutaneous administration might.[45] Since Coumestrol and genistein can act as antiestrogens, markedly inhibiting the utero-vaginotropic effects of estradiol-17β, estrone, and DES,[152] perhaps they may actually provide some protection against estrogen-induced malignancies. Urethane combined with zearalenone or DES was able to induce lymphoma production in mice.[153] Zearalenone, coumestrol, genistein, and formononetin all bind to estrogen receptors in line MCF-7 human breast cancer cells.[46]

The carcinogenic risk of the phytoestrogens is probably related to the extent to which they are present in food, as well as their inherent biological potency. Milk from cows fed rations containing as much as 1925 μg zearalenone per kilogram did not contain any detectable quantities of the compound[154] although alpha and beta zearalenols were detected at levels from 16 to 76 ppb in the milk of a cow treated orally with (³H)-zearalenone.[155] Small amounts of zearalenone (14 μg/kg) have been detected in cornflakes[156] and in corn products such as grits, meal, flour, germ, gluten, starch, and solubles.[157] It has also been detected in corn malt, beers, sour drinks, and sour porridges (see review).[157] Whether the zearalenone contamination of these foods constitutes a hazard must be purely speculative. Reference has already been made to the low oral activity of zearalenone in monkeys.[55] Its oral activity in humans is also probably low, since 75 mg of zearalanol, which is more active than zearalenone,[53] were required to reduce the incidence of hot flashes in women who had submitted to a total abdominal hysterectomy.[158] Previous reference has been made to the small amounts of the isoflavones and coumestans present in food as well as to their low biological activity. It would seem therefore that the low amounts present plus the low oral activity of the phytoestrogens would have to be considered in any assessment of their carcinogenic hazard.

METHODS OF DETECTION AND METABOLISM OF PHYTOESTROGENS

The chemical nature[7] of the isoflavones and methods for their detection[17] have been described. Genistein and biochanin A, when administered intraruminally, are extensively metabolized and eliminated in the urine, the major excretion product being p-ethyl phenol.[159] Less than 1% of the total amount of genistein administered to sheep was excreted in the feces.[40] Intraruminal formononetin, on the other hand, did not significantly increase the concentration of urinary phenols, but was eliminated as daidzein and equol or as a small amount of unchanged formononetin.[159] The chemistry and methods of detection of coumestrol and many of its derivatives have also been described.[44]

The chemical structure of zearalenone was first described by Urry, et al.[160] Its chemical nature and that of many of its derivatives have been reviewed by Shipchandler.[161] Numerous methods for the chemical detection of zearalenone have been developed.[29,30,60,156,162] When ^{14}C-labeled zearalenone was administered orally to rats, 70 to 80% was excreted in the feces and 20 to 30% in the urine. The only significant metabolite found was zearalenol.[98] When (^{3}H)-zearalenone was given *per os* to a lactating cow, after 72 hr, 92% of the radioactivity could be accounted for in the feces which contained 93.2 ppm zearalenone metabolites, zearalenone 43.4 ppm, beta-zearalenol 38.4 ppm, and alpha-zearalenol 15.4 ppm. Radioactivity present in the urine and milk was very low.[155]

SUMMARY

The phytoestrogens, consisting of the isoflavones including biochanan A, daidzein, genistein, genistin, formononetin, pratensein; the coumestans, coumestrol and 4'-O-methylcoumestrol; and the resorcyclic acid lactones, zearalenone and zearalenol, have been shown to occur in a wide variety of plants and plant products. Since seeds such as barley, corn, oats, rice, rye, sesame, sorghum, and wheat, which are commonly used for foods or processed into food products or drinks, can serve as the substrate for the growth of the fungus *Gibberella zeae* which produces zearalenone, this phytoestrogen may be more widely distributed in foods than any of the other phytoestrogens. The signs seen in animals consuming feeds containing phytoestrogens are typical estrogenic responses: hypertrophy of the vulva, vagina, and uterus of mammalian females; the accessory glands of mammalian males; hypertrophy of the mammae and atrophy of the gonads in both sexes of mammals, and enlargement of the oviduct and vent in avian females. The degree to which these signs develop depends on the amount of phytoestrogen present, the length of time of exposure to them, and the species of animal. All these effects are usually temporary and disappear with a change to a diet free of phytoestrogens unless the animals have been exposed to a high level of the compounds for a prolonged period of time. The carcinogenic risk of phytoestrogens may be related to the degree to which they are estrogenic and the extent to which they appear in a particular food item.

REFERENCES

1. **Kahnt, L. C. and Doisy, E. A.**, The vaginal smear method of assay of the ovarian hormones, *Endocrinology*, 12, 760—768, 1928.
2. **Bulbring, E. and Burn, J. H.**, The estimation of oestrin, and male hormone in oily solution, *J. Physiol.*, 85, 320—333, 1935.
3. **Stob, M., Andrews, F. N., and Zarrow, M. X.**, The detection of residual hormone in the meat of animals treated with synthetic estrogens, *Am. J. Vet. Res.*, 15, 319—322, 1954.
4. **Morgan, C. F.**, A comparison of topical and subcutaneous methods of administration of sixteen oestrogens, *J. Endocrinol.*, 26, 317—329, 1963.
5. **Evans, J. A., Varney, R. F., and Koch, F. C.**, The mouse uterine weight method for the assay of estrogens, *Endocrinology*, 28, 747—752, 1941.
6. **Dodds, E. C. and Lawson, W.**, Molecular structure in relation to oestrogenic activity; compounds without a phenanthrene nucleus, *Proc. R. Soc. London*, B125, 222—232, 1938.
7. **Bradbury, R. B. and White, D. E.**, Estrogens and related substances in plants, in *Vitamins and Hormones*, Vol. 12, Harris, R. S., Marrian, G. F., and Thimann, K. V., Eds., Academic Press, New York, 1954, 207—230.
8. **Dodds, C.**, *Biochemical Contributions to Endocrinology*, Stanford University Press, Stanford, Calif., 1957.
9. **Bickoff, E. M., Livingston, A. L., Hendrickson, A. P., and Booth, A. N.**, Relative potencies of several estrogen-like compounds found in forages, *Agric. Food Chem.*, 10, 410—412, 1962.

10. Fisher, A. L., Keasling, H. H., and Schueler, F. W., Estrogenic action of some DDT analogues, *Proc. Soc. Exp. Biol. Med.*, 81, 439—441, 1952.
11. Welch, R. M. and Conney, A. H., Estrogenic activity of DDT and its analogs, *Fed. Proc. Fed. Am. Soc. Exp. Biol.*, 27, 649, 1968.
12. Solomon, J., Cocchia, M. A., Gray, R., Shattuck, D., and Vossmer, A., Uterotrophic effect of delta-9-tetrahydrocannabinol in ovariectomized rats, *Science*, 192, 559—561, 1976.
13. Biggers, J. D., Plant phenols possessing oestrogenic activity, in *The Pharmacology of Plant Phenolics*, Fairbairn, J. W., Ed., Academic Press, New York, 1959, 51—69.
14. Bickoff, E. M., Estrogen-like substances in plants, in *Physiology of Reproduction*, Oregon State University Press, Corvallis, 1961, 93—119.
15. Moule, G. R., Braden, A. W. H., and Lamond, D. R., This significance of oestrogens in pasture plants in relation to animal production, in *Anim. Breeding Abstr.*, 31, 139—157, 1963.
16. Stob, M., Estrogens in foods, in Toxicants Occurring Naturally in Foods, Publication 1354, National Research Council-National Academy of Sciences, Washington, D.C., 1966, 18—23.
17. Bickoff, E. M., Oestrogenic constituents of forage plants, Review Series No 1/1968, Commonwealth Agricultural Bureaux, 1968, 1—39.
18. Stob, M., Estrogens in foods, in Toxicants Occurring Naturally in Foods, 2nd ed., National Research Council-National Academy of Sciences, Washington, D.C., 1973, 550—557.
19. Ferrando, R., Guilleux, M. M., and Guerrillot-Vinet, A., Oestrogenic content of plants as a function of conditions of culture, *Nature (London)*, 192, 1205, 1961.
20. Sondheimer, E., The isolation and identification of 3-methyl-6-methoxy-8-hydroxy-3,4-dihydro iso coumarin from carrots, *J. Am. Chem. Soc.*, 79, 5036, 1957.
21. Bennett, R. D., Ko, S. T., and Heftman, E., Isolation of estrone and cholesterol from the date palm, *Phoenix dactylifera* L., *Phytochemistry*, 5, 231—235, 1966.
22. Sharaf, A. and Nighm, S. A. R., The oestrogenic activity of pomegranate seed oil, *J. Endocrinol.*, 29, 91—92, 1964.
23. Heftmann, E., Ko, S. T., and Bennett, R. D., Identification of estrone in pomegranate seeds, *Phytochemistry*, 5, 1337—1339, 1966.
24. Zondek, B. and Bergmann, E., LXXXIV. Phenol methyl esters as oestrogenic agents, *Biochem. J.*, 32, 641—645, 1938.
25. Costello, C. A. and Lynn, E. V., Estrogenic substances from plants. I. Glycyrrhiza, *J. Am. Pharm. Assoc.*, 39, 177—180, 1950.
26. Zenisek, A. and Bednar, I. J., Contribution to the identification of the estrogen activity of hops, *Am. Perfumer*, 75, 61—62, 1960.
27. Pope, G. S., Gruncy, H. M., Jones, H. E. H., and Tait, S. A. S., The oestrogenic substance (miroestrol) from the tuberous roots of *Pueraria mirifica*, *J. Endocrinol.*, 17, xv—xvi, 1958.
28. Stob, M., Baldwin, R. S., Tuite, J., Andrews, F. N., and Gillette, K. G., Isolation of an anabolic, uterotrophic compound from corn infected with *Gibberella zeae*, *Nature (London)*, 196, 1318, 1962.
29. Stoloff, L., Nesheim, S., Yin, L., Rodricks, J. V., Stack, M., and Campbell, A. D., A multimycotoxin detection method for aflatoxins, ochratoxins, zearalenone, sterigmatocystin, and patulin, *J. Assoc. Off. Anal. Chem.*, 54, 91—97, 1971.
30. Josefsson, B. G. E. and Moller, T. E., Screening method for the detection of aflatoxins, ochratoxin, patulin, sterigmatocystin and zearalenone in cereals, *J. Assoc. Off. Anal. Chem.*, 60, 1369—1371, 1977.
31. Eugenio, C. P., Christensen, C. H., and Mirocha, C. J., Factors affecting production of the mycotoxin F-2 by *Fusarium roseum*, *Phytopathology*, 60, 1055—1057, 1970.
32. Mirocha, C. J., Schauerhamer, B., Christensen, C. M., Niku-Paavola, M. L., and Nummi, M., Incidence of zearalenol (*Fusarium* mycotoxin) in animal food, *Appl. Environ. Microbiology*, 38, 749—750, 1979.
33. Mirocha, C. J., Pathre, S. V., Schauerhamer, B., and Christensen, C. M., Natural occurrence of *Fusarium* toxins in feedstuffs, *Appl. Environ. Microbiol.*, 32, 553—556, 1976.
34. Schroeder, H. W. and Hein, H., Jr., A note on zearalenone in grain sorghum, *Cereal Chem.*, 52, 751—752, 1975.
35. Stoloff, L., Report on mycotoxins, *J. Assoc. Off. Anal. Chem.*, 61, 340—346, 1978.
36. Shotwell, O. L., Goulden, M. L., Bennett, G. A., Plattner, R. D., and Hesseltine, C. W., Mycotoxins. Survey of 1975 wheat and soybeans for aflatoxin, zearalenone, and ochratoxin, *J. Assoc. Off. Anal. Chem.*, 60, 778—783, 1977.
37. Wada, H. and Yuhara, M., Identification of plant estrogens in Chinese milk vetch, soybean and soybean sprout, *Jpn. J. Zootech. Sci.*, 35, 87—91, 1964.
38. Hassan, A., Elghamry, M., and Zayed, S., β-sitosterol as a phytoestrogen, *Naturwissenschaften*, Heft 17, 409—410, 1964.
39. Cheng, E. W., Yoder, L., Story, C. D., and Burroughs, W., Estrogenic activity of some naturally occurring isoflavones, *Ann. N.Y. Acad. Sci.*, 61, 637—736, 1955.

40. Braden, A. W. H., Hart, N. K., and Lamberton, J. A., The oestrogenic activity and metabolism of certain isoflavones in sheep, *Aust. J. Agric. Res.*, 18, 335—348, 1967.
41. Wong, W., Isoflavone contents of red and subterranean clovers, *J. Sci. Food Agric.*, 14, 376—379, 1963.
42. Bickoff, E. M., Booth, A. N., Lyman, R. L., Livingston, A. L., Thompson, C. R., and Deeds, F., Coumestrol, a new estrogen isolated from forage crops, *Science,* 126, 969—970, 1957.
43. Bickoff, E. M., Livingston, A. L., Witt, S. C., Lundin, R. E., and Spencer, R. R., New alfalfa compound identified, isolation of 4'-O-methylcoumestrol from alfalfa, *J. Agric. Food Chem.*, 13, 597—599, 1965.
44. Bickoff, E. M., Livingston, A. L., and Booth, A. N., Estrogenic activity of coumestrol and related compounds, *Arch. Biochem. Biophys.*, 88, 262—266, 1960.
45. Verdeal, K., Brown, R. R., Richardson, T., and Ryan, D. S., Affinity of phytoestrogens for the estradiol-binding proteins and effect of coumestrol on growth of 7,12-dimethylbenz(A) anthracene-induced rat mammary tumors, *J. Natl. Cancer Inst.*, 64(1), 285—290, 1980.
46. Martin, P. M., Horwitz, K. B., Ryan, D. S., and McGuire, W. L., Phytoestrogen interaction with estrogen receptors in human breast cancer cells, *Endocrinology,* 103, 1860—1867, 1978.
47. Underwood, E. J., Shier, F. L., and Peterson, J. E., The effects of prolonged injections of stilboestrol in the ewe, *Aust. Vet. J.*, 29, 206—211, 1953.
48. Shemesh, M., Lindner, H. R., and Ayalon, N., Affinity of rabbit uterine oestradiol receptor of phyto-estrogens and its use in competitive protein-binding radioassay for plasma coumestrol, *J. Reprod. Fertil.*, 29, 1—9, 1972.
49. Shutt, D. A. and Cox, R. I., Steroid and phyto-oestrogen binding to sheep uterine receptors in vitro, *J. Endocrinol.*, 52, 299—310, 1972.
50. Lee, Y. I., Notides, C. A., Tsay, Y., and Kende, D. S., Coumestrol, NDB-norhexestrol, and dansyl-norhexestrol, fluorescent probes of estrogen-binding proteins, *Biochemistry,* 16(4), 2896—2910, 1977.
51. Stob, M., unpublished data.
52. Mirocha, C. J., Christensen, C. M., and Nelson, G. H., Toxic metabolites produced by fungi implicated in mycotoxicoses, *Biotech. Bioeng.*, 10, 469—482, 1968.
53. Katzenellenbogen, B. S., Katzenellenbogen, J. A., and Mordecai, D., Zearalenones: characterization of the estrogenic potencies and receptor interactions of a series of fungal β-resorcyclic acid lactones, *Endocrinology,* 105, 33—40, 1979.
54. Chi, M. S., Mirocha, C. J., Weaver, G. A., and Kurtz, H. J., The acute effect of zearalenone on the White Leghorn female, *Appl. Environ. Microbiol.*, 39, 1026—1030, 1980.
55. Hobson, W., Bailer, J., and Fuller, G. B., Hormone effects of zearalenone in nonhuman primates, *J. Toxicol. Environ. Health,* 3, 43—57, 1977.
56. Kurtz, H. J., Nairn, M. E., Nelson, G. H., Christensen, C. M., and Mirocha, C. J., Histologic changes in the genital tracts of swine fed estrogenic mycotoxin, *Am. J. Vet. Res.*, 30, 551—556, 1969.
57. Beeson, W. M., Andrews, F. N., Perry, T. W., and Stob, M., The effect of orally administered stilbestrol and testosterone on growth and carcass composition of swine, *J. Anim. Sci.*, 14, 475—481, 1955.
58. Stevenson, J. W. and Ellis, N. R., Effects on reproductive functions of diethylstilbestrol administered orally to gilts, *J. Appl. Physiol.*, 5, 549—554, 1953.
59. Mirocha, C. J. and Christensen, C. M., Oestrogenic mycotoxins synthesized by *Fusarium,* in *Mycotoxins,* Purchase, I, F. H., Ed., Elsevier, Amsterdam, 1974, 129—148.
60. Peters, C. A., Photochemistry of zearalenone and its derivatives, *J. Med. Chem.*, 15, 867—868, 1972.
61. Guggolz, J., Livingston, A. L., and Bickoff, E. M., Forage estrogens, detection of daidzein, formononetin, genistein and biochanin A in forages, *Agric. Food Chem.*, 9, 330—332, 1961.
62. Loper, G. M., Accumulation of coumestrol in barrel medic *(Medicago littoralis),* *Crop Sci.*, 8, 317—319, 1968.
63. Sanger, V. L., Engle, P. H., and Bell, D. S., Evidence of estrogenic stimulation in anestrous ewes pastured on ladino clover and birdsfoot trefoil, as revealed by vaginal smears, *Am. J. Vet. Res.*, 19, 228—294, 1958.
64. Siddigui, S., Studies in the constituents of chana (*Cicer arietinum* L.). I. Isolation of 3 new crystalline products of the chana germ, *J. Sci. Indian Res.*, 3, 68—70, 1945.
65. Wong, E., Mortimer, P. I., and Geissman, T. A., Flavonoid constituents of *Cicer arietinum, Phytochemistry,* 4, 89—9, 1965.
66. Francis, C. M., Millington, A. J., and Bailey, E. T., The distribution of oestrogenic isoflavones in the genus *Trifolium, Aust. J. Agric. Res.*, 18, 47—54, 1967.
67. Francis, C. M. and Millington A. J., Varietal variation in the isoflavone content of subterranean clover: its estimation by a microtechnique, *Aust. J. Agric. Res.*, 16, 557—564, 1965.

68. Lyman, R. L., Bickoff, E. M., Booth, A. N., and Livingston, A. L., Detection of coumestrol in leguminous plants, *Arch. Biochem. Biophys.*, 80, 61—67, 1959.
69. Mirocha, C. J., Harrison, J., Nichols, A. A., and McClintock, M., Detection of a fungal estrogen (F-2) in hay associated with infertility in dairy cattle, *Appl. Microbiol.*, 16, 797—798, 1968.
70. Walz, E., Isoflavones and saponin glucosides in *Soja hispida*, *Just. Liebigs Ann. Chem.*, 489, 118—115, 1931.
71. Walter, E. D., Genistin (an isoflavone glycoside) and its aglucone, genistein, from soybeans, *J. Am. Chem. Soc.*, 63, 3273—3276, 1941.
72. Booth, A. N., Bickoff, E. M., and Kohler, G. O., Estrogen-like activity in vegetable oils and mill by-products, *Science*, 131, 1807—1808, 1960.
73. Sharaf, A. and Negm, S., Oestrogenic activity of *Zea mays* oil, *Qual. Plant. Mater. Veg.*, 22, 249—252, 1973.
74. Clevenger, S., Flower pigments, *Sci. Am.*, 210, 84—92, 1964.
75. Ehrlech, P. R. and Raven, P. H., Butterflies and plants, *Sci. Am.*, 216, 104—113, 1967.
76. Francis, C. M. and Hume, I. D., The relationship between lignification and flavonoid production in subterranean clover, *Aust. J. Biol. Sci.*, 24, 1—5, 1971.
77. Floss, H. G. and Mothes, U., On the biosynthesis of furocoumarins in *Pimpinella magna*, *Phytochemistry*, 5, 161—169, 1966.
78. Mirocha, C. J., Christensen, C. M., and Nelson, G. H., Physiologic activity of some fungal estrogens produced by *Fusarium*, *Cancer Res.*, 28, 2319—2322, 1968.
79. Mirocha, C. J., Christensen, C. M., and Nelson, G. H., F-2 (zearalenone) estrogenic mycotoxin from *Fusarium*, in *Microbial Toxins*, Vol. 7, Kadis, S., Ciegler, A., and Ajl, S. J., Eds., Academic Press, New York, 1971, 107—138.
80. Stob, M., Davis, R. L., and Andrews, F. N., Strain differences in the estrogenicity of alfalfa, *J. Anim. Sci.*, 16, 850—853, 1957.
81. Morley, F. H. W. and Francis, C. M., Varietal and environmental variations in isoflavone concentrations in subterranean clover (*Trifolium subterraneum* L.), *Aust. J. Agric. Res.*, 19, 15—26, 1968.
82. Hanson, C. H., Loper, G. M., Kohler, G. O., Bickoff, E. M., Taylor, K. W., Kehr, W. R., Stanford, E. H., Dudley, J. W., Pedersen, M. W., Sorensen, E. L., Carnahan, H. L., and Wilsie, C. P., Variation in coumestrol content of alfalfa as related to location, variety, cutting year, stage of growth, and disease, Tech. Bull. 1333, U. S. Department of Agriculture, Washington, D.C., 1965.
83. Rossiter, R. C. and Beck, A. B., Physiological and ecological studies on the oestrogenic isoflavones in subterranean clover (*T. subterraneum* L.), *Aust. J. Agric. Res.*, 18, 561—573, 1967.
84. Noveroske, R. L., Kuc, J., and Williams, E. B., Oxidation of phloridzin and phloretin related to resistance of *Malus* to *Venturia inaequalis*, *Phytopathology*, 54, 92—97, 1964.
85. Noveroske, R. L., Williams, E. B., and Kuc, J., β-glycosidase and phenoloxidase in apple leaves and their possible relation to resistance to *Venturia inaequalis*, *Phytopathology*, 54, 98—103, 1964.
86. Sherwood, R. T., Olah, A. F., Oleson, W. H., and Jones, E. E., Effect of disease and injury on accumulation of a flavonoid estrogen, coumestrol, in alfalfa, *Phytopathology*, 60, 684—688, 1970.
87. Loper, G. M. and Hanson, C. H., Influence of controlled environmental factors and two foliar pathogens on coumestrol in alfalfa, *Crop Sci.*, 4, 480—482, 1964.
88. Loper, G. M., Hanson, C. H., and Graham, J. H., Coumestrol content of alfalfa as affected by selection for resistance to foliar disease, *Crop. Sci.*, 7, 1189—192, 1967.
89. Loper, G. M., Effect of aphid infestation on the coumestrol content of alfalfa varieties differing in aphid resistance, *Crop Sci.*, 8, 104—106, 1968.
90. Stuthman, D. D., Bickoff, E. M., Davis, R. L., and Stob, M., Coumestrol differences in *Medicago sativa* L. free of foliar disease symptoms, *Crop Sci.*, 6, 333—334, 1966.
91. McNutt, S. H., Purwin, P., and Murray, C., Vulvovaginitis in swine, *J. Am. Vet. Med. Assoc.*, 73, 484, 1928.
92. Pullar, E. M. and Lerew, W. M., Vulvovaginitis of swine, *Aust. Vet. J.*, 13, 28, 1937.
93. Koen, J. S. and Smith, H. C., An unusual case of genital involvement in swine associated with eating moldy corn, *Vet. Med.*, 40, 131—133, 1945.
94. McErlean, B. A., Vulvovaginitis of swine, *Vet. Res.*, 64, 539, 1952.
95. Caldwell, R. W. and Tuite, J., Zearalenone production in field corn in Indiana, *Phytopathology*, 60, 1696—1697, 1970.
96. Caldwell, R. W. and Tuite, J., Zearalenone in freshly harvested corn, *Phytopathology*, 64, 752—753, 1974.
97. Caldwell, R. W., Tuite, J., Stob, M., and Baldwin, R. S., Zearalenone production by *Fusarium* species, *Appl. Microbiol.*, 20, 31—34, 1970.
98. Hidy, P. H., Baldwin, R. S., Greasham, R. L., Keith, C. L., and McMullen, J. R., Zearalenone and some derivatives: production and biological activities, *Adv. Appl. Microbiol.*, 22, 59—82, 1977.

99. Hurd, R. N., Structure activity relationships in zearalenones, in *Mycotoxins in Human and Animal Health,* Rodricks, J. V., Hesseltine, C. W., and Mehlman, M. A., Eds., Pathotox, Park Forest South, Ill., 1977, 379—391.
100. Patton, T. L. and Dmochowski, L., Estrogens. V. Studies on the relationship of estrogenic activity and molecular structure, *Arch. Biochem. Biophys.,* 101, 181—185, 1963.
101. Leavitt, W. W. and Wright, P. A., The plant estrogen, coumestrol, as an agent affecting hypophysial gonadotropin function, *J. Exp. Zool.,* 160, 319—327, 1965.
102. Adams, N. R., Sexual behaviour responses of the ovariectomized ewe to oestradiol benzoate, and their persistent reduction after exposure to phyto-oestrogens, *J. Reprod. Fertil.,* 53, 203—208, 1978.
103. Frank, N. A., Sanger, V. L., Pounden, W. D., Pratt, A. D., and VanKeuren, R., Forage estrogens and their possible influence on bovine mastitis, *J. Am. Vet. Med. Assoc.,* 150, 503—507, 1967.
104. Wright, P. A., Infertility in rabbits induced by feeding ladino clover, *Proc. Soc. Exp. Biol. Med.,* 105, 428—430, 1960.
105. Leavitt, W. W., and Wright, P. A., Effect of legumes on reproduction in mice, *J. Reprod. Fertil.,* 6, 115—123, 1963.
106. Leopold, A. S., Erwin, M., Oh, J., and Browning, B., Phytoestrogens: adverse effects on reproduction in California quail, *Science,* 191, 98—99, 1976.
107. Mirocha, C. J., Pathre, S. V., and Christensen, C. M., Zearalenone, in *Mycotoxins in Human and Animal Health,* Rodricks, J. V., Hesseltine, C. W. and Mehlman, M. A., Eds., Pathotox, Park Forest South, Ill., 1977, 345—364.
108. East, J., The effect of genistein on the fertility of mice, *J. Endocrinol.,* 13, 94—100, 1956.
109. Shutt, D. A., Interaction of genistein with oestradiol in the reproductive tract of the ovariectomized mouse, *J. Endocrinol.,* 37, 231—232, 1967.
110. Carter, M. W., Matrone, G., and Smart, W. W. G., Jr., Effect of genistin on reproduction of the mouse, *J. Nutr.,* 55, 639—645, 1955.
111. Matrone, G., Smart, W. W. G., Jr., Carter, M. W., Smart, V. W., and Garren, H. W., Effect of genistin on growth and development of the male mouse, *J. Nutr.,* 59, 235—241, 1956.
112. Leavitt, W. W. and Meismer, D. M., Effect on female rat development of nonsteroidal oestrogens, *Nature (London),* 218, 181—182, 1968.
113. Noteboom, W. D. and Gorski, J., Estrogenic effects of genistein and coumestrol diacetate, *Endocrinology,* 73, 736—739, 1963.
114. Magee, A. C., Biological responses of young rats fed diets containing genistin and genistein, *J. Nutr.,* 80, 151—156, 1963.
115. Mirocha, C. J., Pathre, S. V., and Christensen, C. M., Chemistry of *Fusarium* toxins, in *Mycotoxic Fungi, Mycotoxins and Mycotoxicoses,* Vol. 1, Wyllie, T. D. and Morehouse, L. G., Eds., Marcel Dekker, New York, 1977, 365—420.
116. Kurtz, H. J. and Mirocha, C. J., Zearalenone (F-2) induced estrogen syndrome in swine, in *Mycotoxic Fungi, Mycotoxins and Mycotoxicoses,* Vol. 2, Wyllie, T. D. and Morehouse, L. G., Eds., Marcel Dekker, New York, 1977, 256—268.
117. Chang, K., Kurtz, H. J., and Mirocha, C. J., Effect of the mycotoxin zearalenone on swine reproduction, *Am. J. Vet. Res.,* 40, 1260—1267, 1979.
118. Bartlett, S., Folley, S. J., Rowland, S. J., Curnow, D. H., and Simpson, S. A., Oestrogens in grasses and their possible effects on milk production, *Nature (London),* 162, 845, 1948.
119. Pope, G. S., McNaughton, M. J., and Jones, H. E. H., Oestrogens in British pasture plants, *J. Dairy Res.,* 26, 196—202, 1959.
120. Oldfield, J. E., Fox, C. W., Bahn, A. V., Bickoff, E. M., and Kohler, G. O., Coumestrol in alfalfa as a factor in growth and carcass quality in lambs, *J. Anim. Sci.,* 25, 167—174, 1966.
121. Stob, M., Beeson, W. M., Perry, T. W., and Mohler, M. T., Effects of coumestrol in combination with implanted and orally administered diethylstilbestrol on gains and tissue residues in cattle, *J. Anim. Sci.,* 27, 1638—1642, 1968.
122. Noble, R. L., Effects of continuous oral administration of aqueous diethylstilbestrol to rats, *J. Endocrinol.,* 1, 128—141, 1939.
123. Hartsook, E. W. and Magruder, N. D., Actions of diethylstilbestrol in the albino rat, *Am. J. Physiol.,* 190, 255—258, 1957.
124. Sullivan, L. W. and Smith, T. C., Influence of estrogens on body growth and food intake, *Proc. Soc. Exp. Biol. Med.,* 96, 60—64, 1957.
125. Browning, C. B., Parrish, D. B., and Fountaine, F. C., Effect of feeding low levels of diethylstilbestrol on gestation and lactation of rats, *J. Nutr.,* 66, 321—332, 1958.
126. Perry, T. W., Stob, M., Huber, D. A., and Peterson, R. C., Effect of subcutaneous implantation of resorcyclic acid lactone on performance of growing and finishing beef cattle, *J. Anim. Sci.,* 31, 789—793, 1970.

127. Dinusson, W. E., Andrews, F. N., and Beeson, W. M., The effects of stilbestrol, testosterone, thyroid alteration and spaying on the growth and fattening of beef heifers, *J. Anim. Sci.*, 9, 321—330, 1950.
128. Burroughs, W., Culbertson, C. C., Kastelic, J., Cheng, E., and Hale, W. W., The effects of trace amounts of diethylstilbestrol in rations of fattening steers, *Science*, 120, 66, 1953.
129. Wallentine, M. V., Drain, J. J., Wellington, G. H., and Miller, J. I., Some effects on beef carcasses from feeding stilbestrol, *J. Anim. Sci.*, 20, 792—795, 1961.
130. Steumpler, A. W. and Burroughs, W., Stilbestrol feeding and growth hormone stimulation in immature ruminants, *J. Anim. Sci.*, 18, 427—436, 1959.
131. Greenman, D. L., Wittliff, J. L., Boyd, P. A., Mehta, R. G., and Jefferson, A. R., Interaction of *Fusarium* mycotoxins with estradiol binding sites in target tissues, *J. Toxicol. Environ. Health*, 3, 348—349, 1977.
132. Christensen, C. M., Nelson, G. H., and Mirocha, C. J., Effect on the white rat uterus of a toxic substance isolated from *Fusarium*, *Appl. Microbiol.*, 13, 653—659, 1965.
133. Mirocha, C. J., Christensen, C. M., and Nelson, G. H., Estrogenic metabolite produced by *Fusarium graminearum* in stored corn, *Appl. Microbiol.*, 15, 497—503, 1967.
134. Shreeve, B. J., Patterson, D. S. P., and Roberts, B. A., Investigation of suspected cases of mycotoxicosis in farm animals in Britain, *Vet. Rec.*, 97, 275—278, 1975.
135. Miller, J. K., Hacking, A., Harrison, J., and Gross, V. J., Stillbirths, neonatal mortality, and small litters in pigs associated with the ingestion of *Fusarium* toxin by pregnant sows, *Vet. Rec.*, 93, 555—559, 1973.
136. Kotsonic, F. N., Smalley, E. B., Ellison, R. A., and Gale, C. M., Feed refusal factors in pure cultures of *Fusarium roseum* "graminearum", *Appl. Microbiol.*, 30, 362—368, 1975.
137. Sharda, C. D. P., Wilson, R. F., Williams, L. E., Swiger, L. A., and Cross, R. F., Mold toxicity in swine and laboratory animals: effect of feeding corn inoculated with pure cultures of *Fusarium roseum* Ohio isolate, *J. Anim. Sci.*, 32, 1169—1173, 1971.
138. Sharma, V. D., Wilson, R. F., and Williams, L. E., Reproductive performance of female swine fed corn naturally molded or inoculated with *Fusarium roseum*, Ohio isolates B and C, *J. Anim. Sci.*, 38, 598—602, 1974.
139. Forsyth, D. M., Yoshizawa, T., Morooka, N., and Tuite, J., Emetic and refusal activity of deoxynivalenol to swine, *Appl. Environ. Microbiol.*, 34, 547—552, 1977.
140. Mirocha, C. J., Schauerhamer, B., and Pathre, S. V., Isolation, detection, and quantitation of zearalenone in maize and barley, *J. Assoc. Off. Anal. Chem.*, 57, 1104—1110, 1974.
141. Browning, C. B., Marion, G. B., Fountaine, F. C., and Gier, H. T., Some effects of feeding diethylstilbestrol to dairy cattle, *J. Dairy Sci.*, 39, 924, 1956.
142. Reuber, H. W., Effects of diethylstilbestrol feeding on the bovine reproductive tract, *Am. J. Vet. Res.*, 19, 585—590, 1958.
143. Hill, H. J. and Pierson, R. E., Repositol diethylstilbestrol as an abortifacient in feedlot heifers, *J. Am. Vet. Med. Assoc.*, 132, 507—512, 1958.
144. Wilson, L. L., Borger, M. L., Peterson, A. D., and Rugh, M. C., and Orley, C. F., Effects of zeranol, dietary protein level and methionine hydroxy analog on growth and carcass characters and certain blood metabolites in lambs, *J. Anim. Sci.*, 35, 128—132, 1972.
145. Noller, C. H., Stob, M., and Tuite, J., Effects of feeding *Gibberella zeae* infected corn on feed intake, body weight gain, and milk production of dairy cows, *J. Dairy Sci.*, 62, 1003—1006, 1979.
146. Chi, M. S., Mirocha, C. J., Kurtz, H. J., Weaver, G. A., Bates, F., Robison, T., and Shimoda, W., Effect of dietary zearalenone on growing broiler chicks, *Poultry Sci.*, 59, 531—536, 1980.
147. Allen, N. K., Mirocha, C. J., Weaver, G., Aakhus-Allen, S., and Bates, F., Effects of dietary zearalenone on finishing broiler chickens and young turkey poults, *Poultry Sci.*, 60, 124—131, 1981.
148. Allen, N. K., Aakhus-Allen, S., and Mirocha, C. J., Effect of zearalenone on reproduction of chickens, *Poultry Sci.*, 59, 1577, 1980.
149. Payne, D. W. and Katzenellenbogen, J. A., Differential effects of estrogens in tissues: a comparison of estrogen receptor in rabbit uterus and vagina, *Endocrinology*, 106, 1345—1352, 1980.
150. Schoental, R., The role of *Fusarium* mycotoxins in the aetiology of tumours of the digestive tract and of certain other organs in man and animals, *Front. Gastrointest. Res.*, 4, 17—24, 1979.
151. Bartholomew, R. M. and Ryan, D. S., Lack of mutagenicity of some phytoestrogens in the Salmonella/mammalian microsome assay, *Mut. Res.*, 78(4), 317—321, 1980.
152. Folman, Y. and Pope, G. S., The interaction in the immature mouse of potent estrogens with coumestrol, genistein and other utero-vaginotrophic compounds of low potency, *J. Endocrinol.*, 34, 215—225, 1966.
153. Bojan, F. and Kertai, P., Induction of lymphomas by urethane in combination with zearalenone (meeting abstract), 5th Meeting of the European Assoc. for Cancer Res., Vienna, Austria, Sept. 9—12, 1979, 52.

154. Shreeve, B. J., Patterson, D. S., and Roberts, B. A., The "carry-over" of aflatoxin, ochratoxin and zearalenone from naturally contaminated feed to tissues, urine and milk of dairy cows, *Food Cosmet. Toxicol.,* 17(2), 151—152, 1979.
155. Mirocha, C. J., Distribution of metabolism of (^{3}H)-zearalenone in a lactating cow, Abstr. 207, 72nd Meeting, American Oil Chemists' Society, May 17—21, 1981.
156. Scott, P. M., Panalaks, T., Kanhere, S., and Miles, W. F., Determination of zearalenone in cornflakes and other corn-based foods by thin layer chromatography, high pressure liquid chromatography, and gas-liquid chromatography/high resolution mass spectrometry, *J. Assoc. Off. Anal. Chem.,* 61, 593—600, 1978.
157. Bennett, G. A. and Shotwell, O. L., Zearalenone in cereal grains, *J. Am. Oil Chem. Soc.,* 56(2), 812—819, 1979.
158. Utian, W. H., Comparative trial of P1496, a new non-steroidal oestrogen analogue, *Br. Med. J.,* 1, 579—581, 1973.
159. Batterham, T. J., Hart, N. K., Lamberton, J. A., and Braden, A. W. H., Metabolism of oestrogenic isoflavones in sheep, *Nature (London),* 206, 509, 1965.
160. Urry, W. H., Wehrmeister, H. L., Hodge, E. B., and Hidy, P. H., The structure of zearalenone, *Tetrahedron Lett.,* 27, 3109—3114, 1966.
161. Shipchandler, M. T., Chemistry of zearalenone and some of its derivatives, *Heterocycles,* 3, 471—520, 1975.
162. Shotwell, O. L., Assay methods for zearalenone and its natural occurrence, in *Mycotoxins in Human and Animal Health,* Rodricks, J. V., Hesseltine, C. W., and Mehlman, M. A., Eds., Pathotox, Park Forest South, Ill., 1977, 403—413.

NATURALLY OCCURRING FOOD TOXICANTS: GOITROGENS

Pavel Langer

A number of organic compounds of different structure and inorganic ions can specifically influence certain steps of intrathyroidal or extrathyroidal metabolism of iodide or thyroid hormones. After a single or short-term administration they depress various thyroid functions without increasing the thyroid weight — from this phenomenon comes the common term *antithyroid compounds*. Maintenance of an effective concentration of these antithyroid drugs for a sufficient time will result in a decrease of thyroid hormone level in blood which will further result in an increase of thyrotropic hormone secretion from the pituitary and this will cause thyroid hypertrophy or goiter. This phenomenon gave rise to another common term for these compounds — *goitrogens*. Theoretically, every antithyroid compound can be goitrogenic under appropriate conditions. Some of them exert their effect as part of a general toxic (e.g., nitriles, cyanide) or metabolic inhibitory action (e.g., antibiotics). However, only a few possessing sufficient antithyroid activity at concentrations which do not have any harmful effects on other tissues have been selected for therapeutic use. Several other compounds are of interest because they are employed primarily as therapeutic agents for "nonthyroid" diseases.

It has been definitely established that some plants representing an important part of human or domestic animal nutrition may contain precursors giving a rise of antithyroid compounds in the organism. In addition, some of these compounds may be transferred to milk or retained in meat which contribute to a further increase of total intake of goitrogenic material by man. These compounds are called *naturally occurring goitrogens*.

The first report on the effect of diet on the development of extremely large goiters came in 1928 when Chesney et al.[1] concluded that goiter in their colony of rabbits was produced by cabbage. The pioneer work on synthetic antithyroid compounds has been done by Astwood,[2,3] who also found the first naturally occurring goitrogen — vinyl-oxazolidine-2-thione.[4] Since that time the problem of naturally occurring goitrogens has been repeatedly reviewed from physiological[5-12,226] or phytochemical view.[12-20,42,66-68]

BIOCHEMISTRY OF NATURALLY OCCURRING GOITROGENS IN PLANTS

Glucosinolates

General

Glucosinolates (mustard oil glucosides or thioglucosides) represent a specific species of natural compounds occurring predominantly in Crucifers, but also in several other families.[14] Their definite structure (Figure 3) was established as S-glucopyranoside of thiohydroximyl-O-sulfate.[21,22] Today, more than 70 glucosinolates are known,[14,16] a brief outline of those most widespread being presented in Tables 1 and 2. The presence of glucosinolates is presumably determined genetically, the seeds containing much higher concentrations than the green parts. Rapeseed — the best understood — contains an average of 35% of oil, 35% of protein, and 1 to 3% of glucosinolates. The same glucosinolates are also found in green parts of the appropriate species, being distributed diffusely throughout the parenchymatous tissue. The glucosides are hydrolyzed by myrosinase (thioglucoside glucohydrolase or thioglucosidase — E.C. 3.2.3.1.) which, in green parts is located in special cells — idioblasts.[227] Thus, the contact of the enzyme with the glucoside occurs only after the disintegration of the tissue. The content of glucosinolates in cabbage — the best understood of Crucifer plants — is presented in Table 2.

Table 1
GOITROGENIC ACTIVITY OF SOME MORE IMPORTANT NATURAL ISOTHIOCYANATES

Glucosinolate (nonchemical names)[a]	R[b]	Aglucone	Goitrogenic activity tested (ref. numbers)
Glucocapparin	CH_3-	Methyl-ITC	139
Sinigrin	$CH_2=CH-CH_2-$	Allyl-ITC	25, 139-142, 157
Gluconapin	$CH_2=CH(CH_2)_2-$	3-Butenyl-ITC	
Glucobrassicanapin	$CH_2=CH(CH_2)_3-$	4-Pentenyl-ITC	
Glucotropaeolin	$C_6H_5-CH_2-$	Benzyl-ITC	
Sinalbin	$p\text{-}HO-C_6H_4-CH_2-$	p-Hydroxy-benzyl-ITC	155
Glucoibervirin	$CH_3-S-(CH_2)_3-$	3-Methyl-thio-propyl-ITC	
Glucoerucin	$CH_3-S-(CH_2)_4-$	4-Methyl-thio-butyl-ITC	
Glucoberteroin	$CH_3-S-(CH_2)_5-$	5-Methyl-thio-pentyl-ITC	
Glucoiberin	$CH_3-SO-(CH_2)_3-$	3-Methyl-sulfinyl-propyl-ITC	
Glucoraphanin	$CH_3-SO-(CH_2)_4-$	4-Methyl-sulfinyl-butyl-ITC	
Glucoallysin	$CH_3-SO-(CH_2)_5-$	5-Methyl-sulfinyl-pentyl-ITC	
Glucocheirolin	$CH_3-SO_2-(CH_2)_3-$	3-Methyl-sulfonyl-propyl-ITC	
Gluconasturtiin	$C_6H_5-(CH_2)_2-$	2-Phenyl-ethyl-ITC	

[a] According to recently proposed nomenclature, the trivial nonchemical names are replaced by names consisting of a name of R- and -glucosinolate (e.g., glucocapparin = methyl-glucosinolate).
[b] For a full structure see Figures 1 to 4.

Table 2
OXAZOLIDINE-2-THIONES DERIVED FROM NATURAL MATERIAL AND THEIR GOITROGENIC ACTIVITY

Glucosinolate (nonchemical name)	Aglucone	Natural occurrence	Ref. Isolation	Ref. Goitrogenic activity
Progoitrin	L-5-Vinyl-oxazolidine-2-thione	Several species of *Brassica*	4, 13, 58, 59	4, 12, 25, 57, 103, 138, 140, 142, 145, 160
Glucoconringiin	L-5-Dimethyl-oxazolidine-2-thione	*Conringia orientalis* *Cochlearia* *Limnanthes*	60, 105	25
Glucobarbarin	L-5-Phenyl-oxazolidine-2-thione	*Barbarea vulgaris* *Reseda luteola*	219, 220	158
Glucocleomin	L-5-Ethyl-methyl-oxazolidine-2-thione	*Cleome spinosa*	221	
Glucosisymbrin	D-4-Methyl-oxazolidine-2-thione	*Sisymbrium austriacum*	222	
Glucosisaustricin	D-4-Ethyl-oxazolidine-2-thione	*Sisymbrium austriacum*	223	
epi-Progoitrin	D-5-Vinyl-oxazolidine-2-thione	*Crambe abyss.*	224	
unknown	L-5-Allyl-oxazolidine-2-thione	*Brassica napus*	225	

Biosynthesis

Some authors suggested that amino acids may be precursors of the aglucone moiety of glucosinolates (Table 1).[22,28] Later, the incorporation of phenylalanine into aromatic isothiocyanates and of glycine into allylisothiocyanate had been reported.[29] In addition, methionine was found to be incorporated to Sinigrin[30] and homomethionine was

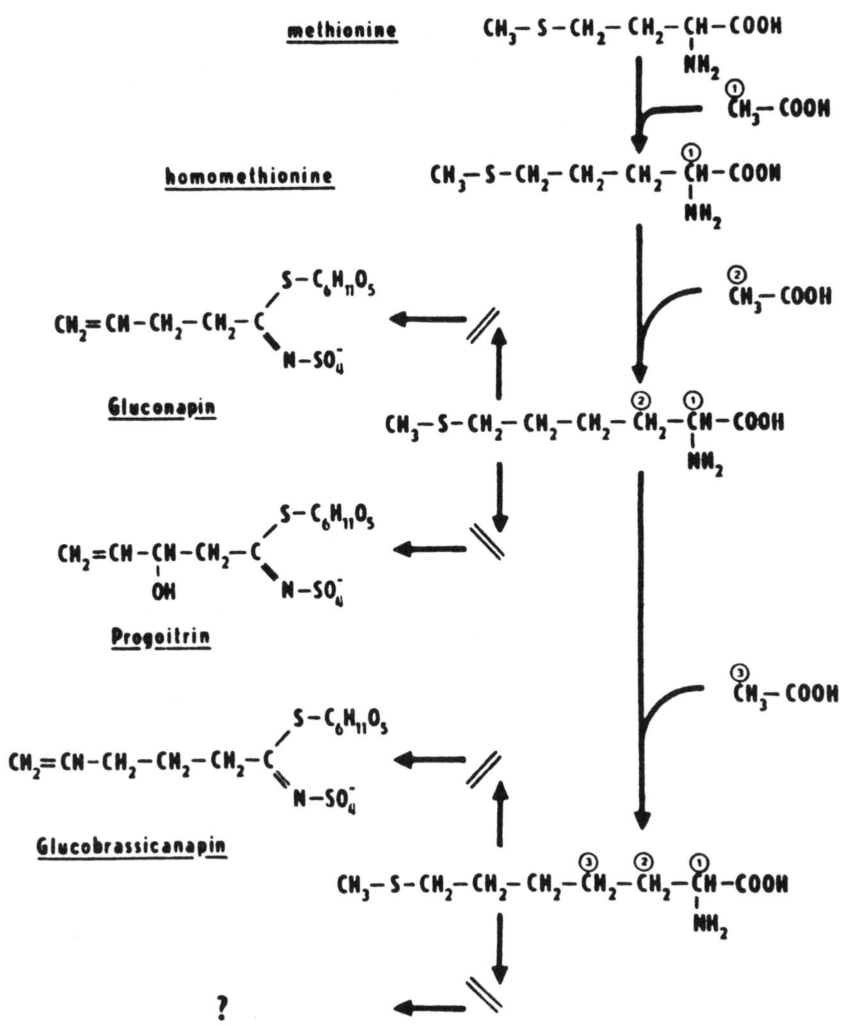

FIGURE 1. Biosynthesis of major glucosinolates in *Brassica napus* L. (From Langer, P. and Greer, M. A., *Antithyroid Substances and Naturally Occurring Goitrogens,* S. Karger, Basel, 1977, 117. With permission.)

suggested to be a direct precursor of the latter glucosinolate when arising from a condensation of methionine and malonic acid.[31] Similar mechanism was reported also for the biosynthesis of Progoitrin (Figure 1).[32] Some problems of glucosinolate biosynthesis have been studied in more detail[33-36] and recently reviewed;[15] the important role of methionine and acetate as sources of the carbon skeleton being stressed (Figure 1). The idea that aldehyde oximes are precursors of glucosinolates (Figure 2) resulted first from the finding of the incorporation of phenylalanine into benzylglucosinolate via phenylacetaldehyde oxime.[37] Such a pathway was later supported and similar biosynthesis of cyanogenic glucosides has been proposed too.[38] The origin of thioglucosyl group was also demonstrated, the thiohydroximide being first glucosilated to form glucothiohydroximic acid (Figure 3) and *N*-sulfate ester being formed.[31] The sulfur moiety of glucosinolate molecule is derived from sulfate or organic sulfur compounds (methionine, cysteine, thioglucose).[40,41] About 80% of labeled sulfur of ^{35}S-labeled methionine, cysteine, and homomethionine was incorporated in the isothiocyanate moiety and 10 to 15% in the sulfate moiety of Sinigrin.[41]

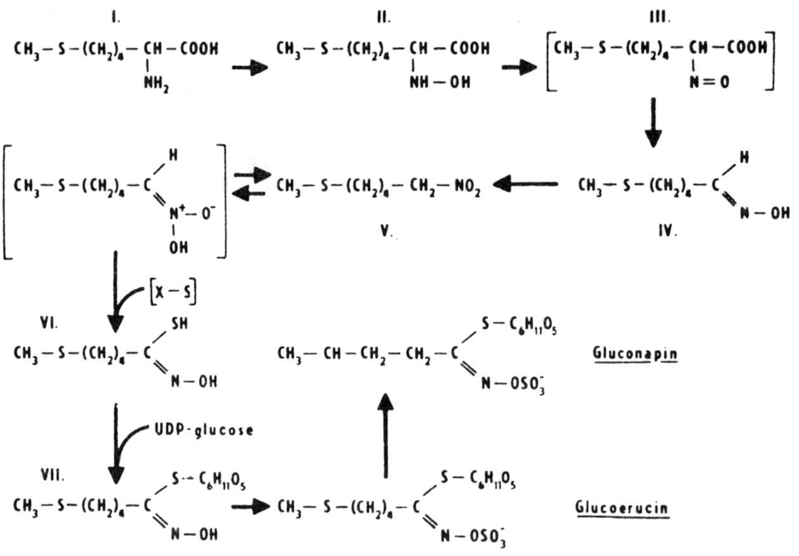

FIGURE 2. Biosynthesis of Gluconapin.[35,36] I. 2-amino-6-(methylthio)-caproic acid, II. 2-(hydroxyamino)-6-(methylthio)-caproic acid, III. 6-(methylthio)-2-nitroso-caproic acid, IV. 5-methyl-thiopentanal oxime, V. 5-(methylthio)-1-nitro-pentane, VI. 5-(methylthio)-pentanethiohydroximic acid; UCP = uridine-5'-diphosphate; PAP = 3'-phosphoadenosine-5'-phosphosulfate. (From Langer, P. and Greer, M. A., *Antithyroid Substances and Naturally Occurring Goitrogens*, S. Karger, Basel, 1977, 119. With permission.)

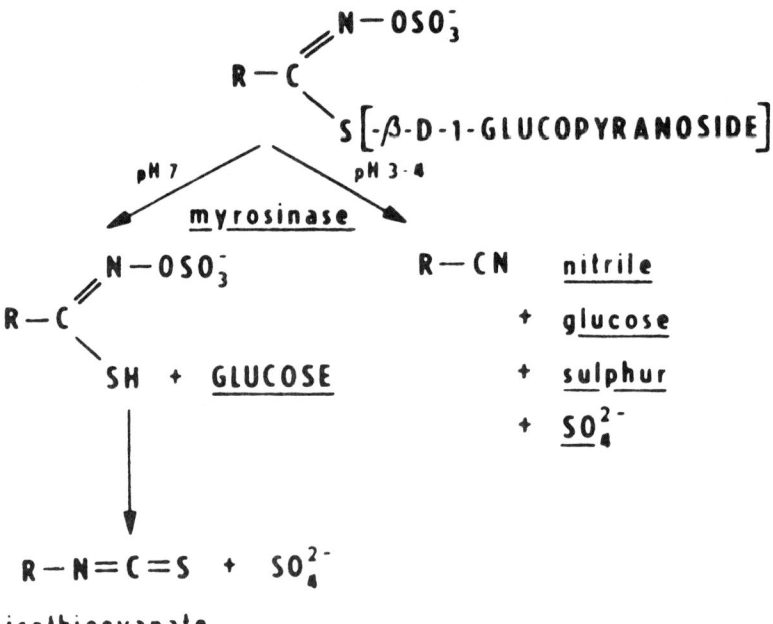

FIGURE 3. Splitting of glucosinolate by myrosinase under various pH. (From Langer, P. and Greer, M. A., *Antithyroid Substances and Naturally Occurring Goitrogens*, S. Karger, Basel, 1977, 80. With permission.)

Enzymatic and Chemical Decomposition Under Different Conditions
Liberation of Isothiocyanates and Nitriles (Table 3)

A variety of pathways for the enzymatic and chemical breakdown of glucosinolates have been described,[42] the appropriate isothiocyanates being one of major products (Table 1). Thus, enzymatic hydrolysis of Sinigrin (allyl-glucosinolate) at pH 7.0 gives allyl-isothiocyanate, D-glucose, and sulfate, whereas in acid medium allyl-cyanide (nitrile) and sulfur are formed instead of isothiocyanate (Figure 3). The nitrile to isothiocyanate ratio during enzymatic hydrolysis of glucosinolates was definitely found to depend on pH,[17,21,43,44] nitriles being almost exclusively formed at acid pH or during cooking by nonenzymic decomposition of natural products (Figure 4). Moreover, the formation of some nitriles would presumably occur when the vegetables reach the acid pH in the stomach, unless the activity of myrosinase has not been destroyed by cooking. The observed multiplicity of alternative pathways for enzymatic hydrolysis of glucosinolates may be partially explained by various physical or chemical conditions and by presumed multiple nature of the enzyme myrosinase which was recently shown to be composed from 3 to 4 isoenzymes.[15] Its striking activation by ascorbic acid[21,45] has recently been explained by a binding of that to an isoenzyme.[15] An epithiospecifier protein was also isolated which appears to be a component of myrosinase and it was suggested that this may be a two protein enzyme system.[46] The formation of various products (e.g., cyanides) due to the nonenzymic decomposition of glucosinolates by the effect of ferrous salts under heating has been reported[47] (Figure 4).

Liberation of Thiocyanate

Thiocyanate may be liberated by enzymatic action either from some specific glucosinolates or under specific conditions — from some glucosinolates usually yielding isothiocyanates.[20,54-56] After a systematic survey, much higher amounts of thiocyanate were detected in the juice pressed from various crushed plants of the *Brassica* genus than in several other species tested (Table 4) and possible interrelations between these findings and the goitrogenic activity were suggested.[48-50] Later various parent glucosides of thiocyanate were found such as Glucobrassicin,[51] Neoglucobrassicin,[52] and Glucobrassicin-1-sulfonate[53] (Figure 5). The content of thiocyanate in some *Brassica* plants is presented in Table 4.

Liberation of Oxazolidine-2-Thiones

5-Vinyl-oxazolidine-2-thione (vinyl-OT, goitrin, L-5-vinyl-2-thiooxazolidone) was isolated from seeds of various *Brassica* and from edible parts of rutabaga *(Brassica napus esculenta)* and its potent antithyroid activity was demonstrated.[4,57] Its parent glucoside — Progoitrin — was found a few years later independently in three laboratories.[13,58,59] The latter two groups reported also an isolation of Glucoconringiin, a parent glucoside of 5-dimethyl-oxazolidine-2-thione (dimethyl-OT), which was actually found as early as 1939,[60] but its biological potency has not been investigated. Alkyl-oxazolidine-2-thiones are apparently formed, after the release of aglucone from the parent glucoside, by the intramolecular Lossen rearrangement when R- group of isothiocyanate has an appropriately located hydroxyl constituent to facilitate ring closure (Figure 6). The scheme of currently known alkyl-oxazolidine-2-thiones and their parent glucosinolates is presented in Table 2. All substances presented were identified first only in seeds except for the identification of vinyl-OT in rutabaga roots. Until the isolation of this compound from cabbage leaves,[61] it was believed that similar compounds do not occur in edible parts plants. Later, however, the content of vinyl-OT in cabbage was measured repeatedly[24,25,62-64] (Table 5). Alternate pathways for a degradation of epi-Progoitrin in seeds of *Crambe abyssinica* have been also demonstrated. Thus, under some specific conditions (increase of temperature and pH, dilution with

Table 3
INDIVIDUAL ISOTHIOCYANATES AND TOTAL, VOLATILE, AND NONVOLATILE GLUCOSINOLATES FOUND IN WHITE CABBAGE BY VARIOUS AUTHORS (mg/kg FRESH WEIGHT)

Isothiocyanate	Mackay et al.,[168] paper and gas chrom.[a]	Clapp et al.,[166] paper chrom.	Bailey[169] et al., gas chrom.[b]	Sedlak,[167] steam dist., paper chrom., UV-spectra[c]	Langer,[25] ether extr., paper chrom., UV-spectra[d]	van Etten et al.,[24] gas-liquid chrom.[e]
Allyl-	Detected	2.9	Detected	16.1 ± 9.6	Detected	4.2—14.5
Methyl-thio-propyl-	—	0.15	—	—	Detected?	0.5—1.5
Methyl-sulfinyl-propyl-	—	0.016	—	38.0 ± 21.8	—	20.1—163.8
Methyl-sulfonyl-propyl-	—	—	—	6.8 ± 0.3	—	—
3-butenyl-	Detected?	Traces	Detected	—	Detected	0.2—18.4
Methyl-thio-butyl-	—	—	—	—	—	0.0—1.4
Methyl-sulfinyl-butyl-	—	—	—	—	—	1.4—118.6
Methyl-sulfonyl-butyl-	—	—	—	—	—	1.2—12.7
Benzyl-	—	—	—	—	—	0.1—2.8
Benzyl-ethyl-	—	—	—	—	—	0.7—6.1
Total glucosinolates[f]	—	—	—	82.3 ± 18.0	4.08	299.0—1288.0
Total volatile aglucons	—	—	—	24.1 ± 15.2	—	—
Total nonvolatile aglucons	—	3.1	—	69.6 ± 26.2	0.50—19.2	—

[a] The presence of 2 to 3 other unidentified isothiocyanates was observed.
[b] The presence of methyl-butyl- and methyl-thio-methyl-ITC was also presumably detected.
[c] A total of ten samples was analyzed, and SD are presented.
[d] The presence of two other unidentified isothiocyanates was observed.
[e] The range of 88 samples analyzed.
[f] Kjaer and Rubenstein[97] found 29 mg/kg, Schuphan[165] found 50-100 mg/kg, and Michajlovskij et al.[106] found 50 mg/kg total glucosinolates by steam distillation and paper chromatography or argentometric titration, respectively.

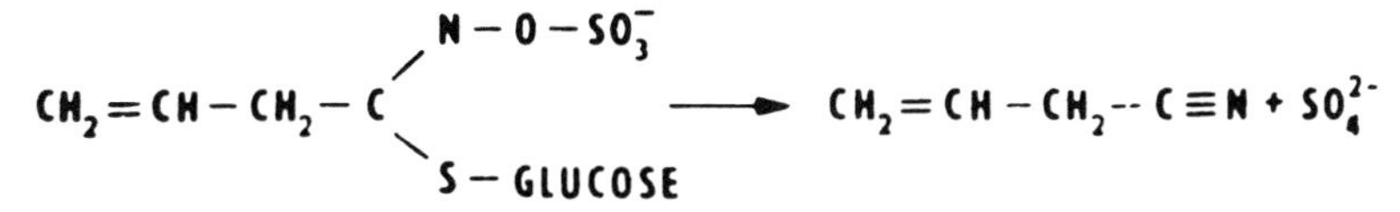

$$CH_2=CH-CH_2-C\begin{subarray}{c}N-O-SO_3^-\\ \\S-GLUCOSE\end{subarray} \longrightarrow CH_2=CH-CH_2-C\equiv N + SO_4^{2-}$$

FIGURE 4. Decomposition of Sinigrin by heating. (From Langer, P. and Greer, M. A., *Antithyroid Substances and Naturally Occurring Goitrogens*, S. Karger, Basel, 1977, 90. With permission.)

water) its conversion into R-goitrin occurred, while after the addition of ferrous ions a formation of a mixture of cyano compounds (1-cyano-2-hydroxy-3-butene and two diasteromeric isomers of 1-cyano-2-hydroxy-3,4-epithiobutane) was reported[65] (Figure 7).

Cyanogenic Glucosides

There exist at least about 2000 species of higher plants distributed among approximately 110 families which are cyanogenic. Out of them only in about 200 species the chemical nature of cyanogen is known,[231] being represented by cyanogenic glucosides or cyanogen lipids. The glucosides contain hydroxynitriles (cyanohydrins) as aglucones and may be found in various anatomical parts such as roots, leaves, stems, flowers, and seeds. Their content is apparently determined genetically and depends on the age of the plant. The known cyanogenic lipids are four in number and occur only in a single family, the Sapindacae.

Among the most important cyanogenic plants belong cassava (manioc), sorghum, white clover, yam, cycad, maize, peas, beans, apricots, prunes, cherries, sugar cane, almonds, bamboo shoots, etc. So far, a total of 30 cyanogenic or pseudocyanogenic glucosides (Table 6) have been isolated and in 23 cases their structure was established.[19,20,66-68]

Similarly, as in the case of glucosinolate aglucones, the hydrocyanic acid, sugar, and aldehyde or ketone are liberated from cyanogenic glucosides after crushing the plant tissue or autolysis due to the action of β-glucosidase or hydroxynitrile lyase (Figure 8). In crushed plant material, however, highly volatile hydrogen cyanide is rapidly lost, while intact or freshly cut plants may contain a sufficiently high amount of cyanogens to be poisonous.

From the viewpoint of goitrogenic activity it should be stated that, in animal organism, cyanide ion is detoxified to thiocyanate which possesses an antithyroid effect. Some varieties of cyanogenic plants are listed as forage crops (white clover, sorghum) or a major source of calories for millions of people (cassava).

Other Miscellaneous or Poorly Defined Compounds

Onion volatiles (disulfides, polysulfides) — An inhibition of thyroid radioiodine uptake in the rat was found following small doses of main volatile compound of food onions — *n*-propyl-disulfide[69] and a number of other natural mono- and disulfides.[70] The same substances have been also incriminated as goitrogenic compounds in cabbage[71] and polysulfides provide a successful sulfur-donor substrate for rhodanese, a thiocyanate-producing animal enzyme.[72]

Soy beans, ground nuts, walnuts, etc. — The goitrogenic activity of soy beans and ground nuts has been reported by a number of investigators.[5,18] Later, goiter was found in babies fed a couple of months with a soy flour baby food.[73,74] This effect was explained as an increased fecal loss of thyroxine due to the increased absorption of this hormone on some yet unknown component of soy flour.[75] A similar mechanism has been suggested for the goitrogenic effect of walnut *(Juglans regia)*[76] and *Araucaria araucana* (pinon).[77] Recently, a peptide was isolated from soy bean flour which inhibits the uptake and organification of iodine by thyroid.[78]

Table 4
THE AMOUNT OF THIOCYANATE IN VARIOUS *BRASSICA* AS FOUND BY VARIOUS AUTHORS (mg SCN⁻/kg FRESH WEIGHT)

Species	Michajlovskij and Langer[48] mean ± SD[a]	Michajlovskij and Langer[49] range	Gmelin and Virtanen[51]	Michajlovskij et al.[106,214]	Josefsson[27]	van Etten et al.[24]
Brassica oleracea L.						
var. *silvestris* L.					200	
var. *acephala* DC					340	
var. *gemmifera* Zenker			100		50	
var. *italica* Planck					200—210	
var. *botrytis* L.	88 ± 41 (38)[a]	30—240 (53)			190—310	
var. *gongyloides* L.	22 ± 6 (44)	15—50 (80)		15—25 (4)	110—140	
var. *sabauda* L.	85 ± 30 (30)	50—540 (59)	270—310	20—28 (38)	180	
var. *capitata* L. alba	31 ± 14 (38)	10—140 (93)	40	20—30 (12)	50—60	15—62 (88)
var. *capitata* L. rubra					50	
var. *cretica*			40			
Brassica napus L.			25—88		80	
Brassica campestris L.					90—100	
Raphanus sativus	6 ± 1 (39)	5—15 (27)				

Note: Numbers in parentheses in body of table indicate the number of samples analyzed.

[a] A brief review of previous data by various authors until 1958 is presented in Reference 48.

ESTIMATION OF GLUCOSINOLATES AND PRODUCTS OF THEIR DECOMPOSITION

General

Since the enzymatic decomposition of glucosinolates starts to proceed immediately after crushing the seeds or plant tissue, it follows that various degrees of actual decomposition may interfere with the estimation of either total glucosinolates or their products. Thus, the inactivation of myrosinase originally present in the material to be analyzed seems essential to obtain data closely related to the true content of the appropriate compounds.

After the inactivation of original myrosinase, the glucosinolates may be extracted and purified by various procedures. Then a known amount of pure myrosinase is added and the complex mixture is incubated under controlled conditions (pH, temperature, time). The total content of glucosinolates may be determined by measuring either the liberated sulfate or glucose and the percentage representation of individual glucosinolates may be calculated from the content of individual aglucones after their decomposition by various methods (see below).

Inactivation of Myrosinase

Various procedures have been described such as repeated extraction of defatted material with boiling 70% methanol,[17] boiling seeds in a mixture of petroleum ether and ethanol (2:1, v/v),[79] boiling in 75% acetone,[80] or dry heating at 90°C for 15 min.[81] Some recent works[82,83] do not use this step any more and start the further analytical procedure from the defatted seed meal.

For green plant material one method is almost always used which consists of the immersion of compact parts into a boiling solution of 70% methanol.[17,24,63,64] This extraction may be repeated 3 times (5 min each). After fine homogenization and filtration of the resulting material, the evaporation of methanol under reduced pressure gives the origin material for further analytical steps.

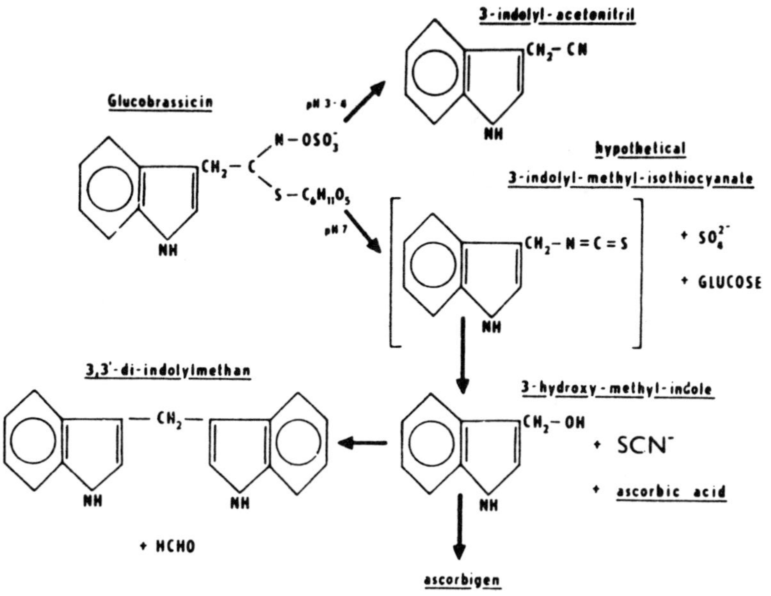

FIGURE 5. Enzymic splitting of Glucobrassicin under various pH. (From Langer, P. and Greer, M. A., *Antithyroid Substances and Naturally Occurring Goitrogens*, S. Karger, Basel, 1977, 82. With permission.)

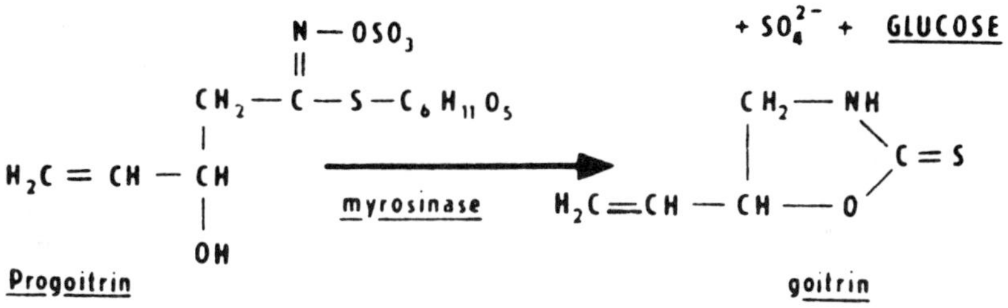

FIGURE 6. Enzymic conversion of Progoitrin into goitrin. (From Langer, P. and Greer, M. A., *Antithyroid Substances and Naturally Occurring Goitrogens*, S. Karger, Basel, 1977, 83. With permission.)

Extraction, Separation, and Identification of Glucosinolates

The individual glucosinolates present in filtered methanol extract may be separated either with the aid of paper chromatography in *n*-butanol to acetic acid to water (4:1:5 or 4:1:3) or with the aid of basic anion exchangers or anionotropic aluminum oxide.[17] Recently, main glucosinolates from a crude extract of rapeseeds were isolated on DEAE-Sephadex A-25 or on arginine coupled to Sephadex G-10.[84] Isoelectric focusing was also used.[85] Glucosinolates from the methanol extract of cabbage were successfully separated on anion exchange resin Dowex® 1-X2.[24]

Incubation of Extracts with Myrosinase Under Optimum Conditions

For the purpose of analysis, the extracts are to be further subjected to enzymatic breakdown which results in a liberation of individual products such as sulfate, glucose, or aglucones into an incubation medium usually consisting of the natural material (defatted seeds, raw extract of green plants, or pure glucosinolates extract), myrosinase in crude[43,86] or purified commercial form, buffer, and ascorbic acid as a catalyst.

Optimum conditions of enzymatic breakdown of glucosinolates were repeatedly

Table 5
THE AMOUNT OF VINYL-OXAZOLIDINE-2-THIONE FOUND IN VARIOUS SPECIES OF *BRASSICA* (mg/kg FRESH WEIGHT)

Species (common names)	Vinyloxazolidine-2-thione (mg kg^{-1})	Ref.
Rape	4—14	143[a]
Turnip	33—69	143[a]
Marrow stem kale	3—9	143[a]
"Rybsen"	24—32	143[a]
"Wasserrübe"	72	143[a]
White cabbage (24 samples)	5—192	25[b]
White cabbage (84 samples)	20—30	167[b]
A number of varieties of *Brassica oleracea*	0—100	
Kale (25 samples)	0—42	214[b]
White cabbage, kale and kohlrabi	15—40	106[d]
White cabbage (84 samples)	3—26	24[e]

[a] Samples from Finland.
[b] Samples from Czechoslovakia.
[c] Samples from Sweden.
[d] Samples from Yugoslavia.
[e] Samples from U.S.

studied.[81,87-89] It was found that there exists a broad optimum for release of aglucones at pH 6 to 9. At 30°C, the enzymatic release of isothiocyanates and oxazolidinethiones is completed in about 30 min. Furthermore, a strict proportionality between the rate of myrosinase action and enzyme concentration was found.[43] Since a strong catalytic action of ascorbic acid on the myrosinase-glucosinolate reaction was described by various authors,[21,43,90] the addition of small amounts of this compound is recommended in all present methods.

Estimation of Total Glucosinolates and Individual Liberated Products

Total glucosinolates — Total glucosinolates originally present may be estimated by measuring the amount of stoichiometrically liberated glucose[24,64,82,84,91] or sulfate.[83] A rapid method for the determination of total glucosinolates based on the conversion of isothiocyanates into thioureas and measurement of specific UV absorbance of thioureas and oxazolidine-2-thiones was recently reported.[82]

Aglucones (thiocyanate, isothiocyanates, oxazolidine-2-thiones) — Before the final quantitative estimation some of the aglucones must be separated, while others may be estimated directly in the mixture. Thus, thiocyanate can be simply measured after protein precipitation by a direct color reaction with Fe^{3+}, Cu^{2+}, or pyridine or by a conversion into cyanogen halide.[27,48,51,92-94] However, because of the presence of several interfering substances in biological material, the adsorption of thiocyanate from interfering compounds on anion exchange resin with subsequent elution or final estimation of separated thiocyanate by gas chromatography[230] has been recently developed. Since the final estimation of isothiocyanates and oxazolidine-2-thiones is based on the measurement of UV-absorption or on paper or gas-liquid chromatography, these compounds must be isolated or extracted from the mixture to obtain relatively pure compounds. The oldest method of separating isothiocyanates from the mixture is a steam distillation of these compounds into an ethanol-ammonia mixture.[26,87,95] Moreover, a number of organic solvents was used for the extraction. Thus, a combined

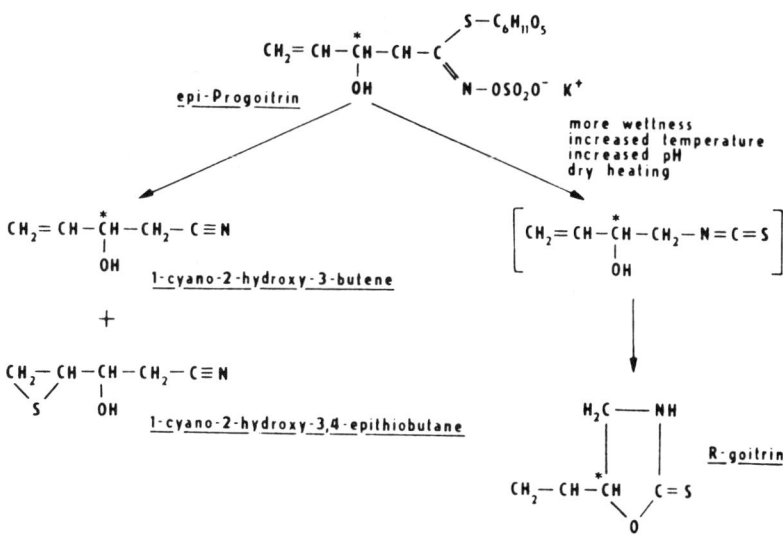

FIGURE 7. Alternate pathways of epi-Progoitrin splitting in wetted seed meal. (From Langer, P. and Greer, M. A., *Antithyroid Substances and Naturally Occurring Goitrogens*, S. Karger, Basel, 1977, 121. With permission.)

extraction with ether and chloroform almost completely removes both isothiocyanates and oxazolidine-2-thiones.[17] Similar results were obtained with repeated ether extraction. Isothiocyanates may be selectively extracted with trimethyl-pentane[96] or isooctane containing 33% of ethanol,[81] while selective extraction of oxazolidine-thione was obtained with ethyl-acetate followed by two-dimensional paper chromatography.[62]

In the presence of ammonia, isothiocyanates are converted into corresponding thioureas. This reaction is quantitative in ethanol,[97] isooctane,[81] and ether.[89] Resulting thioureas may be separated by paper chromatography in water saturated chloroform,[97] butanol to acetic acid to water,[17] to other systems.[98] Recently, however, gas-liquid chromatography is mostly used.[24,63,99-101]

All natural isothiocyanates and oxazolidine-thiones possess a sharp UV-absorption maximum approximately in the range of 240 to 250 nm, the wavelength for the same compound being slightly different in various solvents.[4,43,57,61,62,81,89,102] Moreover, glucosinolates in aqueous solutions show a maximum absorption at 227 nm.[43,58,80,103-105] Under the same conditions, all components of a mixture of various isothiocyanates show the same absorption maximum. However, natural material may contain interfering substances which increase the absorbency at wavelength close to the maximum. Most of these materials may be removed by a preliminary extraction before myrosinase treatment.[89] Moreover, since the molar extinction of thioureas is much higher than that of corresponding isothiocyanate, this shows a higher absorbency compared to the interfering background than the same concentration of the appropriate isothiocyanate.

METABOLISM OF INDIVIDUAL AGLUCONES IN THE ORGANISM

The enzymic decomposition of glucosinolates may happen during the eating of raw plant material or during the preparation of food. However, such decomposition is rarely complete and thus the final uptake of free aglucones depends on the amount liberated from glucosinolates and on the amount removed by water extraction during food processing. Moreover, during prolonged heating of foods the myrosinase may be completely or partially inactivated or a considerable destruction of glucosinolates and aglucones may occur.[106] Finally, intact glucosinolates entering the gastrointestinal tract may be hydrolyzed by the action of thioglucosides from bacterial flora.[7,103,107,108]

Table 6
MOST IMPORTANT CYANOGENIC GLUCOSIDES AND THEIR BOTANICAL DISTRIBUTION

Glucoside	Derived from	Aglucone	Natural occurrence Common names	Natural occurrence Scientific names
Linamarin	Valine, isoleucine, or leucine	α-Hydroxybutyronitrile	Cassava, flux, beans	Compositae, Leguminosae, Euphorbiacae, Linacae, Papaveracae
Lotaustralin		α-hydroxy-α-methylbutyronitrile	See Linamarin	See Linamarin
Acacipetalin		β-dimethyl-α-hydroxyacrylonitrile		Acacia (Leguminosae)
Dihydroacacipetalin				Acacia (Leguminosae), Sapindracae
Cardiospermin				Sapindracae
Prunasin	Phenylalanine	D-mandelonitrile	Almond, apple, apricot, cherry, peach, pear, plum	Caprifoliacae, Leguminosae, Myoporacae, Myrtacae, Polypodiacae, Rosacae, Saxifragacae, Scrophilariacae
Sambunigrin		L-mandelonitrile		Caprifoliacae, Luguminosae, Oleacae
Amygdalin		D-mandelonitrile	See Prunasin	See Prunasin and Rosacae
Vicianin		D-mandelonitrile		Leguminosae, Polypodiacae, Sapotacae
Lucumin				Sapotacae
Holocalin		L-m-hydroxymandelonitrile		Caprifoliacae, Leguminosae
Zierin				Caprifoliacae, Rutacae
Taxiphylin	Tyrosine	D p hydroxy mandelonitrile		Oleacae, Cupressacae, Euphoriacae, Taxacae, Taxodiacae
Dhurrin		L-p-hydroxymandelonitrile	Sorghum	Graminae, Proteacae
Triglochin				Aracae, Juncaginacae, Lileacae

Note: Compiled from References 19, 20, 66, and 68.

Thiocyanate

Thiocyanate in the organism was detected by Treviranus in 1814 who found that human saliva gives a red color with a saturated solution of ferric salts in nitric or sulfuric acids. Thiocyanate was later found in other body fluids such as blood, plasma, milk, urine, and gastric juice.[20]

Endogenous Formation of Thiocyanate

The thiocyanate formed in the animal organism from sulfur donors and cyanide donors through the enzymatic action of rhodanese may be called endogenous thiocyanate in contrast to exogenous thiocyanate originating from foods. Under normal food intake conditions, the regular rate of endogenous thiocyanate formation results in a low and relatively constant level of this ion in plasma and urine,[12] while in fasted rats an increased level of serum thiocyanate was observed.[109]

Rhodanese — Rhodanese in a crude form was isolated by Lang,[110] while Sörbo prepared this enzyme in a crystalline form.[111] Later another transsulfurase was found in

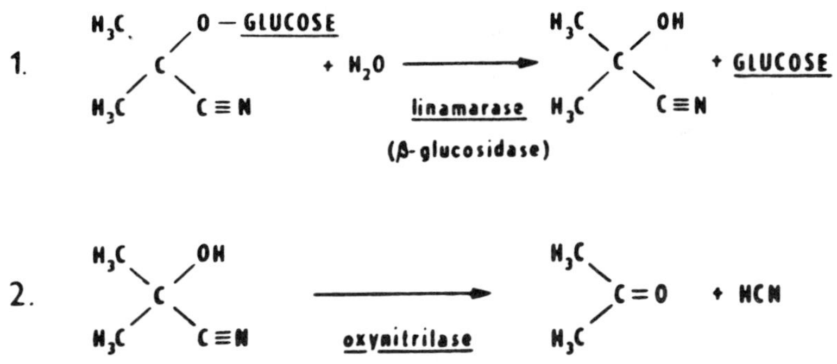

FIGURE 8. Scheme of enzymic splitting of Linamarin. (From Langer, P. and Greer, M. A., *Antithyroid Substances and Naturally Occurring Goitrogens*, S. Karger, Basel, 1977, 80. With permission.)

liver and *Escherichia coli*[112] which participates in a transfer of sulfur from β-mercaptopyruvate (mercaptopyruvate sulfurtransferase). This enzyme was also found in several mammalian tissues as a second enzyme capable of forming thiocyanate. The current terminology for rhodanese is thiosulfate:cyanide sulfur transsulfurase (E.C. 2.8.1.1) and its chemistry, mechanism of action, and biological functions were recently reviewed.[20,72] The mechanism of action of this enzyme was established to be a typical double displacement. It appears that the acquisition of sulfane sulfur atoms (R-SO$_x$S)$^-$ from the donor substrates by enzymic cleavage of sulfur-sulfur bonds is an essential process. Apparently all potential sulfur donors should contain such sulfane sulfur atoms. Finally, a sulfur-rhodanese is formed which further reacts with cyanide ion to produce SCN$^-$. Rhodanese has been found in nearly all tissues of mammals, but the highest concentrations occur in liver, kidney, adrenals, thyroid, and pancreas. The rhodanese activity in mammals is mainly located in mitochondria. In addition, it has been detected in a number of microorganisms, the molecule being simpler than that of mammalian enzyme. Physiological role of rhodanese in the organism is not yet definitely elucidated. Thus, even though the enzyme is rather widely distributed in the tissues, the apparent lack of known substrates makes the cyanide detoxication ineffectual. As recently reviewed,[20] some authors speculate on the role of this enzyme in organic sulfur interconversions.

Sulfur donors — The sulfur for the endogenous formation of thiocyanate is mostly contributed from endogenous sources, one of the most important sources being thiosulfate which occurs in very low concentrations in several tissues.[20] Its formation in thyroid tissue after administering thiourea was also reported.[113] Another sulfur donor may be colloidal sulfur[110] and a number of various persulfides. The origin of thiocyanate sulfur from sulfur-containing amino acids has been repeatedly shown[20] and an increase of urinary thiocyanate excretion in rats following the administration of methylmercaptoimidazole has been reported.[114] Some of the ^{35}S administered ^{35}S-sulfate in rats was found to be excreted by urine as ^{35}S-thiocyanate.[120]

Cyanate donors — In contrast to sulfur donors, the donors of cyanide are predominantly of exogenous origin. A number of observations showed an increase of thiocyanate level in serum and urine after the administration of potassium cyanide.[20] The most important natural source of cyanide is cyanogenic glucosides occurring in a number of plant species (Table 6). In crushed plant tissue, hydrocyanic acid is formed from cyanogenic glucosides due to the action of enzymes. This compound, being highly volatile, is rapidly lost, but intact or freshly cut plants may be an important source of cyanide. Another considerable way the cyanide and cyanogenic compounds enter the human organism is via tobacco smoke. Moreover, cyanide may be produced by some microorganisms.

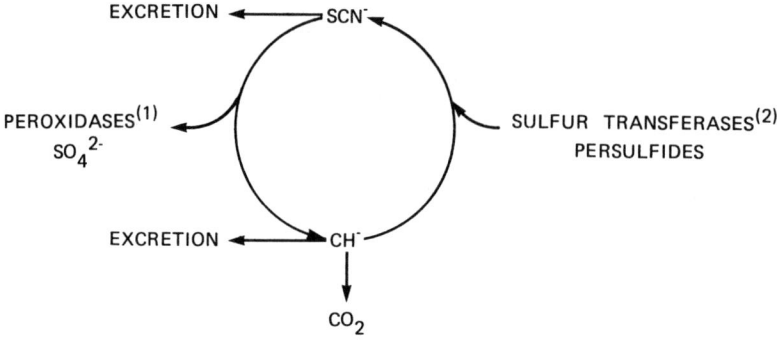

(1) myelo-, thyro-, lacto-peroxidase, hemoglobin
(2) thiosulfate, mercaptopyruvate

FIGURE 9. Wood cycle.[20] (From Wood, J. L., *Chemistry and Biochemistry of Thiocyanic Acid and its Derivatives*, Newman, A. A., Ed., Academic Press, London, 1975, 156—221. With permission.)

Exogenous Preformed Thiocyanate

The thiocyanate originating from plants of *Brassica* family and playing a special role in acute changes of the level of this ion in blood and urine has been called exogenous preformed thiocyanate.[114-117]

Distribution of Thiocyanate in the Organism

There is a close resemblance between thiocyanate, iodide, and chloride space except in the brain, where chloride space is higher. In various anion concentrating tissues (e.g., thyroid, salivary glands, gastric mucosa, mammary glands), the iodide, thiocyanate, and some other univalent anions (perchlorate, fluoroborate, and nitrate) compete for the same binding sites which plays a role in iodine and thyroid hormone metabolism.[118,119] Most of the evidence obtained so far shows that thiocyanate penetrates the cellular membranes of different tissues at different rates, the highest penetration being found in the above-mentioned tissues.[20,121-123]

Metabolic Conversion of Thiocyanate

For a long time, the thiocyanate was considered to be metabolically inert, but later was found that in mammalian organism a part of it may be metabolized to cyanide, sulfate, and possibly to some other products.[20] The formation of ^{35}S-sulfate from ^{35}S-thiocyanate in cow mammary gland[120] and the oxidation of labeled thiocyanate to sulfate in rat thyroid[124,125] were reported, the latter being enhanced by thyrotropin injection.[126] Similarly, the conversion of about 5 to 20% thiocyanate sulfur to sulfate was demonstrated in salivary glands of mice and rats.[127] The excretion of radioactive carbon after the injection of carbon-labeled thiocyanate was reported[128] and cyanide was repeatedly found in blood after the administration of toxic amounts of thiocyanate.[129,130]

The above findings were postulated to be due to lactoperoxidase in salivary glands and thyroid peroxidase in the thyroid.[131] Actually, the oxidation of thiocyanate to cyanide and sulfate by various peroxidase-hydrogen peroxide systems has been repeatedly found.[131-133] It was also established that hemoglobin may function as a peroxidase for the oxidation of thiocyanate by hydrogen peroxide.[131] The summary of described findings reveals the existence of thiocyanate-cyanide cycle or "Wood cycle" (Figure 9), which represents a common pool of thiocyanate and cyanide carbons and, apparently, cyanide originating from other sources may also enter this cycle. However, the oxidation of thiocyanate sulfur to sulfate removes it irreversibly from the thiocyanate pool. Some of the thiocyanate converted into cyanide may be resynthesized through thiosulfate[110] and mercaptopyruvate[133] transsulfurase system.[20]

Thiocyanate Balance

About 4.5% of the labeled sulfur of ^{35}S-thiocyanate was found in the urine of rats as sulfate ion.[135] Some other data support this rate of conversion. Thus, almost quantitative urinary excretion of large doses of thiocyanate was found in rats,[115] while the rate of metabolism was small.[131] However, after small doses of thiocyanate (0.35 μg/100 g diet) were administered to rats for 30 days it was found that, at the end of this period, only about 50% of the administered radioactivity was excreted, 34% of urinary ^{35}S remaining as thiocyanate and the remainder moving chromatographically as sulfate.[120,136] These findings show an apparent discrepancy between large and small doses of thiocyanate in respect to thiocyanate balance. The large doses of this anion apparently result in a saturation of thiocyanate concentrating compartments and of renal reabsorption of thiocyanate which results in excretion of the major portion of such large doses. The loading dose of unlabeled thiocyanate considerably increases the disposal rate of labeled compound.[137] Moreover, a remarkable increase of renal iodide clearance was found after high doses of thiocyanate.

After a single dose there is a rapid distribution of thiocyanate in the extracellular fluid. The initial increase of plasma thiocyanate level depends on the volume of extracellular fluid and subsequent decrease seems to depend on the extracellular fluid turnover rate related to numerous factors such as water balance, kidney function, hormonal regulation of electrolyte and water metabolism, etc.

Isothiocyanates

The plasma thiocyanate level was found to be significantly increased in rats after a long-term[25] or single administration of allylisothiocyanate, but not after methylisothiocyanate. With the aid of ^{35}S-*p*-brom-phenylisothiocyanate, it was found that after paper chromatographic separation of the 1st-day urine about 70% of radioactivity was in the sulfate area, whereas a small amount migrated in the area of stable thiocyanate.[138] After a single dose of this compound, the blood radioactivity reached a maximum at 12 hr and then slowly declined to the 5th day. Similarly, the highest urinary excretion was found on the 1st day, only minute amounts being found on the 5th and 6th days.

The antithyroid effect of isothiocyanates in vitro was demonstrated,[139] which means that the original compound may presumably directly affect the thyroid without being metabolized. As shown before, a certain percentage of the administered isothiocyanate may actually circulate in the organism in unchanged state and this is in agreement with repeated findings of goitrogenic effect of these compounds in vivo.[25,138,140,142]

Another metabolic pathway is mostly hypothetical and is supported only by the antithyroid effect of synthetic compounds which are presumably identical with the hypothetical metabolites. It is well known that, under mild temperature and slightly alkaline conditions isothiocyanates react spontaneously with amino groups which is the basis of Edmann's method of amino acid estimation. The formed thiocarbamyl derivatives, which may be considered as disubstituted thioureas, are spontaneously converted into 2-thiohydantoins. It was presumed that such reactions may also take place in vivo and a number of various thiocarbamyl derivatives and 2-thiohydantoins were synthetized from phenyl- and allyl-isothiocyanates and various amino acids (glycine, tyrosine, aspartic acid, cysteine, valine, and thioglycolic acid). The testing of antithyroid activity showed that the most effective compounds are 3-allyl-2-thiohydantoin and 3-phenyl-2-thiohydantoin, the derivatives with a side chain in position 5 being without effect.[141] It may be of interest to mention that recently some disubstituted thioureas were isolated from some African plants.[205]

Oxazolidine-2-thiones

The transfer of oxazolidine-2-thione (goitrin) to cow milk was repeatedly studied and only minute amounts of the administered pure compound or of that from crushed plants were found in milk.[143] However, the content of goitrin in milk depends on the mode of storage and thermal treatment[62] and increases considerably after hydrogen sulfide treatment of milk.[144]

After the administration of pure goitrin to rats, a compound with a slow mobility in water-saturated chloroform and with an absorption maximum at 240 nm was found in the urine of rats,[145] its antithyroid activity was demonstrated and its structure was determined as L-4-hydroxy-5-vinyl-oxazolidine-2-thione[146] which was later supported.[234] About 15 to 25% of a single dose of 10 mg goitrin has been found in the urine as goitrin plus hydroxy-goitrin.[146]

Thus, the fate of remaining 75% is still not elucidated. Recently a relatively long halflife, i.e., 5.0 to 7.5 days was found, most of the metabolites being excreted in the urine and feces. Moreover, desulfuration of goitrin was found as a new metabolic pathway.[234] The highest accumulation of radioactivity after ^{35}S-goitrin in rats was found in the thyroid, while much less was detected in the liver and kidneys.[148] An increase of sulfhydryl groups in the liver was also found after feeding cabbage.[147]

NATURALLY OCCURRING GOITROGENS AND EXPERIMENTAL GOITER

Cabbage Goiter

The goitrogenic effect of cabbage in rabbits was first observed by Chesney et al.[1] in 1928 and later confirmed in several laboratories.[5,80] However, since some investigators could not repeat the original findings, the goitrogenic properties of cabbage were questioned by Greer,[6] who suggested that the iodine content in cabbage used in several experiments might be less than that in the diet of control groups and thus the "cabbage goiter" might be actually caused by iodine deficiency rather than by some active goitrogen. However, later experiments with a single[116] or long-term feeding of animals with cabbage[25] under controlled iodine intake showed that there exists an active goitrogen.

Antithyroid Effect of Individual Aglucones and Their Decomposition or Metabolic Products

Thiocyanate and Glucobrassicin — Goitrogenic effect of thiocyanate in rats was found after high (up to 50 mg SCN⁻ per rat)[2,149,150] or low doses (0.5 to 16 mg SCN⁻ per rat).[140,142,151,152] Even though a goitrogenic effect of Glucobrassicin per se was postulated,[9] it was later found that antithyroid effect of this glucosinolate is the same as that of equivalent amounts of thiocyanate[117] which means that apparently no additional effect is present in the other parts of Glucobrassicin molecule.

Isothiocyanates — After negative results have been obtained in testing a goitrogenic activity of some naturally occurring isothiocyanates,[153,154] positive findings were reported with p-hydroxybenzyl-isothiocyanate (liberated from Sinalbin) in rabbits[155] and with 3-methyl-sulfonylpropyl-(cheirolin) and n-propyl-isothiocyanate[156] in rats. Later a goitrogenic effect of the most widespread mustard oil in plant kingdom — allyl-isothiocyanate — was repeatedly reported in vivo[114,138,142,157] and in vitro.[139]

Oxazolidine-2-thione — All derivatives of oxazolidine-2-thione (OT) isolated from natural material have not yet been tested, but the goitrogenic potency of vinyl-OT,[4,57,138,142,158] phenyl-OT,[158,159] and dimethyl-OT[25] was repeatedly reported. Even though an effect of extremely small doses of goitrin (vinyl-OT) such as 0.1 to 0.5 μg per rat was reported,[158] this was not confirmed[234] and the lowest dose increasing significantly the thyroid weight after 3 weeks of feeding was established to be about 10[234]

μg^{12} or 40 μg^{12} of the above compound. Among the synthetic derivatives of OT, 3-phenyl- and 4-phenyl-OT and later also 4-ethyl- and 5-methyl-OT, as well as some other compounds,[160] were found to be active.

Nitriles and other products — Even though thyroid hypertrophy after acetonitril (methyl cyanate) administration has been reported,[153] this was recently not confirmed with a mixture of nitriles.[18] However, nitriles originating from cyanogenic glucosides may definitely increase the blood level of thiocyanate and thus affect the thyroid. The antithyroid effects of newly identified products of glucosinolate hydrolysis[65] (Figure 7).

Cyanogenic Glucosides (White Clover and Cassava Goiter)

Some important crops used as cattle feed (New Zealand white clover — *Trifolium repens* L. line seed meal, lima beans) contain cyanogenic glucosides linamrin and lotaustralin. In fact, the goitrogenic effect of line seeds[161] and white clover[162] in sheep has been repeatedly reported. It was found that thiocyanate in the sheep kidney is not handled in the same way as in man or rodents. Since the sheep kidney shows the tendency to retain thiocyanate, this makes a favorable condition for a high increase of thiocyanate level in blood resulting from the detoxication of cyanide, nitriles, or hydrocyanic acid originating from the glucosides.[163]

Identification of Chemical Nature of "Brassica Factor"
Qualitative and Quantitative Composition of Aglucones in Cabbage

Thiocyanate — A range of 10 to 60 mg SCN⁻ per kilogram of cabbage was found in various areas of the world (Table 4).

Isothiocyanates — (Table 3) Several papers reported the content of volatile isothiocyanates in the range of 10 to 100 mg/kg,[25,154,165-167] but also a level of about 3 mg/kg[166] or, recently, up to 120 to 150 mg/kg[24] was found. From the qualitative standpoint, all authors mentioned found allyl-ITC, which was for a long time considered to be a main glucosinolate of cabbage. In addition, 3-butenyl-ITC,[89] ethyl-ITC,[168] 3-methyl-thiopropyl-ITC,[166] 3-methyl-sulfinylpropyl, and 3-methyl-sulfonylpropyl[167] were also reported. With the aid of gas-liquid chromatography, 7 ITC[169] and, recently, 9 ITC were found,[24] among them the highest amount of 3-methyl-sulfinylpropyl (20 to 164 mg/kg), 4-methyl-sulfonylbutyl (2 to 119 mg/kg), and allyl (4 to 146 mg/kg).

5-Vinyl-oxazolidine-2-thione — (Table 5) Several authors[24,25,167,170] reported the content of 0.5 to 25 mg of this compound per kilogram of cabbage.

Additive Antithyroid Effect of Thiocyanate, Allyl-isothiocyanate and Oxazolidine-2-thione May Represent the Chemical Nature of "Brassica Factor"

From several experiments with a long-term feeding (0.5 to 4.0 mg SCN⁻ per rat daily) it was concluded that thiocyanate may represent about 20 to 30% of goitrogenic activity of cabbage.[25,116,140,142,152,157,171] Similar experiments were made with a long-term feeding of rats with 0.5 to 5.0 mg allyl-isothiocyanate[140,142,157] or 10 to 160 μg oxazolidine-2-thione daily.[25,140,142,145] Even though in most cases the administered dose of these compounds was about twice as high as that contained in the amount of cabbage consumed daily, none of these compounds seems fully responsible for the goitrogenic effect of cabbage, the thyroid weight being taken as almost suitable index of total antithyroid activity in long-term experiments, since this represents a final result of a continuous action of a complex of antithyroid effects.

Finally, it was found that the goitrogenic effect of cabbage may be stimulated by a mixture of thiocyanate, allylisothiocyanate, and oxazolidine-2-thione administered in the same amounts as analytically found in the cabbage consumed daily by another group of rats.[25] In 50 groups of animals fed various doses of these 3 substances, it was found that they may exert an additive antithyroid effect.[12,140,142,152]

Mechanism of Antithyroid Action of Individual Aglucones
Thiocyanate

A number of univalent anions whose ionic size is similar to that of iodide (SCN^-, ClO_4^-, Br^-, NO_3^-, BF_4^-) may competitively inhibit the active transport of iodide both in the thyroid and in extrathyroidal iodide concentrating tissues. This effect consists of the inhibition of iodide concentration in some tissues or discharge of concentrated iodide from these tissues (thyroid, salivary glands, mammary glands, gastric mucosa, and a number of other organs such as choroid plexus, ciliary body, small intestine, skin, and hair) which finally results in increasing its supply to the kidneys.

Another effect of thiocyanate consists of a displacement of thyroxine binding to plasma proteins[118,172,173] which results in rapid distribution of thyroxine between plasma and tissues. Actually acute increase of thyroxine flux to the tissues including the pituitary may be found immediately after SCN^- administration,[119] while later a decrease of thyroxine disposal rate takes place. This presumably may exert first the inhibitory effect on the pituitary-thyroid axis and later apparently an increased secretion of TSH takes place which increases the thyroid function.[174] Long-term administration of small doses of thiocyanate to rats was found to result in a mildly positive iodine balance which was claimed to be the same as it would have been if thyroxine had been given.[185]

The inhibition of thyroid peroxidase by thiocyanate has been repeatedly reported[175-177,242] and also changes of biosynthesis of thyroid hormone consisting of the increased monoiodotyrosine/diiodotyrosine (MIT/DIT) ratio and decreased iodothyronine formation.[152] Recently it was observed that the inhibitory effect of SCN^- results from the binding of this anion to the substrate site of thyroid peroxidase.

Isothiocyanates

A scarcity of information shows that isothiocyanates may inhibit the thyroid peroxidase[177] and biosynthesis of thyroid hormone in vivo.[139,140,152]

Oxazolidine-2-thiones

Since naturally occurring oxazolidine-2-thiones possess a thionamide group $S = C - N =$, they belong to strongly active antithyroid compounds showing all effects presumably resembling these of mostly used antithyroid drugs — propylthiouracil and methimazol. Inhibition of thyroid peroxidase activity[177] and of thyroid hormone biosynthesis[152,234] was also demonstrated.

NATURALLY OCCURRING GOITROGENS AND HUMAN THYROID

Short-Term Effects of Foods and Pure Aglucones on Human Thyroid

Brassica plants and milk — A remarkable inhibiting effect of rutabaga on radioiodine uptake by thyroid was found in human volunteers[178] and later a significant decrease of the same measure was observed after 2 weeks of daily ingestion of 500 g raw cabbage.[179] The inhibition of radioiodine uptake in man after the ingestion of milk from cows fed various Cruciferae[180] or after "pasture milk"[181] has been reported, but some other reports could not confirm these findings.[182] Similarly, repeated findings of goitrogenic effect of milk in rats[183-186] were not conclusively confirmed,[187] apparently due to a varying content of goitrogens and iodine in milk. The transfer of thiocyanate from fodder to cow milk was repeatedly reported.[122,123,187] It was stated that SCN^- level in milk may hardly be higher than 10 mg/ℓ[188] and that the milk to plasma ratio in cows is about 1.0.[189] The question of goitrin transfer to milk was not definitely solved probably due to analytical difficulties.[62,143,144]

Thiocyanate — The goitrogenic effect of thiocyanate in patients treated for hypertension by large doses of this drug between about 1935 and 1950 was repeatedly reported,[190] the effective level being more than 5 mg SCN⁻/dℓ. Similar levels of SCN⁻ were later found to inhibit radioiodine uptake by thyroid.[191,192] Moreover, a decrease of radioiodine uptake by thyroid was also reported after considerably smaller doses of SCN⁻, resulting in a level of about 1.2 mg SCN⁻/dℓ.[193] In fact, similar SCN⁻ levels frequently occur in cigarette smokers or even in nonsmokers after repeated intake of *Brassica* plants (i.e., 0.8 to 1.2 mg/dℓ).[114] From this it may be concluded that, under some conditions, thiocyanate itself might interfere with thyroid function in man.

Oxazolidine-2-thione — A decrease of radioiodine uptake in man was found following a single dose of Progoitrin corresponding to about 165 to 670 mg goitrin (L-5-vinyl-oxazolidine-2-thione).[103] Moreover, a depression of radioiodine uptake was also repeatedly found after a single peroral dose of 25 and 50 mg goitrin,[12,182] which corresponds to about 0.5 to 2.0 kg of fresh *Brassica* (see Table 5). However, if we take into account the presence of other goitrogens (i.e., thiocyanate and isothiocyanates), the minimum effective amount of raw plant material might be somewhat less than indicated above.

Exogenous Preformed Thiocyanate as a Tracer of Other Aglucones

During the enzymatic splitting of glucosinolates, the thiocyanate is liberated simultaneously with other aglucones (isothiocyanates and oxazolidine-2-thiones). However, since the chemical estimation of thiocyanate in body fluids is relatively simple compared to the other substances, it may be used as a tracer of these with the exception of thiocyanate originating from cyanogenic glucosides or cigarette smoking. Such a possibility was suggested from the observations of some seasonal and regional variations in serum thiocyanate level (coincident with increased consumption of *Brassica*) in large numbers of inhabitants in Czechoslovakia,[114,194-196] in domestic animals in neighboring Poland,[197] and from the correlations between urinary excretion of thiocyanate (originating from milk and vegetables) on one hand and lactoflavin (originating from milk) or ascorbic acid (originating from vegetables) on the other.[195] An accumulation of thiocyanate in man was also found resulting from the ingestion of small daily doses of *Brassica* for several weeks. This phenomenon might bring some new aspects on the mechanism of action of low dietary intake of goitrogenic compounds.[12,114]

Possible Participation of Naturally Occurring Goitrogens in the Etiology of Endemic Goiter

Endemic goiter — a high frequency incidence of visible or even palpable enlargement of the thyroid in certain territory may be considered a maximum result of action of multiple etiological factors. Among them iodine deficiency appears to be most important. Even though naturally occurring goitrogens do not appear to be one of the major etiological factors in endemic goiter, they may have a significant influence on the thyroid under some specific agricultural, nutritional, geographic, and social conditions in certain areas, presumably causing subclinically impaired thyroid function in a number of inhabitants.

There are few reports on the coincidence between a high consumption of cabbage and goiter incidence[209,210] and other reports on the increased incidence of goiter after malnutrition periods under a high intake of vegetable food during the war.[211,212] In the Adriatic Sea, the island of Krk was found the only one with endemic goiter in inhabitants of its northeastern part, while the southwestern part was almost goiter-free.[213] Later survey showed a high consumption of kale containing high level of thiocyanate and glucosinolates in the goitrous part of the island.[214] Another series of reports on the increasing incidence of goiter in Tasmania among school children after the consumption of increasing amounts of milk from cows fed chou-moellier.[8,180] Even though this observation was later claimed to result from a failure of iodine prophylaxis,[215] this perhaps cannot definitely rule out an increasing role of positive goitrogen under the conditions of continuing iodine deficiency.

Finally, a series of reports on the goitrogenic effect of substances contained in drinking water should be mentioned.[10,218]

Future Perspectives
Cruciferous Seed Meal Problem

Seeds of several Crucifers (rape — *Brassica napus,* turnip rape — *B. campestris,* mustard — *B. juncea* and *B. hirta,* radish — *Raphanus sativus,* flax — *Camelina sativa* and *Crambe abyssinica* or *Crambe hispanica)* play a significant role in the international market as a source of vegetable oil and meal. Out of them rapeseed represents one of the most important and valuable oilseed crops, containing roughly 30 to 40% of oil. Moreover, the residue (rapeseed meal) contains about 40 to 50% of high quality protein with well-balanced amino acid composition. Considering the world production of rapeseed in 1970 to 73 to be about 8 million metric tons,[198] this means about 2.5 million metric tons of oil and the same amount of protein which might cover the optimum protein intake of total world population for about 1 week.

However, there are two circumstances preventing the extensive use of rapeseed products in human and animal nutrition: (1) high content of erucic acid (30 to 50% of total oil) which shows cardiotoxic effects,[198] (2) high glucosinolate content (3 to 8% of meal). Recently, the breeders in Canada[198] and Sweden[206] succeeded in producing rapeseed with low erucic (<1%) and low glucosinolate (<1%), about 4 million acres being seeded in Canada to such new cultivars in 1974.

Since even such "double low" seeds are not virtually free of glucosinolates and since, in other producing areas of the world (Europe, India, China), several high glucosinolate Crucifer crops are grown, some technical means are to be used to improve the quality of meal. Among these, the inactivation of myrosinase by heat appeared to be a cheap and effective way, the remaining glucosinolates being nontoxic per se. However, the use of this method is unrealistic since some intestinal bacteria contain similar enzymes and for this reason some other methods (aqueous acetone or hexane extraction, etc.) are being developed.[207]

In contrast, from some industrial aspects the high content of erucic acid appears to be important, this being used as a lubricant or as a material for further production of plastics, e.g., nylons, perfumes, etc. For such purposes the most valuable appears to be the seed oil of *Crambe abyssinica* containing more than 60% of erucic acid.[204,229] Nevertheless, even in this case, a low glucosinolate content is desirable to improve the nutritional value of seed meals. From this point some recent achievements with a cheap and effective removal of glucosinolate from oil-free and crisped meal by continuing water washing seem to be hopeful.[203]

There are numerous reports on toxic effects of unprocessed rapeseed meal in poultry and livestock, including egg production, fertility, hatchability, growth rate of the progeny, hemorrhagic liver lesions, and liver fibrosis etc.,[18,199-202] while no such effects were recently found with *Crambe* meals detoxified by water extraction[83,203] or with a meal from "double low" rapeseeds (cultivar Tower).[236]

Cassava Problem

Cassava or manioc *(Manihot utilissima Creuz)* is an important cyanogenic plant furnishing the basic food and the major source of calories for about 200 million people in Africa. It contains cyanogenic glucosides Linamarin and Lotaustralin (Table 6) yielding 15 to 400 mg cyanide per kilogram of fresh food. This is reduced by traditional detoxication methods in "purupuru" (to 40 to 60 mg/kg) and "giri" (to 10 mg/kg). The coincidence between a high consumption of cassava, high concentration of thiocyanate in plasma, and endemic goiter in some areas of Nigeria,[208,216] Zaire,[11,217,235,241] and Cameroon[164] was reported. Some other toxic effects of high cyanide consumption (such as neuropathy and amblyopia) also were found.

Fresh Vegetable Problem

It may be previewed that the production and consumption of fresh vegetables including cabbage, cauliflower, kale, turnip, etc. will increase due to some modern aspects on human nutrition including calls for low calorie intake under a relatively sufficient volume and cellulose content of diet. Moreover, most vegetables will be presumably consumed in a fresh or raw state. This means a considerable intake of goitrogens which, however, cannot be removed either by breeding or by extraction since they represent an essential component of natural flavors.

Polychlorinated Biphenyls

Although these compounds do not originate from natural materials, they became persistent and toxic ubiquitous environmental pollutants due to their extensive use for over 40 years in a wide variety of situations.[238] Among several toxic effects of these compounds in animals and man (fatty degeneration and necrosis of hepatocytes, porphyria, degeneration of lymphoid and renal tissue, alterations of reproduction, growth and development), antithyroidal and goitrogenic effects have also been described.[239,240]

Water-Contaminating Goitrogens of Bacterial Origin

Growing evidence shows that some waters may contain organic compounds with thionamide-like goitrogenic activity.[226] The main source of such goitrogenic substances appear to be sedimentary rocks rich in organic matter. Since antithyroid activity has been shown in cultures of *Escherichia coli* isolated from polluted streams of endemic areas and also in cell-free filtrates of these cultures, microorganisms, contaminating such water supplies were implicated as causative factors. Some observations show that these factors may play a considerable role in the etiology of endemic goiter in the areas of iodine deficiency. Thus, under similar intake of iodine, the endemy may be more severe in the areas where a contamination of drinking water may be demonstrated. In addition, an increase of iodine intake by prophylactic measures failed to reduce considerably the prevalence of goiter in some areas where the goitrogens of water origin may occur.

Iodine Prophylaxis

A worldwide experience shows that iodine prophylaxis—a long-term regular intake of small amounts of iodine— may improve the thyroid function in areas with environmental iodine deficiency and may prevent most of the harmful effects of goitrogenic compounds.[237] Even though several problems still remain to be elucidated, it may be concluded that iodine prophylaxis will counteract the action of goitrogens.

REFERENCES

1. Chesney, A. M., Clawson, T. A., and Webster, B., Endemic goitre in rabbits. I. Incidence and characteristics, *Bull. Johns Hopkins Hosp.*, 3, 261—277, 1928.
2. Astwood, E. B., Chemical nature of compounds which inhibit function of thyroid gland, *J. Pharmacol. Exp. Ther.*, 78, 79—89, 1943.
3. Astwood, E. B., Chemotherapy of hyperthyroidism, *Harvey Lect.*, 40, 195—235, 1945.
4. Astwood, E. B., Greer, M. A., and Ettlinger, M. G., L-5-vinyl-2-thiooxazolidone, an antithyroid compound from yellow turnip and from Brassica seeds, *J. Biol. Chem.*, 181, 121—130, 1949.
5. Greer, M. A., Nutrition and goiter, *Physiol. Rev.*, 30, 513—548, 1950.

6. Greer, M. A., Goitrogenic substances in food, *Am. J. Clin. Nutr.*, 5, 440—444, 1957.
7. Greer, M. A., The natural occurrence of goitrogenic agents, *Recent Prog. Horm. Res.*, 18, 187—219, 1962.
8. Clements, F. W., Naturally occurring goitrogens, *Br. Med. Bull.*, 16, 133—137, 1960.
9. Virtanen, A. I., Über die Chemie der Brassica-Faktoren, ihre Wirkung auf die Funktion der Schilddruse und Ubergehen in die Milch, *Experientia*, 17, 241—251, 1961.
10. Gaitan, E., Water-borne goitrogens and their role in the etiology of endemic goitre, *World Rev. Nutr. Diet*, 17, 53—90, 1973.
11. Delange, F. M. and Ermans, A. M., Endemic goiter and cretinism, naturally occurring goitrogens, in *Pharmacological Therapy C,* Vol. 1, Hershman, J. M. and Bray, G. A., Eds., Pergamon Press, London, 1976, 57—93.
12. Langer, P. and Greer, M. A., *Antithyroid Substances and Naturally Occurring Goitrogens,* S. Karger, Basel, 1977.
13. Kjaer, A., Naturligt forekommende isothiocyanater (sennepsolier), *Dan. Tidsskr. Farm.*, 30, 117—135, 1956.
14. Kjaer, A., The natural distribution of glucosinolates: a uniform group of sulfur-containing glucosides, in *Chemistry in Botanical Classification,* Behdz, G. and Santesson, J., Eds., Academic Press, New York, 1973, 229—234.
15. Kjaer, A. and Larsen, P. O., Non-protein amino acids, cyanogenic glucosides and glucosinolates, in *Biosynthesis, A Specialist Periodical Report,* The Chemical Society, London, 1977, 120—135.
16. Ettlinger, M. G. and Kjaer, A., Sulfur compounds in plants, in *Recent Advances in Phytochemistry,* Vol. 1, Mabry, T. J., Alston, R. E., and Runeckles, V. C., Eds., Meredith Co., New York, 1968, 60—144.
17. Gmelin, R., Chemie der S-haltigen Brassica-Inhaltstoffe und ihre Beziehungen zu den Brassica-Faktoren, in *Naturally Occurring Goitrogens and Thyroid Function,* Podoba, J. and Langer, P., Eds., Veda, Bratislava, 1964, 17—34.
18. van Etten, C. H., Goitrogens, in *Toxic Constituents of Plant Foodstuffs,* Liener, I. E., Ed., Academic Press, New York, 1969, 103—142.
19. Eyjolfsson, R., Recent advances in the chemistry of cyanogenic glycosides, in *Progress in the Chemistry of Organic Natural Products,* Vol. 28, Herz, W., Grisebach, H., and Scott, A. I., Eds., Springer-Verlag, Wien, 1970, 74—108.
20. Wood, J. L., *Chemistry and Biochemistry of Thiocyanic Acid and its Derivatives,* Newman, A. A., Ed., Academic Press, London, 1975, 156—221.
21. Ettlinger, M. G., Dateo, G. P., Harrison, B. W., Mabry, T. J., and Thompson, C. P., Vitamin C as a coenzyme: the hydrolysis of mustard oil glucosides, *Proc. Natl. Acad. Sci. U.S.A.*, 47, 1875—1880, 1961.
22. Ettlinger, M. G. and Lundeen, A. J., First synthesis of a mustard oil glucoside: the enzymatic Lassen rearrangement, *J. Am. Chem. Soc.*, 79, 1764—1765, 1957.
23. Radwan, M. N. and Lu, B. C. Y., Solubility of rapeseed protein in aqueous solutions, *J. Am. Oil Chem. Soc.*, 53, 142—144, 1976.
24. van Etten, C. H., Daxenbichler, M. E., Williams, P. H., and Kwolek, W. F., Glucosinolates and derived products in cruciferous vegetables, *Agric. Food Chem.*, 24, 452—455, 1976.
25. Langer, P., Study of chemical representatives of the goitrogenic activity of raw cabbage, *Physiol. Bohemoslov.*, 13, 542—549, 1964.
26. Sedlák, J., Effect of higher sulfate uptake and utilization on the goitrogenicity of winter cabbage, in *Endemic Goitre and Allied Diseases,* Šilink, J. and Černý, J., Eds., Veda, Bratislava, 1966, 229—236.
27. Josefsson, E., Content of rhodanogenic glucosides in some Brassica crops, *J. Sci. Food Agric.*, 18, 492—495, 1967.
28. Kjaer, A., Naturally occurring isothiocyanates and their possible relationship with α-amino acids, *Acta Chem. Scand.*, 8, 1110, 1954.
29. Underhill, E. W. and Chisholm, M. D., Formation of glucotropaeolin from L-phenylalanine-C^{14}-N^{15}, *Biochem. Biophys. Res. Commun.*, 14, 425—430, 1964.
30. Chisholm, M. D. and Wetter, L. R., The administration of methionine-C^{14} and related compounds to horse-radish, *Can. J. Biochem.*, 42, 1033—1040, 1964.
31. Matsuo, M. and Underhill, E. W., A UDP glucose: thiohydroximate glucosyl transferase from Tropaeolum majus L., *Biochem. Biophys. Res. Commun.*, 25, 269—274, 1969.
32. Serif, G. S. and Schmotzer, L. A., Precursor studies of the aglucone of progoitrin, *Phytochemistry,* 7, 1151—1157, 1968.
33. Chisholm, M. D. and Wetter, L. R., The biosynthesis of some isothiocyanates and oxazolidinethiones in rape *(Brassica campestris L.)*, *Plant Physiol.*, 42, 1726—1730, 1967.
34. Kindl, H. and Underhill, E. W., Biosynthesis of mustard oil glucosides, *Phytochemistry,* 7, 745—756, 1968.

35. Josefsson, E., Studies of the biochemical background to differences in glucosinolate content in Brassica napus L., I., *Physiol. Plantarum,* 24, 150—159, 1971.
36. Josefsson, E., Studies on the biochemical background to differences in glucosinolate content in Brassica napus L., II., *Physiol. Plantarum,* 24, 161—175, 1971.
37. Underhill, E. W., Biosynthesis of mustard oil glucosides, conversion of phenylacetaldehyde oxime and 3-phenyl-propionaldehyde oxime to glucotropaeolin and gluconasturtiin, *Eur. J. Biochem.,* 2, 61—63, 1967.
38. Matsuo, M., Incorporation of 4-methyl-thiobutyraldoxime-1-^{14}C, ^{15}N into Sinigrin, *Tetrahedron Lett.,* 38, 4101—4104, 1968.
39. Farnden, K. J. F., Rosen, M. A., and Liljegren, D. R., Aldoximes and nitriles as intermediates in the biosynthesis of cyanogenic glucosides, *Phytochemistry,* 12, 2673—2677, 1973
40. Matsuo, M., On the origin of thioglucoside moiety of Sinigrin, *Chem. Pharm. Bull. Tokyo,* 16, 1128—1129, 1968.
41. Wetter, R. L. and Chisholm, M. D., Sources of sulphur in the thioglucosides of various higher plants, *Can. J. Biochem.,* 46, 931—935, 1968.
42. Kjaer, A., Naturally derived isothiocyantes (mustard oils) and their parent glucosides, in *Fortschritte der Chemie organischer Naturstoffe,* Vol. 18, Zechmeister, L., Ed., Springer-Verlag, Wein, 1960, 122—176.
43. Schwimmer, S., Spectral changes during the action of myrosinase on sinigrin, *Acta Chem. Scand.,* 15, 535—544, 1961.
44. van Etten, C. H. and Daxenbichler, M. E., Formation of organic nitriles from progoitrins in leaves of Crambe abyssinica and Brassica napus, *Agric. Food Chem.,* 19, 194—195, 1971.
45. Henderson, H. M. and McEwen, T. J., Effect of ascorbic acid on thioglucosidases from different crucifers, *Phytochemistry,* 11, 3127—3133, 1972.
46. Tookey, H. L., Crambe thioglucoside glucohydrolase (EC 3.2.3.1.1.): separation of a protein required for epithiobutane formation, *Can. J. Biochem.,* 51, 1654—1660, 1973.
47. Austin, F. I., Gent, C. A., and Wolff, I. A., Degradation of natural thioglucosides with ferrous salts, *J. Agric. Food Chem.,* 16, 752—755, 1968.
48. Michajlovskij, N. and Langer, P., Gehalt einiger Nahrungsmittel an präformiertem Rhodanid, *Z. Physiol. Chem.,* 312, 26—30, 1958.
49. Michajlovskij, N. and Langer, P., Über das Vorkommen präformierten Rhodanids in einigen pflanzlichen Nahrungsmitteln in Hinblick auf jahreszeitliche und regionale Unterschiede, *Z. Physiol. Chem.,* 317, 30—33, 1959.
50. Michajlovskij, N., Nahrungsmittel als Rhodanidträger, in *Naturally Occurring Goitrogens and Thyroid Function,* Podoba, J. and Langer, P., Eds., Veda, Bratislava, 1964, 39—48.
51. Gmelin, R. and Virtanen, A. I., The enzymic formation of thiocyanate (SCN^-) from a precursor(s) in Brassica species, *Acta Chem. Scand.,* 14, 507—510, 1960.
52. Gmelin, R. and Virtanen, A. I., Neoglucobrassicin, ein zweiter SCN^- Precursor vom Indoltyp in Brassica-Arten, *Acta Chem. Scand.,* 16, 1378—1384, 1962.
53. Schraudolf, H., Zur Verbreitung von Glucobrassicin und Neoglucobrassicin in hoheren Pflanzen, *Experientia,* 21, 520—522, 1965.
54. Gmelin, R. and Virtanen, A. I., A new type of enzymatic cleavage of mustard oil glucosides. Formation of allylthiocyanate in *Thalaspi arvense* L. and benzylthiocyanate in *Lepidium ruderale* L., and *Lepidium sativum* L., *Acta Chem. Scand.,* 13, 1474—1475, 1959.
55. Schluter, M. and Gmelin, R., Abnormale enzymatische Spaltung von 4-methyl-thiobutyl-glucosinolat in frisch Pflanzen von Eruca sativa, *Phytochemistry,* 11, 3427—3431, 1972.
56. Saarivirta, M., The formation of benzylcyanamide, benzylthiocyanate, benzylisothiocyanate and benzylamine from benzylglucosinolate in Lepidium, *Planta Medica,* 24, 112—119, 1973.
57. Astwood, E. B., Greer, M. A., and Ettlinger, M. G., The antithyroid factor of yellow turnip, *Science,* 109, 631, 1949.
58. Greer, M. A., Isolation from rutabaga seed of progoitrin, the precursor of the naturally occurring antithyroid compound, *J. Am. Chem. Soc.,* 78, 1260—1261, 1956.
59. Schultz, O. E. and Wagner, W., Senfölglykoside als genuine Muttersubstanzen von natürlich vorkommenden antithyroiden Stoffen, *Arch. Pharm. Berlin,* 289, 597—604, 1956.
60. Hopkins, C. Y., A sulfur containing substance from the seed of Conringia orientalis, *Can. J. Res.,* 16B, 341, 1938.
61. Altamura, M. R., Long, J. R., and Hasselstrom, T., Goitrin from fresh cabbage, *J. Biol. Chem.,* 234, 1847—1849, 1959.
62. Kreula, M. and Kesvaara, M., Determination of L-vinyl-2-thiooxazolidone from plant material and milk, *Acta Chem. Scand.,* 13, 1375—1382, 1959.
63. Daxenbichler, M. E., van Etten, C. H., and Williams, P. H., Glucosinolate products in commercial sauerkraut, *J. Agric. Food Chem.,* 28, 809—811, 1980.

64. van Etten, C. H., Daxenbichler, M. E., Kwolek, W. F., and Williams, P. H., Distribution of glucosinolates in the pith, cambial cortex, and leaves of the head in cabbage, *Brassica oleracea L.*, *J. Agric. Food. Chem.*, 27, 648—650, 1979.
65. Austin, F. L., Gent, C. A., and Wolff, I. A., Degradation of natural thioglucosides with ferrous salts, *J. Agric. Food Chem.*, 16, 752—755, 1968.
66. Montgomery, R. D., The medical significance of cyanogen in plant foodstuffs, *Am. J. Clin. Nutr.*, 17, 103—113, 1965.
67. Conn, E. E., Cyanogenic glucosides, *J. Agric. Food Chem.*, 17, 519—526, 1969.
68. Seigler, D. S., The naturally occurring cyanogenic glucosides, in *Progress in Phytochemistry*, Vol. 4, Reinhold, R., Harborne, J. B., and Swain, T., Eds., Pergamon Press, Oxford, 1977, 83—120.
69. Saghir, A. R., Cowan, J. W., and Salji, J. P., Goitrogenic activity of onion volatiles, *Nature (London)*, 211, 87, 1966.
70. Salji, J. P., Cowan, J. W., and Saghir, A. R., The antithyroid activity of Allium volatiles in the rat — in vitro studies, *Eur. J. Pharmacol.*, 16, 251—253, 1971.
71. Jirousek, L., Zur Frage der Brassica-faktors und des endemischen Kropfes, *Endokrinologie*, 33, 310—321, 1956.
72. Westley, J., Rhodanese, in *Advances in Enzymology*, Vol. 39, Meister, A., Ed., John Wiley & Sons, New York, 1973, 327—368.
73. Shepard, T. H., Pyne, G. E., Kirshwick, J. F., and McLeen, M., Soy bean goiter. Report on three cases, *N. Engl. J. Med.*, 262, 1098—1103, 1960.
74. van Wyk, J. J., Arnold, M. B., Wynn, J. and Pepper, F., Effects of soy-bean product on thyroid function in humans, *Pediatrics*, 24, 752—760, 1959.
75. van Middlesworth, L., Thyroxine excretion, a possible cause of goitre, *Endocrinology*, 61, 570—573, 1957.
76. Linazasoro, J. M., Sanchez-Martin, J. A., and Jimenez-Diaz, C., Goitrogenic effect of walnut and its action on thyroxine excretion, *Endocrinology*, 86, 696—700, 1970.
77. Tellez, M., Gianetti, A., Covarubias, E., and Barzelatto, J., Endemic goiter in Pedregoso (Chile): experimental goitrogenic activity of "Pinon", in *Endemic Goiter*, Stanbury, J. B., Ed., Pan Am. Health Organization, Washington, D.C., 1969, 245—251.
78. Konijn, A. M., Gershon, B., and Guggenheim, K., Further purification and mode of action of a goitrogenic material from soybean flour, *J. Nutrition*, 103, 378—383, 1973.
79. Bachelard, H. S. and Trikojus, V. M., The identification of thioglucosides and their aglucones in weed contaminants of pastures in goitrous areas of Tasmania and Southern Queensland, *Aust. J. Biol. Sci.*, 16, 147—165, 1963.
80. Greer, M. A., The isolation and identification of progoitrin from Brassica seed, *Arch. Biochem. Biophys.*, 99, 369—371, 1962.
81. Appelquist, L. A. and Josefsson, E., Method for quantitative determination of isothiocyanates and oxazolidinethiones in digests of seed meals of rape and turnip rape, *J. Sci. Food Agric.*, 18, 510—519, 1967.
82. Wetter, L. R. and Youngs, C. G., A thiourea-UV assay for total glucosinolate content in rapeseed meals, *J. Am. Oil Chem. Soc.*, 53, 162—164, 1976.
83. Mustakas, G. C., Kirk, L. D., and Griffin, Jr., E. L., Crambe seed processing: removal of glucosinolates by water extraction, *J. Am. Oil Chem. Soc.*, 53, 12—16, 1976.
84. Björkman, R., Preparative isolation and ^{35}S-labelling of glucosinolates from rape seed (*Brassica napus* L.), *Acta Chem. Scand.*, 26, 1111—1116, 1972.
85. Vose, J. R., The fractionation of two glucosinolates from Sinapis alba seed by isoelectric focusing, *Phytochemistry*, 11, 1649—1653, 1972.
86. Neuberg, G. and Schönebeck, O., Über die Verschiedenheit der Sulfatase und Myrosinase, *Biochem. Z.*, 265, 223—236, 1933.
87. Wetter, L. R., The determination of mustard oils in rape-seed meal, *Can. J. Biochem.*, 33, 980—984, 1955.
88. Ettlinger, M. G. and Hodgkins, J. E., The mustard oil rape seed, allylcarbamyl isothiocyanate and synthetic isomers, *J. Am. Chem. Soc.*, 77, 1831—1836, 1955.
89. Langer, P. and Gschwendtova, K., Micro-estimation of major mustard oil and oxazolidinethione in small amounts of plant material, *J. Sci. Food Agric.*, 20, 535—539, 1969.
90. Tsuruo, I. and Hata, T., On the activation mode of the myrosinase by L-ascorbic acid, *Agric. Biol. Chem.*, 31, 27—32, 1967.
91. Lein, K. A. and Schön, W. J., Quantitative Glucosinolatbestimmung aus Halbkörnern von Brassica-arten, *Angew. Bot.*, 43, 87—93, 1969.
92. Barker, M. H., The blood cyanates in the treatment of hypertension, *J. Am. Med. Assoc.*, 106, 762—767, 1936.
93. Aldridge, W. N., The estimation of microquantities of cyanide and thiocyanate, *Analyst*, 70, 474—475, 1945.

94. Johnston, T. D. and Jones, D. I. H., Variation in the thiocyanate content of kale varieties, *J. Sci. Food Agric.*, 17, 70—71, 1966.
95. Wetter, L. R., The estimation of substituted thiooxazolidones in rape-seed meal, *Can. J. Biochem.*, 35, 293—297, 1957.
96. Appelquist, L. A. and Josefsson, E., Studies on the determination of isothiocyanates and vinyl-oxazolidinethione in seeds of rape and turnip rape, *Acta Chem. Scand.*, 19, 1242—1244, 1965.
97. Kjaer, A. and Rubinstein, K., Paper chromatography of thioureas, *Acta Chem. Scand.*, 7, 528—536, 1953.
98. Tapper, B. A. and MacGibbon, D. B., Isolation of 5-allyl-2-thiooxazolidone from *Brassica napus* L., *Phytochemistry*, 6, 749—753, 1967.
99. Heaney, R. K. and Fenwick, G. R., The analysis of glucosinolates in *Brassica* species using gas chromatography. Direct determination of the thiocyanate ion precursors, glucobrassicin and neoglucobrassicin, *J. Sci. Food Agric.*, 31, 593—599, 1980.
100. Josefsson, E. and Akerstrom, L., High-performance liquid chromatographic method for the determination of 5-vinyl-2-oxazolidinethione in milk, *J. Chromatography*, 174, 465—468, 1979.
101. Helboe, P., Olsen, O. and Sørensen, H., Separation of glucosinolates by high-performance liquid chromatography, *J. Chromatography*, 197, 199—205, 1980.
102. Stanovnik, B. and Tisler, M., Prototropic tautomerism of goitrin, *Anal. Biochem.*, 9, 411—416, 1964.
103. Greer, M. A. and Deeney, J. M., Antithyroid activity elicited by the ingestion of pure progoitrin, a naturally occurring thioglucoside of the turnip family, *J. Clin. Invest.*, 38, 1465—1474, 1959.
104. Kjaer, A., Gmelin, R., and Jensen, R. B., β-Methoxybenzyl isothiocyanate, a new natural mustard oil occurring as glucoside (Glucoaubrietin) in *Aubrietia* species, *Acta Chem. Scand.*, 10, 26—31, 1956.
105. Kjaer, A., Gmelin, R., and Jensen, B. R., Glucoconringiin, the natural precursor of 5,5'-dimethyl-2-oxazolidine-thione, *Acta Chem. Scand.*, 10, 432—438, 1956.
106. Michajlovskij, N., Sedlák, J., and Košteková, O., Content of naturally occurring goitrogens in boiled plants of Brassica family, *Endocrinol. Exp.*, 4, 51—61, 1969.
107. Greer, M. A., The significance of naturally occurring antithyroid compounds in the production of goiter in man, *Borden's Rev. Nutr. Res.*, 21, 61—67, 1960.
108. Oginsky, E., Stein, A. E., and Greer, M. A., Myrosinase activity in bacteria as demonstrated by the conversion of progoitrin to goitrin, *Proc. Soc. Exp. Biol. Med.*, 119, 360—364, 1965.
109. Funderburk, C. F. and van Middlesworth, L., Thiocyanate physiologically present in fed and fasted rats, *Am. J. Physiol.*, 215, 147—151, 1968.
110. Lang, K., Die Rhodanbildung im Tierkörper, *Biochem. Z.*, 263, 262—267, 1933.
111. Sörbo, B., Crystalline rhodanse, *Acta Chem. Scand.*, 7, 32—27, 1953.
112. Hylin, J. W., Fiedler, H., and Wood, J. L., Thiocyanate formation by extracts of *Escherichia coli* and of liver, *Proc. Soc. Exp. Biol. Med.*, 100, 165—168, 1959.
113. Maloof, F. and Spector, L., The desulfuration of thiourea by thyroid cytoplasmic particulate fractions, *J. Biol. Chem.*, 234, 949—954, 1959.
114. Langer, P., Serum thiocyanate level in large sections of population as an index of the presence of naturally occurring goitrogens in the organism, in *Naturally Occurring Goitrogens and Thyroid Function*, Podoba, J. and Langer, P., Eds., Veda, Bratislava, 1964, 281—295.
115. Langer, P. and Michajlovskij, N., Präformiertes Rhodanid in Nahrungsmitteln als Hauptursache der Rhodanausscheidung in Harn, *Z. Physiol. Chem.*, 312, 31—36, 1958.
116. Langer, P., Über den Zusammenhang zwischen der Rhodanogenität verschiedener pflanzlichen Nahrungsmitteln und ihren hemmenden Einfluss auf die Radiojodspeicherung durch die Meerschweinchenschilddrüse, *Z. Physiol. Chem.*, 323, 194—198, 1961.
117. Michajlovskij, N. and Langer, P., Identity of the goitrogenic effect of glucobrassicin and the equivalent amount of thiocyanate in rats, *Endocrinol. Exp.*, 1, 229—236, 1967.
118. Michajlovskij, N. and Langer, P., Increase of serum free thyroxine following the administration of thiocyanate and other anions in vivo and in vitro, *Acta Endocrinol., (Kbh.)*, 75, 707—716, 1974.
119. Langer, P., Kokešová, H., and Gschwendtová, K., Acute redistribution of thyroxine after the administration of univalent anions, salicylate, theophylline and barbiturates in rats, *Acta Endocrinol. (Kbh.)*, 81, 516—524, 1976.
120. Funderburk, C. F., Studies of the Physiological Occurrence and Metabolism of Thiocyanate, Thesis, University of Tennessee, Memphis, 1966.
121. Moody, F. G., Water movement through canine stomach during thiocyanate inhibition of gastric acid secretion, *Am. J. Physiol.*, 220, 467—471, 1971.
122. Boulangé, M., Han, K., and Vert, P., Fluctuation saisonière des thiocyanates dans un lait industriel — observations sur cinq années consecutives, *C. R. Soc. Biol.*, 157, 1074—1076, 1963.
123. Michajlovskij, N., Effect of fodder on thiocyanate level in milk (in Slovak), *Biológia*, 16, 459—468, 1961.

124. Maloof, F. and Soodak, M., The inhibition of the metabolism of thiocyanate in the thyroid of the rat, *Endocrinology*, 65, 106—113, 1959.
125. Maloof, F. and Soodak, M., The oxidation of thiocyanate by a cytoplasmic particulate fraction of thyroid tissue, *J. Biol. Chem.*, 239, 1995—2001, 1964.
126. Sanchez-Martin, J. A. and Mitchell, M. L., Effect of thyrotropin upon the intrathyroidal metabolism of thiocyanate-S[35], *Endocrinology*, 67, 325—331, 1960.
127. Logothetopoulos, J. H. and Myant, N. B., Concentration of radioiodide and ^{35}S-thiocyanate by the salivary glands, *J. Physiol.*, 134, 189—194, 1956.
128. Boxer, G. E. and Rickards, J. C., Studies on the metabolism of the carbon of cyanide and thiocyanate, *Arch. Biochem.*, 39, 7—26, 1952.
129. Goldstein, F. and Rieders, F., Formation of cyanide in dog and man following administration of thiocyanate, *Am. J. Physiol.*, 167, 47—54, 1951.
130. Goldstein, F. and Rieders, R., Conversion of thiocyanate to cyanide by an erythrocyte enzyme, *Am. J. Physiol.*, 183, 287—290, 1953.
131. Chung, J. and Wood, J. L., Oxidation of thiocyanate to cyanide catalyzed by hemoglobin, *J. Biol. Chem.*, 246, 555—560, 1971.
132. Sörbo, B. H. and Ljungreen, J. G., Catalytic effect of peroxidase on the reaction between hydrogen peroxide and sulfur compounds, *Acta Chem. Scand.*, 12, 470—476, 1958.
133. Morris, D. R. and Hager, L. P., Mechanism of the inhibition of enzymatic halogenation by antithyroid agents, *J. Biol. Chem.*, 241, 3582—3589, 1966.
134. Fiedler, H. and Wood, J. L., Specificity studies on the beta-mercaptopyruvate cyanide transsulfuration system, *J. Biol. Chem.*, 222, 387—397, 1956.
135. Wood, J. L., Williams, E. F., and Kingsland, N., The conversion of thiocyanate sulfur to sulfate in the white rat, *J. Biol. Chem.*, 170, 251—259, 1947.
136. Funderburk, C. F. and van Middlesworth, L., The effect of thiocyanate concentration on thiocyanate distribution and excretion, *Proc. Soc. Biol. Med.*, 136, 1249—1252, 1971.
137. Ermans, A. M., Delange, F., van der Velden, M., and Kinthaert, J., Possible role of cyanide and thiocyanate in the etiology of endemic cretinism, in *Human Development and the Thyroid Gland*, Stanbury, J. B., Ed., Plenum Press, New York, 1972, 455—473.
138. Langer, P., Some basic observations on the metabolism of naturally occurring goitrogenic compounds, in *Endemic Goitre and Allied Diseases*, Šilink, K. and Černý, J., Eds., Veda, Bratislava, 1966, 197—206.
139. Langer, P. and Greer, M. A., Antithyroid action of some naturally occurring isothiocyanates in vitro, *Metabolism*, 17, 596—605, 1968.
140. Langer, P., Synergic effect of naturally occurring goitrogens on the thyroid gland of rats, *Physiol. Bohemoslov.*, 15, 162—168, 1966.
141. Langer, P., Drobnica, L., and Augustín, J., On the possible mechanism of the antithyroid activity of isothiocyanates, *Physiol. Bohemoslov.*, 13, 450—456, 1964.
142. Langer, P., Antithyroid action in rats of small doses of some naturally occurring compounds, *Endocrinology*, 79, 1117—1122, 1966.
143. Virtanen, A. I., Kreula, M., and Kiesvaara, M., The transfer of L-5-vinyl-2-thiooxazolidone (oxazolidinethione) to milk, *Acta Chem. Scand.*, 12:n580—581, 1958.
144. Arstila, A., Krusius, F. E., and Peltola, P., Studies on the transfer of thio-oxazolidone-type goitrogens into cow's milk in goitre endemic districts of Finland and in experimental conditions, *Acta Endocrinol., (Kbh.)*, 60, 712—718, 1969.
145. Langer, P. and Michajlovskij, N., Studies on the antithyroid activity of naturally occurring L-5-vinyl-2-thiooxazolidone and its urinary metabolite in rats, *Acta Endocrinol., (Kbh.)*, 62, 21—30, 1969.
146. Michajlovskij, N. and Langer, P., Chemical identification and goitrogenic activity of L-5-vinyl-4-hydroxy-2-thiooxazolidone — a metabolite of naturally occurring L-5-vinyl-2-thiooxazolidone, in *Further Advances in Thyroid Research*, Fellinger, K. and Höfer, R., Eds., Vienna Medical Academy, Austria, 1971, 155—162.
147. Sedlák, J., Level of sulfhydryl compounds in rat liver following feeding with goitrogenous and non-goitrogenous cabbage, *Nature (London)*, 186, 892—893, 1960.
148. Peltola, P. and Krusius, F., Distribution of the sulfur-35-labeled goitrogen L-5-vinyl-2-thio-oxazolidone in rat, *Experientia*, 25, 1328—1329, 1969.
149. Förster, W., Zur Frage der thyreostatischen Wirkung von Rhodanese, *Naunyn-Schmiedebergs Arch. Exp. Pathol. Pharmakol.*, 217, 413—429, 1953.
150. Rawson, R. W., Tannheimer, S. F., and Peacock, W., The uptake of radioactive iodine by thyroids of rats made goitrous by potassium thiocyanate and by thouracil, *Endocrinology*, 34, 245—253, 1944.
151. Langer, P., Vergleich der Wirkung von Weisskohl und Rhodanid auf die Rattenschilddrüse, *Z. Physiol. Chem.*, 335, 216—220, 1964.
152. Langer, P., Interrelations between thiocyanate and iodide action on the thyroid in rats, *Rev. Roum. Endocrinol.*, 3, 203—208, 1966.

153. Marine, D., Baumann, E. J., Spence, A. W., and Cipra, A., Further studies on etiology of goiter with particular reference to the action of cyanides, *Proc. Soc. Exp. Biol. Med.*, 29, 772—775, 1932.
154. Jensen, K. A., Conti, J., and Kjaer, A., Volatile isothiocyanates in seeds and roots of various Brassicae, *Acta Chem. Scand.*, 7, 1267—1270, 1953.
155. Wagner-Jauregg, T. and Koch, J., Ernährungsbedingte Schilddrüsenstörungen bei Kaninchen, *Wien. Klin. Wochenschr.*, 58, 448—450, 1946.
156. Bachelard, H. S., McQuillan, M. T., and Trikojus, V. M., An investigation of antithyroid activities of isothiocyanates and derivatives. Observations in fractions of milk from goitrous area, *Aust. J. Biol. Sci.*, 16, 177—191, 1963.
157. Langer, P. and Štolc, V., Goitrogenic activity of allylisothiocyanate — a widespread natural mustard oil, *Endocrinology*, 76, 151—155, 1965.
158. Krusius, F. E. and Peltola, P., The goitrogenic effect of naturally occurring L-5-vinyl- and L-5-phenyl-2-thiooxazolidone in rats, *Acta Endocrinol. (Kbh.)*, 53, 342—352, 1966.
159. Greer, M. A. and Whallon, J., Antithyroid effect of barbarin (Phenyl-thiooxazolidone) a naturally occurring compound from Barbarea, *Proc. Soc. Exp. Biol. Med.*, 107, 802—804, 1961.
160. Faiman, C., Ryan, R. J., and Eichel, H. J., Effect of goitrin analogues and related compounds on the rat thyroid gland, *Endocrinology*, 81, 88—92, 1967.
161. Care, A. D., Goitrogenic properties of linseed, *Nature (London)*, 173, 172—173, 1954.
162. Butler, G. W., Flux, D. S., Petersen, G. B., Wright, E. W., Glanday, A. G., and Johnson, J. M., Goitrogenic effect of white clover (*Trifolium repens* L.), *N.Z. J. Sci. Technol. Sect. A*, 38, 793—802, 1957.
163. Purves, H. D., The search for positive goitrogenic agents, *N.Z. Med. J.*, 80, 489—490, 1974.
164. Aquaron, R., Urinary, salivary and plasma levels of thiocyanate in goitrous and nongoitrous areas of Cameroon after cassava diet, presented at 8th Meeting of Eur. Thyroid Assoc., Abstr. No. 139, Masson et Cie., Paris, 1977.
165. Schuphan, W., Biochemische Stoffbildung bei *Brassica oleracea* L. in Abhängigkeit von morphologischen und endemischen Differenzirungen ihrer Organe, *Z. Pflanzenzücht.*, 39, 127—186, 1958.
166. Clapp, R. C., Long, J. L., Dateo, G. P., Baisseth, R. H., and Hasselstrom, T., The volatile isothiocyanates in fresh cabbage, *J. Am. Chem. Soc.*, 81, 6278—6281, 1959.
167. Sedlák, J., unpublished personal communication.
168. Mackay, D. A. M. and Hewitt, E. J., Comparison of the effect of flavor enzymes from mustard and cabbage upon dehydrated cabbage, *Food Res.*, 24, 253—261, 1959.
169. Bailey, S. D., Bazinet, M. C., Driscoll, J. L., and McCarthy, A. I., The volatile sulfur compound of cabbage, *J. Food. Sci.*, 26, 163—170, 1961.
170. Michajlovskij, N., unpublished personal communication.
171. Langer, P., Über die rhodanogene Wirkung von Allylisothiocyanat, eines der in Pflanzen am häufigsten vorkommenden Senföle, *Z. Physiol. Chem.*, 339, 33—35, 1964.
172. Yamada, T. and Jones, A. E., Effect of thiocyanate, perchlorate and other anions on plasma protein-binding hormone interaction in vitro, *Endocrinology*, 82, 47—53, 1968.
173. Langer, P., Extrathyroidal effect of thiocyanate and propylthiouracil: the depression of the protein-bound iodine level in intact and thyroidectomized rats, *J. Endocrinol.*, 50, 367—372, 1971.
174. Langer, P., Fluctuation of thyroid function following a single and repeated administration of antithyroid drugs, *Endocrinology*, 83, 1268—1272, 1968.
175. Alexander, M. N., Iodide peroxidase in rat thyroid and salivary glands and its inhibition by antithyroid compounds, *J. Biol. Chem.*, 234, 1530—1533, 1959.
176. Hosoya, T., Kondo, Y., and Ui, N., Peroxidase activity in thyroid gland and partial purification of the enzyme, *J. Biochem.*, 52, 180—189, 1962.
177. Suzuki, M. and Langer, P., Effects of naturally occurring goitrogens on some enzymatic activities of pig thyroid subcellular fractions, *Endocrinol. Exp.*, 3, 168—180, 1969.
178. Greer, M. A. and Astwood, E. B., The antithyroid effect of certain foods in man as determined with radioactive iodine, *Endocrinology*, 43, 105—125, 1948.
179. Langer, P. and Kutka, M., Influence of cabbage on the thyroid function in man, in *Naturally Occurring Goitrogens and Thyroid Function*, Podoba, J. and Langer, P., Eds., Veda, Bratislava, 1964, 303—306.
180. Clements, F. W. and Wishart, J. W., A thyroid-blocking agent in the etiology of endemic goitre, *Metabolism*, 6, 623—639, 1956.
181. Greene, R., Farran, H., and Glascock, R. F., Goitrogens in milk, *J. Endocrinol.*, 17, 272—279, 1958.
182. Vilkki, P., Kreula, F. E., and Piironen, E., Studies on the goitrogenic influence of cow's milk on man, *Ann. Acad. Sci. Fenn. Ser. A*, 110, 3—14, 1962.
183. Kilpatrick, R., Broadhead, G. D., Edmons, C. J., Munro, D. S., and Wilson, G. M., Studies on goitre in Sheffield region, in *Advances in Thyroid Research*, Pitt-Rivers., R., Ed., Pergamon Press, London, 1961, 273—278.

184. Munoz-Rodriguez, M., Thiocyanate content in milk as a possible factor of experimental goiter (in Spanish), *Rev. Esp. Fisiol.*, 26, 197—202, 1970.
185. van Middlesworth, L., Dietary aspects of thyroid diseases, *Proc. 2nd Midwest Conference on Thyroid*, University of Missouri, Columbia, 1967, 57—66.
186. Peltola, P., Goitrogenic effect of cow's milk from the goitre district of Finland, *Acta Endocrinol. (Kbh.)*, 34, 131—138, 1960.
187. Virtanen, A. I., Kreula, M., and Kiesvaara, M., Investigations on the alleged goitrogenic properties of milk, *Z. Ernährungswiss.*, Suppl. 3, 23—37, 1963.
188. Virtanen, A. I. and Gmelin, R., On the transfer of thiocyanate from fodder to milk, *Acta Chem. Scand.*, 14, 941—943, 1960.
189. Funderburk, C. F. and van Middlesworth, L., Effect of lactation and perchlorate on thiocyanate metabolism, *Am. J. Physiol.*, 213, 1371—1377, 1967.
190. Danowski, T. S., Clinical endocrinology, *Thyroid*, Vol. 2, Williams & Wilkins, Baltimore, 1962, 219—247.
191. Mitchell, M. L. and O'Rourke, M. E., Response of the thyroid gland to thiocyanate and thyrotropin, *J. Clin. Endocrinol. Metab.*, 20, 47—56, 1960.
192. Mitchell, M. L., O'Rourke, M. E., and Harden, A. B., Differences in the response of euthyroid and hyperthyroid patients to thyro-inhibitory substances, *J. Clin. Endocrinol. Metab.*, 21, 1566—1571, 1961.
193. Reinwein, D. and Irmscher, K., Untersuchung zur Wirkung von Rhodanid auf den Jodstoffwechsel der menschlichen Schilddrüse, *Acta Endocrinol. (Kbh.)*, 49, 629—640, 1965.
194. Šilink, K. and Maršíková, L., Thiocyanate and endemic goitre, *Nature (London)*, 167, 528, 1951.
195. Langer, P., Survey of nutrition and nutritional causes of endemic goitre in some regions in Slovakia (in Slovak), in *Doklady o Preventivnej Starostlivosti v Endokrinologii*, Bárdoš, G., Ed., Veda, Bratislava, 1956, 33—46.
196. Podoba, J., Etiologicaô factors in goitre incidence, in *Endemic Goitre and Allied Diseases*, Šilink, K. and Cerný, K., Veda, Bratislava, 1966, 169—186.
197. Bobek, S. and Pelczarska, A., Thiocyanate level in serum and thyroid in cows from areas with different intensities of goitre in human beings, *Nature (London)*, 198, 1002, 1963.
198. Slinger, S. J., Improving the nutritional properties of rape-seed, *J. Am. Oil Chem. Soc.*, 54, 94A—99A, 1977.
199. Jackson, N., Algerian and French rape-seed meals as a protein source for caged laying hens, with observations on their toxic effects, *J. Sci. Food Agric.*, 21, 511, 1970.
200. March, B. E., Biely, J., and Soong, R., Rape-seed meal in the chicken breeder diet. Effect on production, mortality, hatchability and progeny, *Poultry Sci.*, 51, 1589—1596, 1972.
201. Yamashiro, S., Umemura, T., Bhatnagar, M. K., and David, L., Haemorrhagic liver syndrome of broiler chickens fed diets containing rapeseed products, *Res. Vet. Sci.*, 23, 179—184, 1977.
202. Umemura, T., Yamashiro, S., Bhatnagar, M. K., Moody, D. L., and Slinger, S. J., Liver fibrosis of the turkey on rapeseed products, *Res. Vet. Sci.*, 23, 139—145, 1977.
203. Baker, E. C., Mustakas, G. C., Gumbman, M. R., and Gould, D. H., Biological evaluation of crambe meals detoxified by water extraction on a continuous filter, *J. Am. Oil Chem. Soc.*, 54, 392—396, 1977.
204. Calhoun, W., Crane, J. M., and Stamp, D. L., Development of a low glucosinolate, high erucic acid rapeseed breeding program, *J. Am. Oil Chem. Soc.*, 52, 363—365, 1975.
205. Migirab, S. E., Berger, Y., and Jadot, J., Isothiocyanates, thioures et thiocarbamates isolés de Pentadiplandra brazzeana, *Phytochemistry*, 16, 1719—1721, 1977.
206. Jönsson, R., Breeding for improved oil and meal quality in rape (*Brassica napus* L.) and turnip rape (*Brassica campestris* L.), *Hereditas*, 87, 205—218, 1977.
207. Mukherdjee, K. D., Afzalpurkar, A. B., and Nockrashy, A. S. E., Production of low-glucosinolate rapeseed meals, *Fette Seifen, Anstrichm.*, 78, 306—311, 1976.
208. Nwokolo, C., Ekpechi, O. L., and Nwokolo, U., New foci of endemic goitre in Eastern Nigeria, *Trans. R. Soc. Trop. Med. Hyg.*, 65, 454—479, 1971.
209. Suk, V., Cabbage and goitre in *Carpathian Ruthenia, Anthropologie (Prague)*, 1, 1—6, 1931.
210. Cheng, L. T. and Ku, H. C., A dietary study of the middle class Chinese and Mohamedan in Sungpan, *Contrib. Biol. Lab. Sci. Soc. China Zool. Ser.*, 13, 91—103, 1939.
211. Bastenie, P. A., Diseases of the thyroid in occupied Belgium, *Lancet*, i, 789—791, 1947.
212. Holler, G. and Scholl, F., Ernährungsbedingte Schilddrüsenstörungen beim Menschen, *Wien. Klin. Wochenschr.*, 59, 321—325, 1947.
213. Horvat, A. and Krizmanic, V., The possible role of kale as an etiological factor in endemic goitre on the island of Krk, in *Naturally Occurring Goitrogens and Thyroid Function*, Podoba, J. and Langer, P., Eds., Veda, Bratislava, 1964, 297—301.
214. Michajlovskij, N., Sedlák, J., Jusic, M., and Buzina, R., Goitrogenic substances of kale and their possible relations to the endemic goitre on the Island of Krk, *Endocrinol. Exp.*, 3, 65—72, 1969.

215. Baikie, A. G. and Connolly, R. J., The Tasmanian goitrogen, *Lancet,* i, 47, 1973.
216. Osuntokun, B. O., Epidemiology of tropical nutritional neuropathy in Nigerians, *Trans. R. Soc. Trop. Med. Hyg.,* 65, 454—479, 1971.
217. Delange, F., *Endemic Goitre and Thyroid Function in Central Africa,* S. Karger, Basel, 1974.
218. Gaitan, E. and Island, D. P., Antithyroid and goitrogenic activities in water of endemic goiter areas, presented at 53rd Meeting of American Thyroid Assoc., Cleveland, 1977.
219. Kjaer, A. and Gmelin, R., A new isothiocyanate glycoside (Glucobarbarin) furnishing (-)-5-phenyl-2-oxazolidine-thione upon enzymic hydrolysis, *Acta Chem. Scand.,* 11, 906—907, 1957.
220. Kjaer, A. and Gmelin, R., An isothiocyanate glycoside (Glucobarbarin) of *Reseda luteola* L., *Acta Chem. Scand.,* 12, 1693—1694, 1958.
221. Kjaer, A. and Thomsen, H., Glucocleomin, a new natural glucoside, furnishing (-)-5-ethyl-5-methyl-2-oxazolidinethione on enzymic hydrolysis, *Acta Chem. Scand.,* 16, 591—598, 1962.
222. Kjaer, A. and Christensen, B. W., Glucobenzosisymbrin, a new glucoside present in seeds of *Sisymbrium austriacum, Acta Chem. Scand.,* 15, 1477—1484, 1961.
223. Kjaer, A. and Christensen, B. W., Glucobenzosisaustricin, a new glucoside present in seeds of Sisymbrium austriacum, *Acta Chem. Scand.,* 16, 83—86, 1962.
224. Daxenbichler, M. E., van Etten, C. H., and Wolff, I. A., A new thioglucoside, (R)-2-hydroxy-3-butenylglucosinolate from Crambe abyssinica seeds, *Biochemistry, N. A.,* 4, 318—323, 1965.
225. Tapper, B. A. and MacGibbon, D. B., Isolation of (-)-5-allyl-2-thiooxazolidone from *Brassica napus* L., *Phytochemistry,* 6, 749—753, 1967.
226. Gaitan, E., Goitrogens in the etiology of endemic goitre, in *Endemic Goiter and Endemic Cretinism,* Stanbury, J. B. and Hetzel, B., Eds., John Wiley & Sons, New York, 1980.
227. Iversen, T. H., Baggerud, C., and Beisvaag, T., Myrosin cells in Brasicaceae roots, *Z. Pflanzenphysiol.,* 94, 143—154, 1979.
228. Thürkow, B. and Weuffen, W., Anwendung einer modifizierten Aldridge-Methode zur Eliminierung einiger Aminosauren und Proteinbestandteile als Storfaktoren der Thiocyanatbestimmung in menschlichen und tierischen Seren, *Pharmazie,* 35, 475—478, 1980.
229. Lundquist, P., Mårtenson, J., Sörbo, B., and Öhman, S., Method for determining thiocyanate in serum and urine, *Clin. Chem.,* 25, 678—681, 1979.
230. De Brabander, H. F. and Verbeke, R., Determination of thiocyanate in tissues and body fluids of animals by gas chromatography with electron-capture detection, *J. Chromat.,* 138, 131—142, 1977.
231. Conn, E. E., Cyanogenic compounds, *Ann. Rev. Plant Physiol.,* 31, 433—451, 1980.
232. Olsen, O. and Sørensen, H., Sinalbin and other glucosinolates in seeds of double low rape species and *Brassica napus* cv. Bronowski, *Agric. Food Chem.,* 28, 43—48, 1980.
233. Maeda, Y., Ozawa, Y., and Uda, Y., Steam volatile isothiocyanates of raw and salted cruciferous vegetables, *Nippon Nogei Kagaku Kaishi,* 53, 261—268, 1979.
234. Elfving, S., Studies on the naturally occurring goitrogen 5-vinyl-2-thiooxazolidone, *Ann. Clin. Res.,* 12 (Suppl. 28), 1—47, 1980.
235. Ermans, A. M., Mbulamoko, N. M., Delange, F., and Ahluwalia, R., Eds., *Role of Cassava in the Etiology of Endemic Goitre and Cretinism,* International Development Res. Centre, Ottawa, Canada, 1980.
236. Papas, A., Ingalis, J. R., and Campbell, L. D., Studies on the effects of rapeseed meal on thyroid status in cattle, glucosinoate and iodine content in milk and other parameters, *J. Nutr.,* 109, 1129—1139, 1979.
237. Stanbury, J. B. and Hetzel, B., Eds., Iodine nutrition in health and disease, in *Endemic Goiter and Endemic Cretinism,* John Wiley & Sons, New York, 1980,
238. Kimbrough, R. D., The toxicity of polychlorinated polycyclic compounds and related chemicals, *Crit. Rev. Toxicol.,* 2, 445—498, 1974.
239. Bastomsky, C. H., Goitres in rats fed polychlorinated biphenyls, *Can. J. Physiol. Pharmacol.,* 55, 288—292, 1977.
240. Collins, W. T. and Capen, C. C., Ultrastructural and functional alterations of the rat thyroid gland produced by polychlorinated biphenyls compared with iodide excess and deficiency, and thyrotropin and thyroxine administration, *Virchows Arch. B Cell. Pathol.,* 33, 213—231, 1980.

NITROSAMINES: A REVIEW OF THEIR CHEMISTRY, BIOLOGICAL PROPERTIES, AND OCCURRENCE IN THE ENVIRONMENT

N.T. Crosby

INTRODUCTION

The toxic properties of dimethylnitrosamine (DMN) have been known[1] for around 25 years, following the accidental exposure of workers in an industrial situation where the compound was being used as a solvent. Subsequent toxicological investigations by Barnes and Magee established first of all the potent hepatotoxicity[1] and later the carcinogenic properties[2] of this compound in the rat. These findings stimulated an entirely new area of research into the biochemical actions of a whole family of closely related compounds (N-nitrosamines and N-nitrosamides) as a means of investigating the mechanism of carcinogenesis in animals. Around 100 compounds have now been tested, of which 75 are known[3] to be carcinogenic, in experiments designed to measure the increased incidence of tumors in animals fed diets containing various levels of the suspect compounds. This work is described more fully in the section entitled "Carcinogenicity".

Since these compounds had not been detected in the environment, there was no immediate cause for concern. However, in 1964, when workers[4] in Norway first showed that nitrosamines could occur (or be formed) in fishmeal following their investigations of a liver disease in ruminants and mink, a search for nitrosamines throughout the environment commenced. Particular attention was paid to human food which is known to contain nitrite (or nitrate) and amines, either naturally or by addition during processing, since these are the known precursors of nitrosamines. While some of the earlier results are suspect owing to the nonspecific methods of analysis in use at that time, more recent studies have confirmed that minute quantities of some nitroso compounds can occur in food. A summary of our present knowledge is presented in the section entitled "Foods".

Additional attention has been paid to other areas of the environment following extensive studies of the formation of nitrosocompounds from nitrite and amine *in situ*. The realization that nitrosation reactions could occur, not only during cooking but also within the stomach after ingestion of precursor materials in food, or following administration of drugs, led to a reassessment of the use of nitrite as a food preservative. The possible formation of C-nitroso and S-nitroso compounds from food constituents has also been investigated, although little is known as yet of the public health significance of such compounds. Nitroso compounds have also been reported in tobacco smoke and in urban atmospheres with the result that there is now a world-wide search under way to measure levels of nitroso compounds throughout the environment.

The nitrosamine problem has been reviewed previously in detail by several authors. Of particular importance are the contributions of Crosby,[5] Crosby and Sawyer,[6] Druckrey et al.,[7] Magee and Barnes,[8] Scanlan,[9] Sebranek and Cassens,[10] and Sen.[11] The current review attempts to summarize and assess critically various aspects of the nitrosamine problem outlined above in the light of the more recent findings. For a more detailed study of the experimental data on the analysis, formation in vivo and in vitro, and the occurrence of N-nitroso compounds in the environment, the reader is referred to the Proceedings of Working Conferences held under the auspices of the International Agency for Research on Cancer in 1971,[12] 1973,[13] 1975,[14] 1977,[14a] and 1979.[14b]

CHEMISTRY

Synthesis

As nitroso compounds are potentially hazardous substances, it is essential to take suitable precautions to prevent spillage, inhalation, exposure to the skin, and ingestion etc., particularly during the preparation and manipulation of pure materials or concentrated solutions. Such preparations should not be used by young workers especially, because of the possible cancer risk in later life. Recommendations for the transportation, storage, laboratory use, and disposal of nitrosamines have been made by Groenen and Feron.[15]

N-Nitrosamines are usually prepared from the appropriate secondary amine by nitrosation using sodium nitrite in acidic solution. The reaction can be represented as follows:

$$\begin{array}{c} R_1 \\ R_2 \end{array}\!\!NH + HONO \longrightarrow \begin{array}{c} R_1 \\ R_2 \end{array}\!\!N-N=O + H_2O \qquad (1)$$

The resulting nitrosamine usually separates as a yellowish oil which is then further purified by ether extraction, drying, and fractional distillation *in vacuo*. Detailed practical methods for the preparation of dimethylnitrosamine (DMN) and diethylnitrosamine (DEN) have been given by Vogel,[16] and for some higher members of the series by Pensabene et al.[17] Other nitrosating agents have been proposed, e.g., nitrosyl chloride[18] or nitrosyl tetrafluoroborate.[19] The latter reagent is particularly suitable for the nitrosation of amines that are insoluble in aqueous systems. N-Nitrosamides are obtained similarly by reaction of nitrous acid with the corresponding amide. White[20] compared five methods for the synthesis of N-nitrosamides and preferred the use of nitrogen tetroxide as nitrosating agent. The similarity in structure between the nitrosamines and nitrosamides is illustrated below:

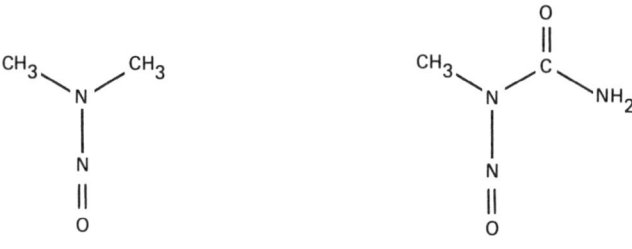

Dimethylnitrosamine   Methylnitrosourea

Kinetics of Nitrosation

The reaction between amines and nitrous acid has been intensively studied. Modern work has been summarized by Ridd,[21] by Mirvish,[22] and by Sander and Schweinsberg.[23] The first, and rate-determining step in the reaction is an electrophilic attack by the nitrosating agent on the free electron pair of the nitrogen atom. In aqueous systems, protons compete with the nitrosating agent so that at any given pH value, the rate of nitrosation falls with increasing basicity of the amine. The rate also varies with the pH value of the medium, being a maximum at pH 3.4 for DMN.[22] The reaction is third order since the rate is proportional to the concentration of amine and the square of the nitrite concentration, as shown in Equations 2 and 3.

$$\text{Rate} = k_1 \times [R_2NH] \times [HNO_2]^2 \qquad (2)$$

$$\text{Rate} = k_2 \times [\text{total amine}] \times [\text{total nitrite}]^2 \qquad (3)$$

In Equation 2, the concentrations of nonionized amine and free nitrous acid vary with pH value and, hence, k_1 is independent of pH. In Equation 3 total concentrations of both amine and nitrite are used so that k_2 (the stoichiometric rate constant) varies with pH, being a maximum at pH 3.4 for DMN; k_2 varies several 1000-fold depending on the basicity of the amine.[24]

In contrast, the optimum pH value for nitrosation of the amino acids proline, hydroxyproline, and sarcosine lies in the range 2.25 to 2.5, and for alkylureas and N-alkylurethanes the rate increases approximately 10-fold for each drop of 1 unit in pH value; no maximum pH value was detected.[24]

Catalysis — The catalytic effects on the nitrosation reaction of certain ions such as halides[21] and thiocyanate[25] have been extensively studied. The order of catalytic activity of the halides is I > Br > Cl; thiocyanate being intermediate between iodine and bromine. The mechanism of this catalytic action is thought to involve formation of covalent nitrosyl derivatives of the type $O = N - X$. Catalysis is more marked at low pH values than in the neutral region where chloride can even exhibit an inhibiting effect.

Inhibition — Any chemical which can react with nitrite will compete with amine for available nitrite and so may act as an inhibitor in the nitrosation reaction. A depressant effect has been demonstrated for ascorbate,[26] and for tannins and milk.[27] The importance of this effect will be studied later.

Effect of temperature — Increase in temperature generally has a marked effect on the rate of a chemical reaction; often the rate increases by a factor of about 2 for every 10° rise in temperature. Quantitatively, the influence of temperature can be expressed by an equation of the form:

$$\text{Log } k = a - \frac{b}{T} \qquad (4)$$

where a and b are constants, k is the rate constant, and T the absolute temperature.

Fan and Tannenbaum[28] studied the effect of low temperatures (down to −40°C) on the nitrosation of morpholine. A surprising enhancement was, however, observed in a frozen buffer system and in milk. This enhancement appears to be a function of overall solute concentration which increases at subfreezing temperatures when water is changed to ice. These results are of importance with regard to frozen foods, fish in particular. The effect of high temperatures used in cooking certain foods will be discussed in the Section entitled "Bacon".

Formation from Primary and Tertiary Amines and Quaternary Ammonium Compounds

The principal product formed in the reaction between a primary aliphatic amine and nitrous acid is a carbonium ion, whereas with aromatic compounds a stable diazonium salt is formed. The reactive carbonium ion can undergo various reactions in producing a variety of deamination products. Under certain conditions nitrosamines are formed,[29] albeit in very low yield. Similarly, the formation of nitrosamines from tertiary amines and quaternary ammonium salts has been demonstrated.[30] Again, the yields obtained are very low. Scanlan et al.[31] showed that the optimum pH value for the conversion of trimethylamine to DMN was pH 3.3, a value very close to the optimum value for the nitrosation of secondary amines. Lijinski et al.[32] have shown that a number of tertiary amines can react with nitrite under suitable conditions to produce nitrosamines. In the case of aminopyrine, a 40% yield was obtained.[33] Lijinski[32] also studied the reaction of nitrous acid with trimethylamine and trimethylamine oxide; compounds known to occur in fish. Up to 50% conversion was achieved after 4 hr at 90°C.

Formation in Vivo
Animal Feeding Trials

In addition to the formation of nitroso compounds in vitro, synthesis by feeding precursor materials (amine + nitrite or nitrate) to animals has also been attempted. The reaction has been monitored both by analysis of stomach contents and by examination of target organs for increased tumor incidence. Thus, Sander and Schweinsberg[23] showed that rats developed esophageal tumors on feeding for several weeks on a diet containing 0.08% sodium nitrite and 0.25% N-methylbenzylamine. Greenblatt et al.[34] induced lung adenomas in mice using nitrite and morpholine, or methylaniline, or piperazine. No tumors developed in animals receiving amine or nitrite alone. Similar results have been obtained with the alkylureas. However, Greenblatt found that the formation of nitroso-N-methylaniline in vivo was only 10% of that predicted from in vitro studies on the basis of the number of lung adenomas produced. Additionally, Greenblatt and Lijinsky[35] failed to induce tumors in mice following the concurrent feeding of nitrite and proline, hydroxyproline, or arginine. Nitrosoproline is, however, thought to be noncarcinogenic.

Alam et al.[36] reported the biosynthesis of N-nitrosopiperidine from piperidine and nitrite in the stomach and isolated intestinal loop of the rat, as well as in the gastric contents in vitro. The fact that synthesis was achieved both in the stomach and in the intestine indicates that the presence of acids is not essential for the formation of nitroso compounds. Later, Alam et al.[37] achieved the same synthesis using nitrate in place of nitrite.

Telling et al.[38] carried out low level feeding studies of pyrrolidine and dimethylamine with nitrite on rats. They found that there was a threshold level below which nitrosamines were not formed in the stomach contents. This threshold level of secondary amine (1000 mg/kg) is greatly in excess of amine levels found in most human foods. The concentration of dietary amine was found to be a more important parameter than concentration of dietary nitrite on subsequent formation of nitrosamines in the animal stomach, in contradiction to the evidence of theoretical kinetic data (Section II A 1). (See section entitled "Kinetics of Nitrosation from Secondary Amines".)

Simulated Food Systems

In order to assess the hazard from *in situ* formation of nitrosamines during passage through the alimentary system, several workers have attempted to simulate conditions occurring in the stomach. Walters et al.[39] treated foods with relatively high levels of nitrite at acidic pH values and, in the case of milk and cheese, some formation of dimethylnitrosamine, nitrosopyrrolidine, and nitrosopiperidine was achieved. Some synthesis was also reported using egg products and tea, but not with lean pork meat or bread. Using concentrations of nitrite closer to those normally encountered in the human stomach, lower conversion to nitrosamines was observed, and then only in the case of cheese.

In contrast, Fiddler et al.[40] studied the effect of sodium nitrite on DMN formation in frankfurters. Concentrations of nitrite at ten times the legal limit produced significant quantities of nitrosamine. The effects of other frankfurter cure ingredients were described in a follow-up paper.[41] Glucono-δ-lactone produced increased quantities of nitrosamine while ascorbate and its optical isomer (erythorbate) inhibited the formation of nitrosamine.

The overall picture which emerges from these studies is that the conversion rate of nitrosamines from precursor materials is low, and coupled with the relatively low concentrations of precursors that are present in the environment, the total yield of nitrosamine is expected to be very small indeed. Competing reactions and the presence of inhibitors will further reduce the yields so that while qualitatively the correlation between in vitro and in vivo studies is good; quantitatively the agreement is less satisfactory.

Drugs, Pesticides, etc.

Lijinski et al.[42] drew attention to the interaction between certain drugs and nitrite resulting in the endogenous synthesis of carcinogenic nitroso compounds. Many drugs contain secondary amines and are taken in relatively high doses over a prolonged period. Under the conditions of test used, DMN was obtained from oxytetracycline and aminopyrine and DEN from disulfiram and nikethamide. Support for these findings was obtained in animal feeding trials.[43] However, Mirvish et al.[44] suggested that ascorbate incorporated with such drugs would reduce the formation of nitrosocompounds, and this was also confirmed in animal feeding trials by Kamm et al.[45] Similar studies involving nitrosoureas have been reported by Ivankovic et al.[46] Scheunig and Ziebarth[47] found that the yield of nitrosamines from drugs in human gastric juice could be as high as 70% under physiological reaction conditions.

Other nitrosatable substances are present in the environment and may react with nitrite to form nitroso derivatives. For example, Ungerer et al.[48] showed that the herbicide N-methyl-N^1 (2-benzothiazolyl)-urea (benzthiazuron) could be nitrosated, and in a later paper[49] a similar reaction with the insecticide carbaryl was described. Yields were, however, only 1 to 2% of theoretical.

Bacterial Production

Sander[50] first reported the action of certain strains of nitrate-reducing bacteria in the formation of nitrosamines. The importance of this discovery was that bacteria catalyzed the nitrosation at pH values close to neutrality; hence, formation of nitrosamines could therefore occur at any site within the body where secondary amines, nitrate (or nitrite), and a suitable bacterial population can coexist. Such conditions might be satisfied in the stomach (for patients suffering from achlorhydria), in the intestine, or in the bladder for patients with urinary tract infections, but not in healthy individuals. These findings have been confirmed by Hawksworth and Hill.[51]

Properties
Physical Properties and Structure

The general formula for the series of compounds known as N-nitrosamines is as follows:

$$\begin{array}{c} R_1 \\ \backslash \\ N-N=O \\ / \\ R_2 \end{array}$$

where R_1 and R_2 may be alkyl, aryl, or alicyclic groups. Since only the nitroso group $>N-N=O$ is common to all compounds, the physical properties vary widely according to the nature of the substituent groups R_1 and R_2. The simple dialkyl nitrosamines are yellowish, nonhygroscopic liquids with high boiling points (150 to 220°C). They are miscible with, and soluble in, a number of organic solvents such as ether, alcohol, chloroform, dichloromethane, and hexane, and also slightly soluble in water. The aromatic nitrosamines are less soluble in water, tend to decompose on distillation at atmospheric pressure, and some are solids at normal temperatures. Some physical properties and molecular formulas of the nitrosamines are summarized in Table 1. Nitrosamines are only weakly basic and can be salted out of aqueous solutions by potassium carbonate. Most of the simple dialkyl nitrosamines are readily volatile in steam and this property has been used to divide nitroso compounds into two classes; the volatile nitrosoamines, and those only slightly or nonvolatile in steam, including the higher alkyl, aryl, or ali cyclic compounds.

X-ray diffraction studies have established[52] the planar nature of the nitroso group which permits overlapping of the σ - π orbitals resulting in a restricted rotation around the N−N bond which has significant multiple bond characteristics. The N−N bond is thus shorter (1.344 Å) than the equivalent bond (1.382 Å) in N-nitrodimethylamine.[53] Ultraviolet and infrared spectra of nitrosamines have been reported by Haszeldine and Jander,[54] and Haszeldine and Mattinson.[55] Further details of the infrared spectra of these compounds and of the assignment of vibrations of the >N−N=O functional group can be found in the work of Williams et al.[56] Mass spectral and other data have been published by Pensabene et al.[17] as well as by other authors (see section entitled "GLC"). Many of the above papers contain additional information on the preparation and properties of nitroso compounds. A few of the more important parameters have been collected together in Table 1. Some properties of the nitrosoureas and nitrosourethans have been given by Mirvish.[57]

Chemical Reactions

The chemical reactions of the nitrosamines are essentially those of the nitroso group itself, e.g., reduction, oxidation, cyclisation and photochemical transformations. The N-nitrosamines are generally more stable than the nitrosamides which undergo hydrolysis at alkaline pH values. The rate of decomposition of N-nitroso compounds has been studied by Fan and Tannenbaum.[58] The chemistry of nitroso compounds has been reviewed by Sidgwick,[59] Smith,[60] Feuer,[61] and by Crosby and Sawyer.[6] Only reactions of analytical significance will be discussed here.

Hydrolysis — The nitroso group is decomposed on heating with strong acid, a reversal of the method of synthesis. Hydrogen bromide dissolved in glacial acetic acid has been used analytically as a denitrosating agent.[62] Aromatic nitrosamines undergo the Fischer-Hepp rearrangement shown below:

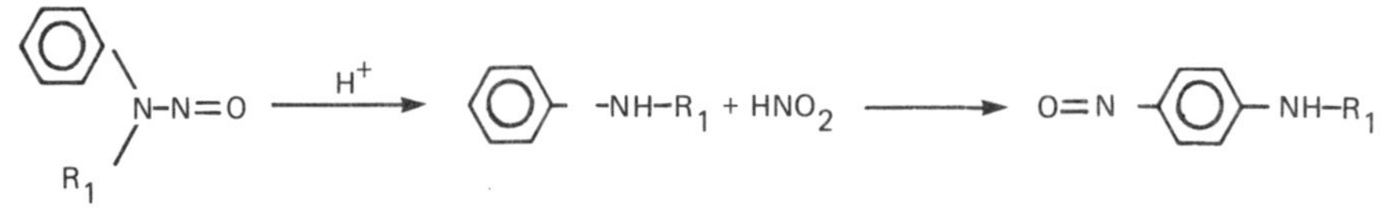

$$\text{Ph-N(R}_1\text{)-N=O} \xrightarrow{H^+} \text{Ph-NH-R}_1 + HNO_2 \longrightarrow O=N-\text{Ph-NH-R}_1 \qquad (5)$$

The Libermann nitroso test for phenols is based on the liberation of nitrous acid from N-nitroso compounds with acid. In the presence of phenol, p-nitrosophenol is first formed, and then indophenol, which is red in acidic solution but turns to blue on dilution and making alkaline.

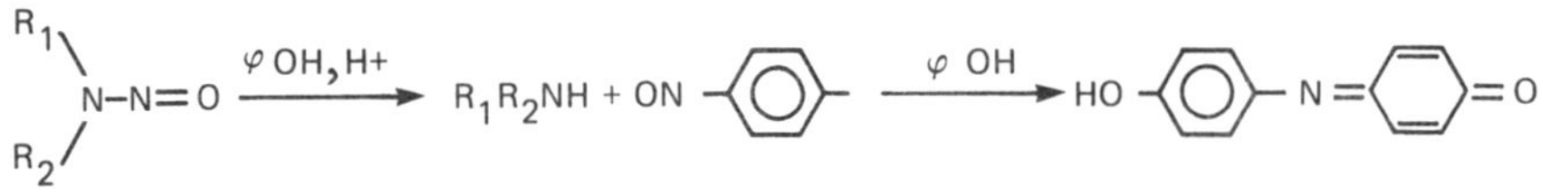

$$\text{R}_1\text{R}_2\text{N-N=O} \xrightarrow{\varphi OH, H^+} R_1R_2NH + ON-\text{Ph} \xrightarrow{\varphi OH} HO-\text{Ph}-N=\text{Ph}=O \qquad (6)$$

Nitrosamines are stable in the presence of dilute acids and frequently distillation at mildly acidic pH values is used to separate nitroso compounds from other more basic nitrogen-containing compounds. The alkylnitrosamides are unstable in alkaline or neutral solutions and decompose to produce the corresponding diazoalkane.

Table 1
SOME CHEMICAL AND PHYSICAL PROPERTIES OF NITROSO COMPOUNDS

Compound	Molecular formula	Molecular weight	Appearance	Properties Density	M.pt./B.pt. (°C)	Refractive index η_d^{20}	Solubility
Dimethylnitrosamine (DMN)	$(CH_3)_2$ N–NO	74	Yellow liquid	d_4^{20} 1.006	b.pt. 151—154°	1.4364	V. sol. water, alcohol, ether
Methylethylnitrosamine	CH_3, C_2H_5 N–NO	88			161°/760 mm, 90°/40 mm		
Diethylnitrosamine (DEN)	$(C_2H_5)_2$ N–NO	102	Pale yellow liquid	d_4^{20} 0.9422	175—177°, 64°/13mm	1.4386	Sol. water, alcohol, ether
Methylpropylnitrosamine	CH_3, C_3H_7 N–NO	102			90°/40 mm		
Methylbutylnitrosamine	CH_3, C_4H_9 N–NO	116			198°/760 mm		
Ethylpropylnitrosamine	C_2H_5, C_3H_7 N–NO	116			104°/44 mm		
Ethylbutylnitrosamine	C_2H_5, C_4H_9 N–NO	130			95°/14 mm		
D-n-propylnitrosamine	$(C_3H_7)_2$ N–NO	130	Golden yellow liquid	d_4^{20} 0.9163	206°, 81°/5 mm	1.4437	Sl. sol. water, sol. alcohol, ether
D-iso-propylnitrosamine	$(C_3H_7)_2$ N–NO	130		d_4^{20} 0.9422	m. pt. 48°, b.pt. 194°		Sl. sol. water, alcohol, ether, benzene
Prepylbutylnitrosamine	C_3H_7, C_4H_9 N–NO	144			103°/13 mm		
Dibutylnitrosamine	$(C_4H_9)_2$ N–NO	158			116°/14 mm		
Diamylnitrosamine	$(C_5H_{11})_2$ N–NO	186			124°/5 mm		
Diphenylnitrosamine	$(C_6H_5)_2$ N–NO	198			m.pt. 144°		Sol. in warm ethanol, benzene
Methylphenylnitrosamine	$CH_3C_6H_5$ N–NO	136	Green/blue plates prisms		m.-pt. 15.2°, 128°/19 mm		Insol. water, sol acetic acid
Ethylphenylnitrosamine	C_2H_5, C_6H_5 N–NO	150		d_4^{20} 1.0874	b.pt. 120°		
Propylphenylnitrosamine	C_3H_7, C_6H_5 N–NO	164			109°/3.5 mm		Insol. water, sol. alcohol, ether, ligroin
Benzylphenylnitrosamine	C_6H_5–CH_2, C_6H_5 N–NO	212	Yellow needles		m. pt. 58°		
Dibenzylphenylnitrosamine	$(C_6H_5$–$CH_2)_2$ N–NO	226			m. pt. 61°		
N-Nitrosopiperidine (PIP)	⬡N–N=O	114			218°/760, 100°/14 mm		
N-Nitrosopyrrolidine	⬠N–N=O	100			214°/760, 98°/12 mm		

137

Table 1 (continued)
SOME CHEMICAL AND PHYSICAL PROPERTIES OF NITROSO COMPOUNDS

Compound	Molecular formula	Molecular weight	Appearance	Density	M.pt./B.pt. (°C)	Refractive index	Solubility
1-Methyl-l-nitroso urea	$H_2N-CO-N(NO)CH_3$	103	Colorless to yellow plates		m.pt. 123—124° (dec.)		Insol. water; v. sol. alcohol, ether, acetone; sol. benzene chloroform
1-Ethyl-l-nitroso urea	$H_2N-CO-N(NO)C_2H_5$	117			m.pt. 99—100°		
N-methyl-N-nitroso urethan	$CH_3\ N(NO)CO-O-C_2H_5$	132			b.pt. 62—64°/70 mm		

Note: Abbrebiations: dec — decomposes; v. sol. — very soluble; sl. sol. — slightly soluble; insol. — insoluble.

Reduction — The nitroso group can be reduced to produce either the corresponding N,N-substituted hydrazine or secondary amine. Zinc or tin with acid, lithium aluminium hydride, or sodium amalgam are the most commonly used reducing agents. More control of the reduction reaction can be achieved using electrochemical processes, and polarographic techniques were widely used in the early days. The electrochemical studies[63] have shown that hydrazines are produced in acidic solution by a 4-electron reduction, while at alkaline pH values, the products are secondary amine and nitrous oxide as follows:

$$R_1R_2N-N-OH^+ + 4e + 4H^+ \longrightarrow R_1R_2N \cdot NH_3^+ + 2H_2O \qquad (7)$$

$$2R_1R_2N-N=O + 4e + 3H_2O \longrightarrow 2R_1R_2NH + N_2O + 4OH^- \qquad (8)$$

Diffusion currents are constant over the range pH 0 to 5, but around pH 7 they drop to a value which is half that in acid solution. In chemical reduction systems, the nature of the products is determined by the pH value of the solution, the concentration and order of addition of the reagents, and the particular nitroso compound present. Reductive transformations have formed the basis of several analytical methods for the determination of nitrosamines.

Oxidation — The oxidation of nitrosamines to nitramines $\left[R_1R_2-N-N\begin{smallmatrix}O\\\\O\end{smallmatrix} \right]$ has been described by Emmons[64] using trifluorperacetic acid, or nitric acid and ammonium persulfate.[65] The reaction generally takes place to around 80 to 90% and has been used as the basis of an analytical method.[66,67] Surprisingly, in view of the powerful oxidizing agents normally selected for this reaction, Althorpe et al.[66] reported that the transformation of nitroso compounds dissolved in hexane could also occur on exposure to sunlight.

Photochemistry — On exposure to UV radiation, the nitroso group is cleaved producing principally a secondary amine and hyponitrous acid.[68] The kinetics of photolysis were examined by Thorburn Burns and Alliston[69] by following the reduction in absorbance at the wavelength of maximum absorption (230 nm). The reaction was first order; halflife being dependent on the individual nitrosamine, irradiation conditions, and other solution parameters. The photosensitivity of nitrosamines has led some workers to recommend that solutions, distillation apparatus, etc. should be wrapped in foil during analysis. These reactions can also be exploited analytically.[7]

BIOLOGICAL PROPERTIES

Acute Toxicity

In general, large doses of the dialkyl nitrosamines given to animals produce severe liver necrosis accompanied by extensive hemorrhage both in the liver and at other sites.[8] The single oral LD_{50} dose for rats has been determined[8] for a number of different compounds and, in general, the required dose increases with the length of the chain in the alkyl group. However, acute toxicity values are of little interest to food chemists except insofar as they may elucidate mechanisms of carcinogenesis, since most foods will only contain minute quantities well below the LD_{50} threshold. The acute toxicity is, however, of importance to laboratory workers who may have to handle pure specimens or concentrated solutions of these compounds. Nitrosamides are particularly damaging to the lungs and skin.

Carcinogenicity

As stated earlier, of 100 nitroso compounds tested so far, some 75 to 80 are known[3,70] to be carcinogenic in animals. Comprehensive reviews of the toxicity and carcinogenicity of these compounds have been published by Preussman,[70] Crosby,[5] and by Magee and Barnes.[8] These studies show that the liver is the main target organ of the symmetrical nitrosamines while unsymmetrical compounds attack the esophagus. However, the response following dosage is frequently complex, being dependent on such factors as compound administered, dosing schedule, route of administration, species and age of animal, diet, and possibly other, as yet unknown, factors. While most compounds are known to be active to varying degrees, a few structures are thought to be inactive. For example, diallyl-, diphenyl-, dibenzyl-, and ethyl tert-butylnitrosamine as well as proline and hydroxyproline derivatives have not exhibited a carcinogenic response under the particular conditions of test selected.[71,72] Almost all the organs of experimental animals have developed tumors following the administration of different nitroso compounds. Montesano and Magee[73] tabulated the sites where tumors have been produced in rats and the number of compounds found to be active at each site. Out of 56 compounds tested, 31 were active at the esophagus-pharynx and 30 at the liver. Other organs affected include the nasal cavities (18), respiratory tract (9), kidney (8), tongue (8), and fore-stomach (6), with other sites affected by 1 or 2 compounds only.

A large number of animal species have now been tested, Schmähl and Osswald[74] examined the carcinogenic activity of DEN in rats, mice, guinea pigs, rabbits, dogs, monkeys, grass parakeets, and pigs. Liver damage was detected in all species following a daily dose of 3 mg/kg of DEN administered in the drinking water. The frequency of liver tumor formation was very high even in the guinea pig, an animal that is normally resistant to chemical carcinogenesis. No tumors were found in the monkey although a positive response has been observed by other workers[75] following dosage over a longer life span. Similarly, Montesano and Magee[73] reported that DMN was carcinogenic in all 10 species tested. Terracini et al.[76] observed a positive response with DMN in rats fed only a single dose. Equally, very low doses were sufficient to produce a tumorigenic response. The incidence of liver tumors among surviving animals after 60 weeks was 1 out of 26 at a dose of 2 mg/kg, and 8 out of 74 at a level of 5 mg/kg.

Metabolism

While most of the experimental evidence for the carcinogenicity of nitrosamines has been obtained using animals, there is no reason to believe that man would not be equally at risk. Supporting evidence has come from a number of studies of the metabolism of nitroso compounds in animals and in man. Nitrosamines themselves may not be carcinogenic but only following metabolism to an active form in vivo, since they generally produce tumors at a site distant from the point of administration. Hence the characteristic organotropism exhibited by nitrosamines could be explained by the existence of suitable enzyme systems in the target organ for the metabolism of the compound to an active form. Magee[77] showed that DMN and DEN are rapidly metabolized in the animal, being uniformly distributed throughout the body tissues with no selective concentration in the liver. None of the original dose could be recovered 4 hr after administration to mice, or 24 hr in the case of rats. Dutton and Heath[78] showed that most of the ^{14}C in labeled DMN is exhaled as $^{14}CO_2$. The metabolism of N-nitrosomorpholine differs[79] from DMN and DEN in that 80% is expelled in the urine. Further experiments using DMN labeled with ^{15}N showed[80] that metabolic products containing nitrogen were excreted in the urea fraction rather than in the liver. Heath[81] later concluded that the toxic metabolite from DMN was a diazoalkane, or a monoalkylnitrosamine, or carbonium ions formed from it.

Parallel experiments using liver tissue slices to study the breakdown of DMN in vitro have been reported.[82] Decomposition of DMN occurred only in the presence of oxygen (or air); tissue that had previously been boiled was inactive. Kidney tissue was active only to a small extent. The effect of DMN on the rate of protein synthesis was investigated by Magee.[83] He found using ^{14}C-labeled amino acids that a significant reduction was observed in the liver but not in the kidney, pancreas, or spleen. Later work[84] established that methylation of nucleic acids present in the liver had occurred and 7-methylguanine was identified in the extracts. Montesano and Magee[85] extended these studies to human liver tissue and concluded that man was about as sensitive as the rat to the carcinogenic action of DMN from their observations of comparable rates of metabolism and similar levels of methylation of nucleic acids.

In conclusion, these experiments on the decomposition of the dialkylnitrosamines suggest that carcinogenesis results from a transformation of the compound to an active metabolite which then interacts by alkylation with cell constituents. 7-Alkyl guanine accounts for 70 to 80% of the total alkylation products identified to date. The importance of the alkylation of cellular constituents for the induction of cancer has been discussed by Swann and Magee.[86]

DETERMINATION IN FOODS

The problems associated with the determination of nitrosamines in foods and other biological systems include sensitivity, specificity, the use of a lengthy and exacting analytical procedure, as well as the fundamental problem that many of the active compounds may be as yet unidentified. The multitude of methods and techniques that have been recommended for the detection and determination of nitroso compounds over the years provides ample evidence of the complexity of the analytical problem.

Many of the earlier methods lacked sensitivity and specificity. Hence, some of the results obtained were probably in error. Recent work has established that nitrosamines do occur in foods but at only very low levels (in the parts per billion or microgram per kilogram range) — (see "Food" section) which increases the analytical difficulties. The necessity for a completely unambiguous identification of the compounds present follows from the hazardous properties of these compounds and the political implications of positive findings in the food supply of a nation. Hence, the emphasis of the current review will be directed towards more recent work in which confirmation techniques have been employed.

For reasons of analytical convenience, nitroso compounds are usually separated into two groups: those compounds that are volatile in steam and those that are involatile. The latter compounds will be discussed separately in the section "Nonvolatile Nitroso Compounds". The volatile compounds have been more extensively studied than the latter compounds and are now adequately characterized. While the division into two groups is somewhat arbitrary, it is based primarily on the fact that many workers use an initial distillation procedure to separate the compounds of interest from the rest of the food matrix. The extract (or distillate) is then further purified by solvent extraction, or chromatographic techniques, and any nitrosamines are then concentrated by reducing the volume of solvent by a factor of around 1000. The final stage in the analytical method is that of identification and measurement. Each of these stages will now be considered in greater detail.

Isolation

The food matrix is a mixture of variable amounts of moisture, fat, protein, and carbohydrate, all built into a complex structure. Methods of extraction will generally separate not only nitrosamines from the matrix but other components also present therein. Moreover, the efficiency of extraction of nitroso compounds from the matrix is generally unknown. Estimates are obtained by means of "spiking" experiments in which small quantities of known compounds are added to the matrix at the start of the analytical procedure and a recovery value is then determined. However, methods of incorporation into the matrix are generally unsatisfactory and may not represent a true replica of the natural situation.

A survey of initial isolation techniques as well as other stages in the analytical procedure has been compiled by Wasserman.[87] Steam distillation of an aqueous slurry of the food has been carried out at alkaline, neutral, and acidic pH values, and at atmospheric or reduced pressures. Eisenbrand et al.[88] determined the yields on distillation of 16 compounds in aqueous solution and found no significant difference between normal or reduced pressures over a wide range of pH values. However, the use of highly alkaline solutions will degrade the food to a greater extent and, subsequently, may increase the problems encountered at the clean-up stage. Telling et al.[89] also found little difference in recoveries of nitrosamines between normal or reduced pressures from aqueous salt solutions, but in the presence of an extract of ham better recoveries were claimed on distillation at reduced pressure. One difference in the experimental conditions used by the two groups of workers was that Eisenbrand et al.[88] distilled a volume as low as 6 mℓ, whereas Telling et al.[89] used 250 mℓ of solution. Operation under reduced pressure requires careful control and makes the procedure even more tedious, but it does produce slightly better recoveries of some of the higher dialkyl compounds. Owing to the possibility of the synthesis of nitrosamines at acidic pH values, the initial distillation should be carried out at alkaline pH values. Further purification may then be achieved by additional distillation at acidic pH values to remove basic compounds without the danger of *in situ* formation of nitroso compounds during the distillation.

Organic solvents such as dichloromethane or diethylether have been proposed[87] for the initial separation of nitroso compounds from foods. Howard et al.[90] used an alkaline methanolic digestion as the first stage of the analysis which produces virtually a total solution of the sample. However, the main use of organic solvents has been as secondary extractants to clean up the initial extract.

Clean-up and Concentration

The initial extract of the food will contain many interfering co-extractants. Solvent partition and chromatographic techniques have been widely used for the removal of such co-extractants. Eisenbrand et al.[91] showed that partition between acetonitrile and *n*-heptane could be used to separate nitrosamines from lipid materials; the lipids being retained in the *n*-heptane phase. Column chromatography using various column packing materials has been described,[87] e.g., acid-treated Celite, ion-exchange resins, silica-gel, polyamide, Florisil, charcoal, and alumina.

Following extraction into an organic solvent, the solvent is then evaporated down to a very small volume to concentrate the nitrosamines prior to examination by thin-layer chromatography (TLC) or by gas-liquid chromatography (GLC). Despite having relatively high boiling points (Table 1) many nitrosamines are appreciably volatile and significant losses can occur at this stage of the method. Most workers have used a Danish-Kuderna evaporator fitted with a micro-Snyder column. Other workers have added *n*-hexane as a retaining solvent during the final stages of the evaporation. Table 2 shows the percentage recovery of four nitrosamines after concentration to varying final volume by evaporation. These results emphasize the critical nature of this stage of the analysis and the care that must be exercised to obtain reproducible and reliable results.

Table 2
RECOVERY OF NITROSAMINES AFTER CONCENTRATION TO A
SMALL VOLUME BY EVAPORATION

Final volume (ml) of dichloromethane solution	% Recovery of nitrosamine			
	Dimethyl-	Diethyl-	Dipropyl-	Dibutyl-
10	92	96	96	98
5	94	96	97	98
2	77	80	83	89
1	76	80	86	94
0.5	63	65	72	85
0.1	36	47	66	88

Identification Techniques

While a wide variety of techniques has been used for the separation and identification of nitrosamines, many of the earlier methods have been shown to be insufficiently selective for a completely unambiguous confirmation of the presence of nitrosamines in conjunction with co-extracted interfering compounds. Polarography and TLC are now no longer used except as initial screening techniques and spectroscopic methods are, in general, insufficiently sensitive to detect the low levels present in foods. A fuller account of these techniques has been published elsewhere.[5]

Gas-Liquid Chromatography (GLC)

GLC is undoubtedly the most widely used technique for the separation of nitrosamines. However, the large diversity of column conditions and stationary phases that has been used point to the difficulties encountered in this type of analysis. Full details of the experimental conditions recommended by various workers can be found in the Proceedings of Working Conferences sponsored by the International Agency for Research on Cancer,[12-14,14a,14b] and will not be repeated here. The operating conditions should be selected to achieve separation not only between individual nitroso compounds but also as far as is possible from other co-extractants which may be present. Figure 1 shows a chromatogram of a meat extract using a flame-ionization detector, in which co-extractants are masking any nitroso compounds which may be present. The extract had previously been subjected to clean-up by distillation and solvent extraction. Hence, while GLC using a flame-ionization detector is a sensitive technique, identification of peaks by a single retention time is an indication only of the *possible* presence of a particular compound. Chromatography on alternative stationary phases differing in polarity, only marginally reduces the uncertainty in the identification.

To overcome this problem, nitrogen-selective detectors have been designed. Westlake and Gunther[92] have reviewed the design of thermionic and conductivity detectors and their application to the analysis of samples for pesticide residues. Howard et al.[90] described a homemade thermionic detector consisting of a flame-ionization assembly modified with a platinum coil coated with potassium chloride for use in the determination of DMN. Other workers have used similar detectors of slightly modified design. Modern forms of the thermionic detector, based on an electrically heated glass bead, are more stable than the earlier types which were compared by Palframan et al.[93]

An alternative type of nitrogen-selective detector has been described by Coulson.[94] This detector can be operated in two modes. Compounds eluted from the gas chromatographic column are either thermally degraded at 400° or catalytically at 800°C to ammonia which is then measured conductimetrically. The sensitivity is increased at the higher temperature, but as all compounds are then decomposed, the selectivity for nitrosamines is decreased. A micro version of this detection system has been described

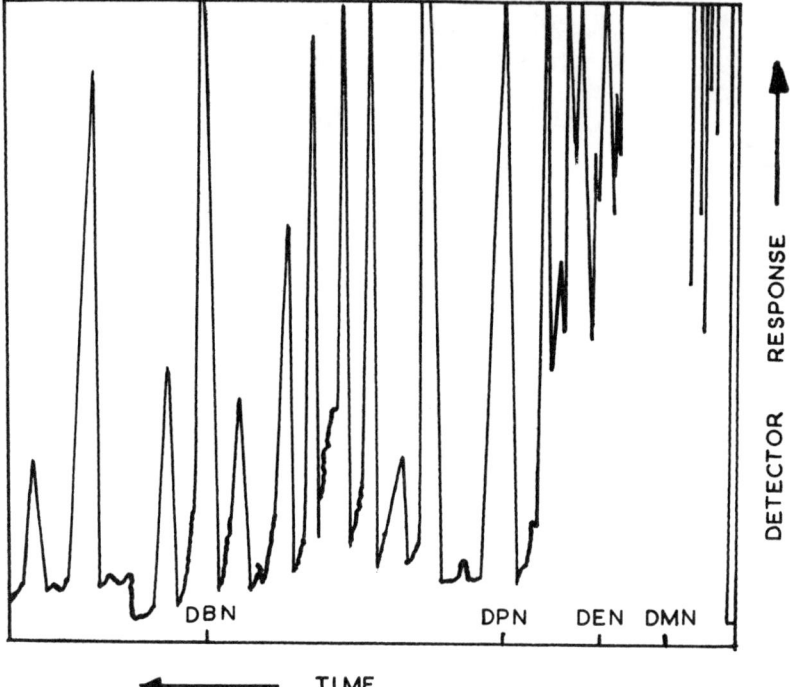

FIGURE 1. Chromatogram of a meat extract obtained using a flame-ionization detector. The retention times of DMN, DEN, DPN, and DBN are shown. (From Crosby, N. T. and Sawyer, R., *Adv. Food Res.,* 22, 1, 1976. With permission.)

by Hall.[95] Gough and Woollam[96] have discussed the use of the Coulson detector for screening purposes. They found that approximately half the number of positive responses obtained with the detector could not be confirmed by subsequent mass spectrometric analysis.

The electron capture detector has also been used for nitrosamine analysis. While this detector is no more sensitive to nitrosamines themselves than the flame-ionization detector, greatly enhanced response can be obtained following conversion of nitrosamines to nitramines or to fluorinated amines.[5] However, despite the use of extensive clean-up methods and the specificity afforded by the chemical conversions employed, confirmation by other techniques is still required.

Mass Spectrometry

The chief use of this technique has been as a detector for gas chromatography and no results are now considered unequivocable unless confirmed by mass spectrometry. However, even this technique is subject to interferences[89,97,98] and, hence, it is important that full details of the mass spectrometric examination used (particularly resolving power) should be given alongside the results. A comprehensive review of mass spectrometric techniques for the determination of *N*-nitroso compounds has been published by Gough.[99]

The combination of a gas chromatograph with a mass spectrometer presents difficulties owing to the operating pressure difference between the two instruments. The coupling has, therefore, to be made through an interface which permits most of the carrier gas from the GC column to be removed without excessive loss of higher molecular weight compounds of interest. A number of reviews of gas chromatography-mass spectrometer separation systems have appeared.[90-102] Gough and Webb[103] described a silicone rubber membrane separator for nitrosamine analysis which permitted the detection of compounds at the 2 mg/ℓ level with a resolution of 7,000. The detection limit could be lowered to 0.2 mg/ℓ by the use of a peak-cutting system. Telling et al.[89] used both molecular ion and NO+ monitoring for the identification of nitrosamines present in meat products, although the molecular ion is about five times more abundant than the NO+ ion. Chemical ionization-mass spectrometric data have been reported and compared with electron impact techniques by Gaffield et al.[104] Alternatively, derivatives of nitrosamines following fluorination or oxidation to nitramines can also be monitored by mass spectrometry.

The mass spectra of N-nitrosoureas and N-nitrosourethanes have been published by Heynes and Roper.[105] Only weak parent ions and no M−NO fragments were observed. The fragmentation pattern produced few ions suitable for analytical characterization.

Thermal Energy Analyzer

A new detector for nitrosamines which is both highly sensitive and highly selective has been described by Fine and Rounbehler.[106] This chemiluminescence analyzer detects the light emitted in the near infrared region produced by the reaction of nitric oxide and ozone and, hence, gives a measure of the nitric oxide produced by the selective catalytic pyrolysis of nitrosamines. Only the minimum sample pretreatment is required and the detector responds to both volatile and nonvolatile nitroso compounds. Hence, this is a group-specific N-nitroso detector which is ideally suitable for sample screening. However, the mechanism of the catalytic cleavage of the N−N bond is not fully understood and it is possible that nitric oxide could be produced from other compounds, e.g., S-nitroso and nitrothiols, nitrones, nitrolic acids, C-nitroso compounds, alkyl nitrites, or nitrates etc.

A simple form of chemiluminescent detector has been described by Gough et al.[107] The application of the equipment to the screening of food extracts for nitroso compounds is also described. Detection limits close to those obtained with mass spectrometry were achieved and quantitative data obtained using both techniques were very similar.[107,108] Chemiluminescent detectors based on the measurement of nitric oxide are obviously more selective than other detectors which respond to all volatile compounds containing nitrogen. However, although the technique is still relatively new, a few instances of erroneous results have already been reported.[109,110]

Collaborative Studies

Collaborative trials of analytical methods for nitrosamine determination in foods have been organized by the International Agency for Research on Cancer. The results of these trials have been reported by Walker and Castegnaro.[111] Samples of canned meat containing added nitrosamines (DMN, DEN, and DBN) at the 20 μg/kg level, and at 5 μg/kg level in a later survey, were examined by a variety of methods generally based on gas chromatography and mass spectrometry by around 13 laboratories. Overall coefficients of variation lay in the range 30 to 50% and no 1 method or technique appeared to be superior to any other. However, the thermal energy analyzer produced much cleaner chromatograms with far fewer interfering peaks, although results were only reported by one laboratory using this technique. The studies confirmed the need for high resolution mass spectrometry to provide conclusive confirmation of identity. Further studies are planned using other commodities such as fish, cooked bacon, cheese, bread, flour, and alcoholic drinks.

OCCURRENCE IN THE ENVIRONMENT

Foods

Studies of the occurrence of nitrosamines in foods have shown that cured meats (especially fried bacon), followed by fish and cheese, represent the major sources of

Table 3
OCCURRENCE OF NITROSAMINES IN FRIED BACON

Sample	Country	No. of samples examined	No. with positives	Nitrosamine	Level (μg/kg)	Ref.
Fried bacon	U.K.	24	6	DMN	<5	112
			9	PYR	1—40	
Uncooked	Canada	1	1	DMN	30	113
Cooked		1	1	DMN, PYR	20, 25	
Fried	U.S.	8	8	PYR	10—108	114
Bacon fat		8	8	PYR	45—207	
Commercial, fried	Canada	12	2	PYR	25—40	115
Fried bacon	U.S.	6	6	PYR	11—38	116
Cook-out fat		6	6	PYR	16—39	
Fried bacon	U.S.	3	3	PYR	2—78	117
Cooked-out fat		3	3	PYR	6—24	
Raw bacon	Netherlands	5	5	DMN, DEN, DBN, PYR, PIP	Up to 1.8	118
Fried bacon		5	5		Up to 55	
Raw	Netherlands	5	0		Up to 4, up to 43	119
		5	2	DMN, DEN		
Uncooked	U.K.	23	0			120
Fried		33	13	DMN	<5	
		33	21	PYR	Up to 200	
Fried	U.K.	50	50	DMN	Up to 5	121
		50	50	PYR	1—20, occasionally up to 200	

volatile nitrosamines in the diet. Reported findings in each of these commodities in recent years have been numerous. A few of the most important papers have been selected and their published results collected together in tabular form. Preference has been given to more recent results where confirmation by mass spectrometry has been reported.

Bacon

Following the first confirmed report[112] of the presence of nitrosamines in bacon by Crosby et al. in 1972, a number of different workers in several countries have obtained similar results (Table 3). A large number of analyses has been made and it is now clear that fried bacon contains N-nitroso pyrrolidine (PYR), usually in the range 1 to 20 μg/kg, but occasionally levels as high as 200 μg/kg have been found.[114,121] DMN is also normally present but at much lower levels (up to 5 μg/kg). In addition, there have been isolated reports of the presence of other nitrosamines in fried bacon, e.g., diethylnitrosamine, N-nitrosopiperidine, and dibutylnitrosamine, usually at levels only just above the limit of detection. Trace amounts of nitrosamines have also been found in uncooked bacon, but always at much lower levels than in the fried product.

The consistent finding of nitrosamines in fried bacon has led several workers to investigate the effects of frying conditions and the variation of some curing parameters on the formation of nitrosamines. Telling et al.[122] showed that levels of DMN were independent of cooking temperature while the PYR content increased significantly as the frying temperature was increased from 140 to 200°C. Pensabene et al.[116] concluded, from experiments with a model system, that PYR formation was at a maximum at 185°C. The amounts of PYR produced using different methods of cooking were also compared; microwave heating gave the lowest levels.

A study[115] has also been made of the effects of initial nitrate and nitrite contents and the conditions of storage of bacon before frying. A high correlation between initial

Table 4
OCCURRENCE OF NITROSAMINES IN CURED MEATS

Food	Country	No. of samples examined	No. with positives	Nitrosamine	Level (μg/kg)	Ref.
Meat products	U.S.	57	1	DMN	5	125
Luncheon meat, salami, chopped ham	U.K.	8	3	DMN, DEN	5	112
Various products	Canada	59	5	DMN	10—80	126
Frankfurters	U.S.	40	3	DMN	11—84	127
Mettwurst sausage	Canada		1	PYR	105	128
spice premix			5	PYR	13—24	
			3	PIP	50—60	129
Various cured meats	Canada	197	19	PYR	3—105	130
			29	DMN	2—35	
			9	DEN	2—25	
Various cured meats	U.K.	75	11	DMN	1—8	120
			1	DEN		
Cured meats	Netherlands	20	2	DEN	3—6	119
			5	DMN		
	Netherlands	29	Most	DMN, DEN, DBN, PIP, PYR	Up to 27	118
Meat products	Netherlands	47	40	DMN, DEN, PIP	16	131
Cured meats	U.K.	75	Most	Volatiles	0.01—10	121
Uncured	U.K.	36	1	DMN	2	
			6		Up to 0.2	

added nitrite levels, and levels of PYR after frying was observed; the correlation with residual nitrite levels immediately before frying being negligible. The distribution of DMN and PYR in the rashers, cooked-out fat, and in the vapors produced during the frying of bacon was determined by Gough et al.[123] They found that the greatest proportion of nitrosamines was lost by volatilization; only 10% of DMN and 25% of PYR remained in the rashers, with 20% DMN and 30% PYR in the cooked-out fat. The origin of the PYR is thought to be from proline by nitrosation and decarboxylation, although the precise mechanism has not been established conclusively. Fiddler et al.[117] found that the lean portion of bacon did not contain PYR when raw, or after frying in a hydrogenated vegetable oil. Hence, PYR appears to be derived from the adipose tissue. Gray and Duggan[124] showed that collagen could be hydrolyzed to release free proline and is, therefore, a potential precursor of PYR. However, other potential precursor materials have also been identified.[9]

Other Meat Products

As can be seen from Table 4, there have been consistent reports of the presence of small quantities of the volatile nitrosamines in a wide range of cured meat products. The effect of processing conditions in frankfurters was studied by Fiddler et al.[133] These authors used an experimentally formulated frankfurter emulsion containing various levels of added nitrite. The frankfurters were lightly smoked for 2 to 4 hr. Tests for residual nitrite concentration showed that about half the added nitrite was still present after processing. The highest level of DMN found was 19 μg/kg and there was some evidence that DMN concentration increased with time of smoking.

Following a survey of meat products, Sen et al.[128] showed that high levels of certain nitrosamines occurred in some meat-cure premixes containing spices and nitrite. The reaction between amines present in the spices and nitrite was apparently taking place even in the dry state as the precursor materials were present in relatively high concentrations. Up to 6000 μg/kg of PYR, 25,000 μg/kg of N-nitrosopiperidine and 900 μg/kg of DMN were found in these products. Black pepper was found to be the source of the N-nitrosopiperidine, while paprika produced PYR. Additions of ascorbate and sodium carbonate to the spice pre-mix reduced, but did not prevent, the formation of nitrosamines.[134] Addition of sodium ascorbate (or its isomer, erythorbate) has been shown by Herring[135] to decrease the amount of PYR formed in bacon on frying. This approach has also been widely tested by in vitro studies and in the formulation of drugs.

Other Foods

There have been a number of reports of the presence of nitrosamines in samples of fish and fishmeal (Table 5). Fazio et al.[136] examined several commercial samples of smoke-processed marine fish and found 4 to 26 μg/kg of DMN in sable, salmon, and shad. Crosby et al.[112] found DMN in the range 1 to 9 μg/kg in samples of fresh, salted, and fried cod; hake, and haddock. Higher levels were reported by Fong and Chan[141] in samples of Cantonese salt-dried fish such as white herring, croaker, yellow croaker, and anchovies. While fish contain higher levels of amines than does meat, the higher levels of nitrosamines in the Cantonese fish were thought to result from contamination of the curing salt used, by salt-tolerant nitrate-reducing staphylococci organisms. More recent studies by Gough et al.,[121] in which 94 samples of fish were analyzed including salted, smoked, pickled, and canned products, showed that DMN was generally present in the range 0.1 to 10.0 μg/kg range. PYR was not normally present even in fried fish.

The occurrence of nitrosamines in cheese was first reported by Crosby et al.[112] in 1972 when levels of DMN up to 4 μg/kg in 6 out of 12 samples were found. These findings were confirmed by other workers from the same laboratory[120,121] when 58 samples including 21 different varieties of cheese were examined. The addition of nitrate during processing had no influence on the presence of DMN in the final product. Levels of DMN detected were again below 5 μg/kg. A wide range of other foods, including cooked complete meals, was analyzed in the same study. No nitrosamines at levels greater than 1 μg/kg were found except in samples of fried bacon, cured meats, and some samples of fish and cheese. In a later paper,[121] the results were used to estimate the weekly intake of volatile nitrosamines from an average U.K. diet. It was concluded that the likely intake of dialkyl nitrosamines from food is about 1 μg/week and the intake of volatile heterocyclic compounds is 3 μg/week.

Air and Water

DMN has been detected in the atmosphere in the vicinity of industrial plants, but at levels usually too low for the identification to be confirmed by mass spectrometry. Levels up to 1 μg/kg, equivalent to an intake of 7.7 μg DMN per day, were observed.[142] N-nitroso compounds were also detected in samples of public drinking water supplies using the thermal energy analyzer coupled to a liquid chromatograph.

Agricultural and Industrial Chemicals

Eisenbrand et al.[49,143] and Sen et al.[144] have examined a number of agricultural products and have shown that, through nitrosation reactions, many of these products can give rise to N-nitroso compounds. Yields of nitroso compounds were generally below 10% of theoretical at a concentration of 10^{-3} M, and decreased markedly as the concentration was lowered even further. In vivo studies demonstrated that similar reactions could take place in the stomach when high concentrations of pesticide residues are present on crops, although the concentrations of nitrite present in the alimentary system are normally well below the values used in these experimental studies.

Table 5
OCCURRENCE OF NITROSAMINES IN FISH AND FISHMEAL

Sample	Country	No. of samples examined	No. with positives	Nitrosamine	Level (µg/kg)	Ref.
Sable						
Raw	U.S.	4	4	DMN	4	136
Smoked		3	3		4—9	
Smoked + NO$_3$		4	4		12—14	
Smoked + NO$_2$		4	4		8—26	
Salmon						
Raw	U.S.	2	0	DMN	ND	136
Smoked		2	1		5	
Smoked + NO$_3$		2	2		16, 17	
Smoked + NO$_2$		2	2		4—6	
Shad						
Raw	U.S.	1	0	DMN	ND	136
Smoked + NO$_3$		1	1		10	
Smoked + NO$_2$		1	1		12	
Cod						
Fresh	U.K.	7	2	DMN	1—4	112
Salted		2	2		1—4	
Fried		7	6		1—9	
Hake						
Frozen	U.K.	4	1	DMN	1—4	112
Fried		2	2		1—9	
Haddock						
Fresh	U.K.	2	0	DMN	ND	112
Fried		1	1		1—4	
Baked		1	1		5—9	
Smoked		1	0		ND	
Fresh fish	U.K.	88	—	DMN	Up to 9	124
Canned fish	U.K.	16	—		Up to 25	
Fish						
Uncooked	U.K.	61	17	DMN	1—5	120,
			6	DMN	5—10	121
Cooked		9	0		ND	
Halibut						
Baked	Canada	1	1	DMN	18	137
Fried		1	1	DMN	15	
Salmon, fried		1	1	DMN	5	
Scallops, fried		1	1	DMN, DEN in scallops	18 (13)	
Cold-smoked, treated sablefish	U.S.	5	4	DMN	10	138
Fishmeal	Norway	—	all	DMN	100—2000	139
	Canada	—	—		350—500	11
Herring meal (untreated)	Canada	13	13	DMN	150—1000	140

Similar nitrosation reactions between drugs and nitrite have been reported by Lijinski.[33,42] Both oxytetracycline and aminopyrine produced DMN at moderately acid pH values and body temperature. The ingestion of milligram quantities of these chemicals as drugs in the presence of nitrite is an added cause for concern, but the formation of nitroso derivatives is readily reduced, or blocked, in the presence of compounds such as ascorbate.[26]

Biological Fluids

Hawksworth and Hill[51] demonstrated the formation of nitroso compounds at sites in the body where nitrates, secondary amines, and nitrate-reducing bacteria coexist.

The urinary tract was identified as the primary source, particularly in patients suffering infection at that point. The role of the bacteria is more than a mere reduction of nitrate to nitrite, followed by nitrosation of the amine with the resulting nitrite, since chemical studies have shown that the nitrosation reaction proceeds only slowly at physiological pH values. Hicks et al.[145] have identified DMN in infected human urine and presented evidence which suggests that there is a link between bladder cancer, chronic urinary tract infections, and the presence of DMN in the urine. No doubt further studies of human and animal body fluids and tissues are required.

Tobacco Smoke Condensates

As early as 1962, Druckrey and Preussmann[146] suggested that nitrosamines might be formed during the burning of tobacco products. Smoking machines have been designed, for other purposes, to simulate the normal smoking process. These enable large numbers of cigarettes to be smoked simultaneously under carefully controlled conditions. The smoke produced is readily trapped and then examined analytically for nitrosamines, although some workers have been concerned at the possible artefactual formation of nitrosamines during, or after, trapping. Precursor materials are likely to be present at low levels only, although little quantitative information is available. Norman and Keith[147] determined the ratio of the various oxides of nitrogen present in the smoke produced from several brands of cigarettes. They found that the main constituent of fresh smoke is nitric oxide (NO) with only traces of the dioxide (NO_2). The concentration of NO varied between 400 and 1000 mg/ℓ depending on the nitrate content of the tobacco. Factors influencing nitrate levels in tobacco have been investigated by Broaddus et al.[148] They found no simple relationship between nitrate content and smoking quality, but the availability of fertilizer nitrogen had a bearing on the nitrate content of the resulting crop. Burley tobaccos were found to have a higher nitrate content than Virginian brands. Very little information is available on the amine content of tobaccos, but the following compounds have been identified:[149,150] anabasine, nornicotine, dimethylamine, pyrrolidine, methylethylamine, diethylamine, piperidine, and proline.

A number of analytical studies of tobacco smoke condensates have been reported. Nitrosamines have been identified in many of these, but findings have seldom been confirmed by mass spectrometry. Rhoades and Johnson[151] found up to 140 ng of DMN per cigarette in the condensate. McCormick et al.[152] identified other nitrosamines as well, e.g., DMN (5 to 180 ng), methylethylnitrosamine (up to 40 ng), DEN (up to 28 ng), PYR (1 to 110 ng), and PIP (up to 9 ng per cigarette). Hoffmann et al.,[153] in a separate study in which isolated compounds were reduced to hydrazones and then estimated by GLC-mass spectrometry, also established the presence of nitrosonornicotine (137 ng), DMN (80 ng), MEN (30 ng per cigarette) with a trace of DEN. The presence of nitrosonornicotine has also been reported by Hecht et al.[154]

NONVOLATILE NITROSO COMPOUNDS

Methods for the identification and estimation of steam-volatile nitroso compounds are now well established. In contrast, progress in the development of methods for nonvolatile compounds has been relatively slow. This stems from the fact that, unlike the volatile group of nitrosamines, there is no simple means of separating nonvolatile compounds from a food matrix that is itself nonvolatile. Additionally, as shown in the section entitled "Formation from Primary and Tertiary Amines, and Quarternary Ammonium Compounds", while nitrosamines may be formed in foods from primary, secondary, and tertiary amines as well as quarternary ammonium compounds, there is little information as to the nature and amounts of these possible precursors in food. Examples of likely compounds are the free amino acids proline, hydroxyproline, and sarcosine, since these compounds do contain nitrosatable secondary amino groups, but there is no well-defined homologous series as with the volatile group of nitrosamines.

One of the earliest attempts to detect nonvolatile nitroso compounds was reported by Walters et al.[155] who adsorbed nitrosamines from aqueous extracts onto activated charcoal columns. Lipid materials interfered and some model compounds were difficult to desorb from the column. The same workers[156] then applied the denitrosation technique, first described by Eisenbrand and Preussmann[62] for volatile compounds, to the determination of nonvolatile compounds, but difficulties were encountered in the separation from the food matrix owing to the large volume of acetic acid which had to be distilled. An alternative approach by the same workers[157] used thionyl chloride for the denitrosation reaction, by which nonvolatile nitrosamines and nitrosamides were converted into volatile derivatives which could then be separated from the food matrix and measured as inorganic nitrite. A wide range of other nitrogen-containing compounds was shown not to interfere, but the technique would work only with dried foods. Fan and Tannenbaum[158] proposed an automatic colorimetric procedure to measure total nonvolatile nitroso compounds. This technique also depended on the release of nitrite from food extracts, but by irradiation with UV light. No interference from C-nitroso compounds, organic and inorganic acids, sugars, nucleoside bases, or amino acids was observed.

The most promising development in the analysis of foods for nonvolatile nitrosamines is undoubtedly the nitroso group-specific detection system described by Fine and Rounbehler,[106] particularly as the detector can now be coupled with both gas chromatographic and liquid chromatographic separation systems.[159] Only minimal clean-up is required prior to analysis since the detector is both highly sensitive and selective.

C-NITROSO COMPOUNDS

The fate of added nitrite during curing, storage, and cooking of meat products has been discussed by several authors.[160] While some of the products formed are well characterized, e.g., nitrosomyoglobin, nitrosothiols, and oxides of nitrogen, not all of the nitrite added can be accounted for in this way. Challis[161] suggested that nitrosation of phenols may occur more readily than the nitrosation of secondary amines and, hence, the competitive nature of the reaction may reduce the amount of N-nitroso compounds formed when phenols are present. As phenols are common constituents of plant materials, and also liquid smoke preparations used in curing, the nitrosation of phenols could occur particularly during the smoke curing of certain processed foods. This aspect has also been studied by Knowles et al.[162] in their work on green and smoked bacon. In the product examined after frying, compounds such as 6-nitro-m-cresol, and 6-nitroso-4-propylguaiacol were identified. They believe that these compounds were present at levels at least one order higher than N-nitroso compounds found in bacon. However, the biological behavior and properties of C-nitroso compounds are largely unknown, hence, the implications of the above findings in relation to public health aspects cannot yet be assessed.

FOOD PRESERVATION AND THE NITROSAMINE PROBLEM

From ancient times, man has had to preserve and conserve his food supply, so that surplus food obtained at harvest can be stored for consumption during periods of shortage with the minimum loss of flavor, texture, and nutrient value. After slaughter of an animal, putrefaction sets in rapidly owing to the action of microorganisms. Preservation implies a change in environmental conditions such as to restrict the growth of such microorganisms.

This can be achieved by alteration of the environmental conditions as far as possible away from the optimum conditions for growth of such spoilage microorganisms without, at the same time, producing unacceptable changes in the chemical constituents of the food, thereby damaging its appearance, taste, or nutrient properties. Reduction in microbiological activity can be achieved in a number of different ways, e.g., (1) the use of lower or higher temperatures than the optimum for microbial growth, (2) a reduction in the moisture content of the foodstuff, (3) the use of chemicals, and (4) a combination of processes (1) to (3). Freezing retards the growth of microorganisms while sterilization using heat destroys active microbes. The latter process involves a compromise between the maximum reduction of microbes with the minimum loss of organoleptic and nutritional qualities. Smoking, in addition to lowering the moisture content of a foodstuff, may also have a bacteriostatic action by means of compounds such as phenols and aldehydes generated in the smoke. Freeze drying and smoking are examples of processes in which temperature and moisture changes occur simultaneously.

The moisture content can also be reduced by increasing the extracellular osmotic pressure as in the process of curing with salts. Addition of salts to meats is also practiced to impart desirable flavor and color characteristics in the final product. However, the most important role of nitrites in meat curing is the protective action against botulinun organisms. The role of nitrites and nitrates in meat curing has been described by Crosby,[5] and by Crosby and Sawyer.[6] Public concern over the use of nitrates and nitrites and the possibility of nitrosamine formation as outlined above has resulted in a reexamination of the use of these compounds for meat curing. In the U.K., the Food Additives and Contaminants Committee recommended that limits should be imposed on the use of nitrates and nitrites in bacon, ham, and pickled meats. These recommendations were implemented[163] in 1971 when limits of 500 mg/kg for nitrate and 200 mg/kg for nitrite were imposed. More recent proposals in the U.S. require bacon to contain 120 ppm of sodium nitrite with 550 ppm sodium ascorbate (or its isomer, sodium erythorbate) in order to minimize the formation of nitrosamines on cooking.

Future regulations[164] will prescribe only 40 ppm of sodium nitrite along with 0.26% potassium sorbate be added to bacon, unless evidence is obtained which shows that these changes would lead to unacceptable hazards from the growth of botulinun organisms or the presence of nitrosamines. In addition, bacon and similar cured-meat products can now be manufactured containing little or no nitrates or nitrites. However, such products will carry a warning label to the effect that they must be stored in a refrigerator (below 40°F) at all times.

CONCLUSIONS

International concern over the presence of nitroso compounds in foods and their formation within the alimentary system and in other parts of the environment has led to increasing restrictions on the use of nitrates and nitrites for food preservation together with the search for alternative agents. The development of analytical methodology has now progressed to the point where satisfactory screening and confirmatory techniques are available so that surveillance programs can be pursued. The significance of the results obtained, particularly in relation to other chemical contaminants in the environment, remains as the most difficult problem yet to be solved.

ACKNOWLEDGMENT

I wish to thank the Government Chemist, Dr. H. Egan, for permission to publish* this review.

---

* Date of submission: July 1978.

REFERENCES

1. Barnes, J. M. and Magee, P. N., Some toxic properties of dimethylnitrosamine, *Br. J. Ind. Med.*, 11, 167, 1954.
2. Magee, P. N. and Barnes, J. M., The production of malignant primary hepatic tumours in the rat by feeding dimethylnitrosamine, *Br. J. Cancer*, 10, 114, 1956.
3. Bogovski, P., N-nitroso compounds in the environment — considerations and prospects, in *Environmental N-nitroso Compounds Analysis and Formation*, Walker, E. A., Bogovski, P., and Griciute, L., Eds., International Agency for Research on Cancer, Sci. Publ. No. 14, Lyon, France, 1976, 3.
4. Ender, F., Harve, G., Helgebostad, A., Koppang, N., Madsen, R., and Ceh, L., Isolation and identification of a hepatotoxic factor in herring meal produced from sodium nitrite preserved herring, *Naturwissenschaften*, 51, 637, 1964.
5. Crosby, N. T., Nitrosamines in foodstuffs, *Residue Rev.*, 64, 77, 1976.
6. Crosby, N. T. and Sawyer, R., N-nitrosamines: a review of chemical and biological properties and their estimation in foodstuffs, *Adv. Food Res.*, 22, 1, 1976.
7. Druckrey, H., Preussmann, R., Ivankovic, S., and Schmähl, D., Organotrope carcinogene Wirkungen bei 65 verschiedenen N-Nitroso-Verbindungen an BD-Ratten, *Z. Krebsforsch*, 69, 103, 1967.
8. Magee, P. N. and Barnes, J. M., Carcinogenic nitroso compounds, in *Advances in Cancer Research*, Vol. 10, Haddow, A. and Weinhouse, S., Eds., Academic Press, New York, 1967, 163.
9. Scanlan, R. A., N-nitrosamines in foods, *Crit. Rev. Food Technol.*, 5, 357, 1975.
10. Sebranek, J. G. and Cassens, R. G., Nitrosamines: a review, *J. Milk Food Technol.*, 36, 76, 1973.
11. Sen, N. P., Nitrosamines, in *Toxic Constituents of Animal Foodstuffs*, Liener, I. E., Ed., Academic Press, London, 1974, 132.
12. Bogovski, P., Preussmann, R., and Walker, E. A., Eds., *N-Nitroso Compounds Analysis and Formation*, International Agency for Research on Cancer, Sci. Publ. No. 3, Lyon, France, 1972.
13. Bogovski, P., Walker, E. A., Eds., *N-Nitroso Compounds in the Environment*, International Agency for Research on Cancer, Sci. Publ. No. 9, Lyon, France, 1974.
14. Walker, E. A., Bogovski, P., and Griciute, L., Eds., *Environmental N-Nitroso Compounds Analysis and Formation*, International Agency for Research on Cancer, Sci. Publ. No. 14, Lyon, France, 1976.
14a. Walker, E. A., Castegnaro, M., Griciute, L., and Lyle, R. E., Eds., *Environmental Aspects of N-Nitroso Compounds*, International Agency for Research on Cancer, Sci. Publ. No. 19., Lyon, France, 1978.
14b. Walker, E. A., Griciute, L., Castegnaro, M., and Börzsöny, M., Eds., *N-Nitroso Compounds: Analysis, Formation and Occurrence*, International Agency for Research on Cancer, Sci. Publ. No. 31, Lyon, France, 1980.
15. Groenen, P. J. and Feron, V. J., Recommendations to work safely with carcinogenic N-nitrosamines, in *N-Nitroso Compounds Newsletter No. 6*, Walker, E. A., Ed., International Agency for Research on Cancer, Lyon, France, 1975, 1.
16. Vogel, A. I., *A Text-book of Practical Organic Chemistry*, 3rd ed., Longman, London, 1956, 426.
17. Pensabene, J. W., Fiddler, W., Dooley, C. J., Doerr, R. C., and Wasserman, A. E., Spectral and gas chromatographic characteristics of some N-nitrosamines, *J. Agric. Food Chem.*, 20, 274, 1972.
18. Fieser, L. F. and Fieser, M., *Reagents for Organic Synthesis*, John Wiley & Sons, New York, 1967, 747.
19. Olah, G., Noszko, L., Kuhn, S. J., and Szelke, M., Preparation of nitrosamines, alkyl nitrites and alkyl nitrates with nitrosyl and nitryl tetrafluoroborate, *Chem. Ber.*, 89, 2374, 1956.
20. White, E. H., The chemistry of the N-alkyl-N-nitrosamides. I. Methods of preparation, *J. Am. Chem. Soc.*, 77, 6008, 1955.
21. Ridd, J. H., Nitrosation, diazotisation and deamination, *Q. Rev. Chem. Soc. (London)*, 15, 418, 1961.
22. Mirvish, S. S., Kinetics of dimethylamine nitrosation in relation to nitrosamine carcinogenesis, *J. Natl. Cancer Inst.*, 44, 633, 1970.
23. Sander, J. and Schweinsberg, F., *In vivo* and *in vitro* experiments on the formation of N-nitroso compounds from amines or amides and nitrate or nitrite, in *N-Nitroso Compounds Analysis and Formation*, Bogovski, P., Preussmann, R., and Walker, E. A., Eds., International Agency for Research on Cancer, Sci. Publ. No. 3, Lyon, France, 1972, 97.
24. Mirvish, S. S., Kinetics of N-nitrosation reactions in relation to tumorigenesis experiments with nitrite plus amines or ureas, in *N-Nitroso Compounds Analysis and Formation*, Bogovski, P., Preussmann, R., and Walker, E. A., Eds., International Agency for Research on Cancer, Sci. Publ. No. 3, Lyon, France, 1972, 104.
25. Boyland, E., Nicie, E., and Williams, K., The catalysis of nitrosation by thiocyanate from saliva, *Food Cosmet. Toxicol.*, 9, 639, 1971.

26. Mirvish, S. S., Wallcave, L., Eagen, M., and Shubik, P., Ascorbate — nitrite reaction. Possible means of blocking the formation of carcinogenic N-nitroso compounds, *Science*, 177, 65, 1972.
27. Bogovski, P., Castegnaro, M., Pignatelli, B., and Walker, E. A., The inhibiting effect of tannins on the formation of nitrosamines, in *N-Nitroso Compounds Analysis and Formation*, Bogovski, P., Preussmann, R., and Walker, E. A., Eds., International Agency for Research on Cancer, Sci. Publ. No. 3, Lyon, France, 1972, 127.
28. Fan, T. Y. and Tannenbaum, S. R., Factors influencing the rate of formation of nitrosomorpholine from morpholine and nitrite. II. Rate enhancement in frozen solutions, *J. Agric. Food Chem.*, 21, 967, 1973.
29. Adamson, D. W. and Kenner, J., The decomposition of the nitrites of some primary aliphatic amines, *J. Chem. Soc. (London)*, 838, 1934.
30. Fiddler, W., Pensabene, J. W., Doerr, R. C., and Wasserman, A. E., Formation of N-nitrosodimethylamine from naturally occurring quaternary ammonium compounds and tertiary amines, *Nature (London)*, 236, 307, 1972.
31. Scanlan, R. A., Lohsen, S. M., Bills, D. D., and Libbey, L. M., Formation of dimethylnitrosamine from dimethylamine and trimethylamine at elevated temperatures, *J. Agric. Food Chem.*, 22, 149, 1974.
32. Lijinski, W., Keefer, L., Conrad, E., and Bogart, R., Nitrosation of tertiary amines and some biologic implications, *J. Natl. Cancer Inst.*, 49, 1239, 1972.
33. Lijinski, W., Reaction of drugs with nitrous acid as a source of carcinogenic nitrosamines, *Cancer Res.*, 34, 255, 1974.
34. Greenblatt, M., Mirvish, S. S., and So, B. T., Nitrosamine studies: induction of lung adenomas by concurrent administration of sodium nitrite and secondary amines in Swiss mice, *J. Natl. Cancer Inst.*, 46, 1029, 1971.
35. Greenblatt, M. and Lijinski, W., Failure to induce tumours in Swiss mice after concurrent administration of amino acids and sodium nitrite, *J. Natl. Cancer Inst.*, 48, 1389, 1972.
36. Alam, B. S., Saporoschetz, I. B., and Epstein, S. S., Formation of N-nitroso-piperidine from piperidine and sodium nitrite in the stomach and the isolated intestinal loop of the rat, *Nature (London)*, 232, 116, 1971.
37. Alam, B. S., Saporoschetz, I. B., and Epstein, S. S., Synthesis of nitroso-piperidine from nitrate and piperidine in the gastrointestinal tract of the rat, *Nature (London)*, 232, 199, 1971.
38. Telling, G. M., Hoar, D., Caswell, D., and Collings, A. J., Studies on the effect of feeding nitrite and secondary amines to Wistar rats, in *Environmental N-Nitroso Compounds Analysis and Formation*, Walker, E. A., Bogovski, P., and Griciute, L., Eds., International Agency for Research on Cancer, Sci. Publ. No. 14, Lyon, France, 1976, 247.
39. Walters, C. L., Newton, B. E., Parke, D. V., and Walker, R., The precursors of N-nitroso compounds in foods, in *N-Nitroso Compounds in the Environment*, Bogovski, P. and Walker, E. A., Eds., International Agency for Research on Cancer, Sci. Publ. No. 9, Lyon, France, 1974, 223.
40. Fiddler, W., Piotrowski, E. G., Pensabene, J. W., Doerr, R. C., and Wasserman, A. E., Effect of sodium nitrite concentration on N-nitrosodimethylamine formation on frankfurters, *J. Food Sci.*, 37, 668, 1972.
41. Fiddler, W., Pensabene, J. W., Kashnir, I., and Piotrowski, E. G., Effect of frankfurter cure ingredients on N-nitrosodimethylamine formation in a model system, *J. Food Sci.*, 38, 714, 1973.
42. Lijinski, W., Conrad, E., and van de Bogart, R., Carcinogenic nitrosamines formed by drug/nitrite interactions, *Nature (London)*, 239, 165, 1972.
43. Lijinski, W., Taylor, H. W., Snyder, C., and Nettesheim, P., Malignant tumours of liver and lung in rats fed aminopyrine or heptamethyleneimine together with nitrite, *Nature (London)*, 244, 176, 1973.
44. Mirvish, S. S., Wallcave, L., Eagen, M., and Shubik, P., Ascorbate-nitrite reaction: possible means of blocking the formation of carcinogenic N-nitroso compounds, *Science*, 177, 65, 1972.
45. Kamm, J. J., Dashman, T., Conney, A. H., and Burns, J. J., Protective effect of ascorbic acid on hepatotoxicity caused by sodium nitrite plus aminopyrine, *Proc. Natl. Acad. Sci.*, 70, 743, 1973.
46. Ivankovic, S., Preussmann, R., Schmähl, D., and Zeller, J. W., Prevention by ascorbic acid of in vivo formation of N-nitroso compounds, in *N-Nitroso Compounds in the Environment*, Bogovski, P. and Walker, E. A., Eds., International Agency for Research on Cancer, Sci. Publ. No. 9, Lyon, France, 1974, 101.
47. Scheunig, G. and Ziebarth, D., Formation of nitrosamines by interaction of some drugs with nitrite in human gastric juice, in *Environmental N-Nitroso Compounds Analysis and Formation*, Walker, E. A., Bogovski, P., and Griciute, L., Eds., International Agency for Research on Cancer, Sci. Publ. No. 14, Lyon, France, 1976, 269.
48. Ungerer, O., Eisenbrand, G., and Preussmann, R., Zur Reaktion von Nitrit mit Pestiziden. Bildung, chemische Eigenschaften und cancerogene Wirkung der N-Nitrosoverbindungen des Herbizids N-methyl-N'-(2-benzothiazolyl)-harnstoff (Benthiazuron), *Z. Krebsforsch.*, 81, 217, 1974.

49. Eisenbrand, G., Ungerer, O., and Preussmann, R., The reactions of nitrite with pesticides. II. Formation, chemical properties and carcinogenic action of the N-nitroso derivative of N-methyl-1-naphthylcarbamate (carbaryl), *Food Cosmet. Toxicol.*, 13, 365, 1975.
50. Sander, J., Nitrosaminosynthese durch Bakterien, *Hoppe-Seyler's Z. Physiol. Chem.*, 349, 429, 1968.
51. Hawksworth, G. M. and Hill, M. J., Bacteria and the N-nitrosation of secondary amines, *Br. J. Cancer*, 25, 520, 1971.
52. Klement, U. and Schmidpeter, A., Reactions of nitrosamines with electrophiles. III. Structure of dimethylnitrosamine copper^{II} chloride, *Angew. Chem. Int. Ed. Engl.*, 7, 470, 1968.
53. Rademacher, P., Stoelevik, R., and Luettke, W., Structure of nitroso- and nitrodimethylamine, *Angew. Chem. Int. Ed. Engl.*, 7, 806, 1968.
54. Haszeldine, R. N. and Jander, J., Studies in spectroscopy. VI. Ultraviolet and infra-red spectra of nitrosamines, nitrites and related compounds, *J. Chem. Soc.*, 2622, 1953.
55. Haszeldine, R. N. and Mattinson, B. J. H., Studies in spectroscopy. IX. Further studies on nitrosamines and nitrites, *J. Chem. Soc.*, p.4172, 1955.
56. Williams, R. L., Pace, R. J., and Jeacocke, G. J., Applications of solvent effects. I. The spectra of secondary nitrosamines, *Spectrochim. Acta*, 20, 225, 1964.
57. Mirvish, S. S., Kinetics of nitrosamide formation from alkylureas, N-alkylurethans, and alkylguanidines: possible implications for the etiology of human gastric cancer, *J. Natl. Cancer Inst.*, 46, 1183, 1971.
58. Fann, T. Y. and Tannenbaum, S. R., Stability of N-nitroso compounds, *J. Food Sci.*, 37, 274, 1972.
59. Sidgwick, N. V., *The Organic Chemistry of Nitrogen*, 3rd ed., reviewed by Millar I. T. and Springall, H. D., Clarendon Press, Oxford, 1966, 339 and 592.
60. Smith, P. A. S., *The Chemistry of Open-Chain Organic Nitrogen Compounds, Volume II: N-Nitroso Compounds*, W. A. Benjamin, New York, 1966, 470.
61. Feuer, H., *The Chemistry of the Nitro and Nitroso Groups, Part I*, Interscience, New York, 1969.
62. Eisenbrand, G. and Preussmann, R., Eine neue Methode zur Kolorimetrischen Bestimmung von Nitrosaminen nach Spaltung der N-Nitrosogruppe mit Bromwasserstoff in Eisessig, *Arzneim. Forsch.*, 20, 1513, 1970.
63. Lund, H., Electro-organic preparations. III. Polarography and reduction of N-nitrosamines, *Acta Chem. Scand.*, 11, 990, 1957.
64. Emmons, W. D., Peroxytrifluoracetic acid. I. The oxidation of nitrosamines to nitramine, *J. Am. Chem. Soc.*, 76, 3468, 1954.
65. Chute, W. J., Herring, K. G., Toombs, L. E., and Wright, G. F., Catalysed nitration of amines. I. Dinitroxydiethylamine, *Can. J. Res.*, 26B, 89, 1948.
66. Althorpe, J. D., Goddard, D. A., Sissons, D. J., and Telling, G. M., The gas chromatographic determination of nitrosamines at the picogram level by conversion to their corresponding nitramines, *J. Chromatogr.*, 53, 371, 1970.
67. Sen, N. P., Gas-liquid chromatographic determination of dimethylnitrosamine as dimethylnitramine at picogram levels, *J. Chromatogr.*, 53, 301, 1970.
68. Chow, Y. L., Photolysis of N-nitrosamines, *Tetrahedron Lett.*, 34, 2333, 1964.
69. Thorburn Burns, D. and Alliston, G. V., Some studies on the photolytic decomposition stage in the estimation of N-nitrosamines, *J. Food Technol.*, 6, 433, 1971.
70. Preussmann, R., Toxicity of nitrite and nitrosamines, *Proc. Int. Symp., Nitrite in Meat Products*, Zeist-Krol, B. and Tinbergen, B. J., Eds., Centre for Agricultural Publishing and Documentation, Pudoc, Wageningen, 1974, 217.
71. Druckrey, H., Preussmann, R., and Schmähl, D., Carcinogenicity and chemical structure of nitrosamines, *Acta Unio Int. Contra Cancrum*, 19, 510, 1963.
72. Greenblatt, M. and Lijinski, W., Failure to induce tumours in Swiss mice after concurrent administration of amino acids and sodium nitrite, *J. Natl. Cancer Inst.*, 48, 1389, 1972.
73. Montesano, R. and Magee, P. N., Comparative metabolism *in vitro* of nitrosamines in various animal species including man, in *Chemical Carcinogenesis Essays*, Montesano, R. and Tomatis, L., Eds., International Agency for Research on Cancer, Sci. Publ. No. 10, Lyon, France, 1974, 39.
74. Schmähl, D. and Osswald, H., Carcinogenesis in different animal species by diethylnitrosamine, *Experientia*, 23, 497, 1967.
75. Kelly, M. G., O'Hara, R. W., Adamson, R. H., Gadekar, K., Botkin, C. C., Reese, W. H., and Kerber, W. T., Induction of hepatic cell carcinomas in monkeys with N-nitrosodiethylamine, *J. Natl. Cancer Inst.*, 36, 323, 1966.
76. Terracini, B., Magee, P. N., and Barnes, J. M., Hepatic pathology in rats on low dietary levels of dimethylnitrosamine, *Br. J. Cancer*, 21, 559, 1967.
77. Magee, P. N., Toxic liver injury. The metabolism of dimethylnitrosamine, *Biochem. J.*, 64, 676, 1956.
78. Dutton, A. H. and Heath, D. F., Demethylation of dimethylnitrosamine in rats and mice, *Nature (London)*, 178, 644, 1956.

79. Stewart, B. W. and Magee, P. N., Metabolism and some biochemical effects of N-nitrosomorpholine, Biochem. J., 126, 21P, 1972.
80. Heath, D. F. and Dutton, A. H., The detection of metabolic products from dimethylnitrosamine in rats and mice, Biochem. J., 70, 619, 1958.
81. Heath, D. F., The decomposition and toxicity of dialkylnitrosamines in rats, Biochem. J., 85, 72, 1962.
82. Magee, P. N. and Vandekar, M., Toxic liver injury. The metabolism of dimethylnitrosamine in vitro, Biochem. J., 70, 600, 1958.
83. Magee, P. N., Toxic liver injury. Inhibition of protein synthesis in rat liver by dimethylnitrosamine in vivo, Biochem. J., 70, 606, 1958.
84. Magee, P. N. and Farber, E., Toxic liver injury and carcinogenesis. Methylation of rat-liver nucleic acids by dimethylnitrosamine in vivo, Biochem. J., 83, 114, 1962.
85. Montesano, R. and Magee, P. N., Metabolism of dimethylnitrosamine by human liver slices in vitro, Nature (London), 228, 173, 1970.
86. Swann, P. F. and Magee, P. N., Nitrosamine induced carcinogenesis. The alkylation of nucleic acids of the rat by N-methyl-N-nitrosourea, dimethylnitrosamine, dimethylsulphate and methyl methane sulphonate, Biochem. J., 110, 3, 1968.
87. Wasserman, A. E., A survey of analytical procedures for nitrosamines, in N-Nitroso Compounds Analysis and Formation, Bogovski, P., Preussmann, R., and Walker, E. A., Eds., International Agency for Research on Cancer, Sci. Publ. No. 3, Lyon, France, 1972, 10.
88. Eisenbrand, G., Hodenberg, A., and Preussmann, R., Trace analysis of nitroso compounds. II. Steam distillation at neutral, alkaline and acid pH under reduced and atmospheric pressure, Z. Analyt. Chem., 251, 22, 1970.
89. Telling, G. M., Bryce, T. A., and Althorpe, J., Use of vacuum distillation and gas chromatography-mass spectrometry for determination of low levels of volatile nitrosamines in meat products, J. Agric. Food Chem., 19, 937, 1971.
90. Howard, J. W., Fazio, T., and Watts, J. O., Extraction and gas chromatographic determination of N-nitrosodimethylamine in smoked fish: application to smoked nitrite-treated chubb, J. Assoc. Off. Anal. Chem., 53, 269, 1970.
91. Eisenbrand, G., Marquardt, P., and Preussmann, R., Trace analysis of N-nitroso compounds. I. Liquid-liquid distribution in acetonitrile/heptane as a clean up method, Z. Analyt. Chem., 247, 54, 1969.
92. Westlake, W. E. and Gunther, F. A., Advances in gas chromatographic detectors illustrated from application to pesticide residue evaluation, Residue Rev., 18, 175, 1967.
93. Palframan, J. F., MacNab, J. A., and Crosby, N. T., An evaluation of the alkali flame ionisation detector and the Coulson electrolytic conductivity detector in the analysis of N-nitrosamines in foods, J. Chromatogr., 76, 307, 1973.
94. Coulson, D. M., Electrolytic conductivity detector for gas chromatography, J. Gas Chromatogr., 3, 134, 1965.
95. Hall, R. C., A highly sensitive and selective microelectrolytic conductivity detector for gas chromatography, J. Chromatogr. Sci., 12, 152, 1974.
96. Gough, T. A. and Woollam, C. J., Techniques for the screening of foodstuffs for volatile nitrosamines, in Environmental N-Nitroso compounds Analysis and Formation, Walker, E. A., Bogovski, P., and Griciute, L., Eds., International Agency for Research on Cancer, Sci. Publ. No. 14, Lyon, France, 1976, 85.
97. Dooley, C. J., Wasserman, A. E., and Osman, S., A contaminant in N-nitrosodimethylamine confirmation by high resolution mass spectrometry, J. Food Sci., 38, 1096, 1973.
98. Gough, T. A. and Webb, K. S., A method for the detection of traces of nitrosamines using combined gas chromatography and mass spectrometry, J. Chromatogr., 79, 57, 1973.
99. Gough, T. A., The determination of N-nitroso compounds by mass spectrometry, a review, Analyst, 103, 785, 1978.
100. Simpson, C. F., Gas chromatography-mass spectroscopy interfacial systems, Crit. Rev. Anal. Chem., 3, 1, 1972.
101. Fenselau, C., Gas chromatography mass spectrometry. Report on the state of the art, Appl. Spectros., 28, 305, 1974.
102. McFadden, W. H., Techniques of Combined Gas Chromatography/Mass Spectrometry, Wiley Interscience, New York, 1973.
103. Gough, T. A. and Webb, K. S., The use of a molecular separator in the determination of trace constituents by combined gas chromatography and mass spectrometry, J. Chromatogr., 64, 201, 1972.

104. Gaffield, W., Fish, R. H., Holmstead, R. L., Poppiti, J., and Yergey, A. L., Chemical ionization-mass spectrometry of nitrosamines, in *Environmental N-Nitroso Compounds Analysis and Formation,* Walker, E. A., Bogovski, P., and Griciute, L., Eds., International Agency for Research on Cancer, Sci. Publ. No. 14, Lyon, France, 1976, 11.
105. Heynes, K. and Roper, H., Analytik von N-Nitroso Verbindungen. 2. Mitt. Trennung und Quantitative Bestimmung von homologen N-Nitroso-N-alkylharnstoffen und N-Nitroso-N-alkylurethanen durch schnelle hochdruckflussigkeits — chromatographie, *J. Chromatogr.,* 93, 429, 1974.
106. Fine, D. H. and Rounbehler, D. P., Trace analysis of volatile N-nitroso compounds by combined gas chromatography and thermal energy analysis, *J. Chromatogr.,* 109, 271, 1975.
107. Gough, T. A., Webb, K. S., and Eaton, R. F., Simple chemiluminescent detector for the screening of foodstuffs for the presence of volatile nitrosamines, *J. Chromatogr.,* 137, 293, 1977.
108. Gough, T. A., Webb, K. S., Pringuer, M. A., and Wood, B. J., A comparison of various mass spectrometric and a chemiluminescent method for the estimation of volatile nitrosamines, *J. Agric. Food Chem.,* 25, 663, 1977.
109. Gough, T. A. and Webb, K. S., Positive interferent in the chemiluminescent detection of nitrosamines, *J. Chromatogr.,* 154, 234, 1978.
110. Gough, T. A. and Webb, K. S., The mass spectrometric and chemiluminescent detection of picogram amounts of N-nitrosodimethylamine, Annual Meeting of the Am. Soc. for Mass Spectrometry and Allied Topics, St. Louis, Mo., May 1978.
111. Walker, E. A. and Castegnaro, M., New data on collaborative studies on analysis of volatile nitrosamines, in *Environmental N-Nitroso Compounds Analysis and Formation,* Walker, E. A., Bogovski, P., and Griciute, L., Eds., International Agency for Research on Cancer, Sci. Publ. No. 14, Lyon, France, 1976, 77.
112. Crosby, N. T., Foreman, J. K., Palframan, J. F., and Sawyer, R., Estimation of steam-volatile N-nitrosamines in foods at the 1 μg/kg level, *Nature (London),* 238, 342, 1972.
113. Sen, N. P., Donaldson, B. A., Iyengar, J. R., and Panalaks, T., Nitrosopyrrolidine and dimethylnitrosamine in bacon, *Nature (London),* 241, 473, 1973.
114. Fazio, T., White, R. H., Dusold, L. R., and Howard, J. W., Nitrosopyrrolidine in cooked bacon, *J. Assoc. Off. Anal. Chem.,* 56, 919, 1973.
115. Sen, N. P., Iyengar, J. R., Donaldson, B. A., and Panalaks, T., Effect of sodium nitrite concentration on the formation of nitrosopyrrolidine and dimethylnitrosamine in fried bacon, *J. Agric. Food Chem.,* 22, 540, 1974.
116. Pensabene, J. W., Fiddler, W., Gates, R. A., Fagan, J. C., and Wasserman, A. E., Effect of frying and other cooking conditions on nitrosopyrrolidine formation in bacon, *J. Food Sci.,* 39, 314, 1974.
117. Fiddler, W., Pensabene, J. W., Fagan, J. C., Thorne, E. J., Piotrowski, E. G., and Wasserman, A. E., The role of lean and adipose tissue on the formation of nitrosopyrrolidine in fried bacon, *J. Food Sci.,* 39, 1070, 1974.
118. Stephany, R. W., Freudenthal, J., and Schuller, P. L., Quantitative and qualitative determination of some volatile nitrosamines in various meat products, in *Environmental N-Nitroso Compounds Analysis and Formation,* Walker, E. A., Bogovski, P., and Griciute, L., Eds., International Agency for Research on Cancer, Sci. Publ. No. 14, Lyon, France, 1976, 343.
119. Groenen, P. J., Jonk, R. J. G., van Ingen, C., and ten Noever de Brauw, M. C., Determination of eight volatile nitrosamines in thirty cured meat products with capillary gas chromatography-high-resolution mass spectrometry: the presence of nitrosodiethylamine and the absence of nitrosopyrrolidine, in *Environmental N-Nitroso Compounds Analysis and Formation,* Walker, E. A., Bogovski, P., and Griciute, L., Eds., International Agency for Research on Cancer, Sci. Publ. No. 14, Lyon, France, 1976, 321.
120. Gough, T. A., McPhail, M. F., Webb, K. S., Wood, B. J., and Coleman, R. F., An examination of some foodstuffs for the presence of volatile nitrosamines, *J. Sci. Food Agric.,* 28, 345, 1977.
121. Gough, T. A., Webb, K. S., and Coleman, R. F., Estimate of the volatile nitrosamine content of U.K. food, *Nature (London),* 272, 161, 1978.
122. Telling, G. M., Bryce, T. A., Hoar, D., Osborne, D., and Welti, D., Progress in the analysis of volatile N-nitroso compounds, in *N-Nitroso Compounds in the Environment,* Bogovski, P. and Walker, E. A., Eds., International Agency for Research on Cancer, Sci. Publ. No. 9, Lyon, France, 1974, 12.
123. Gough, T. A., Goodhead, K., and Walters, C. L., Distribution of some volatile nitrosamines in cooked bacon, *J. Sci. Food Agric.,* 27, 181, 1976.
124. Gray, J. I. and Duggan, L. R., Formation of N-nitrosopyrrolidine from proline and collagen, *J. Food Sci.,* 40, 484, 1975.
125. Fazio, T., White, R. H., and Howard, J. W., Analysis of nitrite and/or nitrate processed meats for N-nitrosodimethylamine, *J. Assoc. Off. Anal. Chem.,* 54, 1157, 1971.
126. Sen, N. P., The evidence for the presence of dimethylnitrosamine in meat products, *Food Cosmet. Toxicol.,* 10, 219, 1972.

127. Wasserman, A. E., Fiddler, W., Doerr, R. C., Osman, S. F., and Dooley, C. J., Dimethylnitrosamine in frankfurters, *Food Cosmet. Toxicol.,* 10, 681, 1972.
128. Sen, N. P., Miles, W. F., Donaldson, B. A., Panalaks, T., and Iyengar, J. R., Formation of nitrosamines in a meat curing mixture, *Nature (London),* 245, 104, 1973.
129. Panalaks, T., Iyengar, J. R., and Sen, N. P., Nitrate, nitrite and dimethylnitrosamine in cured meat products, *J. Assoc. Off. Anal. Chem.,* 56, 621, 1973.
130. Panalaks, T., Iyengar, J. R., Donaldson, B. A., Miles, W. F., and Sen, N. P., Further survey of cured meat products for volatile N-nitrosamines, *J. Assoc. Off. Anal. Chem.,* 57, 806, 1974.
131. Groenen, P. J., de Cock-Bethbeder, M. W., Jonk, R. J. G., and van Ingen, C., Further studies on the occurrence of volatile N-nitrosamines in meat products, in *Proc. Int. Symp., Nitrite in Meat Products,* Tinbergen, B. J. and Krol, B., Eds., Centre for Agricultural Publishing and Documentation, Wageningen, The Netherlands, 1977, 227.
132. Eisenbrand, G., Janzowski, C., and Preussmann, R., Analysis, formation and occurrence of volatile and non-volatile N-nitroso compounds; recent results, in *Proc. Int. Symp., Nitrite in Meat Products,* Tinbergen, B. J. and Krol, B., Eds., Centre for Agricultural Publishing and Documentation, Wageningen, The Netherlands, 1977, 155.
133. Fiddler, W., Piotrowski, E. G., Pensabene, J. W., Doerr, R. C., and Wasserman, A. E., Effect of sodium nitrite concentration on N-nitrosodimethylamine formation in frankfurters, *J. Food Sci.,* 37, 668, 1972.
134. Sen, N. P., Donaldson, B. A., Charbonneau, C., and Miles, W. F., Effect of additives on the formation of nitrosamines in meat curing mixtures containing spices and nitrite, *J. Agric. Food Chem.,* 22, 1125, 1974.
135. Herring, H. K., Effect of nitrite and other factors on the physico-chemical characteristics and nitrosamine formation in bacon, in *Proc. Meat Ind. Res. Conf.,* University of Chicago, 1973, 47.
136. Fazio, T., Damico, J. N., Howard, J. W., White, R. H., and Watts, J. W., Gas chromatographic determination and mass spectrometric confirmation of N-nitrosodimethylamine in smoke-processed marine fish, *J. Agric. Food Chem.,* 19, 250, 1971.
137. Iyengar, J. R., Panalaks, T., Miles, W. F., and Sen, N. P., A survey of fish products for volatile N-nitrosamines, *J. Sci. Food Agric.,* 27, 527, 1976.
138. Gadbois, D. F., Ravesi, E. M., Lundstrom, R. C., and Maney, R. S., N-nitrosodimethylamine in cold-smoked sablefish, *J. Agric. Food. Chem.,* 23, 665, 1975.
139. Skaare, J. U. and Dahle, H. K., Gas chromatographic determination and mass spectrometric confirmation of N-nitrosodimethylamine in fish meal, *J. Chromatogr.,* 111, 426, 1975.
140. Hurst, R. E., Dimethylnitrosamine levels in untreated herring meals, *J. Sci. Food Agric.,* 27, 600, 1976.
141. Fong, Y. Y. and Chan, W. C., Dimethylnitrosamine in Chinese marine salt fish, *Food Cosmet. Toxicol.,* 11, 841, 1973.
142. Fine, D. H., Rounbehler, D. P., Belcher, N. P., and Epstein, S. S., N-nitroso compounds in air and water, in *Environmental N-Nitroso Compounds Analysis and Formation,* Walker, E. A., Bogovski, P., and Griciute, L., Eds., International Agency for Research on Cancer, Sci. Publ. No. 14, Lyon, France, 1976, 401.
143. Eisenbrand, G., Ungerer, O., and Preussmann, R., Formation of N-nitroso compounds from agricultural chemicals and nitrite, in *N-Nitroso Compounds in the Environment,* Bogovski, P. and Walker, E. A., Eds., International Agency for Research on Cancer, Sci. Publ. No. 9, Lyon, France, 1974, 71.
144. Sen, N. P., Donaldson, B. A., and Charbonneau, C., Formation of nitrosodimethylamine from the interaction of certain pesticides and nitrite, in *N-Nitroso Compounds in the Environment,* Bogovski, P. and Walker, E. A., Eds., International Agency for Research on Cancer, Sci. Publ. No. 9, Lyon, France, 1974, 75.
145. Hicks, R. M., Walters, C. L., Elsebai, I., El Aassar, A-B., El Merzabani, M., and Gough, T. A., Demonstration of nitrosamines in human urine: preliminary observations on a possible etiology for bladder cancer in association with chronic urinary tract infections, *Proc. R. Soc. Med.,* 70, 413, 1977.
146. Druckrey, H. and Preussmann, R., Zur Enstehung carcinogener Nitrosamine am Beispiel des Tabakrauches, *Naturwissenschaften,* 49, 498, 1962.
147. Norman, V. and Keith, C. H., Nitrogen oxides in tobacco smoke, *Nature (London),* 205, 915, 1965.
148. Broaddus, G. M., York, J. E., and Moseley, J. M., Factors affecting the levels of nitrate nitrogen in cured tobacco leaves, *Tob. Sci.,* 9, 149, 1965.
149. Boyland, E., Roe, F. J. C., and Gorrod, J. W., Induction of pulmonary tumours in mice by nitrosonornicotine, a possible constituent of tobacco smoke, *Nature (London),* 202, 1126, 1964.
150. Neurath, G. B., Nitrosamine formation from precursors in tobacco smoke, in *N-Nitroso Compounds Analysis and Formation,* Bogovski, P., Preussmann, R., and Walker, E. A., Eds., International Agency for Research on Cancer, Sci. Publ. No. 3, Lyon, France, 1972, 134.

151. Rhoades, J. W. and Johnson, D. E., N-Dimethylnitrosamine in tobacco smoke condensate, *Nature (London)*, 236, 307, 1972.
152. McCormick, A., Nicholson, M. J., Baylis, M. A., and Underwood, J. G., Nitrosamines in cigarette smoke condensate, *Nature (London)*, 224, 237, 1973.
153. Hoffmann, D., Rathkamp, G., and Liu, Y. Y., Chemical studies on tobacco smoke. XXVI. On the isolation and identification of volatile and non-volatile N-nitrosamines and hydrazines in cigarette smoke, in *N-Nitroso Compounds in the Environment,* Bogovski, P. and Walker, E. A., Eds., International Agency for Research on Cancer, Sci. Publ. No. 9, Lyon, France, 1974, 159.
154. Hecht, S. S., Ornaf, R. M., and Hoffmann, D., Determination of N'-Nitrosonornicotine in tobacco by high speed liquid chromatography, *Anal. Chem.,* 47, 2046, 1975.
155. Walters, C. L., Johnson, E. M., and Ray, N., Separation and detection of volatile and non-volatile N-nitrosamines, *Analyst,* 95, 485, 1970.
156. Johnson, E. M. and Walters, C. L., The specificity of the release of nitrite from N-nitrosamines by hydrobromic acid, *Anal. Lett.,* 4, 483, 1971.
157. Lunt, T. G., Fueggle, D. G., and Walters, C. L., The estimation of total nonvolatile nitrosamines and nitrosamides in microgram amounts, *Anal. Lett.,* 6, 369, 1973.
158. Fan, T. Y. and Tannenbaum, S. R., Automatic colorimetric determination of N-nitroso compounds, *J. Agric. Food Chem.,* 19, 1267, 1971.
159. Fine, D. H., Huffman, F., Rounbehler, D. P., and Belcher, N. M., Analysis of N-nitroso compounds by combined high-performance liquid chromatography and thermal energy analysis, in *Environmental N-Nitroso Compounds Analysis and Formation,* Walker, E. A., Bogovski, P., and Griciute, L., Eds., International Agency for Research on Cancer, Sci. Publ. No. 14, Lyon, France, 1976, 43.
160. *Proceedings of the International Symposium on Nitrite in Meat Products,* Krol, B. and Tinbergen, B. J., Eds., Central Institute for Nutrition and Food Research TNO, Zeist, Sept. 10, 1973; Wageningen, 1974; and Wagengen, Sept. 7, 1976.
161. Challis, B. C., Rapid nitrosation of phenols and its implications for health hazards from dietary nitrites, *Nature (London),* 244, 466, 1973.
162. Knowles, M. E., Gilbert, J., and McWeeny, D. J., Nitrosation of phenols in smoked bacon, *Nature (London),* 249, 672, 1974.
163. Preservatives in Food Regulations 1975, Statutory Instrument 1975, No. 1487, Her Majesty's Stationery Office, London.
164. U.S. Federal Register, May 9, 1978, FR Document 78-13469.

POLYCYCLIC AROMATIC HYDROCARBONS IN FOODS*

John W. Howard and Thomas Fazio

INTRODUCTION

More than a decade ago, Tilgner[1] in his discussion of carcinogens in food stated: "...higher aromatic polycyclic aromatic hydrocarbons (PAH) of which benzo(a)pyrene is but one, have become ubiquitous and may become contaminants under various circumstances". This important class of pollutants has been shown to occur in water, air, food, and soil as well as such diverse sources as tobacco smoke, automobile and engine exhausts, high boiling petroleum distillates, carbon black, coal tar, pitch, rubber tires, etc.

The vast majority of studies conducted thus far in the environmental area concentrated on the determination of benzo(a)pyrene, one of the most potent PAH carcinogens. While these investigations demonstrated that this compound is ubiquitous in the environment, Andelman and Suess noted that it constitutes only between 1 and 20% of the total carcinogenic PAH.[2] In his assessment of the situation, Suess commented that only a few investigators have sought a variety of carcinogenic PAH in the same environment sample.[3] Furthermore, the measurement and sampling techniques and the analytical methodology of various researchers are not always mentioned. Thus, these limiting factors must be considered in assessing carcinogenic PAH in the environment. Haenni[4] and Tilgner and Daun[5] suggest that only a small fraction of the potential compounds in this class have been recognized, identified, and toxicologically evaluated. In their study of PAH content of sediments taken from the coastal waters at Buzzards Bay, Mass., Giger and Blumer concluded that the complexity of the isolated aromatic fraction was indicative of the presence of tens of thousands of aromatic compounds, mostly of unknown structure and biological activity.[6]

With the development of analytical procedures in the 1960s, a large volume of data on the presence of PAH in foodstuffs has been accumulated on a worldwide basis; however, as discussed above, much of the work has been concerned only with the determination of benzo(a)pyrene. PAH have been reported in smoked fish and meats, grilled and roasted foods, root and leaf vegetables, vegetable oils, grains, plants, fruits, seafoods, whiskies, etc. The sources of such contamination include curing smokes, contaminated soils, polluted air and water, modes of cooking or preparation of foods, food additives, food processing, and endogenic or biosynthesis by plants and microorganisms. Aside from smoke-cured foods, charcoal-broiled meats, and possibly environmental pollution, Haenni indicated that the most common sources of PAH as potential food contaminants were food additives of petroleum origin.[4] However, in a subsequent review several years later, Haenni and Fischbach[7] offered the opinion that more attention should be directed toward contamination of food crops from soils, air, ground waters, etc. Suess, in his assessment of the environmental load and cycle of PAH, concluded that there is prevailing evidence for the natural occurrence of these compounds which he attributes to endogenic synthesis (by microorganisms, phytoplankton, algae, and highly developed plants), volcanic activity, open burning of forests, etc. (not ignited by man), and natural seepage of petroleum.[3] He points out, however, that such contributions of PAH are small compared to man-induced and/or man-controlled combustion processes which include the burning of coal, production of coke in the iron and steel industry, catalytic cracking of petroleum, heating and

* This chapter is reprinted with permission from *J. Assoc. Off. Anal. Chem.*, 63(5), 1077—1104, 1980.

power generation, emissions from transportation vehicles, asphalt paving, and coal tar pitch. In addition, contamination of waterways by oil spills, marine transportation, and industrial wastes is another factor, although its contribution is considered insignificant compared to land-based, high-temperature processes. The author states, however, that the impact of such contamination on the aquatic environment should not be underestimated since the chemical halflife of PAH may be much longer in water than in the atmosphere. Tilgner commented that evidence is mounting that environmental contamination of agricultural raw materials is being caused by contaminated air, water, and soil.[8] He concluded that air pollution seems to be the most potent food contaminant.

As indicated above, the occurrence of PAH in food should be viewed as a part of the much larger problem on the formation of these compounds in the environment. It is also apparent that the findings of PAH in air, water, and soil are being given much more relevance with respect to their contamination of the food supply. The purpose of this report is to update and to consolidate the findings on PAH in food and other products of food additive significance. For the convenience of the reader we have included previously published reviews on the presence of PAH in foods.[1-5,8-14]

ANALYSES OF FOODS

Haenni in 1968 comprehensively discussed the development of analytical aids to the control of potential PAH contaminants in food additives and in foods by the use of ultraviolet specification within specific wavelength ranges.[4] Such specifications are currently employed to control the content of these contaminants in products of petroleum origin such as waxes, mineral oils, petrolatums, and other products of food additive significance. The basic principles of analytical control as developed for U.S. regulatory requirements have been adopted in ensuing years by a number of other nations.[7]

With respect to the determination of individual PAH in environmental samples, there have been a number of publications of methods and findings of these compounds in air, water, soil, etc. While this information may be relevant to the contamination of food, it should be recognized that the substrates involved are very different from the complex compositions of foodstuffs. Thus, the use of these methods for trace analysis of foods is in question until their application is established. In 1970, Schaad reviewed various chromatographic separation procedures including column, paper, thin layer, and gas chromatography.[15]

As Haenni[4] noted, PAH most often occur in environmental samples as a minute fraction of a complex mixture of hydrocarbons and it is the exception rather than the rule to find only one of these compounds or only two occurring together. It is therefore of major importance that the methodology employed in such analyses include separation techniques for the determination and subsequent identification of individual PAH. This is particularly true in regulatory work where the analyst must be able to separate and unequivocally identify the carcinogenic from the noncarcinogenic types. For example, one of the most significant difficulties is the resolution of the so-called benzpyrene fraction consisting of the carcinogen benzo(a)pyrene, its isomer benzo(e)pyrene, benzo(k)fluoranthene, and perylene. (Benzo(b)fluoranthene, which also has been found in food, should be included with the above compounds.) At a joint meeting in 1968 of the International Union Against Cancer (UICC) and International Agency for Research on Cancer (IARC) on Environmental Carcinogens, the Joint Working Group specified that an acceptable method should be capable of separating *at least* benz(a)anthracene, benzo(a)pyrene, benzo(e)pyrene, benzo(g,h,i)perylene, pyrene, benzo(k)fluoranthene, and coronene.[16,17] Based on more recent findings of PAH in environmental samples, this listing would probably be extended appreciably if a Working Group were convened today.

Most of the studies conducted on environmental samples during the 1960s utilized ultraviolet and fluorescence techniques to estimate the PAH content. In an early review, Gunther and Buzzetti[9] discussed the analytical problems associated with the isolation and characterization of these compounds. In subsequent work further refinement of these isolative procedures and the aforementioned determinative techniques resulted in the development of analytical procedures which were capable of accurately measuring a wide variety of PAH in various products including foods as discussed below. With respect to fluorescence, Shabad reported that, in Russia, Dikun employs a luminescence technique which is carried out at low temperatures and gives the fine structure of the PAH under analysis.[10] Dikun has collaborated with the present authors in several studies on the analysis of PAH in foods and obtained excellent results. However, exact details of the isolation and the technique were not made available to us.

An assessment of the literature reveals that only a few methods for determining PAH in foods have been subjected to collaborative study and accepted on a national and/or international basis. Collaborative studies of a method specific for benzo(a)pyrene and a general procedure for PAH have been conducted under the auspices of the Association of Official Analytical Chemists (AOAC) and the International Union of Pure and Applied Chemistry (IUPAC).[18,19] Very briefly, these procedures involve an initial saponification of the product in ethanolic potassium hydroxide, followed by a partition step between dimethyl sulfoxide and an aliphatic solvent and column chromatography on pretreated Florisil. Thin layer chromatography (TLC) on cellulose (immobile phase, 20% dimethylformamide in ethyl ether; mobile phase, isooctane) and cellulose acetate (21% acetylated; ethanol-toluene-water [17:4:4 v/v/v]) is then employed as the separative technique with ultraviolet and fluorescence spectrophotometric procedures being used for determination of the hydrocarbons. In the study of the benzo(a)pyrene method (with cellulose acetate TLC used alone), smoked ham and fish samples were fortified at 4 and 10 µg/kg. Standard deviations of the data obtained with the use of the 2 determinative techniques ranged from 3.15 to 13.6%. The method was adopted as an AOAC official first action method in 1968 and was accepted as a recommended method by IUPAC in 1972.[18,20,21] The study of the general method for PAH was conducted on ham samples fortified with benzo(a)pyrene, benzo(e)pyrene, benz(a)anthracene, and benzo(g,h,i)perylene at a level of 10 µg/kg. Statistical evaluation of the data obtained from collaborators in Canada, England, the Federal Republic of Germany, and the U.S. showed standard deviations between and within laboratories ranging from 7.4 to 12.7%. The procedure was adopted as an official method in 1972 and has been accepted by the IUPAC Commission at its Madrid 1975 meeting as a recommended method.[19,20,22]

Grimmer and Böhnke in 1975 described a method for determining PAH in high-protein foods, oils, and fats.[23] The protein-rich foods (meat, poultry, fish, yeast) are initially saponified in methanolic potassium hydroxide, whereas oil and fatty products soluble in methanol or cyclohexane (without a residue) are processed directly. The PAH are concentrated by liquid-liquid extraction (methanol-water-cyclohexane, N,N-dimethylformamide-water-cyclohexane) and by column chromatography on Sephadex LH20. The compounds are separated and determined by gas-liquid chromatography (GLC) (5% OV-101 on Gas-Chrom Q) using a flame ionization detector. This latter method has been subjected to collaborative study, and a report has been published.[22] Sunflower oil and meat were fortified at levels of approximately 10 µg/kg with each of the following compounds: chrysene, benzo(b)fluoranthene, benzo(a)pyrene, benzo(e)pyrene (not used in the sunflower oil study), perylene, dibenz(a,j)anthracene, indeno(1,2,3-cd)pyrene, benzo(g,h,i) perylene. The coefficients of variation obtained on statistical evaluation of the data ranged from 9.4 to 24.5% for the sunflower oil and from 7.1 to 27% for the meat product. The Commission on Food Additives,

IUPAC, considered it a useful screening procedure and it was so accepted as a recommended method at the Paris meeting in 1976.[22] As noted by the Commission, the procedure depends solely on relative retention times for identification of the contaminants, and thus, findings must be regarded as tentative until confirmation by independent adequate means such as mass spectrometry, ultraviolet, and fluorescence. Grimmer and Böhnke have pointed out that the OV-101 column employed is not effective in the separation of some important PAHs, such as benz(a)anthracene from chrysene and triphenylene, and the benzofluoranthenes.[23] The authors stated that the use of OV-17 packing and capillary columns will improve the resolution of some of these compounds. An additional term of import in the analyses of PAH in food mentioned in the above report is that "to isolate these compounds quantitatively from insoluble samples (meat, fish, etc.), hydrolysis is an absolute necessity". Studies by the above authors indicated that only about 30% benzo(a)pyrene and other PAH were extractable from fish with methanol, whereas an alkaline hydrolysis of the fish protein yielded an additional 60% of the PAH compounds. It was concluded that the compounds were linked adsorptively to high molecular structures not destroyed by methanol.

As assessed by Janini et al. in 1975, applications of capillary GLC have been reported in the analysis of PAH and related compounds in cigarette smoke and in air and automobile exhausts.[24-28] Various other workers have investigated and/or utilized GLC for analysis of environmental samples; however, as stated by Janini, the technique has been used with varying degrees of success in which columns for specific narrow ranges of PAH have been developed.[29-34] Janini also noted that no liquid phase has been reported which wholly meets the aforementioned recommendations of the UICC/IARC Joint Working Group. With exception of the Grimmer and Böhnke study above, none of these procedures have been applied to food.[23]

Gouw et al.[35] studied the separation of 44 PAH using short (10 m) glass capillary columns coated with SE-52. Problems were encountered in the resolution of the benzpyrene fraction, the benzfluoranthenes, and the chrysene-triphenylene-benz(a)anthracene types. Janini and his associates described the results of their GLC studies of PAH with nematic liquid crystals, using a flame ionization detector.[24,36,37] This technique, although not applied as yet to environmental samples, does appear to have potential in achieving separations of some of the important PAH (16 to 21-carbon PAH) if column bleed and stability can be controlled. Initial studies of an N,N'-bis(p-methoxybenzylidene)-a,a'-bi-p-toluidine (BMBT) nematic liquid crystal showed good separations of the following PAH compounds which are more difficult to resolve: pyrene-fluoranthene; benz(a)anthracene — chrysene — triphenylene; benzo(k)fluoranthene — perylene — benzo(a)pyrene; and dibenz(a,h) anthracene-benzo(g,h,i)perylene.[24] In subsequent work, however, the authors found that BMBT exhibited measurable column bleed over prolonged operating periods at elevated temperatures.[36] In the same article they reported the synthesis of a new liquid crystal, BBBT, the bis-p-butoxy homolog of BMBT, which provided the aforementioned separations with significantly diminished column bleed. Unfortunately, it was found that this crystal could not be used effectively in the analysis of higher molecular weight PAH (22 to 24 carbons) because of excessive solute retention and broad elution peaks.

In their most recent publication, Janini et al. report having synthesized N,N'-bis(p-phenylbenzylidene)-a,a'-bi-p-toluidine (BPhBT) and N,N'-bis-(p-hexyloxybenzylidene)-a,a'-bi-p-toluidine (BH × BT).[37] Both of these liquid crystals as well as a 1:1 mixture of the 2 products were found to yield optimum separations of the PAH compounds mentioned above. The authors state that the low bleed levels and high efficiency characteristics observed for BPhBT and 1:1 BPhBT-BH × BT packed columns have warranted their application as liquid phases in GC-MS systems. It was also found that the BPhBT phase could be used to resolve 22-carbon pentacyclic arenes (dibenzanthracenes) and 24-carbon hexacyclic arenes (dibenzpyrenes). Burchill et al.[38] also reported the results of their work with the aforementioned liquid crystals. These authors state that limited column life was experienced during their work on PAH in coal gases. Temperatures maintained at 250°C for an extended period (even 1 day) tended to destroy the column with resultant changes in retention times and responses. Janini found that column deterioration for liquid crystals can be retarded by placing a 1 in. plug of preconditioned 5% SE-30 packing at both ends of the column.[37]

Winkler et al.[39] described a method for the determination of PAH in maize. After initial Soxhlet extraction and separations on silica gel and Sephadex LH 20 columns, the PAH are determined by capillary gas chromatography using SE-54 and glass columns 50 m long.

The technique of high pressure liquid chromatography (HPLC) offers promise as an effective tool for separation and analysis of PAH. As Krstulovic et al.[40] pointed out, nonvolatile, thermally labile compounds can be readily be analyzed by this technique without derivatization. Furthermore, samples are not destroyed in the analysis and it is possible to collect fractions for subsequent analyses by other techniques. In addition, the very sensitive fluorescence and ultraviolet characteristics of these compounds can be utilized with HPLC.

A review of the literature reveals that the majority of studies conducted thus far with this technique have been concerned with the separation of standard compounds and/or with applications to the analyses of air particulates on various columnar materials. These analyses include investigation of HPLC using reverse phase,[41-43] adsorption,[44] and complexation[45-48] packing materials with ultraviolet or fluorescence detectors. During the past several years, workers in this area have tended to use chemically bonded phases or reverse phases such as octadecylsilane (ODS).[49,50] For example, Dong et al., in their work with ODS Zorbax, studied 2 synthetic PAH mixtures.[49] While good separations of selected compounds were obtained, analyses of the chromatograms shown for the two mixtures and an air sample indicate that difficulties are encountered in the separation of benzo(e)pyrene, perylene, benzo(k)fluoranthene-benzo(b)fluoranthene, triphenylene-crysene-benz(a)anthracene, and various other higher molecular weight arenes. However, separation of benzo(a)pyrene was achieved and the authors note that improved separations of benz(a)anthracene-chrysene can be obtained with ODS Permaphase packing.

Ives and Giuffrida[51] reported on the separation of 18 PAH using Durapak OPN and 40% cellulose acetate. Of particular importance in this study was the separation on the cellulose acetate of benzo(a)pyrene from benzo(e)pyrene and perylene; the latter two compounds were partially resolved. Benzo(b)fluoranthene was separated from benzo(e)pyrene and benzo(a)pyrene, but not from chrysene; the latter compound was resolved from benz(a)anthracene. With respect to the Durapak packing, difficulties were encountered in the separation of the members of the benzo(a)pyrene fraction; however, some of the arenes not resolved by the cellulose acetate were separated on the Durapak column. On the basis of the results, the authors concluded that there was a need to utilize more than one system in order to obtain resolution of the various PAH involved.

Klimisch, in reference to the work of Kirkland on the maximum number of effective plates per second achieved in HPLC columns with silica gel, suggested that it would be more promising to separate the isomeric benzpyrenes using a system with high selectivity rather than columns with high numbers of effective plates per second.[52,53] Klimisch found that excellent separation of benzo(a)pyrene from other members of the fraction could be achieved with the use of 45% cellulose acetate columns. Three solvent systems were employed: ethanol-dichloromethane (2:1); ethanol-toluene (2:1); and ethanol-1,2-dichloroethane (2:1). The best separations were obtained with the first two systems; however, the latter system shortened analysis time and still gave quantitative results.

At the present time there are only a few published articles on the application of HPLC to PAH analysis of foods. In 1976, Guerrero et al.[54] employed HPLC (μ Bondapak/C_{18} column, acetonitrile-water, 75 + 25) for the determination of benzo(a)pyrene and benzo(g,h,i)perylene in clams taken from waters where oil spills had occurred. No data were given in the report as to separation of other PAH from the compounds determined with the Bondapak column. In 1977, Hunt et al.[50] compared two siloxane bonded phases, 2-phthalimido-propyltrichlorosilane (PPS) and ODS-Partisil 5 in their study of PAH content of mussels. The authors indicate that some useful separations (16 compounds were studied) were obtained with the PPS column, which was found superior to the Partisil material. Based on the relative retention times and chromatograms, it would appear that the benzo(a)pyrene fraction [benzo(a)pyrene, benzo(e)pyrene, benzo(k)fluoranthene and perylene] was not completely resolved. Panalaks[55] has published his findings of PAH in smoked and charcoal-broiled food using HPLC as the determinative method. A Vydac ODS packing was employed with a mobile phase of 87% (v/v) methanol-water. Review of the chromatograms included indicated that difficulties were encountered in the resolution of various PAH including benz(a)anthracene and members of the benzo(a)pyrene fraction.

The majority of the investigations conducted thus far with HPLC suffer from the fact that the authors did not use sufficient compounds or, more aptly, were not selective enough in choosing the more important compounds in their work. Thus it is difficult in some cases to assess the capabilities of the column materials employed. Novotny et al., in their assessment of various chemically bonded phases, point out "that many PAH isomers are still unresolved..." and call for further approaches that should be designed on the development of detailed analytical knowledge.[5] It is obvious, then, that a more concerted effort needs to be made in this area which offers some specific advantages with respect to PAH analysis.

During the last several years, mass spectrometry and the combination of gas chromatography-mass spectrometry (GC-MS) have been applied extensively in detailed and in some cases quantitative analyses of PAH in air particulates, petroleum products, marijuana and tobacco smoke condensates, marine sediments, etc.[6,56-61] The use of high-resolution (capillary) columns in some of these studies along with the development of effective isolative techniques has had a significant impact on the separation and identification of hitherto unresolved toxicologically important isomers. For example, Lee et al.[60] reported the isolation of over 150 PAH compounds from marijuana and tobacco smoke condensates, using combined capillary GC-MS. Giger and Blumer developed isolative procedures applicable to the analyses of PAH in marine sediments.[6] A combination of ultraviolet, visible, and mass spectrometric techniques have demonstrated the complexity of the PAH fraction in the marine environment.

Up to the present time, mass spectrometric techniques (primarily probe) have been used on an occasional basis in the analysis of PAH in foods, primarily to aid in the identification of a specific carcinogen isolated from a product. Pancirov and Brown[62] modified the procedure of Howard et al. and applied it to the analysis of various marine tissues. Gas chromatography, ultraviolet spectrophotometry, and mass spectrometry were employed in this study; however, information on the column packings used is not included.

Grimmer and Böhnke used GC-MS in their profile analyses of the PAH content of various foodstuffs.[23] The authors indicate that all of the samples contained more than 100 PAH; however, detailed information on the confirmation of these compounds by MS is not described. As a result of research and demonstrated applications, it can be expected that capillary GC-MS will find much greater use in the analyses of PAH in foods in the near future. Aside from the need to confirm the identities of reported carcinogens in the environment, it is important to bring these specialized techniques to bear on the definitive characterization of the PAH contaminants in the food supply.

SMOKED FOODS

Numerous studies have been conducted on the PAH content of curing smokes and the reader is referred to reviews by Tilgner,[63] Draudt,[64] Sikorski and Tilgner,[65] and Tilgner and Daun.[5] Much of the research has been concerned with attempts to control or eliminate the PAH content and was conducted outside the U.S. Tilgner and Daun[5] stated that over 25 PAH have been identified in curing smoke and approximately 40 others have not been characterized.

Investigations have been conducted on a world-wide basis with respect to determination of PAH in smoked foodstuffs. As shown in Table 1, various levels of benzo(a)pyrene have been reported in a wide variety of smoked products.[66-90] The differences in hydrocarbon content may be ascribed to the many variables involved in the smoking process including the type of generator, combustion temperature, and degree of smoking.[64] With respect to surface deposition of the smoke constituents, Tilgner[63] and Gorelova et al.[91] stated that the PAH compounds will migrate into the interior of the food, the extent of migration being dependent upon the character of the product and its storage time.

The majority of the earlier findings were reported by European and Russian investigators. These initial studies were no doubt prompted by the hypothesis that a correlation might exist between a high incidence of stomach cancer in some population groups (Icelandic and Baltic fishermen) and the presence of PAH compounds in smoked foods. Both Dungal[92] and Voitelovich et al.[68] claimed that such a correlation did exist; however, some investigators felt that the data were not sufficient to warrant such a conclusion.[93]

Some of the highest levels of benzo(a)pyrene have been found in smoked fish as reported by Russian and Japanese investigators. For example, Voitelovich et al.[68] and Petrun and Rubenchik[71] reported findings ranging from 1.7 to 60 µg/kg. Shabad,[10] in his review of studies in the U.S.S.R., did not comment on these data; however, he stated that the technology of smoking had been altered to use special smoke liquids which were free of benzo(a)pyrene and did not induce tumors when tested on animals.

Masuda and Kuratsune in 1971 reported finding levels of benzo(a)pyrene of up to 37 µg/kg[78] in their analyses of Japanese smoked dried fish products. The fish products included Katsuobushi, Sababushi, and Urumebushi made, respectively, from bonito, mackerel, and sardines. Katsuobushi is prepared from broiled boned bonito flesh, by smoking through intermittent exposure to wood smoke for 1 or 2 weeks and drying in the sun. The product is stored in wooden boxes for about a week to permit mold growth and the drying and molding processes are then repeated a few times. The Sababushi and Uremebushi are prepared from flesh of mackerel and sardines by a similar process but with less smoking and no storing for mold production. These authors found 16 PAH including 12 with 4 to 5 condensed rings and a number of carcinogenic types including benzo(a)pyrene as mentioned above. They believe that these products probably comprise one of the foods most heavily contaminated with PAH in the world. The relationship between the high PAH content of these foods (consumed frequently but not in large quantities) and the high incidence of gastric cancer in Japan was considered by the authors, who judged that it is inconclusive in the absence of epidemiological studies. Shirotori[79] confirmed Masuda and Kuratsune's findings in Katsuobushi and also reported levels of benzo(a)pyrene of 7.4 to 31.3 µg/kg in nori, a seaweed food.[79]

Toth[76] and Toth and Blaas[80] reported levels of 9 to 55 µg/kg of benzo(a)pyrene and 13 other PAH in 6 Yugoslavian smoked meats. However, the authors state that from their experimental sausage-making tests, the benzo(a)pyrene content could be reduced to not over 1 µg/kg. As would be expected, products smoked for long periods to a black color contained higher levels of the PAH.

Table 1
LEVELS OF BENZO(A)PYRENE FOUND IN SMOKED FOODS

Food product	Levels (μg/kg)	Country	Ref.
Sausage and fish	1.7—10.5	Czechoslovakia	66
Fish and mutton	0.3—2.1	Iceland	67
Fish	1.7—53	Russia	68
Fish	7	Russia	69
Sausage and fish	0.1—1.4	Russia	70
Fish	4.2—60	Russia	71
Fish (salmon)	2.6—3.0	Italy	72
Wurstel	0.4—1.0	Italy	72
Bacon	1.6—4.0	Italy	72
Salami	2.0—2.8	Italy	72
Sardines	1.8	Italy	72
Provola (cheese)	4.1—6.2	Italy	72
Haddock, salmon	0.3, 1.0	U.S.	73
Herring, sturgeon	1.0, 0.8	U.S.	74, 75
Ham	3.2	U.S.	74, 75
Ham, belly fat	1.0—14	Germany	76
Fish	0.05—5.7	Russia	77
Katsuobushi (bonito), Sabushi (mackerel), Urumebushi (sardines)	2—37	Japan	78
Katsuobushi (bonito)	8.7—27.2	Japan	79
Nori (seaweed food)	7.4—31.3	Japan	79
Meats	9—55	Yugoslavia	76, 80
Fish	11.5	Poland	81
Fish, mutton (commercially smoked)	1.0	Iceland	82
Mutton (home smoked)	23	Iceland	
Hot sausage	0.8	U.S.	83
Ham	1.0	U.S.	83
Turkey fat	2.1	U.S.	83
White fish	4.3	U.S.	83
Whiting	6.9	U.S.	83
Chubs	1.3	U.S.	83
Cod	4.5	U.S.	83
Meats (bologna, frankfurters, salami, pepperoni, sausages, hams, bacon, beef, pork)	0.2—2.0	Canada	84
Fish (herring, canned, oysters)	0.5—15	Canada	84
Cheese, Gouda	0.5	Canada	84
Bacon	1.2—3.6	U.S.	85
Cured meats, sausage, fish, cheese	<6	Italy	86
Sausages (mutton), bologna	0—0.15	Norway	87
Fish, oysters	0—9	New Zealand	88
Meat	<0.5	New Zealand	88
Beef	18.8—24.1	U.S.	89
Pork	25.8—31.6	U.S.	89
Lamb	8.8—12.3	U.S.	89
Turkey	ND	U.S.	89
Frankfurters	ND	U.S.	90
Salmon steak	ND	U.S.	90

Thorsteinsson[82] compared the PAH content of foods after traditional home smoking and commercial smoking in Iceland. The home-smoked meat (mutton) contained as much as 23 μg benzo(a)pyrene per kilogram and corresponding high amounts of other PAH, including benz(a)anthracene. Samples of meat hung just above the stove showed as high as 107 μg benzo(a)pyrene per kilogram. In contrast, levels of the latter compound did not exceed 1 µg/kg in meat and fish smoked commercially. This author also concluded that 60 to 75% of the benzo(a)pyrene occurred in the superficial layers of the meat products and that protective coverings including loose cotton fabric and cellophane reduced the PAH content of the smoked meats significantly. The latter covering provided almost full protection against benzo(a)pyrene penetration. These studies are in agreement with the findings of Rhene and Bratzler[85] who studied the formation and distribution of benzo(a)pyrene in smoked bologna and bacon. The latter authors also found that cellulose casing significantly reduced the benzo(a)pyrene content in the bologna and that with or without casing, the penetration of the compound did not exceed 1.4 to 1.6 mm from the surface. With respect to the cooking of the smoked bacon, at least half of the PAH was found in the fat drippings.

In comparison to the numerous studies conducted by foreign workers, data on smoked foods in North America are meager. Genest and Smith[94] in Canada analyzed various smoked fish, frankfurters, and cheeses, but benzo(a)pyrene was not detected; however, the detection limits of the method employed ranged only from 10 to 50 µg/kg. Lijinsky and Shubik[73] reported the presence of benzo(a)pyrene at levels of 0.3 and 1.0 µg/kg and other PAH in 2 samples of smoked fish.[72]

In 1966, the Food and Drug Administration (FDA) developed methods (detection limits of 2 µg/kg and below) for determination of PAH in smoked foods and applied them to various smoked and unsmoked foodstuffs.[74,75] Levels of benzo(a)pyrene of up to 3.2 µg/kg noted that pyrene and fluoranthene were found in all of the products examined including the unsmoked samples. In follow-up investigations, the FDA and U.S. Department of Agriculture developed a cooperative program.[83] Assorted foods and related samples were analyzed for benzo(a)pyrene, and 32 out of 60 of these products contained the hydrocarbon. Levels reported for 21 samples were below 1 µg/kg; greater amounts were isolated from the remaining 11 samples. In the smoked products, levels of benzo(a)pyrene did not exceed 7.0 ppb (smoked whiting), which was well below some of the values reported in the literature by Russian and European workers. These data were not unexpected at the time since Draudt (1963) had stated that lightly smoked products are common in the U.S. in contrast to some countries in which foods are heavily smoked for preservative purposes.[64]

In his most recent study, Panalaks,[84] using high pressure liquid chromatography, completed the analyses of 70 smoked food products commercially available in Canada. PAH were detected in 70% of the samples. Levels of benzo(a)pyrene were from 0.1 to 15 µg/kg. It is also noteworthy that the reported benz(a)anthracene content ranged from 0.2 to 30 µg/kg. The latter compound was found in both smoked and unsmoked oysters. With respect to the Panalaks study, it appears to the reviewers that some follow-up studies should be conducted, particularly with respect to the reports that 7,12-dimethylbenz(a)anthracene is present in smoked and unsmoked oysters and several other PAH, not previously found in foods, are present in the various products analyzed. Further confirmation of identity would be desirable.

Doremire et al.[89] fluorometrically examined charcoal-grilled meats for benzo(a)pyrene and found levels ranging from not detectable (ND) to 133 ppb. Concentrations of benzo(a)pyrene appear to be proportional to the fat content of the meat product. Lijinsky and Ross[95] explained this phenomenon by the theory that the rendered fat falls on the hot coals and is pyrolyzed, giving rise to benzo(a)pyrene formation, which is then deposited on the meat surface.

FATS AND OILS

D'Arrigo[13] did a tabulated review on the presence of PAH in vegetable oils and fats, animal oils and fats, and by-products of oils such as margarines and soaps. The author surveyed the variations in PAH content and attributed the differences in findings to technological treatments of oils and fats, heating, usage of solvents, refining, and oxidation.

The detection of PAH, including pyrene, benzo(e)pyrene, and benzo(a)pyrene, in edible vegetable oils was first reported by Jung and Morand in the early 1960s.[96-98] Subsequent studies by Ciusa et al. indicated the presence of phenanthrene, pyrene, fluoranthene, benz(a)anthracene, chrysene, and perylene in pressed and refined olive oils.[99] Higher levels were detected in the rectified products; however, no benzo(a)pyrene was isolated. In 1966, Borneff and Fabian published a method for isolation of PAH in fats and oils.[100] Estimated levels of up to 1 µg benzo(a)pyrene per kilogram were reported for vegetable oils (up to 20 µg total PAH, carcinogenic types per kilogram). The authors indicated that heating destroyed about 70% of the PAH originally present in the oils. No PAH were found in pork fat. Howard et al.[101] described a quantitative method and its application to the analyses of soybean, cottonseed, corn, olive, safflower, and peanut oils processed in the U.S. With the exception of safflower oil (only three samples) trace quantities of PAH, including benzo(a)pyrene, were found in at least one of each type of oil analyzed. Levels of benzo(a)pyrene ranged from 0.4 to 1.5 µg/kg. In subsequent investigations, Howard et al.[102] attempted to establish the source of the contamination. Analyses of 15 commercial hexanes used in the solvent extraction of edible oils were conducted on the thesis that they were contributing the residues. Although nine of the samples contained polycyclics, no carcinogens were detected. However, analysis of various crude oil samples not subjected to solvent extraction did reveal the presence of benzo(a)pyrene. The authors concluded that the results of the studies indicated that the contamination occurred in the initial processing operation, or was present in the original starting material as suggested by reports in the literature.

Subsequent reports by Grimmer and Hildebrandt[103] and Biernoth and Rost[104] in Germany confirmed the presence of PAH compounds in both refined and crude oils. In examination of crude rapeseed, sunflower, palm kernel, palm, peanut, cottonseed, soybean, linseed, and coconut oils for polycyclics, the former authors found the highest concentration (43.7 µg/kg) of benzo(a)pyrene in oil from smoke-dried coconut, while sunflower seed and palm kernel oils contained 10.6 and 4.1 µg/kg, respectively.[103] It is noteworthy that other carcinogenic types, benz(a)anthracene and dibenz(a,h)anthracene, were also isolated from the aforementioned products. Grimmer and Hildebrandt also concluded that hexane solvents were not the source of the contamination. Benzo(a)pyrene (0.9 to 29 µg/kg) and other PAH including benz(a)anthracene and dibenz(a,h)anthracene were found by Biernoth and Rost in their study of refined coconut oils.[104] These latter authors also indicated that although the PAH content of the oils was reduced to only a small extent by bleaching earths, treatment with activated charcoal and subsequent deodorization was an effective means of removing the PAH from the oils.

Fabian analyzed fats and oils of vegetable and animal origin with findings as high as 20 to 100 µg of carcinogenic types per kilogram (3 to 18 µg/kg benzo(a)pyrene) in various margarines and coconut oil, but these compounds were not found in butter or lard.[105-107] The author stated that levels could be reduced to 2 to 4 µg/kg by treatment with steam and activated carbon. In a study of margarine and mayonnaise, Fritz[108] and Franzke and Fritz[109] found 0.2 to 0.6 µg of benzo(a)pyrene and 6 other PAH per kilogram; they also reported 11 PAH including benzo(a)pyrene, 1.9 and 0.5 µg/kg, in crude and refined safflower oils, respectively. Similar findings were published by Grigorenko et al.[110] who found 1 to 5 µg/kg in sunflower oils. In subsequent work levels of 0.5 to 2 µg of benzo(a)pyrene per kilogram of soybean, cottonseed, and sunflower oils were reported by the latter authors.[111]

In a more recent study[112] in New Zealand, Swallow analyzed various vegetable oils and animal fats. Variable concentrations of PAH were found in all of the 7 vegetable oils examined: the highest levels of benzo(a)pyrene (9 μg/kg) were present in a peanut product. Concentrations up to 15 μg of the same hydrocarbon per kilogram were reported in used beef drippings, which is the main fat used for commercial frying in New Zealand. The author stated that the amounts of PAH in butter and margarine were minimal.

In his assessment, Tilgner[8] stated that it is most probable "...that the contamination of vegetable fats occurs either through reabsorption by plants grown in contaminated soils or by surface contamination from polluted air — both being contributory factors in oilseeds. The contaminants may find their way from the contaminated vegetable raw material into crude and refined oils. The contamination does not originate during the solvent extraction and processing operations." As discussed in the following section on "Plants", there is considerable disagreement on the source(s) of such contamination.

PLANTS

The presence of PAH has been demonstrated in a wide variety of plants from diverse sources. In 1969, Guddal first reported the isolation of anthracene, pyrene, and fluoranthene from chrysanthemum roots grown in contaminated soil near a gas works plant.[113] The author concluded that the PAH were resorbed by the plant since follow-up investigations of roots grown in uncontaminated soils and not exposed to smoke from the factory were not found to be contaminated with the hydrocarbons. These findings stimulated interest in the PAH content of soils and plants as well as their possible endogenous formation in all plants and microorganisms. Andelman and Suess have noted that the question of endogenous formation arose because of the apparent ubiquity of the hydrocarbon in the environment, particularly in a wide variety of materials which were not likely to have been associated with pyrolytic processes.[2] Blumer, in 1961, reported levels of benzo(a)pyrene of from 40 to 1300 μg/kg and other PAH in soil taken from Connecticut and Massachusetts forests located away from cities and industrial complexes.[114] The author postulated that the contaminants were derived from the pyrolysis of wood or alternatively from organisms which contribute their organic matter to soils. Borneff and Fischer[115] described findings of 100 μg of fluorescent PAH per kilogram in lake phytoplankton; 13 compounds including benzo(a)pyrene were identified. The concept of bacterial synthesis of PAH and subsequent translocation to plants was seconded by Mallet[116] in France who found varying levels of benzo(a)pyrene in tree leaves and in decaying matter under trees.

In a series of articles during the 1960s, various German workers presented evidence that PAH are absorbed and synthesized by plants. Doerr, in 1965, reported that barley roots in soil or water cultures absorbed benzo(a)pyrene with subsequent transferral to the shoots.[117] Graf and Diehl[118] isolated 8 PAH from various plant leaves (including salad greens, cauliflower, potatoes, carrots, apples, apricots, edible mushrooms, and wheat and rye grains) at levels of 8 to 40 μg/kg. In the same paper, the authors also described the results of their studies with wheat and rye grown hydroponically in carcinogen-free nutrient solutions in the presence and absence of light. The seedlings contained 10 to 20 μg of benzo(a)pyrene per kilogram of dried material in contrast to the seeds, in which only traces of the carcinogen were found. The investigators concluded that the hydrocarbon was synthesized by the plants both in the presence and absence of light. In another series of experiments, the authors fertilized 5 different plant varieties with 10 μg of benzo(a)pyrene/ℓ and observed a distinct increase in vegetation. Borneff et al.[119,120] also concluded that the endogenous formation of carcinogens in plants occurs. This conclusion was based on the results observed in laboratory culture studies of fresh water algae in which the extracted algae contained 10 to 50 μg carcinogenic PAH per kilogram. Knorr and Schenk, in 1968, discussed their laboratory studies of various bacteria which indicated that benzo(a)pyrene had been accumulated through synthesis in amounts of 2 to 6 μg/kg of dried material.[121]

Based on their own investigations and an analysis of the results of others, Schmidt and Fritz[122] concluded that benzo(a)pyrene and other PAH occur in edible plants to a considerable extent. These authors cited Graf's experiments indicating that PAH are synthesized by plants as essential materials in their metabolic processes. They suggested that these findings indicate that foodstuffs of plant origin which are consumed in great quantities may in fact be the primary source of ingested PAH, rather than smoked, roasted, or heated products, which had been the most suspect sources.

Hancock et al.[123] conducted studies on leaves of plants grown near a railroad station and another site close to an airport. A comparison of pyrene to benzo(a)pyrene ratios suggested that most of the PAH found on leaves were products of plant biochemical synthesis. In his recent review of the "Environmental Load and Cycle of PAH", Suess[3] concluded that "...the existence of a natural background concentration of PAH has now been well established. It consists of PAH biosynthesized on a worldwide scale by plants and microorganisms on land and in the water and formed during open burning of forests and prairies not ignited by man. Volcanic activity is an additional source".

Tilgner[8] noted that a strong relationship appears to exist between air pollution and the occurrence of benzo(a)pyrene in grain and vegetables. For example, grain samples from the heavily industrialized Ruhr district in Germany were found by Grimmer and Hildebrandt[124] to contain approximately 10 times more PAH than samples taken from Lower Saxony and Holstein District remote from industry.

Grimmer and Hildebrandt[125] also conducted studies on four different types of vegetables grown simultaneously in the same field. The benzo(a)pyrene content found varied considerably, e.g., tomatoes 0.22 μg/kg, leeks 6.6 μg/kg, spinach 7.4 μg/kg, and kale 20 μg/kg. Salad greens grown close to Hamburg contained levels of PAH five to six times greater than that grown in a suburban area. In subsequent work, Grimmer[126] was of the opinion that "in the appraisal of the amount of carcinogenic hydrocarbons ingested by man quite new criteria are apparent. Neither smoked foods or grilled meat but vegetables and salads contain the largest amounts of PAH."

Gunther et al.[127] reported the presence of about 125 mg/kg of anthracene and 6 unidentified PAH in the rinds of oranges grown in atmosphere-polluted areas in the U.S., but not in fruit harvested in uncontaminated locations. Bolling[128] studied the effects of location and of drying with combustion gases on the benzo(a)pyrene content of cereals. Wheat, corn, oats, and barley grown in industrial areas showed a fourfold to tenfold higher contamination than crops from more remote areas. Drying with combustion gases increased the contamination of the grain threefold to tenfold; coke as fuel caused much less contamination than oil.

Hutt et al.[129] reported that PAH are deposited on grains dried by direct heating with fuel oil. The use of fuel oils produced levels between 140 and 250% of the initial benzo(a)pyrene content. Levels of benzo(a)pyrene found ranged from 3 to 18 ppb and higher in dried grains.

Various Russian investigators reported the contamination of plants by PAH. Shabad et al.[130] stated that, on the basis of available data, there are at least three routes of PAH passage into plants: air deposition, adsorption from soil, and synthesis. The results of their studies have led them to believe that air deposition is the principal route of contamination. According to the authors the PAH "penetrates into the soil mainly from air spread across the layers into the water, and passes into plants, fodder, and finally into human food". With respect to the minimal "background" quantities of

PAH, Shabad et al. believe that natural synthesis cannot be ruled out; however, the problem requires further study under well-controlled and fully air-tight conditions. Shcherbak[131,132] also stated that pollution of plants may occur from sedimentation of atmospheric dust and soot or by migration of the carcinogens into the plants from polluted soils. Shabad and Cohan[133] concluded that the main source of contamination of soil is from air particulates. They indicated that migration or resorption of PAH into plants was dependent on the PAH level in the soil and the type of plant. Less benzo(a)pyrene was found in grain plants (wheat, etc.).

Several other investigators have refuted the biosynthesis of PAH by plants. By careful exclusion of contaminated air from developing plants (lettuce, soybean, rye, and tobacco), Grimmer and Duevel[134] demonstrated that they were free of the PAH found in plants from the same lots of seeds exposed to the atmosphere in fields or greenhouses. Schamp and van Wassenhove[135] stressed the necessity for extreme precautions in isolation of benzo(a)pyrene from extracts of plants and bitumens; otherwise false positives can occur. In their analyses, Wagner and Siddiqi[136] found that an increase in benzo(k)fluoranthene in summer wheat and rye paralleled an increase in its concentration in the soil. These workers also reported 4.8 to 8.6 μg of benzo(a)pyrene per kilogram and 24.6 to 76.8 μg of benzo(k)fluoranthene (dry basis) per kilogram in young wheat plants. Hertel et al.[137] have reported 0.12 to 0.54 mg of benzo(a)pyrene per kilogram in commercial wheat.

WATER ENVIRONMENT — SEAFOODS

Kraybill[138] stated that PAH are ubiquitous in the aquatic environment and may present the greatest carcinogenic insult. Andelman and Suess[2] surveyed the literature on the incidence and significance of PAH in the water environment. The above reviewers[2,3] also discussed sources of contamination of the waterways including industrial and domestic effluents, atmospheric particulates, oil spills, marine transportation, and biosynthesis by plants and microorganisms.

Most of the early studies on PAH in the aquatic environment were conducted outside the U.S. Two Russian workers, Ilnitsky and Varshavskaya,[139] reviewed some of the literature up to 1952 with respect to water contamination with benzo(a)pyrene. These authors concluded that the benzo(a)pyrene was increasingly polluting natural waters. Bornff co-workers in Germany have investigated fresh water as well as the effectiveness of various treatments for removal of the contaminants.[140-145] These reports give the total PAH contents found at that time (1960s) in samples taken from various rivers and lakes in Germany. PAH found in surface waters were 0.065 to 3 μg/ℓ; in plants and sediments were 700 μg/kg for phytoplankton and up to 55 mg/kg for suspended solids; in ground waters were 0.045—0.14 μg/ℓ; and in pure waters were up to 0.025 μg/ℓ. According to these investigators, it is through the discharge of urban and domestic sewage, the release of industrial wastes, rain water, and leaching of the pollutants of industrial origin from vegetation and soils that the compounds enter natural waters and thereby contaminate public water supplies. In experimental studies Saccini-Cicatelli[146,147] has observed that tubifex worms placed in benzo(a)pyrene-contaminated water took up as much as 88.2 mg of the hydrocarbon per kilogram and retained up to 350 μg/kg when placed in pure water. As discussed in the previous section under "Plants," Knorr and Schenk and Borneff et al. reported the synthesis of benzo(a)pyrene by bacteria and algae, respectively.[119-121] Andelman and Suess[2] noted finding PAH in phytoplankton, in river sediments and suspended solids, and in worms and pointed out that these aqueous biota serve as food for edible fish. They also indicated that benzo(a)pyrene has been detected in fish taken from European rivers in which these biota were reported to be contaminated.

Table 2
LEVELS OF BENZO(a)PYRENE FOUND IN MARINE LIFE AT VARIOUS GEOGRAPHIC LOCATIONS

Source	Marine life	Level of benzo(a)pyrene (μg/kg dry wt)	Ref.
Greenland	Plankton	5.5	149
	Algae	60	149
	Codfish	15	149
	Mollusk	60	149
	Mussel	18 (shell) 55 (body)	149
French coasts	Plankton	5—400	150, 151
	Shrimp, oyster, mussel, mollusk, crab	1.5—90	152
	Oyster, lower shell	70	
	Oyster, upper shell	112	153
	Mussel	16—22	156
Italian coasts	Plankton	6.1—21.2	154
	Algae	2.2	154
	Mussel	11 (shell) 130, 540 (body)	154
	Mollusk	2.4	154
	Sardine	65	154
U.S. (California)	Thatched barnacles	Present	157, 158
	Goose barnacle	Present	158
U.S. (Virginia)	Oyster	2—6	159
U.S. (Alabama)	Oyster (shell)	24	153
U.S. (Maine)	Clam	3	90

The majority of the early studies of PAH in the marine environment were performed by Mallet and colleagues in France.[148-155] The results of these investigations and other early studies conducted off the coasts of France, Italy, Greenland, and the U.S. indicated the presence of benzo(a)pyrene at varying levels in flora and fish as summarized in Table 2.[2,154,156-159] According to Mallet and Sardou[150], plankton may be able to fix PAH from exogenous sources and marine fauna may be contaminated regardless of whether in polluted or unpolluted locations. With respect to sources of PAH in marine sediments, Andelman and Suess[2] included surface effluents, ships, volcanic debris, and activity of organisms (including bacteria). The same authors also noted that the benzo(a)pyrene contamination of marine life off the unpopulated coast of Greenland is of the same order as that found off French coasts, thus indicating the ubiquity of benzo(a)pyrene in the oceans. They suggested that endogenous synthesis in flora may be the source of contamination in remote areas.

In 1976, Suess concluded that the ability of marine organisms to concentrate PAH had been demonstrated; however, there is still some controversy with respect to their capacity to degrade the hydrocarbons.[3] The author has stressed that "...while some aquatic microorganisms will degrade PAH, their actual existence and bioactivity depend on their surrounding environmental conditions. Changes in salinity, temperature, sunlight, and wave action directly affect growth rate and metabolism." In the same article it is also noted that the more highly developed aquatic fauna may contribute to such degradation in that some of the mammalian metabolic pathways were found to involve oxidases and other enzymes needed for degrading of the PAH. However, there is insufficient information as to how widespread these systems are. Thus, while a number of investigations have shown a significant degradation of PAH in some marine fish and invertebrates, other researchers were unable to demonstrate their oxidation in some benthic marine invertebrates, phytoplankton, and some zooplankton within a period of 1 month. Zobell[160] summarized information on sources and biodegradation related to marine pollution.

The PAH contamination of marine life in U.S. coastal waters (Table 2) was first investigated by Shimkin[157] and Koe and Zechmeister[158] who isolated benzo(a)pyrene from thatched barnacles off the coast of California. Cahnmann and Kuratsune[159] reported estimated levels of 2 to 6 μg of benzo(a)pyrene and other PAH per kilogram (estimated total level about 1200 μg/kg) in oysters collected from Norfolk, Va., an area moderately contaminated with petroleum oils. These workers assumed that the quantities of hydrocarbons in oysters vary with their habitat, based on findings of other investigators who showed variations in the levels of the compounds, and in composition of the hydrocarbon mixture, depending upon the environment.[157,158,161]

During the 1970s, considerable attention was focused on the occurrence of oil spills and the effects on the marine environment. For detailed information the reader is referred to the "Workshop on the Input, Fate and Effects of Petroleum in the Marine Environment" sponsored by the National Academy of Sciences (NAS) in 1973 in Airlie, Va.[162] This workshop estimated that approximately 6 million tons of petroleum hydrocarbons enter the oceans annually, the major contributors being marine transportation and urban runoff, with 2.1 and 1.9 million tons/annum (Mt/a), respectively. Coastal refineries, industrial and domestic together, were estimated to contribute 0.8 Mt/a, natural seepages and atmospheric fallout each adding another 0.6 Mt/a. On the basis of the reported benzo(a)pyrene concentration in crude oil being about 1 mg/kg, NAS[162] concluded that about 6 tons of petroleum-linked benzo(a)pyrene enter the oceans each year. In assessing this contamination, Suess[3] noted that the contribution to the total environmental load is insignificant in comparison to that from land-based, high-temperature processes and constitutes only about 0.1%. Ketchum[163] stated that although oil spills are spectacular events and attract the most public attention, they constitute only about 10% of the total amount of oil entering the marine environment. According to this author, the other 90% originates from the normal operation of oil-carrying tankers, other ships, offshore production, refinery operations, and the disposal of oil-waste material.

Blumer et al.[164] and Ehrhardt[165] suggested that marine organisms nonselectively accumulate petroleum hydrocarbons in amounts present in the water and, that once accumulated, the hydrocarbons (in particular the aromatic hydrocarbons) are retained in the tissues for long periods of time, being depurated only very slowly. Anderson,[166] on the other hand, in controlled studies of oysters and clams placed in water-fuel oil mixtures followed by depuration in clean waters, reported that both aromatic and saturated hydrocarbons are released from tissues relatively rapidly. For example, maintenance of the shellfish in clean water for periods from 24 to 52 days was sufficient to cleanse the tissues of detectable levels of hydrocarbons. Lee et al.[167] have exposed mussels to mineral oil and various tagged hydrocarbons, ^{14}C-heptadecane, ^{14}C-naphthalene, and ^{3}H-benzo(a)pyrene. It was found that the mussels rapidly accumulated the hydrocarbons, but when they were transferred to uncontaminated water, 80 to 90% of the hydrocarbons were lost from the mussels in a 2-week period.

Blumer et al.[164] discussed the extent of the pollution problem associated with an oil spill in Buzzards Bay, Mass. Contamination of edible shellfish with oil resulted and persisted for a number of months after the incident, as did the pollutant in the marine sediments. The gas chromatographic technique employed by the authors did not permit separation and identification of specific PAH; however, the chromatograms showed clear evidence of higher PAH in the oysters and scallops. As referred to earlier, Giger and Blumer[6] analyzed sediments from Buzzards Bay and found 12 PAH; however,

Table 3
LEVELS OF PAH (μg/kg)[a] FOUND IN
OYSTERS TAKEN FROM U.S. WATERS

Compounds	Aransas Bay	Galveston Bay	
		Approved	Closed
Benzo(b)fluoranthene	0.3	1.2	2.2
Benzo(k)fluoranthene	—[b]	0.1	0.4
Benzo(e)pyrene	0.2	1.2	2.1
Chrysene	0.5	0.2	0.6
Fluoranthene	1.7	3.0	7.8
Pyrene	0.9	1.8	6.5
Perylene	—	0.7	1.0
Phenanthrene	—	—	2.2

[a] Average values.
[b] Not found.

mass spectral analyses of the remaining complex mixture indicated that many more condensed ring compounds of unknown structure and biological activity were present.

Fazio and others[168] obtained data on PAH levels in oysters in Aransas and Galveston Bays (U.S.). The Galveston Bay area was suspected of being contaminated with petroleum hydrocarbon residues. The results are summarized in Table 3. Samples were taken as follows: 5 samples of suspected contamination from closed areas in Galveston Bay, 13 samples from approved areas in Galveston Bay, and 2 samples designated as controls from Aransas Bay approximately 150 mi outside of the suspected contamination area. No benzo(a)pyrene was found in any of the samples; however, slightly higher levels of PAH were found in the oysters taken from the closed area. With few exceptions, the hydrocarbon types isolated from the three harvested areas were essentially the same.

Fazio and Howard in 1975 also conducted, under contract, a survey of retail market and growing area oysters for the presence of PAH. The sampling consisted of 25 eastern oysters (*Crassostrea virginica*) from the Chesapeake Bay area, 25 from the Baltimore retail market, 25 from the Galveston Bay area, and 25 from the Galveston retail market. The results of these analyses showed no detectable levels of benzo(a)pyrene in the Chesapeake Bay area or retail market samples (Baltimore and Galveston). The oil-polluted areas of Galveston Bay showed levels of benzo(a)pyrene as high as 9.4 ppb, while oysters taken from approved (noncontaminated) areas did not contain any detectable levels. Pyrene and fluoranthene were detected in all of the samples from all sources at levels up to 157 ppb.

Dunn and Stick[169] in Canada described their findings of elevated levels of benzo(a)pyrene (up to 21.5 μg/kg) in mussels growing near and on creosoted timbers in Vancouver coastal waters. The same authors[170] also studied the release of the above hydrocarbon from environmentally contaminated mussels transferred from a polluted area into clean circulating water. The amount of benzo(a)pyrene, initially 45 μg/kg wet weight, declined approximately exponentially over the 6 weeks of the experiment with a reported overall half-life of 16 days. It was concluded that short depuration periods of 1 to 3 days commonly used to eliminate bacterial contamination from edible shellfish before marketing would have little effect on the tissue content of benzo(a)pyrene in mussels.

In a study of 19 mainland and 6 island stations situated throughout the Southern California Bight, Dunn, and Young[171] found that even in a heavily populated coastal area, baseline levels of benzo(a)pyrene in mussels are at or near the limits of detectability (0.1 μg/kg) of the analytical method employed. These researchers have pointed out that their data are in contrast to the results reported by European workers who found substantial contamination of marine organisms (biosynthesis) taken from remote and presumably unpolluted areas. The former authors concluded that the geographical distribution and low baseline levels of benzo(a)pyrene in mussels support a human rather than a biogenic origin of benzo(a)pyrene contamination of marine organisms.

Pancirov and Brown[62] investigated the extent of PAH contamination in various samples of shell- and fin fish along the U.S. eastern seaboard and various other locations in the U.S. and Canada. Ten PAH including benzo(a)pyrene, benz(a)anthracene, and chrysene were isolated from the edible marine tissues. Only the oyster and crab samples taken from Long Island Sound and Raritan Bay waters exposed to municipal and industrial wastes were found to contain levels of the PAH above 2 μg/kg. The authors noted that in comparison with other foodstuffs neither shellfish nor fin fish show unusually high amounts of PAH. Based on their findings of pyrene at much higher relative concentrations than its methyl isomers, the authors offered the opinion that the hydrocarbon contamination is not of petroleum origin but rather is due to combustion sources. This opinion is based on published data on the PAH content of petroleum, which show that the methyl derivatives of pyrene significantly outnumber the parent compound. However, it is pointed out that this line of reasoning does not take into account the possibility of preferential metabolism of the hydrocarbons with side chains or the difference in the rate and extent of accumulation of these compounds in marine tissues.

Brown and Pancirov[172] reported baseline levels of PAH for five species of fish (flounder, scup, black sea bass, butterfish, red hake) and one species of shellfish (sea scallops) obtained from the Baltimore Canyon area. With the start of exploration and possible production of oil and/or gas off the east coast of the U.S. there was concern that environmental damage might result. Levels of benz(a)anthracene and benzo(a)pyrene ranged from 0.3 to 20 ppb and <1 to 11 ppb, respectively.

COOKING AND HEATING OF FOODS

The formation of PAH in food as the result of the preparation procedures employed has also received attention. Kuratsune[173] found benzo(a)pyrene in the charred material scraped from biscuits heated over a gas burner, whereas the compound was not detected in the char taken from broiled sardines heated in the same manner. PAH have also been identified in coffee soots, a by-product produced in the commercial roasting of coffee beans and in roasted coffee.[174,175]

According to Fritz,[176] the greater part of benzo(a)pyrene together with other PAH such as anthranthrene, coronene, indenopyrene, and various benzofluoranthenes is found in the coffee membrane and tar. In normal roasted beans, the levels of benzo(a)pyrene ranged from 0.3 to 0.5 μg/kg. This compound was also found at levels of 0.47 to 0.7 μg/kg in malt and barley, the raw materials for malt-coffee and coffee substitutes. Roasting of malt in a coal-fired furnace resulted in its formation at approximately 15.8 μg/kg (mean value), whereas the roasting of malt-coffee and a coffee substitute in a gas-fired roaster produced 0.9 and 1.0 μg/kg, respectively. Masuda et al.[177] reported the presence of 18 PAH in the smoke and scorches from fish broiled in either a gas or electric broiler; the gas-broiled fish contained more PAH than those cooked in the electric broiler. In the same report, these authors also indicated that roasted barley used in the preparation of Mugicha (a Japanese drink prepared by infusing roasted unhulled barley in hot water) contained several PAH, but not carcinogenic types.

Various investigators have studied the pyrolytic behavior of carbohydrates, fats, and proteins and the resultant formation of PAH.[178-180] Davies and Wilmshurst[178] heated starch in the absence of air and at atmospheric pressure with the following results: at 370 to 390°C, benzo(a)pyrene was found at a level of 0.7 µg/kg in the distillation residue; at 650°C, 17 µg/kg were formed.[178] Similar studies were conducted by Masuda et al.[179] on various carbohydrates, amino acids, and fatty acids. No PAH were found at 300°C, but 19 hydrocarbons including benzo(a)pyrene were detected in the above products at 500 and 700°C. Halaby and Fagerson[180] pyrolyzed a number of lipids and minor constituents such as carotene and cholesterol in a tube furnace at 400 to 700°C under nitrogen. At 700°C, pyrolysis of lipids produced approximately 100 µg/kg concentrations of PAH. Benzo(a)pyrene was produced in all samples heated at the above temperature. At 400°C, the relatively low levels made identification difficult, but in general those compounds found at 700°C were present. The authors stated that about 10 times as much PAH is produced by pyrolysis of cholesterol as from other lipid materials, but lower levels are found in beta-carotene after pyrolysis.

The production of PAH in the grilling of meat has also received attention. Seppilli and Scassellati-Sforzolini[181] analyzed grilled beef and noted the presence of various PAH. Lijinsky and Shubik[182] reported levels of 5 to 8 µg benzo(a)pyrene per kilogram in charcoal-broiled steaks and 10.5 µg/kg in barbecued ribs. Other carcinogenic compounds of interest found in this work included benz(a)anthracene and dibenz(a,h)anthracene. The authors concluded that the fat or other carbon-hydrogen-oxygen containing compounds in the meat were the probable pyrolysis sources of the hydrocarbons. Malanoski et al.[83] have assayed barbecued pork and beef and reused cooking oil with findings of 1.4 to 4.5 µg benzo(a)pyrene per kilogram.

The effect of variations in methods of cooking on the content of benzo(a)pyrene and other PAH in meat was discussed by Lijinsky and Ross.[183] This investigation confirmed that the production of PAH in charcoal broiling was dependent on the fat content and the proximity of the food to the heat source. For example, levels of benzo(a)pyrene as high as 50 µg/kg were found in thick T-bone steaks cooked close to the coals for long periods, whereas concentrations were considerably reduced in samples prepared (to the same end point) at a greater distance from the heat source. It was the conclusion of the authors that if the production of carcinogens is to be minimized the method of cooking should avoid contact of the food with the flames, the food should be cooked for longer periods at lower temperatures, and the meat used should have a minimum of fat.

In his study of cooked foods, Fritz[184] found that roasting, frying, or deep frying resulted in negligible quantities of endogenous carcinogens, while exogenous treatment with flue gas increased the hydrocarbons, especially benzo(a)pyrene. The findings support those of Halaby and Fagerson on the pyrolysis of fats at 400°C mentioned above. Fritz, in other studies of heated foodstuffs, reported the following levels of benzo(a)pyrene:

1. <0.5 µg/kg in baked bread and biscuits and burnt crust
2. <1 µg/kg in malt-coffee and barley coffee substitutes roasted in a gas-fired roaster, but >15.8 µg/kg when the products were roasted in a coal-fired roaster
3. 0.3 to 0.5 µg/kg in normal roasted coffee, and
4. none in oils and lard when cooked at normal temperatures[185-187]

Ballschmieter[188] examined roasted peanuts and concluded that there was no significant problem since levels were <1 µg of the 8 PAH determined per kilogram. In a comparison of drying of wheat and rye in indirect vs. direct driers (in the latter the combustion gases are in contact with the grain), Fornal et al.[189] reported levels of PAH to be several-fold higher in the direct dried cereals as compared to those treated with the indirect process. Rohrlich and Suckow[190] found that the drying of wheat over a light fuel oil flame increased the benzo(a)pyrene deposition from approximately 6- to 130-fold depending on the degree of exposure.

In addition to studies of smoked foods in Iceland cited above, Thorsteinsson and Thordarson[191] investigated singed foods, such as sheep heads and seabirds, which are Icelandic dietary items. According to the authors, the fuel formerly used was peat, dry sheep manure, scrap wood, or coal, but in recent years diesel oil, propane, and acetylene gas have come into use at least for commercial singeing. With propane or acetylene-oxygen fuel, the singed products were essentially free of PAH. When coal or diesel oil was used as fuel, up to 28 µg of benzo(a)pyrene per kilogram was found in the singed sheep heads. Even higher levels, 99 µg/kg, occurred in the seabirds singed over coal. It should be noted that concentrations of benz(a)anthracene and other PAH were also found in the latter samples. Thorsteinsson and Thordarson pointed out that the district in northern Iceland where consumption of singed birds is particularly high is among the highest in that country with respect to the incidence of gastric cancer.

YEASTS

Much of the analytical work conducted on yeast can be ascribed to the interest in production of single cell proteins on petroleum substrates. Although such products are produced in Europe and other countries, production in the U.S. has been slow to develop. McGinnis and Norris[192] have attributed this to the absence of carcinogenic properties of petroleum-grown yeast in his animal feeding studies. Scrimshaw[194] has also dismissed the view that such products constitute a potential hazard.

Shabad et al.[10] reported the finding of 10 to 20 µg benzo(a)pyrene per kilogram in hydrolyzed yeasts (grown in a special cellulose medium) employed as a cattle feed in Russia. Further investigations revealed that technical ammonium sulfate salts produced by the treatment of coal gas with sulfuric acid had been added to the nutrient medium for cultivation of the hydrolyzed yeast. Analyses of these salts indicated the presence of benzo(a)pyrene at 1000 to 1400 µg/kg.

McGinnis and Norris[192] discussed their analytical studies of yeast grown on n-hydrocarbons and dextrose. The dextrose-grown yeast was not found to contain any highly condensed ring aromatics apart from pyrene and fluoranthene. However, benzo(a)pyrene (range of 1.1 to 5.9 µg/kg) and other PAH such as benz(a)anthracene were found in 3 of the 4 n-hydrocarbon-grown yeasts analyzed. (The exception was an n-hydrocarbon sample pretreated with silica gel). In a subsequent study, McGinnis[195] analyzed the n-hydrocarbon substrates used for fermentation; however, pyrene, fluoranthene, and some substituted phenanthrenes and pyrenes were the only compounds isolated. The author concluded that the contamination of the yeast with the aforementioned carcinogenic PAH could not be traced to the n-hydrocarbon source.

In the development of their gas chromatographic method for PAH in foods, Grimmer and Böhnke[23] discussed the application of their procedure to yeast, meat, smoked fish, and unrefined sunflower oil. The authors state that all of the samples were found to contain more than 100 PAH (characterized by mass spectrometry), of which only the main components were determined: phenanthrene, anthracene, fluorene, fluoranthene, pyrene, benz(a)anthracene, chrysene, benzofluoranthenes, benzo(a)pyrene, benzo(e)pyrene, perylene, dibenzanthracenes, indeno(1,2,3-cd)pyrene, benzo(g,h,i) perylene, anthanthrene, and coronene.

Truhaut and Ferrando[196] have compared the levels of three PAH found in various

European commercial yeasts and two samples grown experimentally on petroleum substrates. The content of the commercial products ranged from 0 to 13.2 μg benzo(a)pyrene per kilogram and from 0 to 9.7 μg benzo(g,h,i)perylene per kilogram. No dibenz(a,h) anthracene was detected. With respect to the 2 alkane yeasts, the results obtained were 0.6 to 2.5 μg benzo(a)pyrene per kilogram, 0 to 1.3 benzo(g,h,i)perylene per kilogram, and 0.1 to 0.5 dibenz(a,h)anthracene per kilogram. The authors indicate, however, that these compounds were not detected in subsequent analysis of yeast samples (petroleum substrate) taken from actual commercial production.

Santoro et al. analyzed yeasts grown on n-paraffins and molasses by gas-liquid chromatography with a column containing liquid crystals as stationary phase.[197] Yeasts grown on n-paraffins showed traces of benz(a)anthracene and chrysene (1 to 10 ppb) and yeasts grown on molasses showed levels of 15.2 ppb benz(a)anthracene, 24.8 ppb of benzo(a)pyrene, and 41.0 ppb of chrysene. The authors claim that the presence of PAH in molasses is probably due to the manner in which this product is processed.

LIQUID SMOKE FLAVORS

Smoke flavors are used in this country and others to impart a smoked flavor to foods. The advantages of the use of these products over conventional or direct smoking methods have been discussed by various workers,[5,64,198] Tilgner and Daun[5] noted the reduction in processing costs; however, they also remarked that there are over 40 patents in various countries that are mostly based upon wood distillation procedures yielding so-called liquid smoke with typical and unacceptable aroma and flavor. The authors recommended more fundamental studies to clarify the varying complex interaction phenomena occurring in the food after addition of the concentrate. Hollenbeck[199,200] described his manufacturing process in detail and stated that the major benefit to be derived is flavor reproducibility.

Various investigators in the U.S. and abroad analyzed smoke flavors for PAH. Lijinsky and Shubik,[73] in the analyses of 2 aqueous flavors, isolated various hydrocarbons including pyrene, fluoranthene, benzo(g,h,i)perylene, chrysene, benz(a)anthracene, carbazole, and an unidentified compound with ultraviolet and fluorescence spectra almost identical to those of benzo(a)pyrene. White et al.[201] determined PAH in liquid smoke flavors and the resinous condensates that settle out of the aqueous products on standing. Of 7 aqueous flavors analyzed, 4 were free of PAH; the other 3 contained from 2 μg of pyrene per kilogram to 35 μg of phenanthrene per kilogram, with intermediate levels of anthracene, fluoranthene, and triphenylene. One of these flavors contained the apparent benz(a)pyrene (2 μg/kg) as reported by Lijinsky and Shubik;[182] it was shown to be 4-methylbenzo(a)pyrene, the only carcinogen found. The 4 resinous condensates contained relatively high levels of benzo(a)pyrene (25 to 3800 μg/kg) plus a number of uncharacterized fluorescent compounds. The authors concluded that there was a need to assure the efficient removal of the resinous condensates from the aqueous flavors before they were used in foods.

In his 1967 review, Shabad discussed the work of his Russian colleagues, Gorelova et al.[202] and Prokofieva[203] in this area.[10] It is stated that the technology of food smoking was altered and that special smoking liquids were in use which had been found to be free of benzo(a)pyrene and did not induce tumors when fed to animals. In a later publication, Gorbatov et al.,[204] also of the U.S.S.R., compared liquid smokes for use in cured meats with respect to chemical composition and quality. These workers mentioned the desirability of removing the carcinogenic hydrocarbons and residual tars from the products before use. These hydrocarbons and tars may be removed by distillation or possibly by filtration through cellulose pulp as described by Hollenbeck. With reference to the latter process, Gorbatov et al. noted that Hollenbeck admitted that the pulp is not effective for the removal of all carcinogens.

Gorbatov et al.[204] also indicated that "the proper procedure for the production of liquid smokes from condensates, including purification steps, depends on the use to which the liquid smoke is to be put. Thus, liquid smokes intended for surface treatment only, do not require the removal of certain ingredients which must be eliminated if the liquid smoke is to be incorporated internally." As an example, the authors state that liquid smoke for the surface treatment of certain sausages must contain those substances that provide the desired product color (tars and certain carbohydrate compounds). The authors concluded that "this new technology ... will require additional research and development work in order to perfect it for commercial use". This research would include improvement of separation and purification techniques for the flavoring and components from wood pyrolyzates.

Toth and Blaas[80] in Germany reported the examination of 15 commercial liquid smoke preparations for benzo(a)pyrene. The results of this study indicate that 12 of the products contained <1 μg/kg; however, the 3 remaining preparations contained 8 to 15 μg/kg. The authors concluded that the majority of the flavors would impart less benzo(a)pyrene to meat than the conventional smoking process and thus would not present a health risk. No information is presented on the resinous or the oil-soluble content of these products.

BEVERAGES

Masuda et al.[205] discussed the contamination of whiskies with PAH. They point out that Scotch whisky is made from malted barley prepared by exposure of sprouted barley to smoke generated by burning peat, in contrast to American bourbon whisky aged in white oak barrels charred internally. Five brands of bourbon, eight brands of Scotch, and two brands of Japanese whisky were analyzed. The presence of phenanthrene, pyrene, or fluoranthene was detected in all of these products. Benz(a)anthracene and chrysene were detected in two kinds of whiskey, a Japanese and a Scotch, while benzo(a)pyrene, benzo(b)fluoranthene, and benzo(e)pyrene were found in one Scotch. Concentrations of these hydrocarbons were extremely low, ranging from 0.03 to 0.08 μg/ℓ.

Malanoski et al.[83] also analyzed samples of bourbon and Scotch; however, benzo(a)pyrene was not detected.

CONCLUSIONS

The results of the studies cited in this review emphasize the extent of the occurrence of trace quantities of polycyclic aromatic hydrocarbons (PAH) in our environment. These contaminants, some of which possess carcinogenic activity, have been shown to occur in water, air, food, and soil, as well as such diverse sources as tobacco smoke, automobile and engine exhausts, high boiling petroleum distillates, carbon black, coal tar, pitch, and rubber tires. Assessment of the potential health hazard has been of great concern in recent years, but has been hampered by the slow development of rapid and specific multicomponent procedures for determining PAH in complex food and environmental matrices.

During the last decade, significant progress has been made in the development of multi-residue procedures for the analysis of benzo(a)pyrene and other PAH in food at the low microgram per kilogram (parts per billion) levels. Some of these methods have been studied collaboratively and with various modifications have been shown to be applicable to the analysis of a wide variety of products. However, the multi-residue methods are lengthy, which tends to preclude their use as effective monitoring tools. Obviously, further efforts should be directed toward the simplification of these procedures. The basic extraction techniques have been developed and proven for a wide variety of foods; however, the intermediate cleanup and final separative procedure should be further assessed in light of recent advances. Many of the reports reviewed in this paper do not even contain data which would permit an assessment of the reliability (recovery and/or reproducibility) of the reported data. Although the values discussed are those reported, they must be judged in the light of their consistency with the remainder of the literature.

As evidenced in this review, much of the effort has been expended on the accumulation of data on the benzo(a)pyrene content of foods, which constitutes only between 1 and 20% of the total carcinogenic PAH in the environment.[3] Grimmer and Böhnke commented that most investigators have relied on methods that measure only benzo(a)pyrene content in food, although other PAH are also present in higher concentrations.[23] There is an obvious need for further research to develop a more complete picture of the PAH contamination in foods. In conducting such studies it is essential that we include those carcinogenic PAH which have been recently isolated and characterized in the environment. For example, cyclopenta(c,d)pyrene has been recently isolated from some furnace carbon blacks, soot, engine exhausts, and coal tar pitch.[206,207] In addition, in the analysis of environmental samples including foods, more emphasis needs to be placed on the use of confirmatory techniques. This applies not only to compounds tentatively identified as being present, based on retention times, but also to the characterization of other moieties (potential PAH), which are carried through the cleanup procedures and cast off or ignored as impurities or background interferences. As stated by Schechter, "Data reported without application of suitable confirmatory techniques may not only be worthless, but what is worse, incorrect information may be seriously misleading and may be unrectifiable." This statement, made in 1968 about pesticide residues,[208] applies even more appropriately to carcinogenic residues, which frequently are determined at levels of a few parts per billion or less.

Although the large body of information on PAH in smoked and grilled foods reported in prior reviews continues to be expanded, there appears to be an increasing interest in environmental and indigenous factors as sources of contamination. Various investigators have reported the presence of benzo(a)pyrene and other PAH in foodstuffs of plant origin. Since these foods are consumed in great quantity, these workers have suggested that such plants may in fact be the primary source of ingested PAH rather than smoked or heated products. At this time, three routes of PAH contamination have been considered: air deposition, absorption from soil and water, and biochemical synthesis. There appears to be at least general agreement that available data support the first two routes; however, there is considerable controversy concerning the synthesis route. Questions of false positives have also arisen with respect to these plant analyses. Obviously, a concerted effort is needed to provide reliable and conclusive data so that a proper assessment can be made with respect to the PAH contamination of food crops.

New potential sources of PAH contamination have been recognized as marine oil spills and discharges from refineries into estuarine waters. With the increase in the transport of foreign crude oils and off-shore drillings to meet consumption demands, a large portion of our ecosystem has been contaminated by petroleum products from oil spills, refineries, seepages, and other sources. The potential health hazard associated with the consumption of commercial species of shellfish (oysters, mussels, and clams) contaminated by petroleum products must be assessed for the presence of PAH compounds which are carcinogenic. At the present time, there is not sufficient information to come to any definitive conclusions as to whether or not a health hazard exists. Studies as to the fate of petroleum in the marine environment and the uptake and depuration of marine organisms are at present limited and controversial. Fish and lobsters have been shown to metabolize most petroleum hydrocarbons within 2 weeks, but metabolism in lower organisms is slower and the pathways are poorly understood. Some organisms such as mussels and oysters have been shown to eliminate most absorbed petroleum hydrocarbons when placed in clean water. The length of time required to depurate fully has been variable. NAS in 1975 reported that although their information was limited, the effect of soil contamination on human health appears not to be cause for alarm.[162] They do not recommend eating contaminated seafood but, in most cases, because of the taste factor, not many will be tempted to do so. The authors do not agree that an organoleptic yardstick should be used as the criterion for estimating low levels of potential carcinogenic polycyclic aromatic hydrocarbons. More research is needed on all aspects of the marine pollution problem before we can make reasonably accurate predictions, estimations, and recommendations concerning the dangers of oil pollution to commercially important shellfish industries and concerning the public health hazards arising from the consumption of petroleum-contaminated shellfish.

Even though great strides have been made in identifying potential health hazards, much still needs to be learned about the occurrence or accumulation of PAH in our total environment. Therefore, more research is needed to develop accurate data with respect to the many facets of our total environment, so that the overall public health hazard may be effectively evaluated and controlled.

REFERENCES

1. Tilgner, D. J., Carcinogens in foods, *Food Manuf.*, 43(6), 37—42, 1968.
2. Andelman, J. B. and Suess, M. J., PAH in the water environment, *Bull. W.H.O.*, 43, 479—508, 1970.
3. Suess, M. J., The environmental load and cycle of PAH, *Sci. Total Environ.*, 6, 239—250, 1976.
4. Haenni, E. O., Analytical control of PAH in food and food additives, *Residue Rev.*, 24, 42—78, 1968.
5. Tilgner, D. J. and Daun, H., PAH (polynuclears) in smoked foods, *Residue Rev.*, 27, 19—41, 1969.
6. Giger, W. and Blumer, M., PAH in the environment: isolation and characterization by chromatography, visible, ultraviolet, and mass spectrometry, *Anal. Chem.*, 46, 1663—1671, 1970.
7. Haenni, E. O. and Fischbach, H., Trace PAH analysis, the contribution of chemistry to food supplies, IUPAC, Butterworths, London, 1974, 209—225.
8. Tilgner, D. J., Food in a carcinogenic environment, *Food Manuf.*, 87, 47—50, 1970.
9. Gunther, F. A. and Buzzetti, F., Occurrence, isolation and identification of polynuclear hydrocarbons as residues, *Residue Rev.*, 9, 90—113, 1965.
10. Shadbad, L. M., Studies in the U.S.S.R. on the distribution, circulation, and fate of carcinogenic hydrocarbons in the human environment and the role of their disposition in tissues in carcinogenesis: a review, *Cancer Res.*, 27, 1132—1137, 1967.
11. Howard, J. W. and Fazio, T., A review of PAH in foods, *J. Agric. Food Chem.*, 17, 527—531, 1969.
12. Saito, T., Contents of polycyclic hydrocarbon in natural products, *Kagaku To Seibutsu*, 8(3), 178—185, 1970.
13. D'Arrigo, V., Idrocarburi policiclici aromatici nelle sostanze grasse, *Quad. Merceol.*, 10, 151—179, 1971.
14. Lo, M. T. and Sandi, E., Polycyclic aromatic hydrocarbons in foods, *Residue Rev.*, 69, 35—86, 1978.
15. Schaad, R., Chromatographie (Karzinogener) Polyzyklischer Aromatischer Kohlenwasserstoffe, *Chromatogr. Rev.*, 13, 61—82, 1970.
16. UICC (International Union Against Cancer) Tech. Rep. Series, Vol. 4, Lyons, France, 1970.
17. IARC Internal Tech. Rep. No. 71/002, Lyons, France, 1971.
18. Howard, J. W., Fazio, T., and White, R. H., Collaborative study of a method for benzo (a) pyrene in smoked foods, *J. Assoc. Off. Anal. Chem.*, 51, 544—548, 1968.

19. Fazio, T., White, R. H., and Howard, J. W., Collaborative study of the multicomponent method for PAH in foods, *J. Assoc. Off. Anal. Chem.*, 56, 68—70, 1973.
20. *Official Methods of Analysis*, 12th ed., AOAC, Arlington, Va., 1975, 385—388.
21. IUPAC Inform. Bull. Tech. Rep. No. 4, Geneva, Switzerland, 1972.
22. Recommended methods for PAH in food, *Pure Appl. Chem.*, 50, No. 11/12, 1978.
23. Grimmer, G. and Böhnke, H., PAH profile analysis of high protein foods, oils and fats by gas chromatography, *J. Assoc. Off. Anal. Chem.*, 58, 725—732, 1976.
24. Janini, G., Johnston, K., and Zielinski, W., Use of a nematic liquid crystal for gas-liquid chromatographic separation of polyaromatic hydrocarbons, *Anal. Chem.*, 47, 670—674, 1975.
25. Carugno, N. and Rossi, S., Evaluation of polynuclear hydrocarbons in cigarette smoke by glass capillary columns, *J. Gas Chromatogr.*, 5, 103—106, 1967.
26. Grob, K., High resolution gas chromatographic analysis of cigarette smoke, *Chem. Ind. (London)*, 248—252, 1973.
27. Grimmer, G., Hildebrandt, A., and Böhnke, H., Probenahme und Analytik Polyclischer Aromatischer Kohlenwasserstoffe in Kraftfahrzengabgasen, *Erdoel Kohle*, 25, 443—447, 531—536, 1972.
28. Grimmer, G. and Böhnke, H., Bestimmung des Gesamtgehaltes aller Polycylischen Aromatischen Kohlenwasserstoffe in Luftstaub und Kraftfahrzengabgas mit der Capillar-Gas-Chromatographie, *Z. Anal. Chem.*, 261, 310—314, 1972.
29. Cantuti, V., Cartoni, G., Liberti, A., and Torri, A. G., Improved evaluation of polynuclear hydrocarbons by gas chromatography, *J. Chromatogr.*, 17, 60—65, 1965.
30. DeMaio, L. and Corn, M., Gaschromatographic analysis of PAH with packed columns, *Anal. Chem.*, 38, 131—133, 1966.
31. Bhatia, K., Gas chromatographic determination of PAH, *Anal. Chem.*, 43, 609—610, 1971.
32. Frycha, J., Evaluation of the separation of phenanthrene, anthracene, and carbazole in pure tar products by gas-solid chromatography, *J. Chromatogr.*, 65, 341—344, 1972; Separation of polynuclear aromatic hydrocarbons by gas-solid chromatography on graphitized carbon black deposited on Chromosorb W, *J. Chromatogr.*, 65, 432—434, 1972.
33. Lane, D., Moe, H., and Katz, M., Analysis of polynuclear aromatic hydrocarbons, some heterocyclics and aliphatics with single gas chromatograph column, *Anal. Chem.*, 45, 1776—1778, 1973.
34. Zane, A., Separation of some polynuclear aromatic hydrocarbons by gas-solid chromatography on graphitized carbon black, *J. Chromatogr.*, 38, 130—133, 1968.
35. Gouw, T., Whittemore, I., and Jentoft, R., Versatile short capillary column in gas chromatography, *Anal. Chem.*, 42, 1394—1399, 1970.
36. Janini, G., Muschik, G., and Zielinski, W., N,N'-Bis(p-butoxybenzylidene)-α,α'-bi-p-toluidine: thermally stable liquid crystal for unique gas-liquid chromatographic separations of polycyclic aromatic hydrocarbons, *Anal. Chem.*, 48, 809—813, 1976.
37. Janini, G., Muschik, G., Schroer, J., and Zielinski, W., Gas-liquid chromatographic evaluation and gas chromatography/mass spectrometry application of new high temperature liquid crystal stationary phases for PAH separations, *Anal. Chem.*, 48, 1879—1883, 1976.
38. Burchill, P., Herod, A., and James, R., A comparison of some chromatographic methods for estimation of PAH in pollutants, *Carcinogenesis*, 3, 35—45, 1978.
39. Winkler, E., Buchele, A., and Muller, O., Method for the determination of PAH in maize by capillary column gas-liquid chromatography, *J. Chromatogr.*, 138, 151—164, 1977.
40. Krstulovic, A., Rosie, D., and Brown, P., Selective monitoring of PAH by high pressure liquid chromatography with a variable wavelength detector, *Anal. Chem.*, 48, 1383—1386, 1976.
41. Schmit, J., Henry, R., Williams, R. C., and Dieckmann, J. F., Applications of high speed reversed-phase liquid chromatography, *J. Chromatogr. Sci.*, 9, 645—651, 1971.
42. Vaughan, C., Wheals, B., and Whitehouse, M., Use of pressure-assisted liquid chromatography in the separation of polynuclear hydrocarbons, *J. Chromatogr.*, 78, 203—210, 1973.
43. Wheals, B., Vaughan, C., and Whitehouse, M., Use of chemically modified microparticulate silica and selective fluorimetric detection for the analyses of polynuclear hydrocarbons by high-pressure liquid chromatography, *J. Chromatogr.*, 106, 109—118, 1975.
44. Strubert, W., Separation of fused ring aromatics on silica gel, detection of nanogram or ppb amounts, *Chromatographia*, 6, 205—206, 1973.
45. Jentoft, R. and Gouw, T., Separation of PAH by high resolution liquid-liquid chromatography, *Anal. Chem.*, 408, 1787—1790, 1968.
46. Karger, B., Martin, M., Loheac, J., and Guiochon, G., Separation of polyaromatic hydrocarbons by liquid-solid chromatography using 2,4,7-trinitrofluorenone impregnated Corasil I columns, *Anal. Chem.*, 45, 496—500, 1973.
47. Vivilecchia, R., Thiebaud, M., and Frei, R., Separation of polynuclear azoheterocyclics by high-pressure liquid chromatography using silver-impregnated adsorbent, *J. Chromatogr. Sci.*, 10, 411—416, 1972.

48. Lochmuller, C. and Amoss, C. W., 3-(2,4,5,7-Tetranitrofluorenimino) propyl-diethoxysiloxane, highly selective, bonded π-complexing phase for high-pressure liquid chromatography, *J. Chromatogr.*, 108, 85—93, 1975.
49. Dong, M., Locke, D., and Ferrand, E., High pressure liquid chromatographic method for routine analysis of major parent PAH in suspended particulate matter, *Anal. Chem.*, 48, 368—371, 1976.
50. Hunt, D. C., Wild, P., and Crosby, N. T., Phthalimidopropylsilane — A new chemically bonded stationary phase for the determination of polynuclear aromatic hydrocarbons by high pressure liquid chromatography, *J. Chromatogr.*, 130, 320—323, 1977.
51. Ives, N. and Giuffrida, L., Liquid chromatography on PAH, *J. Assoc. Off. Anal. Chem.*, 55, 757—761, 1972.
52. Klimisch, H. J., Determination of PAH. Separation of benzpyrene isomers by high pressure liquid chromatography on cellulose acetate columns, *Anal. Chem.*, 45, 1900—1962, 1973.
53. Kirkland, J. J., High-performance liquid chromatography with porous silica microspheres, *J. Chromatogr. Sci.*, 10, 593—599, 1972.
54. Guerrero, H., Biehl, E., and Kenner, C., High pressure liquid chromatography of benzo(a)pyrene and benzo(g,h,i)perylene in oil-contaminated shellfish, *J. Assoc. Off. Anal. Chem.*, 59, 989—992, 1976.
55. Panalaks, T., Determination and identification of PAH in smoked and charcoal-broiled food products by high pressure liquid chromatography, *J. Environ. Sci. Health Bull.*, No. 4, 229—315, 1976.
56. Novotny, M., Lee, M., and Bartle, K., The methods for fractionation, analytical separation and identification of polynuclear aromatic hydrocarbons in complex mixtures, *J. Chromatogr. Sci.*, 12, 606—612, 1974.
57. Lee, M., Novotny, M., and Bartle, K., Gas chromatography/mass spectrometry and nuclear magnetic resonance determination of polynuclear aromatic hydrocarbons in airborne particulates, *Anal. Chem.*, 48, 1566—1572, 1976.
58. Bartle, K., Lee, M., and Novotny, M., High resolution GLC (gas-liquid chromatography) profiles of urban air pollutant polynuclear aromatic hydrocarbons, *Int. J. Environ. Anal. Chem.*, 3, 349—356, 1974.
59. Lee, M., Bartle, K., and Novotny, M., Profiles of the polynuclear aromatic fraction from engine oils obtained by capillary-column gas-liquid chromatography and nitrogen-selective detection, *Anal. Chem.*, 47, 540—543, 1975.
60. Lee, M., Novotny, M., and Bartle, K., Gas chromatography/mass spectrometric and nuclear magnetic resonance spectrometric studies of carcinogenic polynuclear aromatic hydrocarbons in tobacco and marijuana smoke condensates, *Anal. Chem.*, 48, 405—416, 1976.
61. Lao, R., Thomas, R., Cja, H., and Dubois, L., Application of gas chromatography-mass spectrometer-data processor combination to the analysis of the PAH content of airborne pollutants, *Anal. Chem.*, 46, 908—915, 1973.
62. Pancirov, R. and Brown, R., Polynuclear aromatic hydrocarbons in marine tissues, *Environ. Sci. Technol.*, 11, 989—992, 1977.
63. Tilgner, D. J., Smoke curing processes, *Fleischwirtschaft*, 10, 649—657, 1958.
64. Draudt, H. N., The meat smoking process: a review, *Food Technol.*, 17, 85—90, 1963.
65. Sikorski, Z. E. and Tilgner, D. J., Über Raucherrauchverfahren, I. Mitteilung jetziger Stand der chemischen Rauscherrauchanalyse, *Z. Lebensm. Unters.*, 124, 274—283, 1964.
66. Dobes, M. K., Hopp, J., and Sula, J., Examination of smoked food for the presence of benzo(a)pyrene, *Cesk. Onkol.*, 1, 254—266, 1954; thru *Chem. Abstr.*, 49, 4199, 1954—55.
67. Bailey, E. and Dungal, N., Polycyclic hydrocarbons in Icelandic smoked food, *Br. J. Cancer*, 12, 348—350, 1958.
68. Voitelovich, F., Dikun, P. P., and Shabad, L., Comparative study of malignant tumor frequency in Tookoom District of the Latvian SSR, *Vopr. Onkol.*, 3, 351—357, 1957.
69. Gorelova, N. D., Content of 3,4-benzo(a)pyrene in sprats cured with smoke from a friction smoke generator or smoke generator PSM vniro, *Vopr. Onkol.*, 9(8), 77—80; thru *Chem. Abstr.*, 59, 15862, 1963.
70. Gorelova, N. D. and Dikun, P. P., 3,4-Benzopyrene content of sausage and smoked fish prepared using fuel gas and coke, *Gig. Sanit.*, 30(7), 120—122; thru *Chem. Abstr.*, 63, 10574e, 1965.
71. Petrun, A. S. and Rubenchik, B. L., Possibility of carcinogenic 3,4-benzopyrene in electrostatically smoked fish, *Vrach. Delo*, 2, 93—95; thru *Chem. Abstr.*, 64, 20517h, 1966.
72. Mannelli, G., The presence of benzopyrene in smoked foods, *Ann. Fac. Econ. Commer.*, 4(2), 467—472, 1966.
73. Lijinsky, W. and Shubik, P., The detection of PAH in liquid smoke and some foods, *Toxicol. Appl. Pharmacol.*, 7, 337—343, 1965.
74. Howard, J. W., Teague, R., White, R., and Fry, B. E., Extraction and estimation of PAH in smoked foods. I. General method, *J. Assoc. Off. Anal. Chem.*, 49, 595—611, 1966.

75. Howard, J. W., White, R. H., Fry, B. E., and Turicchi, E., Extraction and estimation of PAH in smoked foods. II. Benzo(a)pyrene, *J. Assoc. Off. Anal. Chem.*, 49, 611—617, 1966.
76. Toth, L., PAH in smoked ham and belly fat, *Fleischwirtschaft*, 51, 1069—1070, 1971.
77. Dikun, P. P., Drasnitskaya, N. D., Shendrikova, I. A., Gretskaya, O. P., Emshanova, A. V., and Lapshin, I. I., 3,4-Benzopyrene levels in smoked fish subjected to drying with gas combustion products, *Vopr. Onkol.*, 15(3), 79—82, 1969.
78. Masuda, Y. and Kuratsune, M., PAH in smoked fish, "Katsuobushi", *Gann*, 62, 27—30, 1971.
79. Shirotori, T., Contents of 3,4-benzopyrene in common Japanese foods, *Tokyo Kasei Daigaku Kenkyu Kiyo*, 12, 47—53, 1972.
80. Toth, L. and Blaas, W., Effect of smoking technology on the content of carcinogenic hydrocarbons in smoked meat products, *Fleischwirtschaft*, 52, 1121—1123, 1972.
81. Wierzchowski, J. and Gajewska, R., Determination of 3,4-benzopyrene in smoked fish, *Bromatol. Chem. Toksykol.*, 5, 481—486, 1972.
82. Thorsteinsson, T., Polycyclic hydrocarbons in commercially and home-smoked food in Iceland, *Cancer*, 23, 455—457, 1969.
83. Malanoski, A. J., Greenfield, E. L., Barnes, C. J., Worthington, J. M., and Joe, F. L., Jr., Survey of PAH in smoked foods, *J. Assoc. Off. Anal. Chem.*, 51, 114—121, 1968.
84. Panalaks, T., Determination and identification of PAH in smoked and charcoal-broiled food products by high pressure liquid chromatography and gas chromatography, *J. Environ. Sci. Health Bull.*, No. 4, 299—315, 1976.
85. Rhene, K. and Bratzler, L., Benzo(a)pyrene in smoked meat products, *J. Food Sci.*, 35, 146—149, 1970.
86. Lucisano, A., DeBattistis, P., and Marzadori, F., Determination of 3,4-benzopyrene in smoked foodstuffs, *Vet. Ital.*, 24, 232—240, 1973.
87. Fretheim, K., Carcinogenic PAH in Norwegian smoked meat sausages, *J. Agric. Food Chem.*, 24, 976—979, 1976.
88. Swallow, W., Survey of PAH in selected foods and food additives available in New Zealand, *N.Z. J. Sci.*, 19, 407—413, 1976.
89. Doremire, M. E., Harmon, G. E., and Pratt, D. E., 3,4-Benzopyrene in charcoal grilled meats, *J. Food Sci.*, 62, 203—206, 1979.
90. Joe, F. L., Roseboro, E. L., and Fazio, T., Survey of some market basket commodities for polynuclear aromatic hydrocarbon content, *J. Assoc. Off. Anal. Chem.*, 62, 615—620, 1979.
91. Gorelova, N. K., Dikun, P. P., Solinke, V. A., and Emshanova, A. V., The 3,4-benzopyrene content of fish smoked by different processes, *Vopr. Onkol.*, 6(1), 33—37; thru *Chem. Abstr.*, 55, 4814h, 1960—61.
92. Dungal, N., The special problem of stomach cancer in Iceland, *J. Am. Med. Assoc.*, 178, 789—798, 1961.
93. Kraybill, H. F., A synopsis of information and data on PAH in the environment, including carcinogenicity assessment, unpublished report to the National Cancer Institute, 1973.
94. Genest, C. and Smith, D., A simple method for the detection of benzo(a)pyrene in smoked foods, *J. Assoc. Off. Agric. Chem.*, 57, 894—897.
95. Lijinsky, W. and Ross, A. E., Production of carcinogenic polynuclear hydrocarbons in the cooking of food, *Food Cosmet. Toxicol.*, 5, 343—351, 1967.
96. Jung, J. and Morand, P., Presence dans differentes huiles vegetales d'une substance donnant le spectre de fluorescence du benzo-3,4-pyrene, *Comptes Rendus*, 254, 1489—1491, 1962.
97. Jung, L. and Morand, P., Presence de pyrene, de benzo-1, 2-pyrene et benzo-3,4-pyrene dans differentes huiles vegetales, *Comptes Rendus*, 257, 1638—1640, 1963.
98. Jung, L. and Morand, P., Interpretation des spectres de fluorescence des huiles vegetales, *Ann. Fals. Exp. Chim.*, 57, 17—25, 1964.
99. Ciusa, W., Nebbia, G., Bruccelli, A., and Volpones, E., Identification of PAH present in olive oils, *Riv. Ital. Sostanze Grasse*, 42, 175—179; thru *Chem. Abstr.*, 63, 10184b, 1965.
100. Borneff, J. and Fabian, B., Kanzerogene Substanzen in Speisefett und -ol, *Arch. Hyg. Bakteriol.*, 150, 485—512, 1966.
101. Howard, J. W., Turicchi, E. W., White, R. H., and Fazio, T., Extraction and estimation of PAH in vegetable oils, *J. Assoc. Off. Anal. Chem.*, 49, 1236—1244, 1966.
102. Howard, J. W., Fazio, T., and White, R. H., PAH in solvents used in extraction of edible oils, *J. Agric. Food Chem.*, 16, 72—76, 1963.
103. Grimmer, G. and Hildebrandt, A., Content of polycyclic hydrocarbons in crude vegetable oils, *Chem. Ind.*, 2000—2002, 1967.
104. Biernoth, G. and Rost, H.E., The occurrence of PAH in coconut oil and their removal, *Chem. Ind.*, 2002—2003, 1967.
105. Fabian, B., Carcinogenic substances in edible fat and oil. IV. Investigations of margarine, vegetable fat and butter, *Arch. Hyg. (Berlin)*, 152, 231—237, 1968.

106. Fabian, B., Carcinogenic substances in edible fat and oil. V. Investigations on differently prepared fried sausages, *Arch. Hyg. (Berlin)*, 152, 251—254, 1968.
107. Fabian, B., Carcinogenic substances in edible fat and oil. VI. Further investigations on margarine and chocolate, *Arch. Hyg. (Berlin)*, 153, 21—24, 1969.
108. Fritz, W., 3,4-Benzopyrene and other polyaromatics in margarine and mayonnaise, *Nahrung*, 12, 495—496, 1968.
109. Franzke, C. and Fritz, W., Über das Vorkommen von 3,4-benzpyrene neben anderen polycyclischen aromatischen Kohlenwasserstoffen in Pflanzenfetten, *Fette Seifen Anstrichm.*, 71, 23—24, 1969.
110. Grigorenko, L. T., Dikun, P. P., Kalinina, I. A., Mironova, A. N., and Rzhehkin, V. P., 3,4-Benzopyrene level in sunflower and cottonseed oils, *Prikl. Biokhim. Mikrobiol.*, 6(2), 142—150, 1970.
111. Grigorenko, L. T., Dikun, P. P., Kalinina, I. A., and Mironova, A. N., Effect of industrial hydrogenation and alkaline neutralization of vegetable oils on the content in them of 3,4-benzopyrene, *Tr. Vses. Nauchno Issled. Inst. Zhirov*, 28, 243—247, 1971.
112. Swallow, W., Survey of PAH in selected foods and food additives available in New Zealand, *N.Z. J. Sci.*, 19, 407—412, 1976.
113. Guddal, E., Isolation of PAH from the roots of *Chrysanthemum vulgare*, Bernh. *Acta Chem. Scand.*, 13, 834—835, 1969.
114. Blumer, M., Benzopyrenes in soils, *Science*, 134, 474—475, 1961.
115. Borneff, J. and Fischer, R., Determination of PAH in the phytoplankton of a lake, *Arch. Hyg. Bakteriol.*, 146, 334—335; thru *Chem. Abstr.*, 58, 1179h, 1962—63.
116. Mallet, L., Pollution of soil and vegetation with 3,4-benzopyrene type hydrocarbons, *Congr. Expertise Chim.*, Vol. Spec. Conf. Commun. 4th, Athens, 301—307; thru *Chem. Abstr.*, 66, 84240b, 1964, 1967.
117. Doerr, R., Alkaloid and benzopyrene uptake by intact plant roots, *Naturwissenschaften*, 52(7), 166; thru *Chem. Abstr.*, 62, 16635a, 1965.
118. Graf, W. and Diehl, H., Über den naturbedingten normale kanzergener polyzyklischer Aromatic und seine Ursache, *Arch. Hyg. Bakteriol.*, 150, 249—259, 1966.
119. Borneff, J., Selenka, F., Kunte, H., and Maximos, A., Experimental studies on the formation of PAH in plants, *Environ. Res.*, 2, 22—29, 1968.
120. Borneff, J., Selenka, F., Kunte, H., and Maximos, A., The synthesis of benzo(a)pyrene and other PAH in plants, *Arch. Hyg.*, 152, 279—282, 1968.
121. Knorr, M. and Schenk, D., About the question of synthesis of polycyclic aromatics by bacteria, *Arch. Hyg.*, 152, 282—285, 1968.
122. Schmidt, F. and Fritz, W., Zur Genese des Magenkrebses. II. Die bedeutung kanzerogener Kohlenwasserstoffe in Nahrungsmitteln., *GBK Metteil.*, 5, 15—30, 1968.
123. Hancock, J. L., Applegate, H. G., and Dodd, J. D., Polynuclear aromatic hydrocarbons on leaves, *Atmos. Environ.*, 4, 363—370, 1970.
124. Grimmer, G. and Hildebrandt, A., Der Gehalt polycyklischer Kohlenwasenstoffe in verschiedenen Gemusesorten und Salaten, *Dtsch. Lebensm. Rundsch.*, 61, 237—239, 1965.
125. Grimmer, G. and Hildebrandt, A., Der Gehalt polycyklischer Kohlenwasenstoffe in Brotgetreide verschiedener Standorte, *Z. Krebsforsch.*, 67, 272—277, 1965.
126. Grimmer, G., Cancerogene Kohlenwasserstoffe in der Umgebung des Menschen, *Dtsch. Apoth. Ztg.*, 108, 529, 1968.
127. Gunther, F. A., Buzzetti, F., and Westlake, W., Residue behavior of polynuclear hydrocarbons on and in oranges, *Residue Rev.*, 17, 81—104, 1967.
128. Bolling, H., Carcinogenic substances in cereals dried with combustion gas, *Tec. Molitoria*, 15(24), 137; thru *Chem. Abstr.*, 62, 16878h, 1964.
129. Hutt, W., Meiering, A., Delschlagerr, W., and Winkler, E., Grain contamination in drying with direct heating, *Can. Agric. Eng.*, 20(2), 103—107, 1978.
130. Shabad, L. M., Cohan, Y., Ilnitsky, A., Khesina, A., Shcherbak, N., and Smirnov, G., The carcinogenic hydrocarbon benzo(a)pyrene in the soil, *J. Natl. Cancer Inst.*, 47, 1179—1191, 1971.
131. Shcherbak, N. P., Effect of oil products refinery ejections on soil and plant contamination, *Gig. Sanit.*, 7, 93—96, 1968.
132. Shcherbak, N. P., Fate of benzo(a)pyrene in soil, *Vopr. Onkol.*, 15(4), 75—79, 1969.
133. Shabad, L. M. and Cohan, Y. L., The contents of benzo(a)pyrene in some crops, *Arch. Geschwulstforsch.*, 40(3), 237—243, 1972.
134. Grimmer, G. and Duevel, D., Biosynthetic formation of polycyclic hydrocarbons in higher plants. VIII. Carcinogenic hydrocarbons in the human environment, *Z. Naturforsch.*, 25, 1171—1175, 1970.
135. Schamp, N. and Van Wassenhove, F., Determination of benzo(a)pyrene in bitumen and plants, *J. Chromatogr.*, 69, 421—425, 1972.
136. Wagner, K. H. and Siddigi, I., Storage of 3,4-benzofluoranthene in summer wheat and summer rye, *Z. Pflanzenernaehr. Bodenk.*, 130(3), 241—243, 1971.

137. **Hertel, W., Suchow, P., and Rohrlich, M.**, 3,4-Benzopyrene in grain and ground-grain products. I. Determinations of 3,4-benzopyrene in grain and grain products, *Getreide Mehl*, 20(9), 65—67, 1970.
138. **Kraybill, H. F.**, Distribution of chemical carcinogens in aquatic environments, *Prog. Exp. Tumor Res.*, 20, 3—34, 1976.
139. **Ilnitsky, A. P. and Varshavskaya, S. N.**, Water as a factor in spreading carcinogens in the environment, *Gig. Sanit.*, 29(9), 78—86, 1964.
140. **Borneff, J. and Fischer, F.**, Carcinogenic substances in water and soil. VIII., *Arch. Hyg.*, 146, 1—16, 1962.
141. **Borneff, J.**, Carcinogenic substances in water, *Muench. Med. Wochenschr.*, 105, 1237—1242, 1963.
142. **Borneff, J. and Kunte, H.**, Carcinogenic substances in water and soil. XIV., *Arch. Hyg.*, 147, 401—409, 1963.
143. **Borneff, J.**, Carcinogenic substances in water and soil, *Arch. Hyg.*, 148, 1—11, 1964.
144. **Borneff, J.**, Carcinogenic substances in water, soil and plants, *Landarzt*, 40, 109—112, 1964.
145. **Borneff, J. and Kunte, H.**, Carcinogenic substances in water and soil. XVII. About the origin and evaluation of PAH in water, *Arch. Hyg.*, 149, 226—243, 1965.
146. **Saccini-Cicatelli, M.**, Storage of BP in tubifex worms, *Boll. Pesca. Piscic. Idrobiol.*, 20, 245—250, 1965; thru *Chem. Abstr.*, 66, 1730n, 1967.
147. **Saccini-Cicatelli, M.**, Accumulation of BP in tubifex, *Boll. Soc. Ital. Biol. Sper.*, 42, 957—959; thru *Chem. Abstr.*, 66, 2680z, 1967.
148. **Mallet, L., Tendron, M., and Plessis, V.**, Investigations for (benzpyrene-type) carcinogenic hydrocarbons in the water and marine deposits of estuaries and their occurring biota, *Ann. Med. Leg.*, 40, 168—171, 1960.
149. **Mallet, L., Perdriau, A., and Perdriau, J.**, Pollution of benzopyrene type polycyclic hydrocarbons of the western region of the Arctic Ocean, *C. R. Acad. Sci. (Paris)*, 256, 3487—3489; thru *Chem. Abstr.*, 59, 1404h, 1963.
150. **Mallet, L. and Sardou, J.**, Investigation on the presence of the BP-type PH in the plankton environment of the region of the Bay of Villefranche, *C. R. Acad. Sci. (Paris)*, 258, 5264—5267; thru *Chem. Abstr.*, 61, 8666a, 1964.
151. **Mallet, L. and Lami, R.**, Investigation on pollution of plankton by benzpyrene-type polycyclic hydrocarbons in the Rance Estuary, *C. R. Soc. Biol. (Paris)*, 158, 2261—2262, 1964; thru *Chem. Abstr.*, 63, 2744a, 1965.
152. **Mallet, L.**, Investigation for benzpyrene-type polycyclic hydrocarbons in the fauna of marine environments (the Channel, Atlantic and Mediterranean), *C. R. Acad. Sci. (Paris)*, 253, 168—170, 1961; thru *Chem. Abstr.*, 56, 4539f, 1962.
153. **Mallet, L. and Schneider, C.**, Presence of benzpyrene-type polycyclic hydrocarbons in geological and archeological levels, *C. R. Acad. Sci. (Paris)*, 259, 675—677; thru *Chem. Abstr.*, 61, 14404f, 1964.
154. **Boucart, J. and Mallet, L.**, Marine pollution of the shores of the central region of the Tyrrhenian Sea (Bay of Naples) by benzpyrene-type polycyclic hydrocarbons, *C. R. Acad. Sci. (Paris)*, 260, 3729—3734, 1965; thru *Chem. Abstr.*, 62, 15901b, 1965.
155. **Mallet, L. and Priou, M.**, Retention of BP-type PH by the marine sediments, fauna and flora of the Bay of Saint Malo, *C. R. Acad. Sci. (Paris)*, 264, 969—971, 1967; thru *Chem. Abstr.*, 66, 108064a, 1967.
156. **Greffard, J. and Meury, J.**, Carcinogenic hydrocarbon pollution in Toulon Harbor, *Cah. Oceanogr.*, 19, 457—468, 1967; thru *Chem. Abstr.*, 68, 2369—2370, 1968.
157. **Shimkin, M., Koe, B. K., and Zechmeister, L.**, An instance of the occurrence of carcinogenic substances in certain barnacles, *Science*, 113, 650—651, 1951.
158. **Koe, B. and Zechmeister, L.**, The isolation of carcinogenic and other PAH from barnacles. Part II. The goose barnacle, *Arch. Biochem.*, 41, 396—403, 1952.
159. **Cahnmann, H. and Kuratsune, M.**, Determination of PAH in oysters collected in polluted water, *Anal. Chem.*, 29, 1312—1317, 1957.
160. **Zobell, C. E.**, Sources and biodegradation of carcinogenic hydrocarbons, Proceedings of Convention on Prevention and Control of Oil Spills, U.S. Coast Guard, American Petroleum Institute and the Environmental Protection Agency (American Petroleum Institute, Washington, D.C.), 1971.
161. **Zechmeister, L. and Koe, B.**, The isolation of carcinogenic and other PAH from barnacles, *Arch. Biochem.*, 35, 1—11, 1952.
162. **National Academy of Sciences**, Inputs, fate and effects of petroleum in the marine environment, A report of the Ocean Affairs Board, National Academy of Sciences, Washington, D.C., 1975.
163. **Ketchum, B. H.**, Oil in the marine environment, *Background papers for a Workshop on Inputs, Fates, and Effects of Petroleum in the Marine Environment*, Vol. II, National Academy of Sciences, Washington, D.C., 1973, 709—738.
164. **Blumer, M., Souza, G., and Sass, J.**, Hydrocarbon pollution of edible shellfish by an oil spill, *Mar. Biol.*, 5, 195—202, 1970.

165. **Ehrhardt, M.,** Petroleum hydrocarbons in oysters from Galveston Bay, *Environ. Pollut.,* 3, 257—271, 1972.
166. **Anderson, J. W.,** Uptake and depuration of specific hydrocarbons from oil by the bivalves, *Background papers for a Workshop on Inputs, Fates, and Effects of Petroleum in the Marine Environment,* Vol. II, National Academy of Sciences, Washington, D.C., 1973, 609—708.
167. **Lee, R. F., Sauerkeber, R., and Benson, A.,** Petroleum hydrocarbons; uptake and discharge by the marine mussel, *Mytilus edulis, Science,* 177, 344—346, 1972.
168. **Fazio, T.,** Unpublished data, Food and Drug Administration, Washington, D.C., 1971.
169. **Dunn, B. and Stick, H.,** Monitoring procedures for chemical carcinogens in coastal waters, *J. Fish. Res. Board Can.,* 33, 2040—2046, 1976.
170. **Dunn, B. and Stick, H.,** Release of the carcinogen benzo(a)pyrene from environmentally contaminated mussels, *Bull. Environ. Contam. Toxicol.,* 15, 398—401, 1976.
171. **Dunn, B. and Young, D.,** Baseline levels of benzo(a)pyrene in Southern California mussels, *Mar. Pollut. Biol.,* 7, 231—234, 1976.
172. **Brown, R. A. and Pancirov, R. J.,** Polynuclear aromatic hydrocarbons in Baltimore Canyon fish, *Environ. Sci. Technol.,* 13, 878—879, 1979.
173. **Kuratsune, M.,** Benzo(a)pyrene content of certain pyrogenic materials, *J. Natl. Cancer Inst.,* 16, 1485—1496, 1956.
174. **Kuratsune, M. and Hueper, W. C.,** PAH in coffee soots, *J. Natl. Cancer Inst.,* 20, 37—51, 1958.
175. **Kuratsune, M. and Hueper, W. C.,** PAH in roasted coffee, *J. Natl. Cancer Inst.,* 24, 463—469, 1960.
176. **Fritz, W.,** Zur Bildung cancerogener Kohlenwasserstoffe bei der thermischen Behandlung von Lebensmitteln. 2. Mitt das Rosten von Bohnenkaffee und Kaffee-Ersatzstoffen, *Nahrung,* 12, 799—804, 1968.
177. **Masuda, Y., Mori, K., and Kuratsune, M.,** PAH in common Japanese foods. I. Broiled fish, roasted barley, shoyu, and caramel, *Gann,* 57, 133—142, 1966.
178. **Davies, W. and Wilmshurst, J. R.,** Carcinogens formed in the heating of foodstuffs. Formation of 3,4-benzopyrene from starch at 370°-390°C, *Br. J. Cancer,* 14, 295—299, 1960.
179. **Masuda, Y., Mori, K., and Kuratsune, M.,** PAH formed by pyrolysis of carbohydrates, amino acids, and fatty acids, *Gann,* 58, 69—74, 1967.
180. **Halaby, G. A. and Fagerson, I. S.,** PAH in heat-treated foods; Pyrolysis of some lipids, beta-carotene, and cholesterol, *Proc. 3rd Int. Symp. Food Sci. Technol.,* 820—829, 1970.
181. **Seppilli, A. and Scasellati-Sforzolini, G.,** Sulla presenza di idrocarburi policiclici cancerigeni nelle carni cotte alla graticola, *Boll. Soc. Ital. Biol. Sper.,* 39, 110, 1963.
182. **Lijinsky, W. and Shubik, P.,** Polynuclear hydrocarbon carcinogens in cooked meat and smoked food, *Ind. Med. Surg.,* 34, 152—154, 1965.
183. **Lijinsky, W. and Ross, A. E.,** Production of carcinogenic polynuclear hydrocarbons in cooking of food, *Food Cosmet. Toxicol.,* 5, 343—347, 1967.
184. **Fritz, W.,** Contamination of foods with carcinogenic hydrocarbons during processing and cooking, *Arch. Geschwulstforsch.,* 40, 81—90, 1972.
185. **Fritz, W.,** Zur Bildung Cancerogener Kohlenwasserstoffe bei der thermischen Behandlung von Lebensmitteln. 2. Mitt das Rosten von Bohnenkaffee und Kaffee-Ersatzstoffen, *Nahrung,* 12, 799—804.
186. **Fritz, W.,** Zur Bildung Cancerogener Kohlenwasserstoffe bei der thermischen Behandlung von Lebensmitteln. 3. Mitt das Backen von Brot und Biskuits, *Nahrung,* 12, 805—808.
187. **Fritz, W.,** Zur Bildung Cancerogener Kohlenwasserstoffe bei der thermischen Behandlung von Lebensmitteln. 4. Mitt der Einflub des Frittiernes, *Nahrung,* 12, 809—811, 1968.
188. **Ballschmieter, H. M. B.,** Uber polycyclische aromatishe Kohlenwasserstoffe in gerosteten Erdnussen, *Fette Seifen Anstrichm.,* 71, 521—523, 1969.
189. **Fornal, J., Fornal, L., and Babuchowski, L.,** 3,4-Benzopyrene in dried cereals, *Przegl. Zbozowo Mlyn.,* 14(12), 445—447, 1970.
190. **Rohrlich, M. and Suckow, P.,** 3,4-Benzopyrene in grain and grain-meal products. II. Effect of drying, storage, and processing on the 3,4-benzopyrene content in grain and grain-meal production, *Getreide Mehl,* 20(12), 90—93, 1970.
191. **Thorsteinsson, T. and Thordarson, G.,** Polycyclic hydrocarbons in singed food in Iceland, *Cancer,* 21, 390—392, 1968.
192. **McGinnis, E. L. and Norris, M. S.,** Determination of four- and five-ring condensed hydrocarbons. I. Analysis of polynuclear aromatic hydrocarbons in yeast produced by growth on both *n*-hydrocarbon and dextrose feeds, *J. Agric. Food Chem.,* 23, 221—225, 1975.
193. **Takata, T.,** From normal paraffin to proteins, *Hydrocarbon Process,* 48(3), 99—103, 1969.
194. **Scrimshaw, N. S.,** Symposium on single-cell proteins for animal feeding, Brussels, Belgium, Protein-Calorie Advisory Group (PAG) of the United Nations System, Summary; PAG ad hoc Working Group, Single Cell Proteins, March 31, 1976.

195. McGinnis, E. L., Determination of four- and five-ring condensed hydrocarbons. II. Analysis of polynuclear aromatic compounds in n-paraffin feed oil for yeast fermentation, *J. Agric. Food Chem.*, 23, 226—229, 1975.
196. Truhaut, R. and Ferrando, R., The toxicological aspects of single cell proteins used in animal feeding, *Proc. Protein-Calorie Advisory Group (PAG) Symposium,* Brussels, Belgium, 1976, 38—48.
197. Santoro, A., Modica, R., Paglialunga, S., and Bartosek, I., *Toxicol. Lett.*, 3, 85—93, 1979.
198. Tilgner, D. J., Smoke condensate obtained from naturally occurring smoke, *Fleischwirtschaft*, 46, 501, 1966.
199. Hollenbeck, C. M., Aqueous smoke solution for use in foodstuffs and method for producing same, U.S. Patent 3,106,473 (Red Arrow Products Corp.), 1963.
200. Hollenbeck, C. M., Fresh, balanced smokiness for a wide range of food products, *Food Process.*, 25, 136—138, 1964.
201. White, R. H., Howard, J. W., and Barnes, C. J., Determination of PAH in liquid smoke flavors, *J. Agric. Food Chem.,* 19, 143—146, 1971.
202. Gorelova, N. K., Dikun, P. P., and Lapshin, I. I., Detection of 3,4-benzpyrene in liquids used for smoking foodstuffs processed with them, *Vopr. Onkol.,* 5, 341—345, 1969.
203. Prokofieva, O. G., The study of the carcinogenic activity of some liquids used in the smoking industry, *Vopr. Onkol.,* 8, 95—96, 1962.
204. Gorbatov, V., et al., Liquid smokes for use in cured meats, *Food Technol.,* 25, 71—77, 1971.
205. Masuda, Y., Mori, K., Hirohata, T., and Kuratsune, M., Carcinogenesis in the esophagus. III. PAH and phenols in whiskey, *Gann,* 57, 549—557, 1966.
206. Wallcave, L., Gas chromatographic analysis of PAH in soot samples, *Environ. Sci. Technol.,* 3, 948, 1969.
207. Gold, A., Carbon black adsorbates: separation and identification of a carcinogen and some oxygenated polyaromatics, *Anal. Chem.,* 47, 1469—1472, 1975.
208. Schechter, M. S., Editorial: The need for confirmation, *Pestic. Monit. J.,* 2, 1, 1968.

Toxic Plants

MUSHROOM POISONING

Kenneth F. Lampe

INTRODUCTION

In 1973, in the second volume of his *The Use of Fungi as Food and In Food Processing*, W. D. Gray, reflecting the surge of interest of that time, devoted nearly half of the text to poisonous and hallucinogenic mushrooms.[1] This interest has continued unabated, so that in less than half a decade the mechanism of action of hepatotoxicity of *Amanita phalloides* and the deliriant action of *Amanita muscaria* have become clarified, the toxin responsible for the alcohol-sensitizing activity of *Coprinus atramentarius* identified, the toxin producing the late-onset renal damage following the ingestion of certain species of *Cortinarius* characterized and synthesized, and the hallucinogenic toxins of certain species of *Gymnopilus* determined. During this period there were two major symposiums on toxic mushrooms in Europe,[2,3] and two book-length monographs and a summary review on this subject have appeared in the U.S.[4,5]

During this time, also, there has been an increasing concern for the health hazards to agricultural workers posed by commercial mushroom cultivation with numerous articles appearing on the syndrome of "mushroom worker's lung" as well as reports on the toxic fumes produced during processing of *Gyromitra esculenta*. An awareness has developed only recently of the potential possessed by some of the more desirable edible species to produce testicular damage in man (*Coprinus*) or carcinomas of the lung, liver, and intestine (*Gyromitra*).

The sudden demand for new mushroom tastes and a trend toward the ingestion of uncooked vegetables in the previously predominantly mycophobic North America is already beginning to result in puzzling intoxications for which there is no European counterpart. So undoubtedly this review, too, will require a major updating in a very few years.

DIAGNOSIS OF SYSTEMIC MUSHROOM POISONING BY SYMPTOMS

It is possible to divide virtually all systemic mushroom intoxications into two main groups depending on the duration of the latent period between the consumption of the mushroom and the appearance of symptoms. Those that produce signs of toxicity within 2 hr of ingestion, or immediately after the consumption of alcohol, are rarely considered to be of serious consequence, requiring only conservative, symptomatic management. Intoxications characterized by a later onset, usually six or more hours after ingestion, are associated with serious intoxications with a grave prognosis.

Each group may be further subdivided by its characteristic presenting symptoms.[7] In this rapid onset group this may be: mushrooms whose response is primarily gastroenteric irritation resulting in nausea, abdominal discomfort, diarrhea, and sometimes vomiting; mushrooms evoking sweating and other signs of parasympathetic hyperactivity; the psilocybin-containing species which produce delirium or hallucinations not associated with sleep or the deliriant mushrooms associated with sleep or coma (the pantherine syndrome); and mushrooms not producing any adverse effects unless alcohol also is consumed. In the delayed onset category are: *Gyromitra esculenta*, which produces headache, nausea, and fatigue about 6 to 8 hr after ingestion; the *Amanita phalloides* group which produce severe emesis and diarrhea approximately 12 hr after ingestion; and those producing a marked increase in fluid consumption and urination 3 or more days after ingestion, belonging to the *Cortinarius* group.

Naturally, all attempts should be made to obtain a specimen of the offending mushroom and to have it identified. Since it is not always possible to accomplish this rapidly, if at all, then the details concerning the preparation of the mushroom may provide additional aid in the differential diagnosis, and may even eliminate mushrooms as the etiology of an illness. Von Clarmann gives a useful checklist for the adult patient.[8] In an abbreviated and modified form, this includes the following: Was more than one kind of mushroom ingested? How were the mushrooms stored between collection and preparation and what was their condition at the time of preparation? Were the mushrooms eaten raw, sauteed, or prepared in boiling water as in a soup or stew? If prepared by simply boiling in water, was the cooking water discarded or ingested? At what time were the mushrooms eaten? Were they eaten again later and, if so, were they reheated? When and what was the first sign of illness? Are all persons who ate the mushrooms ill? Are persons in the group who ate none of the mushrooms ill? Was alcohol drunk with the meal or within a day following the meal?

SYSTEMIC MUSHROOM INTOXICATIONS WITH RAPID ONSET

Simple Gastroenteric Irritants

There are a number of recent books and papers listing those mushrooms found in North America whose principle adverse response is gastroenteritis,[1,4,9-17] but little is actually known of their chemistry or toxicology.[9] Toxicological observations and chemical studies reported for some of the more commonly encountered mushrooms in this category are shown in Table 1. There is a great deal of variation in response between subjects as well as to the geographic origin of the mushroom, and its mode of preparation. All produce varying degrees of abdominal discomfort within 3 hr of ingestion. Some may produce a persistent emesis and diarrhea which, particularly in younger children, may result in severe dehydration, electrolyte loss, and hypovolemic shock. The importance of fluid and electrolyte replacement in children must be emphasized. Mushrooms eaten by adults will almost invariably have been cooked, a process that markedly reduces or even inactivates some gastroenteric irritants. It has been suggested that many childhood fatalities following the ingestion of normally "nontoxic" mushrooms are secondary to uncompensated fluid and electrolyte losses resulting from profound emesis and diarrhea in response to gastroenteric irritants in the raw mushroom.[18] Otherwise, the management is entirely symptomatic as for gastritis of any other etiology.

Sweat-Inducing Mushrooms

Muscarine (Figure 1) and some of its physiologically active isomers are present in varying concentrations in a number of species of mushrooms, but usually only reach clinically significant levels in certain species of *Inocybe, Clitocybe,* and *Omphalotus*.[19,20] Although *Amanita muscaria* and *A. pantherina* contain muscarine, the concentrations are usually too low to produce clinically observable effects.

The toxic response is not affected by cooking. The symptoms of parasympathetic stimulation evoked by muscarine are usually evident within 15 to 30 min after ingestion. There appears to be a dose-response relationship as to the appearance of any particular effect, the most sensitive being profuse sweating. As the quantity of muscarine increases, one also may observe nausea, vomiting, and abdominal pain. More severe intoxications produce blurred vision, salivation, lacrimation, rhinorrhea, and diarrhea. Tremors, dizziness, and bradycardia are only rarely seen.

This is the only class of mushroom for which atropine is indicated. It should be given in sufficient dosage until symptoms are abolished or until dryness of the mouth is induced. The symptoms will abate, even without treatment, in 2 hr. Despite the discomfort, intoxications by muscarine-containing species should rarely cause concern.

Table 1
COMMONLY ENCOUNTERED GASTROENTERIC IRRITANT-CONTAINING MUSHROOMS

Group A: Mushrooms Most Commonly Encountered in Poisoning Incidents which may Result in Severe Intoxications

Chlorophyllum molybdites (Meyer ex Fr.) Mass. (*Lepiota morgani* Sacc.)
  Poisoning: 21—29
  Chemistry and toxicology: 30—32
  Identification in gastric washings: 33, 34
Entoloma lividum (Bull. ex St-Amans) Quél. (*Rhodophyllus lividus* Quél.
  R. sinuatus Sing.)
  Poisoning: 35—37
Tricholoma pardinum Quél.
  Poisoning: 35, 38
Omphalotus olearius (DC. ex Fr.) Sing. (*Clitocybe illudens* (Schw.) Sacc.,
  Pleurotus olearius (DC. ex Fr.) Gill.)
  Poisoning: 39—43
  Chemistry: 44
Paxillus involutus (Batsch ex Fr.) Fr.
  Poisoning: 45—47

Group B: Mushrooms Generally Encountered in Mild or Transient Intoxications

Agaricus arvensis Schaeff. ex Secr. var. *palustris* A. H. Smith and
  A. hondensis Murr.
  Poisoning: 48
Boletus pulcherrimus Thiers & Halling (*B. eastwoodiae* (Murr.) Sacc. & Trotter)
  Poisoning: 49
Boletus miniatoolivaceus Frost var. *sensibilis* Peck (*B. sensibilis* Peck)
  Poisoning: 50
Boletus luridus Schaeff. ex Fr.
  Poisoning: 4
Boletus satanas Lenz
  Poisoning: 51
Gomphus floccosus (Schw.) Sing.[a] (*Cantharellus floccosus* Schw.)
  Poisoning: 48
  Chemistry: 52—54
Gyromitra ambigua (Karst.) Harmaja
  Poisoning: 55 (as *G. infula* (Schaeff. ex Fr.) Quél.), 56
Hebeloma crustuliniforme (Bull. ex St-Amans) Quél.
  Poisoning: 57
Lactarius glaucescens Crossland
  Poisoning: 58
Lactarius torminosus (Schaeff. ex Fr.) S.F. Gray
  Poisoning: 40, 59
Pholiota aurea (Fr.) Kummer (*Togaria aurea* W. G. Smith; *Phaeolepiota aurea*
  Marie ex Konr. & Maubl.)
  Poisoning: 60, 61
Pholiota squarrosa (Müller ex Fr.) Kummer
  Poisoning: 62 (but considered edible by most)
Ramaria formosa (Fr.) Quél.
  Poisoning: 11, 40
Russula species
  Poisoning: 36 (see also 63)
Tricholoma irium (Fr.) Kummer (*Clitocybe irina* (Fr.) Bigelow & A. H. Smith
  Poisoning: 38
Verpa boehemica (Kromb.) Schroet.
  Poisoning: 60, 61, 64

Note: Numbers indicate references in which information on aspects of these mushrooms can be found.

[a] Intoxications may have a delayed onset (6 to 8 hr).

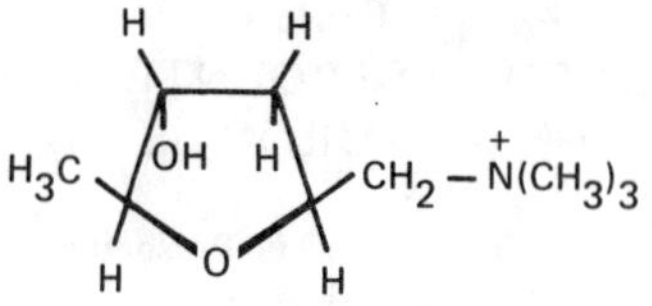

FIGURE 1. Muscarine.

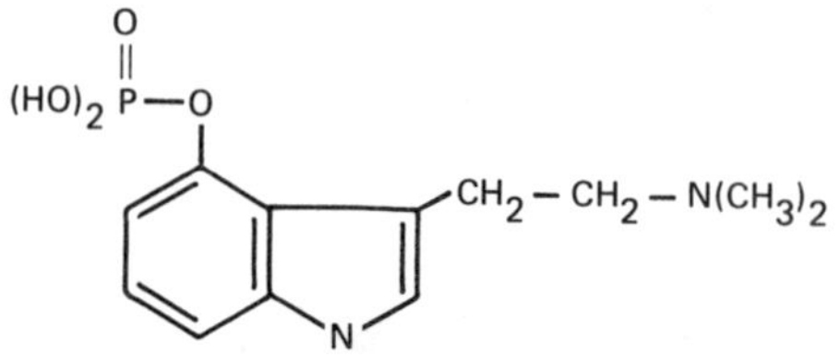

FIGURE 2. Psilocybin.

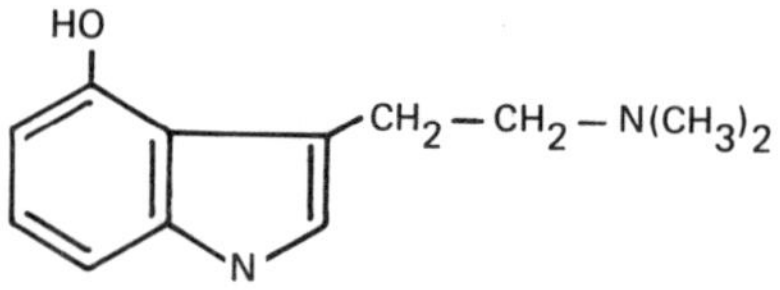

FIGURE 3. Psilocin.

Mushrooms Inducing Delirium or Hallucinations
Psilocybin-Containing Mushrooms

During 1953, Valentina and R. Gordon Wasson investigated reports that the Indians in Mexico employed hallucinogenic mushrooms to evoke divinatory revelations.[65-67] Most of these mushrooms were later identified by Heim[68,69] to be species of *Psilocybe*. The active hallucinogen from one of these mushrooms, *P. mexicana* Heim, was isolated by Hofmann et al.,[70] who also determined its chemical structure and prepared it synthetically.[71,72] It was named psilocybin (Figure 2). A related substance, which is usually also present but only in lesser concentration, was named psilocin (Figure 3). These compounds were later shown to be present in other hallucinogenic species of the genera *Psilocybe, Panaeolus, Copelandia, Gymnopilus, Conocybe*,[19] and *Pluteus*.[210]

The clinical response to these mushrooms does not differ from that using psilocybin; however, the psychological component is determined by dose, prior experience with psychoactive substances, and the mood and personality of the subject. Intoxication by these mushrooms is almost always deliberate. The temporal sequence of onset of different clinical effects[73,74] and the frequency of occurrence of various effects[75] have been determined using psilocybin in experimental volunteers. Most subjects reported dizziness or unsteadiness, weakness, drowsiness, altered temperature sensation, difficulty in focusing, and changes in mood. With higher dosage, objects appeared altered in shape or color, there were changes in hearing acuity, paresthesias in the extremities, depersonalization, a dreamlike state, and visual hallucinations. The overall duration of effect was usually 2 to 4 hr.

Although psilocin is sensitive to oxidation, psilocybin is relatively stable, so considerable activity is retained in dried mushrooms. The active component may be extracted by boiling water. The hallucinatory oral dose in the nontolerant adult is 6 to 12 mg.

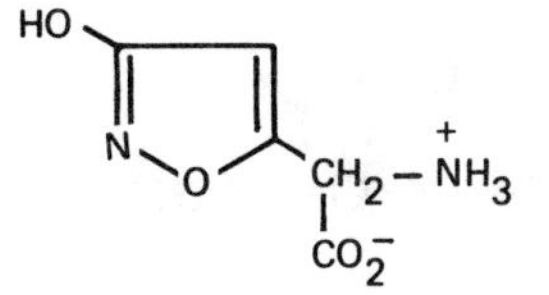

FIGURE 4. Ibotenic acid.

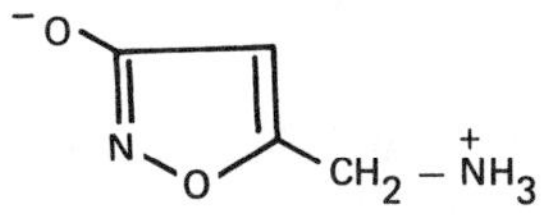

FIGURE 5. Muscimol.

Generally this dosage requires the consumption of a large number of mushrooms, depending upon species, growing conditions, and geographic origin.[13,76-78] The accidental poisoning of small children is therefore unlikely unless substantial quantities of the mushrooms have been inappropriately gathered and cooked for food. There have been a few reports[79,80] of mydriasis, hyperthermia, loss of conciousness, convulsions, and death in small children. Therapeutic intervention is rarely sought or required for adults. The clinical effects may be terminated, however, by the administration of diazepam or a phenothiazine.

Deliriant Mushrooms Associated with Sleep or Coma (The Pantherine Syndrome)

Intoxications of this type are related almost entirely to *Amanita pantherina* (DC. ex Fr.) Secr. and *A. muscaria* (L. ex Fr.) Hooker. Numerous reports of such poisonings following the consumption of these mushrooms for food are in the older literature. More recently, intoxications have become associated with the deliberate ingestion of these mushrooms, particularly *A. muscaria*, for its deliriant action. Despite its species name, *A. muscaria* usually contains only traces of muscarine, but an occasional strain may induce sweating and other evidences of parasympathetic activity. The principle toxins of these species, ibotenic acid (Figure 4) and muscimol (Figure 5) were elucidated independently by Boden et al.,[81,82] Takemoto et al.,[83,84] and by Müller and Eugster.[85] Both compounds have been examined singly as pure substances in man.[86-90] Cooking does not affect activity markedly, but the dried mushroom gradually loses activity.

Pharmacologically, muscimol acts as a GABA receptor agonist.[91-96] It is presumed that ibotenic acid is decarboxylated in vivo to muscimol, which is the active form. Symptoms usually appear within 20 to 90 min after ingestion. Mild intoxications are characterized by drowsiness and an inconsistently appearing gastroenteritis. After about 1 hr, there is drowsiness and dizziness which may be associated with sleep. This may be followed by elation, increased motor activity, tremors, visual illusions, delusions, and even delirium. This pattern may alternate with periods of drowsiness or sleep. A complex neurological picture may be observed in severely poisoned children,[97] which may progress to coma and convulsions.

Poisoning in adults is rarely severe. In children, however, the intoxication may persist for 6 to 9 hr and airway management and anticonvulsive medication may be required. Except in those rare cases exhibiting marked parasympathetic hyperactivity, atropine should not be administered. Despite suggestions in the literature, physostigmine is ineffective for terminating the deliriant action. In most instances, no therapeutic intervention other than protective care should be tendered.

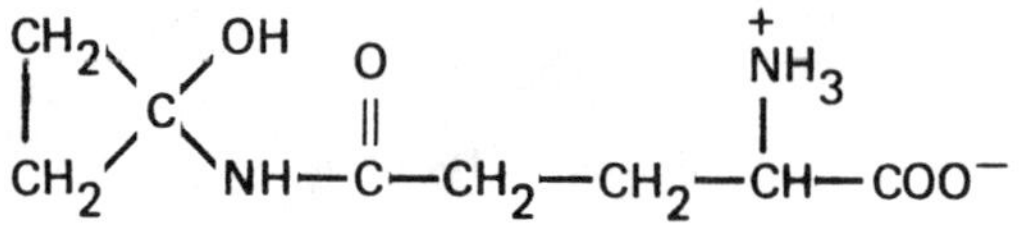

$$\begin{array}{c}CH_2\\ |\\ CH_2\end{array}\!\!\!>\!\!C\!\!<\!\!\begin{array}{c}OH\\ \\ NH\end{array}\!\!-\!\!\overset{\overset{\displaystyle O}{\|}}{C}\!-CH_2-CH_2-\overset{\overset{\displaystyle \overset{+}{N}H_3}{|}}{CH}-COO^-$$

FIGURE 6. Coprine.

Mushrooms Inducing Sensitivity to Alcohol

Various mushrooms are capable of inducing a marked sensitivity to alcohol. This effect is encountered most commonly with *Coprinus atramentarius* Fr., which is a particularly desirable edible mushroom. However, if alcohol is consumed up to approximately 72 hr after the ingestion of ths species, the individual may experience flushing, hypotension, tachycardia and palpitations, paresthesias, severe nausea and vomiting, and an intense headache. This mushroom contains the prototoxin coprine (Figure 6), the structure of which was determined independently by Lindberg et al.[98] and by Hatfield and Schaumberg.[99] The coprine content of fresh *C. atramentarius* (European) is about 160 mg/kg.[98] This substance is converted in the body[100] into 1-aminocyclopropanol and thence to the active toxin, cyclopropanone hydrate (Figure 7).[101]

The pharmacological actions of coprine have been investigated only in animals.[100-103] The active metabolite, cyclopropanone hydrate, reversibly inhibits the low K_m acetaldehyde dehydrogenase of the liver. This results in the accumulation of acetaldehyde in the blood during alcohol metabolism. It is the elevated acetaldehyde level which is responsible for the clinically observable response. The pharmacokinetics of the coprine response has not been studied in man. In rats, the sensitizing effect becomes maximal about 4 hr after administration of coprine and declines to negligible activity in 144 hr.[103] Coprine differs from disulfiram, the acetaldehyde dehydrogenase inhibitor used therapeutically in chronic alcoholism, in that coprine does not affect dopamine-β-decarboxylase,[103] so the cardiovascular response to these substances differs in respect to the change of heart rate following alcohol consumption. Coprine is a more potent sensitizer than disulfiram.

The manifestations of acetaldehyde accumulation following alcohol consumption in the sensitized individual persists for about 2 to 3 hr. Therapeutic intervention usually is not required.

Following the subacute oral administration of coprine to male rats (200 mg/kg/day, 14 days) and dogs (25 and 75 mg/kg/day, 28 days), severe changes can be found in the germ cells with accompanying degenerative changes in the testes and epididymides.[104] This is apparently a direct effect which does not involve the Leydig or Sertoli cells. These results suggest a potential risk of human testicular damage from the consumption of relatively large quantities of *Coprinus atramentarius* during its fruiting season.

Coprine also has been isolated from *C. quadrifidus* Peck, *C. variegatus* Peck, and *C. insignis* Peck.[102] Other mushrooms reported by Benedict[9] to produce a similar alcohol-sensitizing activity include *Clitocybe clavipes* (Fr.) Kumer,[105] *Boletus luridus* Schaeff. ex Fr., and *Verpa bohemica* (Krombh.) Schroet. None of these were found to contain coprine,[102] so their activity in this regard requires further investigation.

SYSTEMIC MUSHROOM INTOXICATIONS WITH DELAYED ONSET

Gyromitra esculenta

In 1883, Bostroem compiled 151 cases of human poisoning from the European literature attributed to this mushroom which included 59 fatalities.[106] Franke et al.[107] extended this survey up to 1965. Intoxications resulting from the ingestion of this species are seen most frequently in eastern Europe and only occasionally elsewhere.

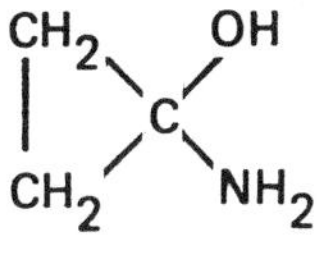

FIGURE 7. 1-Aminocyclopropanol and cyclopropanone hydrate. Figure 8. Gyromitrin. Figure 9. Monomethylhydrazine.

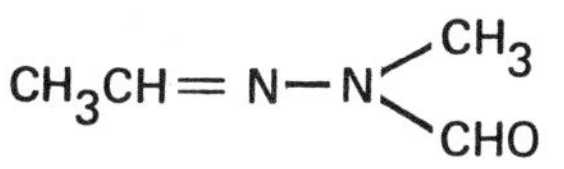

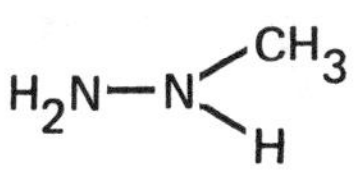

Gyromitra esculenta (Pers. ex Fr.) Fr. contains a number of hydrazones, the first of which was characterized by List and Luft.[108,109] This prototoxin, named gyromitrin (Figure 8), is the *N*-methyl-*N*-formyl hydrazone of acetaldehyde. Additional homologs, in which the acetaldehyde is replaced by other aldehydes, now also are known to be present. These include the derivatives of pentanal, 3-methylbutanal, and hexanal.[110,111] All of these compounds readily hydrolyze to form the active toxin, monomethylhydrazine (Figure 9).

Intoxications are characterized by a sudden onset of symptoms usually appearing about 6 to 8 hr after ingestion. The initial clinical signs are a feeling of fatigue, severe headache, sometimes dizziness, and a feeling of fullness of actual abdominal discomfort. This is often accompanied by persistent vomiting. In most cases, the intoxication will become no more severe, the patient recovering completely in 2 to 6 days. In more serious cases, acute and sometimes fatal hepatitis may develop.

Since hydrazine interferes with the action of pyridoxine, the daily intravenous administration of this vitamin should be instituted. The clinical features and management of *Gyromitra esculenta* poisoning does not differ, in this respect, from that for the management of the acute overdosage of the antitubercular agent isoniazid. In children, the early gastroenteric phase of the intoxication may require fluid and electrolyte replacement.

Gyromitrin and the other hydrazones present, as well as monomethylhydrazine itself, all are removed readily from the mushroom by boiling water. Thus, it has been recommended that the mushroom be boiled in water and the cooking water discarded. This treatment removes 99.5% of the toxins within 10 min.[112] Monomethylhydrazine is volatile with steam. There is a clinical report of a cook seized with headache and vomiting following inhalation of vapors from cooking mushrooms.[113] This volatility of the toxin is of considerable significance for employee health during the preparation and drying of these mushrooms for commerce.[114] Neither air-dried or canned preparations of *G. esculenta*, mostly originating from Poland and Russia, have ever been reported to cause illness.[37] The content of gyromitrin in dried mushrooms is about 3 mg/kg[115] compared to 1.2 to 1.6 g/kg in fresh specimens.[112,116] The quantities of the other hydrazones remaining after drying or boiling have been determined also.[117]

It has been shown that monomethylhydrazine, when administered chronically in the drinking water, significantly increases the incidence of lung tumors in mice[118] and malignant histiocytomas of the liver and tumors of the cecum in the hamster.[119] A similar experiment in mice[120] and hamsters[121] employing gyromitrin resulted in benign hepatomas, liver cell carcinomas, adenomas of the gall bladder, cholangiomas, and cholangiocarcinomas. It has been suggested that the hepatocarcinogenicity of the *N*-methyl-*N*-formylhydrazine formed from hydrolysis of gyromitrin can be ascribed to its cytochrome P-450 mediated oxidation, through a hydroxylamine intermediate, to a nitrosamide carcinogen.[122] Probably *G. esculenta* should no longer be classified as an edible species because of the potential carcinogenicity to man from the residues of hydrazones and monomethylhydrazine which may be retained in the mushroom even after appropriate preparation to prevent acute systemic toxicity.

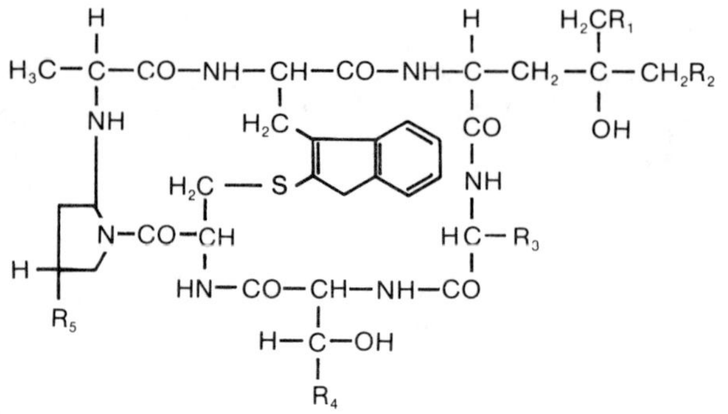

```
                    H              H    H₂CR₁
                    |              |    |
          H₃C—C—CO—NH—CH—CO—NH—C—CH₂—C—CH₂R₂
              |        |           |    |
              NH       H₂C         CO   OH
                        \          |
                    H₂C—S          NH
                     \  /          |
                      \/           HC—R₃
                  N—CO—CH          |
              H  /        HN—CO—CH—NH—CO
               \/             |
               R₅             H—C—OH
                              |
                              R₄
```

	R₁	R₂	R₃	R₄	R₅
Phalloidin	•OH	•H	•CH₃	•CH₃	•OH
Phalloin	•H	•H	•CH₃	•CH₃	•OH
Phallisin	•OH	•OH	•CH₃	•CH₃	•OH
Phallacidin	•OH	•H	•CH(CH₃)₂	•COOH	•OH
Phallacin	•H	•H	•CH(CH₃)₂	•COOH	•OH
Phallisacin	•OH	•OH	•CH(CH₃)₂	•COOH	•OH

FIGURE 10. Phallotoxins.

The *Amanita phalloides* Group

Excluding eastern Europe, nearly all fatal mushroom intoxications are due to certain species of *Amanita*. These include *A. phalloides* (Fr.) Secr., *A. verna* (Bull. ex Fr.) Vitt., *A. virosa* Secr., *A. bisporigera* Atk., and *A. ocreata* Peck. The *Amanita* toxins are also found in significant concentration in *Galerina autumnalis* (Pk.) A.H. Sm. and Sing., *G. marginata* (Batsch. ex Secr.) Kühner, and *G. venenata* A.H. Smith. There is chromatographic evidence but no quantitative data for the occurrence of these toxins in *Lepiota helveola* Bres., *L. brunneoincarnata* Chodat and Martin, *L. subincarnata* Lg.,[123] and in *Conocybe filaris* Fr.[124]

There are two classes of orally active toxins in the *A. phalloides* group, both of which are thermostable, cyclic polypeptides. One of these, the phallotoxins, are cyclic heptapeptides (Figure 10). Although of considerable biochemical interest, they have too low a mammalian toxicity to be considered of clinical significance and thus will not be described since they have been reviewed recently elsewhere.[5,6] *A. virosa* also contains monocyclic peptides which are toxicologically equivalent to the phallotoxins. The amatoxins, which are responsible for all of the observable clinical actions, are cyclic octapeptides (Figure 11). Except in *A. phalloides*, some or all of the phallotoxins of amatoxins may be absent in a particular collection of one of the other species. Amaninamide has been found only in *A. virosa*.[125] The relative abundance of these toxins has been determined for European specimens of *A. phalloides*, *A. verna*, *A. virosa*, and *G. marginata*[126-129] and for American specimens of *Amanita*[130,211] and *G. autumnalis*.[131]

A number of procedures for clinical application have been developed for the rapid chemical identification of amatoxin-containing mushrooms or for the detection of amatoxins in body fluids. These include a spot test applicable to fresh or dry mushrooms,[132] separation of the amatoxins in mushroom samples by thin-layer chromatography followed by spectrophotometric verification of the toxin,[133] examination of mushroom spores in gastric aspirate,[134] radioimmunoassay of serum, urine, or gastric aspirate;[135] and RNA-polymerase competition binding assay of these biological fluids.[136]

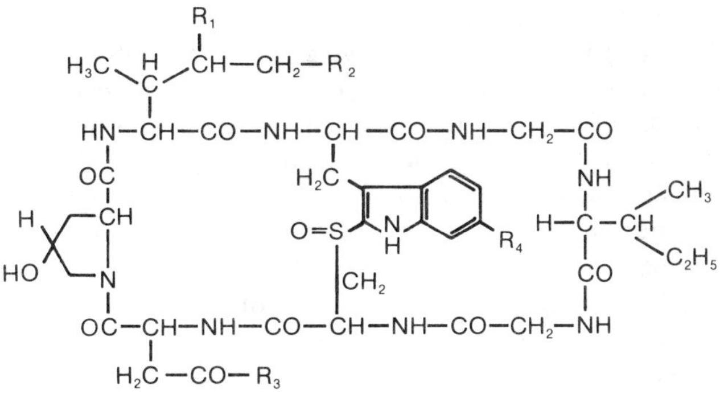

[Chemical structure diagram of amatoxins]

	R₁	R₂	R₃	R₄
α - Amanitin	•OH	•OH	•NH$_2$	•OH
β - Amanitin	•OH	•OH	•OH	•OH
γ - Amanitin	•CH	•H	•NH$_2$	•OH
ε - Amanitin	•OH	•H	•OH	•OH
Amanin	•OH	•OH	•OH	•H
Amanullin	•H	•H	•NH$_2$	•OH
Amaninamide	•OH	•OH	•NH$_2$	•H

FIGURE 11. Amatoxins.

Poisonings produced by mushrooms of the *A. phalloides* group are characterized by a prolonged latent period, usually about 12 hr, between the ingestion of the mushroom and the first appearance of symptoms. Initially there is nausea and a painful colic accompanied by persistent vomiting and a profuse, watery diarrhea. Over the subsequent few hours this gradually resolves and the patient enters a symptom-free period. This interphase is of unpredictable duration but has been as much as 3 to 5 days. This is succeeded by a serious, sometimes fatal, hepatitis. Rarely, this may be associated with renal failure.

Examination of the liver and kidney cells shows vesicular-like damage to the cell nucleus. The disruption of the nucleus appears quite rapidly and can be demonstrated within 1 to 2 hr after the administration of amatoxins to an experimental animal.[137] It was shown that amatoxins acted by binding to and inhibiting RNA polymerase II, preventing the elongation of messenger RNA, thereby disrupting the continuous synthesis of protein required for maintenance of the cell. The early studies have been reviewed recently.[138-140] Although the underlying biochemical deficit is well established, considerable investigation still is required to complete our understanding of the alterations in structure and molecular composition of the amatoxin-poisoned liver cell nucleus.[141-144]

During the initial phase of poisoning from mushrooms of this group, appropriate attention is mandatory for the replacement of fluid and electrolyte loss secondary to the profuse diarrhea and persistent vomiting. An adequate urine flow during the first phase of the intoxication also may enhance the elimination of the amatoxins.[145] If the patient can tolerate the oral administration of activated charcoal in water, this should be given at intervals to reduce the enterohepatic cycling of the amatoxins.

The principal manifestation will be the rapid development of a severe hepatic insufficiency. An increase of serum transaminase levels is the most useful indicator of the extent of liver damage and should be used to monitor the severity and progress of the intoxication. Other blood chemistries (alkaline phosphotase, LDH, bilirubin, glucose, BUN, creatinine), clotting factors, body weight, and mental status examination (tests for constructional apraxia) should be made daily. The values of lactic dehydrogenase will be increased significantly with a marked elevation in isoenzyme fractions 4 and 5.[146] After a transient increase in blood glucose, hypoglycemia becomes marked as stored glycogen is exhausted. All clotting factors of hepatic origin fall simultaneously. A return toward normal of fibrinogen and Factor V is the first sign of recovery and always indicates survival.[147] Jaundice may appear, but it is not a consistent finding. Neurologic and mental changes reflect the degree of hepatic encephalopathy.

Unsupported patients have a mortality rate greater than 50%, with an annual worldwide total of several hundred.[148] In contrast, early and vigorous supportive therapy can reduce this to less than 5%.[149]

Treatment is entirely supportive and does not differ from that for acute viral hepatitis and fulminant hepatic coma. If the management has been successful, the patient improves rapidly after about a week. Examination of survivors shows complete recovery of liver function. If kidney function was disturbed, its recovery tends to be much more prolonged with a persistent histological deficit.

Because of the high morbidity of *Amanita phalloides* group intoxications, many drugs and procedures have been introduced to supplement the basic management. These have included high-dosage vitamin therapy, maintenance of elevated blood glucose levels, various lipotropic factors, adrenocortical steroids, blood exchange transfusions, dialysis, and sex hormones.[138] Two of these of current, if controversial interest, are thioctic acid (α-lipoic acid) and high-dosage penicillin G therapy.

Thioctic acid had been of some interest in the late 1950s as an ancillary agent to be used in liver necrosis due to exogenous toxins. In 1963, Kubička credited the drug with benefiting a series of some 40 *A. phalloides*-poisoned patients in his care.[150] He outlined his management of the patient as follows.[151] The patient is lavaged and given an enema. Fluid and electrolytes are replaced. The SGOT and SGPT and serum bilirubin are determined twice daily and used as an index for thioctic acid therapy. From the beginning of the intoxication, the patient is given 75 mg/day of thioctic acid as a continuous infusion. If the transaminases show an increase, the dosage is immediately elevated to 300 mg/day and continued at this level until the SGOT and SGPT start to decrease. If coma intervenes, the dosage is further elevated to 500 mg/day. During this period the patient also receives glucose, thiamine, and ascorbic acid.

This therapy received considerable early support in Europe, but its use there, outside of Italy and central Europe, has begun to decline. In the U.S., on the other hand, it is becoming popular.[3,4,146] Unfortunately, there is little experimental work in control animals to verify its value. Hopefully, this will be conducted in the near future. Recently, Kubička and his co-workers have cautioned that thioctic acid should not be considered as an amatoxin antidote, but rather that it is a vitamin-like agent that makes it possible for the liver cell to survive, by catalysis of the Krebs cycle and the respiratory enzymes within the cell for the critical period of 5 to 10 days until regeneration of the mitochondria can take place.[152,153]

Floersheim investigated a number of compounds, including penicillin G, for their ability to reduce mortality in *A. phalloides*-poisoned animals.[154-157] It was postulated that the effective drugs, such as penicillin, acted by displacing the amatoxins that were bound to serum albumin, thus permitting their free excretion by the kidney. It has been shown subsequently that the amatoxins do not bind to this serum protein,[158] so the beneficial action of penicillin, if any, cannot be ascribed to that mechanism. Its use as an adjunct in *A. phalloides* poisonings is currently popular in Europe;[159-161] the usual procedure being to give 250 mg/kg/day penicillin G by continuous infusion for 3 to 10 days. It is hoped, too, that the value of this procedure will be given critical experimental evaluation in the near future.

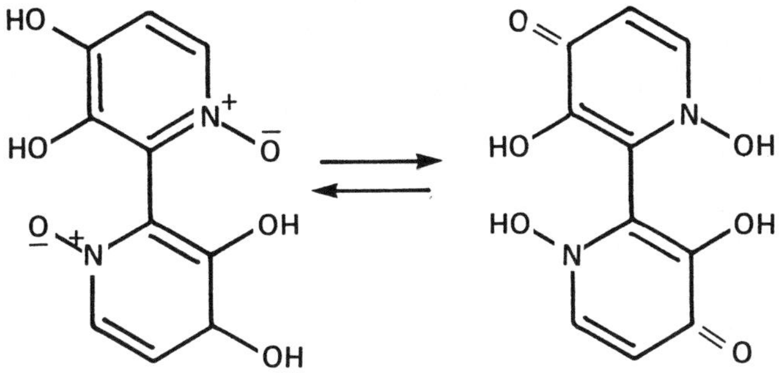

FIGURE 12. Orellanine.

The *Cortinarius* Group

A few species of the large genus *Cortinarius* have the remarkable effect of producing kidney failure some 3 to 17 days after the mushroom ingestion.[162] These unusual intoxications were first described for *Cortinarius orellanus* Fr. in Poland,[163] and more recently for that species in Germany,[164] France,[165,166] Czechoslovakia,[167,168] and Switzerland.[169] Similar intoxications have been seen with *C. speciosissimus* Kühn and Romagnesi in Finland[170-172] and England,[173] and with *C. gentilis* Fr. in Finland.[174]

Toxicity is not affected by cooking or drying of these mushrooms. A structure for the toxin, orellanine (Figure 12), has been proposed[175] but has been challenged.[213] The mechanics of the renal injury are unknown.

The first observable effect is a marked increase in liquid intake, during which the patient may drink several liters a day. This is followed by nausea, emesis, constipation, headaches, muscular pains, and chills. Initially there is a corresponding increase in urinary output, but this is followed by renal failure which is ultimately responsible for the death of the patient. Postmortem examination shows renal tubular necrosis, fatty degeneration of the liver, and intestinal inflammation. Nonfatal poisonings are characterized by a prolonged course of recovery requiring several months. Treatment is entirely symptomatic.

UNCLASSIFIED TOXIC MUSHROOMS

There are a great number of mushrooms which can only be listed as "suspected" because there are insufficient clinical case reports to have attracted the attention of investigators. Indeed, a major factor is inadequate reporting of intoxications. In some instances it may have been impossible to obtain a specimen of the offending mushroom for identification. There is also the problem of the great variability in toxicity, so that a species growing in one part of a country may produce sickness, whereas in another section of the same country may be eaten with relish. Part of this is due to variability in growing conditions. It may well be that there are various chemical strains of mushrooms which cannot be differentiated on the basis of gross or microscopic examination. It is also suspected that certain mushrooms are capable of forming hybrids, as for example, the presumably harmless *Amanita gemmata* (Fr.) Gill. with toxic *A. pantherina* (DC. ex Fr.) Secr.[176]

Hypholoma fasciculare (Huds. ex Fr.) Karst. (*Naematoloma fasciculare* Karst.), for example, seems to be edible, although not particularly desirable, in some locations and dangerously toxic elsewhere. Reported cases up to 1963 have been reviewed by Wasiljkow.[177] In a typical case,[178,179] there is an intermediate latent period of 5 to 6 hr after ingestion until the onset of vomiting and diarrhea. Albuminuria is present. The symptoms gradually abate over a few days. In a fatal case,[180] the onset was similar, but this was followed by a symptom-free period, followed in turn by a fulminant hepatitis. Other than some brief work reported by Nishihara et al.,[181] no systematic attempt has been made to isolate or identify the toxin.

Quite a number of similarly intriguing areas of potential research interest could be cited. A sample of the diversity these afford are: *Scleroderma aurantium* Pers., which has been reported to cause tetany and paresthesias;[182] *Stropharia coronilla* (Bull. ex Fr.) Quél., which was tried by two adolescents seeking hallucinogic activity who developed "bone pain";[183] *Verpa bohemica* (Krombh.) Schroet., listed in Table 1, also has been reported to cause significant motor incoordination;[184] and *Omphalotus olearius* (DC. ex Fr.) Sing., also listed in Table 1, can produce a variety of sensory disturbances and paresthesias as well as acting as a relatively potent muscle relaxant.[185]

HYPERSENSITIVITY TO MUSHROOMS

Food (Idiosyncratic or Acquired)

There is considerable variation in response to mushrooms. Part of this depends upon the age of the individual, the geographic source of the mushroom, and on its mode of preparation. Mushrooms that may be enjoyed in large quantity by some members of a family may cause severe reactions in others. The adverse reaction may be expressed as any combination of the following from simple abdominal discomfort, diarrhea, headache, bronchiolar wheezing, rhinorrhea, malaise, to severe, colicky pain and vomiting.[1,184,186] Ramsbottom[187] made note of this: "Some are made ill by the smallest portion of fungus which is perfectly harmless to others. The idiosyncracy varies: a particular species only may cause trouble, or it may be many, or all . . . The phenomenon is not more frequent with fungi than with several common foods, but its manifestation usually creates more alarm, particularly if perchance there is not that psychological sense of safety which purchase bestows." These idiosyncratic reactions have been explained by differences in metabolism, or gastrointestinal absorption, or to an acquired allergic sensitivity. One interesting case of a selective intolerance to the edible *Agaricus campestris* L. ex Fr. (*Psalliota campestris* Kummer), manifested as diarrhea, was shown to be due to a genetic intestinal deficiency of trehalase and could be duplicated by giving the patient trehalose, a sugar contained in that mushroom.[188,189]

Lung (Extrinsic Asthma and "Mushroom Worker's Lung")

The early work on fungus spores as allergens has been reviewed by Ainsworth.[190] Of considerable recent interest is a condition among industrial mushroom workers who develop acute respiratory distress, cough, pain, dyspnea, elevated temperature, severe headache, nausea, vomiting, weight loss, and other clinical signs. This condition was described first by Bringhurst and Gershon-Cohen,[191] and has been reported subsequently by a number of other investigators.[192-202] Currently it is classified as a hypersensitive allergic alveolitis due to an inhaled antigen (Type II allergy). A variety of organic dusts can be responsible depending upon the mushroom involved. In the case of one species, *Pleurotus ostreatus* (Jacq. ex Fr.) Kummer, it was demonstrated by precipitating antibodies (Ouchterlony test)[199] and later by immunofluorescence testing[202] that it was the mushroom spores themselves which carried the offending antigen.

Workers employed in the preparation of dried mushroom soup from *Agaricus bisporus* (J. Lange) Pilát (*Psalliota hortensis* of this reference) presented with rhinorrhea, dyspnea, and wheezing. Some, but not all, demonstrated immediate skin tests and a fall in FEV_1 of over 30% following bronchial challenge (Type I allergy).[203] The workers gave a history of an even more pronounced discomfort during their prior manufacturing exposure of some years earlier to *Boletus edulis* Bull. ex Fr. It is possible that mushroom spores may be responsible for unexplained post-frost cases of asthma and allergic rhinitis.[214]

Hemolytic Reactions

Hemolytic reactions following mushroom ingestion, sometimes complicated by secondary renal failure, are occasionally reported. These may have different underlying mechanisms. In the case reported by Szepietowski and Ratajczak,[204] in which *Gyromitra esculenta* (Pers. ex Fr.) Fr. was involved, it may be presumed that there may have been an inborn genetic deficiency of glucose-6-phosphate dehydrogenase activity, since such hemolytic reactions are associated in patients treated with isoniazid, which is a hydrazine derivative similar to the known toxins in *G. esculenta*.

On the other hand, an immunohemolytic reaction was suspected in the case of *Boletus luteus* Linn. ex Fr.[205] and was certainly demonstrated with *Paxillus involutus* (Batsch ex Fr.) Fr.[206] This latter mushroom expresses toxicity in a number of forms (see references in Table 1), but it is not clear how many of these may involve a hypersensitivity response.

Dermatitis

The medical literature is remarkable for the paucity of reports of allergic contact dermatitis due to mushrooms. In 1941, Hellerström reported on two patients, one sensitive to *Boletus edulis* Linn. ex Fr. and the other sensitive to *B. luteus*, and also to *Lactarius deliciosus* Linn. ex Fr., and to *Clavaria flava* Schaef. ex Fr.[207] There is apparently only one other report, which describes a contact dermatitis in a "commercial mushroom" grower.[208] The mushroom is not further identified, but may refer to *Agaricus brunnescens* Peck.

Not all cutaneous problems in mushroom workers should be ascribed to hypersensitivity, of course. After an intensive study following an outbreak of fingernail splitting in a group of workers in which the mushroom itself, yeasts, fungal infections such as *Aspergillus*, *Mucor*, and *Trichosporon*; sterilizants, and pesticides were eliminated as the possible etiologies, it was found that a recently introduced plastic bag used to contain the growing medium was the actual culprit.[209]

MUTAGENICITY

Carcinomas of the liver, lung, and intestine produced by *Gyromitra esculenta* in animals already have been discussed. Additional species of some common edible mushrooms were examined by Ames test.[215] *Agaricus bisporus*, *Boletus edulis*, four species of *Lactarius* (*L. necator*, *L. torminosus*, *L. helvus*, and *L. rufus*), and the Japanese shiitake (*Lentinus edodes*) were mutagenic to tester strains sensitive to base-pair substitution mutagens, and *L. necator*, *L. rufus*, and *B. edulis* also exhibited frame-shift activity. Metabolic activation was not required and the mutagenic activity could be detected in boiled mushroom extracts. The significance of this finding as a human health hazard will depend on isolation and characterization of the mutagenic substances and their evaluation in mammalian species.

REFERENCES

1. Gray, W. D., *The Use of Fungi as Food and in Food Processing, Part II*, CRC Press, Boca Raton, Fla., 1973, 159—192, 205—209.
2. Bertelli, A., Fournier, E., Frimmer, M., and Gorinin, S., Eds., *Clinical and Experimental Aspects of Fungal Poisoning, Current Problems in Clinical Biochemistry*, Vol. 7, Han Huber, Bern, 1977.
3. Faulstich, H., Kommerell, B., and Wieland, Th., Eds., *Amanita Toxins and Amanita Poisoning*, Witzrock, New York, 1980.

4. Lincoff, G. and Mitchel, D. H., *Toxic and Hallucinogenic Mushroom Poisoning*, Van Nostrand Reinhold, New York, 1977.
5. Rumack, B. H. and Salzman, E., Eds., *Mushroom Poisoning: Diagnosis and Treatment*, CRC Press, Boca Raton, Fla., 1978.
6. Lampe, K. F., Toxic fungi, *Ann. Rev. Pharmacol. Toxicol.*, 19, 85, 1979.
7. Lampe, K. F., Mushroom poisoning in children updated, *Paediatrician*, 6, 289, 1977.
8. von Clarmann, M., Pilzvergiftung, *Fortschr. Med.*, 82, 508, 1964.
9. Benedict, R. G., Mushroom toxins other than *Amanita*, in *Microbial Toxins*, Vol. 8, Kadis, S., Ciegler, A., and Ajl, S. J., Eds., Academic Press, New York, 1972, 281.
10. Tyler, V. E., Jr., Poisonous mushrooms, *Prog. Chem. Toxicol.*, 1, 339, 1963.
11. Miller, O. K., Jr., *Mushrooms of North America*, E. P. Dutton, New York, 1972.
12. Menser, G. P., *Hallucinogenic and Poisonous Mushroom Field Guide*, And/Or Press, Berkeley, Calif., 1977.
13. Haard, R. and Haard, K., *Poisonous and Hallucinogenic Mushrooms*, 2nd ed., Cloudburst Press, Brackendale, B. C., 1977.
14. Groves, J. W., Edible and Poisonous Mushrooms of Canada, Res. Branch Can. Dept. Agric., Publ. 1112, Ottawa, 1962.
15. Smith, A. H., *The Mushroom Hunter's Field Guide*, University of Michigan Press, Ann Arbor, 1966.
16. Smith, A. H., *A Field Guide to Western Mushrooms*, University of Michigan Press, Ann Arbor, 1975.
17. Guzmán, G., *Identificación de los hongos comestibles, venenosos, y alucinantes*, Editorial Limusa, Mexico, 1977.
18. Lampe, K. F., Mushroom poisoning in the young child, *Paediatrician*, 2, 83, 1973.
19. Chilton, W. S., Chemistry and mode of action of mushroom toxins, in *Toxic and Hallucinogenic Mushroom Poisoning*, Van Nostrand Reinhold, New York, 1977, 87.
20. Stadelmann, R. J., Müller, E., and Eugster, C. H., Über die Verbreitung der steromeren Muscarine innerhalb der Ordnung der *Agaricales*, *Helv. Chim. Acta*, 59, 2432, 1976.
21. Blount, E. A., A personal experience with mushroom poisoning, *Med. Record (1866—1922)*, 60, 815, 1901.
22. Chestnut, V. K., Poisonous properties of the green-spored *Lepiota*, *Asa Gray Bull.*, 8, 87, Plate V, 1900.
23. Child, G. P., The inability of Coprini to sensitize man to ethyl alcohol, *Mycologia*, 44, 200, 1952.
24. Graff, P. W., The green-spored *Lepiota*, *Mycologia*, 19, 322, 1927.
25. McCarter, G. R. B., Mushroom poisoning in Rhodesia: with a report of a case of poisoning due to *L.morganii*, *Centr. Afr. J. Med.*, 5, 412, 1959.
26. Smith, C. O., *Lepiota morgani* in Southern California, *Mycologia*, 28, 86, 1936.
27. Webster, H., A rash mycophagist, *Rhodora*, 17, 30, 1915.
28. Blayney, D., Rosenkranz, E., and Zettner, A., Mushroom poisoning from *Chlorophyllum molybdites*, *West. J. Med.*, 132, 74, 1980.
29. Levitan, D., Macy, J. I., and Weisman, J., Mechanisms of gastrointestinal hemorrhage in a case of mushroom poisoning by *Chlorophyllum molybdites*, *Toxicon*, 19, 179, 1981.
30. Eilers, F. I. and Nelson, L. R., Characterization and partial purification of the toxin of *Lepiota morgani*, *Toxicon*, 12, 557, 1974.
31. Floch, H., Labarbe, C., and Roffi, J., Etude expérimentale de la toxicité de la Lépiote de Morgan, *Rev. Mycol.*, 31, 317, 1966.
32. Torrelio, M. and Izquierdo, J., Cholinergic-like effects of *Chlorophyllum molybdites* (Meyer. ex Fr.) Mass. (Agaricaceae), *Arch. Int. Pharmacodyn. Ther.*, 185, 185, 1970.
33. Eilers, F. I. and Barnard, B. L., A rapid method for the diagnosis of poisoning caused by the mushroom *Lepiota morgani*, *Am. J. Clin. Pathol.*, 60, 823, 1973.
34. Weresub, L. K., Congo red for instant distinction between poisonous *Lepiota molybdites* and edible *L. brunnea*, *Can. J. Bot.*, 49, 2059, 1971.
35. Alder, A. E., Erkennung und Behandlung der Pilzvergiftung, *Dtsch. Med. Wschr.*, 86, 1121, 1961.
36. Ford, W. W., Poisonous mushrooms, in *Legal Medicine and Toxicology*, Peterson, F., Ed., W. B. Saunders, Philadelphia, 1923, 817.
37. Heim, R., *Les Champignons Toxiques et Hallucinogenes*, N. Boubee & Cie, Paris, 1963.
38. Smith, A. H., *Tricholoma irinum* in Michigan, *Mich. Bot.*, 1, 51, 1962.
39. Farlow, W. G., Poisoning by *Argaricus illudens*, *Rhodora*, 1, 43, 1899.
40. Fischer, O. E., Mushroom poisoning, in *The Gilled Mushrooms (Agaricaceae) of Michigan*, Kauffman, C. H., Ed., originally publ. 1918, reprinted Dover, New York, 1971.
41. Maretić, Z., Poisoning by the mushroom *Clitocybe olearia* Maire, *Toxicon*, 4, 263, 1967.
42. Maretić, Z., Russell, R. E., and Golobić, V., Twenty-five cases of poisoning by the mushroom *Pleurotus olearius*, *Toxicon*, 13, 379, 1975.
43. Seaver, F. J., Poisoning with *Clitocybe illudens*, *Mycologia*, 31, 110, 1939.

44. Carey, S. T., *Clitocybe illudens*: its cultivation, chemistry, and classification, *Mycologia*, 66, 951, 1974.
45. Bschor, F. and Mallach, H. J., Vergiftungen durch den Kahlen Krempling (*Paxillus involutus*) eine geniessbare Pilzart, *Archiv. Toxikol.*, 20, 82, 1963.
46. Schmidt, O., Kremplingsvergiftung in Meiningen, *Z. Pilzkd.*, 29, 54, 1963.
47. Sikorski, M., Marciniak, J., and Gliniecka, M., Zatrucie krowiakiem podwiniétym (olszówka), *Pol. Tyg. Lek.*, 29, 1165, 1974.
48. Smith, A. H., *Mushrooms in their Natural Habitats*, Sawyer's, Portland, Ore., 1949.
49. Kienholz, J. R., A poisonous *Boletus* from Oregon, *Mycologia*, 26, 275, 1934.
50. Collins, F. S., A case of Boletus poisoning, *Rhodora*, 1, 21, 1899.
51. Moeschlin, S., *Poisoning, Diagnosis and Treatment*, Grune & Stratton, New York, 1965, 599.
52. Carrano, R. A. and Malone, M. H., Pharmacologic study of norcaperatic and agaric acids, *J. Pharm. Sci.*, 56, 1611, 1967.
53. Henry, E. D. and Sullivan, G., Phytochemical evaluation of some cantharelloid fungi, *J. Pharm. Sci.*, 58, 1497, 1969.
54. Miyata, J. T., Tyler, V. E., Jr., Brady, L. R., and Malone, M. H., The occurrence of norcaperatic acid in *Catharellus floccosus*, *Lloydia*, 29, 43, 1966.
55. Wells, V. L. and Kempton, P. E., Studies on the fleshy fungi of Alaska. II., *Mycologia*, 60, 888, 1968.
56. Harmaja, H., Another poisonous species discovered in the genus *Gyromitra*: *G. ambigua*, *Karstenia*, 15, 36, 1976.
57. Price, H. W., Mushroom poisoning due to *Hebeloma crustuliniforme*, *Am. J. Dis. Child.*, 34, 441, 1927.
58. Charles, V. K., Mushroom poisoning caused by *Lactaria glaucescens*, *Mycologia*, 34, 112, 1942.
59. Goldman, H., Ueber Vergiftungen mit dem Giftpilze *Agaricus torminosus*, *Wien. Klin. Wschr.*, 14, 279, 1901.
60. Wells, V. L. and Kempton, P. E., *Togaria aurea* in Alaska, *Mycologia*, 57, 316, 1965.
61. Wells, V. L. and Kempton, P. E., Studies on the fleshy fungi of Alaska. I., *Lloydia*, 30, 258, 1967.
62. Shaffer, R. L., Poisoning by *Pholiota squarrosa*, *Mycologia*, 57, 318, 1965.
63. McIlvaine, C. and Macadam, R. K., *One Thousand American Fungi*, 2nd rev. ed., Bowen-Merill, 1902; reprinted with nomenclatural changes by R. L. Shaffer, Dover, New York, 1973.
64. Simons, D. M., The mushroom toxins, *Del. Med. J.*, 43, 177, 1971.
65. Wasson, R. G., The hallucinogenic mushrooms of Mexico: an adventure in ethnomycological exploration, *Trans. N.Y. Acad. Sci. Ser. II.*, 21, 325, 1959.
66. Wasson, R. G., The hallucinogenic fungi of Mexico: an inquiry into the origins of the religious idea among primitive peoples, *Bot. Mus. Leafl. Harv. Univ.*, 19, 137, 1961.
67. Wasson, R. G., The hallucinogenic mushrooms of Mexico and psilocybin: a bibliography, *Bot. Mus. Leafl. Harv. Univ.*, 20, 25, 1962.
68. Heim, R., Les champignons divinatoires recueillis par Mme. Valentina Pavlovna Wasson et M. R. Gordon Wasson au cours de leurs missions de 1954 et 1955 dans les pays mije, mazatèque, zápotèque et nahua du Mexique méridional et central, *C. R. Acad. Sci. (Paris)*, 242, 1389, 1956.
69. Heim, R., *Les Champignons Toxiques et Hallucinogenes*, N. Boubee & Cie, Paris, 1963.
70. Hofmann, A., Heim, R., Brack, A., and Kobel, H., Psilocybin, ein psychotroper Wirkstoff aus dem mexikanischen Rauschpilz *Psilocybe mexicana* Heim, *Experientia*, 14, 107, 1958.
71. Hofmann, A., Frey, A., Ott, H., Petrzilka, Th., and Troxler, F., Konstitutionsaufklärung und Synthese von Psilocybin, *Experientia*, 14, 397, 1958.
72. Hofmann, A., Heim, R., Brack, A., Kobel, H., Frey, A., Ott, H., Petrzilka, Th., and Troxler, F., Psilocybin und Psilocin, zwei psychotrope Wirkstoffe aus mexikanischen Rauschpilzen, *Helv. Chim. Acta*, 42, 1557, 1959.
73. Hollister, L. E., Prusmack, J. J., Paulsen, J. A., and Rosenquist, N., Comparison of three psychotropic drugs (Psilocybin, JB-329, and IT-290) in volunteer subjects, *J. Nerv. Ment. Dis.*, 131, 428, 1960.
74. Hollister, L. E., Clinical, biochemical and psychologic effects of psilocybin, *Arch. Int. Pharmacodyn. Ther.*, 130, 42, 1961.
75. Hollister, L. E. and Hartman, A. M., Mescaline, lysergic acid diethylamide and psilocybin: comparison of clinical syndromes, effects on color perception and biochemical measures, *Comp. Psychiatr.*, 3, 235, 1962.
76. Guzmán, G., Ott, J., Boydston, J., and Pollock, S. H., Psychotropic mycoflora of Washington, Idaho, Oregon, California and British Columbia, *Mycologia*, 68, 1267, 1976.
77. Pollock, S. H., The *Psilocybin* mushroom pandemic, *J. Psychedelic Drugs*, 7, 73, 1975.
78. Hatfield, G. M., Valdes, L. J., and Smith, A. H., The occurrence of psilocybin in *Gymnopilus* species, *Lloydia*, 41, 140, 1978.
79. Heim, R., Hofmann, A., and Tscherter, H., Sur une intoxication collective à syndrome psilocybien causée en France par un *Copelandia*, *C.R. Acad. Sci. Ser. D*, 262, 519, 1966.

80. McCawley, E. L., Brummett, R. E., and Dana, G. W., Convulsions from *Psilocybe* mushroom poisoning, *Proc. West. Pharmacol. Soc.*, 5, 27, 1962.
81. Bowden, K., Drysdale, A. C., and Mogey, G. A., Constituents of *Amanita muscaria*, *Nature (London)*, 206, 1359, 1965.
82. Bowden, K. and Drysdale, A. C., A novel constituent of *Amanita muscaria*, *Tetrahedron Lett.*, 12, 727, 1965.
83. Takemoto, T., Nakajima, T., and Yokobe, T., Structure of ibotenic acid, *Yakugaku Zasshi*, 84, 1232, 1964.
84. Takemoto, T., Nakajima, T., and Sakuma, R., Isolation of a flycidal constituent "ibotenic acid" from *Amanita muscaria* and *A. pantherina*, *Yakugaku Zasshi*, 84, 1233, 1964.
85. Müller, G. F. R. and Eugster, C. H., Muscimol, ein pharmakodynamish wirksamer Stoff aus *Amanita muscaria*, *Helv. Chim. Acta*, 48, 910, 1965.
86. Johnston, G. A. R., Curtis, D. R., de Groat, W. C., and Duggan, A. W., Central actions of ibotenic acid and muscimol, *Biochem. Pharmacol.*, 17, 2488, 1968.
87. König-Bersin, P., Waser, P. G., Langemann, H., and Lichtensteiger, W., Monamines in the brain under the influence of muscimol and ibotenic acid, two psychoactive principles of *Amanita muscaria*, *Psychopharmacologia*, 18, 1, 1970.
88. Theoblad, W., Büch, O., Kunz, H. A., Krupp, P., Stenger, E. G., and Heimann, H., Pharmakologische und experimentalpsychologische Untersuchungen mit 2 Inhaltsstoffen des Fliegenpilzes (*Amanita muscaria*), *Arzneim-Forsch.*, 18, 311, 1968.
89. Waser, P. G., The pharmacology of *Amanita muscaria*, in Ethnopharmacologic Search for Psychoactive Drugs, Efron, D. H., Ed., U.S. Public Health Service Publ. No. 1645, 1967, 419.
90. Chilton, W. S., The course of an intentional poisoning, *McIlvainea*, 2, 17, 1975.
91. Biggio, G., Brodie, B., Costa, E., and Guidotti, A., Mechanisms by which diazepam, muscimol, and other drugs change the content of cGMP in cerebellar cortex, *Proc. Natl. Acad. Sci. U.S.A.*, 74, 3592, 1977.
92. Brehm, L., Hjeds, H., and Krogsfaard-Larsen, P., The structure of muscimol, GABA analogue of restricted configuration, *Acta Chem. Scand.*, 26, 1298, 1972.
93. Johnston, G. A. R., Muscimol and the uptake of γ-aminobutyric acid by rat brain slices, *Psychopharmacologia*, 22, 230, 1971.
94. Naik, S. R., Guidotti, A., and Costa, E., Central BGABA receptor agonists: comparison of muscimol and baclofen, *Neutropharmacology*, 15, 479, 1976.
95. Walker, R. J., Woodruff, G. N., and Kerkut, G. A., The effect of ibotenic acid and muscimol on single neurons of the snail, *Helix aspersa*, *Comp. Gen. Pharmacol.*, 2, 168, 1971.
96. Andén, N.-E., Grabowska-Andén, M., and Wachtel, H., Effects of the GABA receptor agonist muscimol on the turnover of brain dopamine and on the motor activity of rats, *Acta Pharmacol. Toxicol.*, 44, 191, 1979.
97. Pfefferkorn, W. and Kirsten, G., Beitrag zum Pantherina — Syndrom in Kindesalter — Pantherpilzvergiftung, *Kinderaerztl. Praz.*, 35, 355, 1967.
98. Lindberg, P., Bergman, R., and Wickberg, B., Isolation and structure of coprine, the *in vivo* aldehyde dehydrogenase inhibitor of *Coprinus atramentarius*: synthesis of coprine and related cyclopropane derivatives, *J. Chem. Soc. Perkin Trans.*, I, 1977, 684.
99. Hatfield, G. M. and Schaumberg, J. P., Isolation and structural studies of coprine, The disulfiramlike constituent of *Coprinus atramentarius*, *Lloydia*, 38, 489, 1975.
100. Tottmar, O. and Lindberg, P., Effects on rat liver acetaldehyde dehydrogenases *in vitro* and *in vivo* by coprine, the disulfiram-like constituent of *Coprinus atramentarius*, *Acta Pharmacol. Toxicol.*, 40, 476, 1977.
101. Wiseman, J. S. and Abeles, R. H., Mechanism of inhibition of aldehyde dehydrogenase by cyclopropanone hydrate and the mushroom toxin coprine, *Biochemistry*, 18, 427, 1979.
102. Hatfield, G. M. and Schaumberg, J. P., The disulfiram-like effects of *Coprinus atramentarius* and related mushrooms, in *Toxic and Hallucinogenic Mushroom Poisoning*, Van Nostrand Reinhold, New York, 1977, 181.
103. Carlsson, A., Henning, M., Lindberg, P., Martinso, P., Trolin, G., Waldeck, B., and Wickberg, B., On the disulfiram-like effect of coprine, the pharmacologically active principle of *Coprinus atramentarius*, *Acta Pharmacol. Toxicol.*, 42, 292, 1978.
104. Jönsson, M., Lindquist, N. G., Plöen, L., Ekvärn, S., and Kronevi, T., Testicular lesions of coprine and benzcoprine, *Toxicology*, 12, 89, 1979.
105. Cochran, K. W. and Cochran, M. W., *Clitocybe clavipes*: antabuse-like reaction to alcohol, *Mycologia*, 70, 1124, 1978.
106. Bostroem, E., Ueber die Intoxicationen durch die essabare Lorchel. (Stockmorchel. *Helvella esculenta*.) Eine experimentelle Untersuchung, *Dtsch. Arch. Klin. Med.*, 32, 209, 1883.
107. Franke, S., Freimuth, U., and List, P. H., Über die Giftigkeit der Frühjarslorchel *Gyromitra (Helvella) esculenta* Fr., *Archiv. Toxikol.*, 22, 293, 1967.

108. List, P. H. and Luft, P., Gyromitrin, das Gift der Fruehjahrslorchel, *Gyromitra (Helvella) esculenta* Fr., *Tetrahedron Lett.*, 20, 1893, 1967.
109. List, P. H. and Luft, P., Gyromitrin, das Gift der Fruehjahrslorchel, *Arch. Pharmazie*, 301, 294, 1968.
110. Pyysalo, H., Some new toxic compounds in false morels, *Gyromitra esculenta, Naturwissenschaften*, 62, 395, 1975.
111. Pyysalo, H., Indentification of volatile compounds in seven edible fresh mushrooms, *Acta Chem. Scand.*, B30, 235, 1976.
112. Pyysalo, H., Tests for gyromitrin, a poisonous compound in false morel *Gyromitra esculenta, Z. Lebensm. Unters. Forsch.*, 160, 325, 1976.
113. Stuhlfauth, K. and Jung, F., Vergiftung mit Lorcheln *(Helvella esculenta), Samml. Vergiftungsfallen,* (A998), 86, 1952—54.
114. Biskupek, H., Badanie zatruć przemyslowych piestrzenenicakasztanowata — *Gyromitra esculenta* Pers. ex Fr. na przykladach zaobserwowanych w Polsce. Cześć III — Badania chemiczne lotnej substancji toksyczney, *Bromat. Chem. Toksykol.*, 4, 373, 1971.
115. Schmidlin-Mészáros, J., Gyromitrin in Trockenlorcheln *(Gyromitra esculenta sicc.), Mitt. Geb. Lebensmittelunters. Hyg.*, 65, 453, 1974.
116. List, P. H. and Luft, P., Nachweis und Gehaltsbestimmung von Gyromitrin in frischen Lorcheln, *Arch. Pharmazie*, 302, 143, 1969.
117. Pyysalo, H. and Niskanen, A., On the occurrence of N-methyl-N-formylhydrazones in fresh and processed false morel, *Gyromitra esculenta, J. Agric. Food Chem.*, 25, 644, 1977.
118. Toth, B., Hydrazine, methylhydrazine and methylhydrazine sulfate carcinogensis in Swiss mice. Failure of ammonium hydroxide to interfere in the development of tumors, *Int. J. Cancer*, 9, 109, 1972.
119. Toth, B. and Shimizu, H., Methylhydrazine tumorigenesis in Syrian golden hamsters and the morphology of malignant histiocytomas, *Cancer Res.*, 33, 2744, 1973.
120. Toth, B. and Nagel, D., Tumors induced in mice by N-methyl-N-formylhydrazine of the false morel *Gyromitra esculenta, J. Natl. Cancer Inst.*, 60, 201, 1978.
121. Toth, B. and Patil, K., Carcinogenic effects in the Syrian golden hamster of N-methyl-N-formylhydrazine of the false morel mushroom *Gyromitra esculenta, J. Cancer Res. Clin. Oncol.*, 93, 109, 1979.
122. Braun, R., Greeff, U., and Netter, K. J., Indications for nitrosamide formation from the mushroom poison gyromitrin by rat liver microsomes, *Xenobiotica*, 10, 557, 1980.
123. Gérault, A. and Girre, L., Recherches toxicologiques sur le genre *Lepiota* Fries, *C.R. Acad. Sci. Ser. D*, 280, 2841, 1975.
124. Brady, L. R., Benedict, R. G., Tyler, V. E., Stuntz, D. E., and Malone, M. H., Identification of *Conocybe filaris* as a toxic basidiomycete, *Lloydia*, 38, 983, 1965.
125. Buku, A., Wieland, Th., Bodenmüller, H., and Faulstich, H., Amaninamide, a new toxin of *Amanita virosa* mushrooms, *Experientia*, 36, 33, 1980.
126. Faulstich, H., Georgopoulos, D., and Bloching, M., Quantitative chromatographic analysis of toxins in single mushrooms of *Amanita phalloids, J. Chromatogr.*, 79, 257, 1973.
127. Faulstich, H., Georgopoulos, D., Bloching, M., and Wieland, Th., Analysis of the toxins of amanitin-containing mushrooms, *Z. Naturforsch. Teil C*, 29, 86, 1974.
128. Seeger, R. and Stijve, T., Amanitin content and toxicity of *Amanita verna* Bull., *Z. Naturforsch. Teil C*, 34, 330, 1979.
129. Stijve, T. and Seeger, R., Determination of α-, β-, and γ-amanitin by high performance thin-layer chromatography in *Amanita phalloides* (Vaill. ex Fr.) Secr. from various origin, *Z. Naturforsch. Teil C*, 34, 1133, 1979.
130. Yocum, R. and Simons, D., Amatoxins and phallotoxins in *Amanita* species of the northeastern United States, *Lloydia*, 40, 178, 1977.
131. Johnson, B. E. C., Preston, J. F., and Kimbrough, J. W., Quantitation of amanitins in *Galerina autumnalis, Mycologia*, 68, 1248, 1976.
132. Beutler, J. A. and Vergeer, P. P., Amatoxins in American mushrooms: evaluation of the Meixner test, *Mycologia*, 72, 1142, 1980.
133. Andary, C., Enjalbert, F., Privat, G., and Mandrou, B., Dosage des amatoxines par spectrophotométrie directe sur chromatogramme chez *Amanita phalloides* Fries (Basidiomycetes), *J. Chromatogr.*, 132, 525, 1977.
134. Gillman, L., Identification of common poisonous mushrooms, in *Toxic and Hallucinogenic Mushroom Poisoning*, Van Nostrand Reinhold, New York, 1977, 27.
135. Busi, C., Fiume, L., Costantino, D., Langer, M., and Vesconi, F., Amanita toxins in gastroduodenal fluid of patients poisoned by the mushroom, *Amanita phalloides, N. Engl. J. Med.*, 300, 800, 1979.
136. Brown, A. and Garrity, G. M., Detection and quantitation of amanitin using an RNA-polymerase competition binding assay, *Toxicon*, 18, 702, 1980.
137. Fiume, L. and Laschi, R., Lesioni ultrastrutturali prodotte nelle cellule parenchimali epatiche dalla falloidine e dalla α-amanitina, *Sperimentale*, 115, 288, 1965.

138. **Lampe, K. F.**, Pharmacology and therapy of mushroom intoxications, in *Toxic and Hallucinogenic Mushroom Poisoning*, Van Nostrand Reinhold, New York, 1977, 125.
139. **Lindell, N. J.**, Inhibitors of mammalian RNA polymerases, *Pharmacol. Ther. A*, 2, 195, 1977.
140. **Roeder, R. G., Golomb, M. W., Jaehning, J. A., Ng, S. Y., Parker, C. S., Schwartz, L. B., Sklar, V. E. F., and Weinmann, R.**, Animal nuclear RNA polymerases, in *Receptors and Hormone Action*, Vol. I, O'Malley, B. W. and Birnbaumer, L., Eds., Academic Press, New York, 1977, 195.
141. **Brasch, K. and Sinclair, G. D.**, The organization, composition and matrix of hepatocyte nuclei exposed to α-amanitin, *Virchows Archiv B Cell Pathol.*, 27, 193, 1978.
142. **Novello, F., Pession-Brizzi, A., and Derenzini, M.**, Nuclear protein synthesis in regenerating rat liver. Selective histone inhibition by α-amanitin, *Exp. Cell Res.*, 112, 219, 1978.
143. **Barsotti, P. and Marinozzi, V.**, A morphological study on the early changes in hepatocyte nuclei induced by low doses of α-amanitin, *J. Submicr. Cytol.*, 11, 13, 1979.
144. **Barsotti, P., Derenzini, M., Novello, F., Pession-Brizzi, A., and Marinozzi, V.**, Pretreatment of rats with cycloheximide prevents hepatocyte nuclear fragmentation induced by α-amanitin, *Biol. Cellulaire*, 39, 159, 1980.
145. **Vesconi, S., Langer, M., and Constantino, D.**, Mushroom poisoning and forced diuresis, *Lancet*, 2, 854, 1980.
146. **Becker, F. M., Tong, T. G., Bartter, F., Boerner, U., Roe, R. L., Scott, R. T. A., and MacQuarrie, M. B.**, Diagnosis and treatment of *Amanita phalloides*-type poisoning, *West. J. Med.*, 125, 100, 1976.
147. **Meili, E. O., Frick, P. G., and Strub, P. W.**, Coagulation changes during massive hepatic necrosis due to *Amanita phalloides* poisoning, *Helv. Med. Acta*, 35, 304, 1970.
148. **Wieland, O.**, Changes in liver metabolism induced by the poisons of *Amanita phalloides*, *Clin. Chem. N.Y.*, 11, 323, 1965.
149. **Cavalli, P. L., Ragni, R., and Zuccaro, G.**, L'avvelenamento da funghi. Problemi terapeutici, *Arch. Sci. Med. (Torino)*, 125, 690, 1968.
150. **Kubička, J.**, Neue Möglichkeiten in der Behandlung von Vergiftungen mit dem Grunen Knollenblatterpilz — *Amanita phalloides*, *Mykol. Mitteil.*, 7, 92, 1963.
151. **Kubička, J.**, Rozbor smrtelných otrav houbami léčených kyselinou thioktovou, *Casopis Lek. Cesk.*, 108, 790, 1969.
152. **Čuřík, R., Veselský, J., and Kubička, J.**, Jaterní biopsie u ženy na vrcholu masívní otravy muchomůrko želenou — *Amanita phalloides*. Elektronmikroskopický nález, *Cas. Lek. Cesk.*, 115, 1399, 1976.
153. **Veselský, J., Kubička, J., and Čuřík, R.**, Aktuální poznámky k otravám muchomůrkou zelenou — *Amanita phalloides* (Fr.) Link., *Cesk. Mykol.*, 32, 1, 1978.
154. **Floersheim, G. L., Schneeberger, J., and Bucher, K.**, Curative potencies of penicillin in experimental *Amanita phalloides* poisoning, *Agents Actions*, 2, 138, 1971.
155. **Floersheim, G. L.**, Antidotes to experimental α-Amanitin poisoning, *Nature (London) New Biol.*, 236, 115, 1972.
156. **Floersheim, G. L.**, Curative potencies against α-amanitin poisoning by cytochrome C., *Science*, 177, 808, 1972.
157. **Floersheim, G. L.**, Experimentelle Grunlagen zur Therapie von Vergiftungen durch den grünen Knollenblätterpilz *(Amanita phalloides)*, *Schweiz. Med. Wochenschr.*, 108, 185, 1978.
158. **Fiume, L., Sperti, S., Montanaro, L., Busi, C., and Costantino, D.**, Amanitins do not bind to serum albumin, *Lancet*, 1, 1111, 1977.
159. **Bismuth, C., Crabie, P., and Guyon, A.**, Bisalbuminémie transitoire sous béta-lactamines lors d'intoxications phalloidiennes, *Nouv. Presse Med.*, 5, 1696, 1976.
160. **Moroni, F., Fantozzi, R., Masini, E., and Mannaioni, P. F.**, A trend in the therapy of *Amanita phalloides* poisoning, *Arch. Toxicol.*, 36, 111, 1976.
161. **Bozza Marubini, M., Ghezzi, R., Giampiccoli, G., Maritano, M., and Sottili, S.**, The treatment of *Amanita phalloides* poisoning in man with the methods of Floersheim-Galmarini, *Clinical and Experimental Aspects of Fungal Poisoning, Current Problems in Clinical Biochemistry*, Vol. 7, Van Huber, Bern, 1977, 156.
162. **Favre, H., Leski, M., Christeler, E., Vollenweider, E., and Chatelant, F.**, Le *Cortinarius orellanus*: un champignon toxique provoquant une insuffisance rénale aiguë retardé, *Schweiz. Med. Wschr.*, 106, 1097, 1976.
163. **Grzymala, S.**, Etude clinique des intoxications par les champignons du genre *Cortinarius orellanus* Fr., *Bull. Med. Leg. Toxicol. Med.*, 8, 60, 1965.
164. **Färber, D. and Feldmeier, S.**, Die Orellanus-Pilzvergiftung im Kindesalter, *Anasth. Prax*, 13, 87, 1977.
165. **Marichal, J.-F., Triby, F., Wiederkehr, J.-L., and Carbiener, R.**, Insuffisance rénale chronique après intoxication par champignons de type *Cortinarius orellanus* Fries, *Nouv. Presse Med.*, 6, 2973, 1977.

166. Brousse, A., Herve, J. P., Leguy, P., Cledes, J., and Leroy, J. P., L'intoxication par champignons de type *Cortinarius orellanus*. Une cause rare d'insuffisance rénale, *Nouv. Presse Med.*, 10, 1940, 1981.
167. Bouška, I., Reháneck, L., Veselský, J., and Čuřík, R., Diagnostické problémy při otravě houbou pavučincem plyšovým (*Cortinarius orellanus* Fr.) s nefrotuckám účinkem, *Soud. Lek.*, 24, 27, 1979.
168. Středová, M., Krautová, H., Šellenberg, P., Henrink, J., and Marek, J., Otrava houbami z rodu pavučinec *(Cortinarius), Vnitrnl Lek.*, 24, 822, 1978.
169. Favre, H., Leski, M., Christeler, P., Vollenwieder, E., and Chatelanat, F., Le *Cortinarius orellanus*: un champignon toxique profiquant une insuffisance rénale aiguë retardee, *Schweiz. Med. Wschr.*, 106, 1097, 1976.
170. Hulmi, S., Sipponen, P., Forsström, J., and Vilska, J., Seitikkisienen aiheuttama vakava munuaisvaurio, *Duodecim*, 90, 1044, 1974.
171. Nieminen, L. and Pyy, K., Sex differences in renal damage induced in the rat by the Finnish mushroom, *Cortinarius speciosissimus, Acta Pathol. Microbiol. Scand. Sect. A.*, 84, 222, 1976.
172. Nieminen, L., Möttönen, M., Tirri, R., and Ikonen, S., Nephrotoxicity of *Cortinarius speciosissimus*: a histological and enzyme histological study, *Exp. Pathol.*, 11, 239, 1975.
173. Short, A. I. K., Watling, R., MacDonald, M. K., and Robson, J. S., Poisoning by *Cortinarius speciossimus, Lancet*, 2, 942, 1980.
174. Möttönen, M., Nieminen, L., and Heikkilä, H., Damage caused by two Finnish mushrooms, *Cortinarius specioissimus* and *Cortinarius gentilis* on the rat kidney, *Z. Naturforsch.*, 30c, 668, 1975.
175. Antokowiak, W. and Gessner, W., The structures of orellanine and orelline, *Tetrahedron Lett.*, 21, 1931, 1979.
176. Tyler, V. E., Jr., Chemotaxonomy in the basidiomycetes, in *Evolution in the Higher Basidiomycetes*, Peterson, R. H., Ed., University of Tennessee, Knoxville, 1971.
177. Wasiljkow, B. P., Die Vergiftungsfälle des Büscheligen Schwefelkopfes, *Hypholoma fasciculare* (Fr.) Quel., *Schweiz. Z. Pilzk.*, 41, 117, 1963.
178. Mortara, M. and Martinetti, L., Vergiftung durch *Hypholoma fasciculare* Fries (Schwefelkopf, Bitterschwamm), *Arch. Toxikol.*, 15, 390, 1954—55.
179. Mortara, M. and Martinetti, L., Un raro avvelenamento da funghi: l'avvelenamento da *Hypholoma fasciculare, Med. Int.*, 63, 180, 1955.
180. Herbich, J., Lohwag, K., and Rotter, R., Tödliche Vergiftung mit dem grünblättrigen Schwefelkopf, *Arch. Toxikol.*, 21, 310, 1966.
181. Nishihara, M., Lin, C. C., Furukawa, I., and Nakanishi, S., Chemical studies on poisonous mushroom. I. A preliminary experiment on the isolation of poisonous ingredients in *Hypholoma fasciculare, Doshisha Eng. Rev.*, 9(1), 36, 1958.
182. Stevenson, J. A., *Scleroderma* poisoning, *Mycologia*, 53, 438, 1961.
183. Thomas, H. W., Mitchel, D. H., and Rumack, B. W., Poisoning from the mushroom *Stropharia coronilla* (Bull. ex Fr.) Quél., *J. Ark. Med. Soc.*, 73, 311, 1977.
184. Simons, D. M., The mushroom toxins, *Del. Med. J.*, 43, 177, 1971.
185. Maretić, Z., Russell, R. E., and Golobić, V., Twenty-five cases of poisoning by the mushroom *Pleurotus olearius, Toxicon*, 13, 379, 1975.
186. Dearness, J., The personal factor in mushroom poisoning, *Mycologia*, 3, 75, 1911.
187. Ramsbottom, J., *Poisonous Fungi*, Penguin Books, London, 1945.
188. Bergoz, R. and Righetti, A., Intolérance aux champignons par malabsorption sélective du tréhalose: un syndrome rare et inédit, *Schweiz Med. Wschr.*, 100, 1244, 1970.
189. Bergoz, R., Trehalose malabsorption causing intolerance to mushrooms — Report of a probable case, *Gastroenterology*, 60, 909, 1971.
190. Ainsworth, G. C., Fungus spores as allergens, *Medical Mycology*, Pitman & Sons, London, 1952, 74.
191. Bringhurst, L. S. and Gershon-Cohen, J., Respiratory disease of mushroom workers, *J. Am. Med. Assoc.*, 171, 101, 1959.
192. Sakula, A., Mushroom-worker's lung, *Br. Med. J.*, 3, 708, 1967.
193. Jackson, E. and Welch, K. M. A., Mushroom worker's lung, *Thorax*, 25, 25, 1970.
194. Craig, D. B. and Donevan, R. E., Mushroom-worker's lung, *Can. Med. Assoc. J.*, 102, 1289, 1970.
195. Nicholson, D. P., Extrinsic allergic pneumonias, *Am. J. Med.*, 53, 131, 1972.
196. Chan-Yeung, M., Grzybowski, S., and Schonell, M. E., Mushroom worker's lung, *Am. Rev. Resp. Dis.*, 105, 819, 1972.
197. Lockey, S. D., Sr., Mushroom worker's pneumonitis, *Ann. Allergy*, 33, 282, 1974.
198. Stewart, C. J., Mushroom worker's lung — two outbreaks, *Thorax*, 29, 252, 1974.
199. Noster, U., Hausen, B. M., Felten, G., and Schulz, K. H., Pilzzüchterlunge durch Speisepilzsporen, *Dtsch. Med. Wschr.*, 101, 1241, 1976.
200. Stolz, J. L., Arger, P. H., and Benson, J. M., Mushroom worker's lung disease, *Radiology*, 119, 61, 1976.

201. Stolz, J. L. and Arger, P. H., Respiratory disease due to mushrooms: mushroom worker's lung, in *Toxic and Hallucinogenic Mushroom Poisoning*, Van Nostrand Reinhold, New York, 1977, 187.
202. Noster, U., Schulz, K. H., and Hausen, B. M., Immunfluoreszenz-Test in der Diagnostik der "Pilzzüchterlung", *Dtsch. Med. Wschr.*, 103, 655, 1978.
203. Symington, I. S., Kerr, J. W., and McLean, D. A., Type I allergy in mushroom soup processors, *Clin. Allergy*, 11, 43, 1981.
204. Szepietowski, T. and Ratajczak, T., Ostra niewydolność nerek po zatruciu piestrzenica, *Pol. Tyg. Lek.*, 26, 1551, 1971.
205. Bobrowski, H., Ostra niewydolność nerek w przebiegu ostrego nabytego zespolu hemolityczego u osoby uczulonej na grzyb maslak *(Boletus luteus)*, *Pol. Tyg. Lek.*, 21, 1864, 1966.
206. Schmidt, J., Hartmann, W., Würstlin, A., and Deicher, H., Akutes Nierenversagen durch immunhämolytische Anämie nach Genuss des Kahlen Kremplings *(Paxillus involutus)*, *Dtsch. Med. Wschr.*, 96, 1188, 1971.
207. Hellerström, S., Sensitization to edible mushrooms, *Acta Derm. Venerol.*, 22, 331, 1941.
208. Hopkins, H. H., Mushroom dermatitis, *Md. State Med. J.*, 1, 504, 1952.
209. Schubert, B., Minard, J.-J., Baran, R., Verret, J.-L., and Schnitzler, L., Onychopathie des champignonnistes, *Ann. Derm. Venereol.*, 104, 627, 1977.
210. Saupe, S. G., Occurrence of psilocybin/psilocin in *Pluteus salicinus* (Pluteaceae), *Mycologia*, 73, 781, 1981.
211. Beutler, J. A. and Der Marderosian, A. H., Chemical variation in *Amanita, J. Natl. Prod.*, 44, 422, 1981.
212. Faulstich, H., Buku, A., Bodenmüller, H., and Wieland, Th., Virotoxins: actin-binding cyclic peptides of *Amanita virosa* mushrooms, *Biochemistry*, 19, 3334, 1980.
213. Kürnsteiner, H. and Moser, M., Isolation of a lethal toxin from *Cortinarius orellanus* Fr., *Mycopathologia*, 74, 65, 1981.
214. Check, W. A., Common mushroom spores may cause asthma and hay fever in fall, *JAMA*, 247, 2071, 1982.
215. von Wright, A., Knuutinen, J., Lindroth, S., Pellinen, M., Widén, K.-G., and Seppä, E.-L., The mutagenicity of some edible mushrooms in the Ames test, *Food Chem. Toxic.*, 20, 265, 1982.

CHEMICAL SUBSTANCES IN PLANTS TOXIC TO ANIMALS

Gillian A. Cooper-Driver

INTRODUCTION

Plants have been used as medicinals since time immemorial.[1,2] Man must have soon realized that the beneficial effects of the plants concerned were dose related. If one consumed too much of a medicinal herb at any one time the "cure" might be worse than the original malady, even resulting in death.

The deliberate use of plants as ritual poisons is well documented by the ancient Greeks (e.g., hemlock 700 B.C.) and the deleterious effects of certain plants, even when eaten in very small quantities, to both man and animals well known. Equally developed at that time was the knowledge that the essential principles (medicinal or toxic) could be extracted from the plant by macerating or boiling in water. This knowledge was encoded in ancient pharmacopoeias and extended and refined in the medieval herbals. But it was not until the beginning of the 19th century that the compounds responsible for pharmacological activity were finally obtained in a pure state and their physiological activity studied in detail.

The first compound obtained in this way by Sertuner in 1803 was the alkaloid morphine from the opium poppy. By the end of the century, thousands of so-called "natural products" had been isolated and the determination of their structure and the basis of their physiological or toxic action occupied the attention of the best chemists, physiologists, and pharmacologists in the world.

By far the largest number of natural products come from plants, and since they apparently have no known role in the organism's primary metabolism they are referred to as "secondary products".[3,4] While it now seems clear that some of these compounds do have a regulatory function in plant metabolism, their major role appears to lie in the defense of the plant against herbivores and pathogens.[5,6]

Over 10,000 known low molecular weight secondary compounds have now been isolated from higher plants and fungi and those which are toxic to animals, including man, fall into the following categories;[2,7] alkaloids, proteins and amino acids; terpenoids; glycosides including cyanogenic glycosides, glucosinolates, cardiac glycosides and saponins; polyketides; and other miscellaneous groups such as inorganic and photosensitive compounds.[2,7,8]

Pharmaceutical chemists have demonstrated that considerable heterogeneity in toxicity exists within most classes of these compounds and have established structure-activity relationships within each group. Toxicological evaluation generally utilizes the lethal dose (LD) as an index and quotes toxicity in forms of LD_{50}, the concentration at which half the experimental animals die. Lethality provides a measure of comparison among different substances whose mechanism and sites of action may be markedly different.

Due to the very large number of toxic compounds found in plants, only a few representatives from each group will be described in any detail. References, however, are provided for those requiring more detailed information.

ALKALOIDS (TABLE 1)

The alkaloids, of which nearly 6000 are known, are a group of structurally varied compounds which are difficult to classify in a simple manner.[10-15] All contain nitrogen, mainly as part of a heterocyclic ring, and many also possess other complex ring struc-

Table 1
ALKALOIDS IN PLANTS TOXIC TO ANIMALS

Alkaloid type True	Name	Occurrence Family[18]	Species	Common name	Toxicity[a]	Symptoms
Pyrrolidine	Nicotine	Solanaceae	*Nicotiana tabacum* L.	Tobacco	LD$_{50}$ 50—60 mg/kg orally rats	Carcinogenic, vomiting, diarrhea, respiratory failure
Tropane	Atropine, hyoscyamine, scopolamine	Solanaceae	*Atropa belladona* L. *Datura stramonium* L. *Hyoscyamus niger* L.	Belladonna Jimson weed Henbane	LD/kg orally rats	Flushed skin, dilated pupils, dry mouth, delirium; death from respiratory failure
	Scopolamine	Solanaceae	*Scopolina carniolica* L. *Datura metel* L.	Jimson weed	LD$_{50}$ 17 mg/kg i.v. rats	
	Cocaine	Erythroxlaae	*Erythroxylon cocoa* Lam.	Cocaine	LD$_{50}$ 17.5 mg/kg i.v. rats	
Pyrrolizidine	Amsinckine	Boraginaceae	*Amsinckia intermedia* Fisch. and Mey	Tarweed		Hepatocarcinogenic, liver toxicity and atrophy often resulting in death
	Heliotrine, lasiocarpine	Boraginacca	*Heliotropium europaeum* L.	Heliotrope		
	Monocrotaline Retrorsine	Leguminosae Compositae (Asteraceae)	*Crotalaria spectabilis* Roth *Senecio jacobaea* L.	Rattle box Stinking willie	MLD 100 mg/kg	
Pyridine-piperidine	Coniine	Umbelliferae	*Conium maculatum* L.	Poisonous hemlock		Vomiting, diarrhea, inflammation of the gastrointestinal tract, mental confusion, convulsions, death
	Lobeline Pseudopelletierine	Campanulaceae Punicaceae	*Lobelia inflata* L. *Punia granatum* L.	Indian tobacco Pomegranate		

Class	Alkaloid	Family	Species	Common name	LD50	Symptoms
Quinolizidine	Cytisine	Leguminosae (Fabaceae)	*Laburnum anagyroides* Medik.	Golden rain	LD₅₀ 4 mg/kg s.c. dogs	Gastrointestinal disorders, irregular pulse and coma
	Lupinine Sparteine	Leguminosae (Fabaceae)	*Lupinus* sp.	Lupin		
	Sparteine Isosparteine	Leguminosa (Fabaceae)	*Cytisus scoparius* Link.	Scotch broom	MLD 120 mg/kg s.c. mice	
Isoquinoline	Berberine	Berberidacea (Hydrastidaceae)	*Hydrastis canadensis* L.	Goldenseal	LD₅₀ 24.3 mg/kg i.p. mice	Gastrointestinal disorders, death
	Sanguinarine	Papaveraceae	*Sanguinaria canadensis*	Bloodroot		
	Papaverine, morphine, codeine, thebaine	Papaveraceae	*Papaver somniferum* L.	Opium poppy	LD₅₀ 750 mg/kg orally rats	
	Herberine, protopine, sanguinarine, dihydosanguinarine	Papaveraceae	*Argemone mexicana* L.	Mexican poppy		
	Chelidonine, chelerythrine, sanguinarine, berberine, protopine	Papaveraceae	*Chelidonium majus* L.	Celandine poppy		
	Apomorphine, protoberine, protopine	Fumariaceae	*Corydalis caseana* Gray	Fitweed	LD₅₀ 80 mg/kg i.v. dogs	
	Calycanthine D-tubo-cuccurarine	Famariaceae Calycanthaceae Menispermaceae	*Dicentra canadensis* (Goldie) Walp. *Calycanthus fertalis* L. *Chondodendron tomentosum* R and P.	Squirrel-corn Caroline allspice Pareira	Highly toxic	Respiratory paralysis and hypotension
Indole	Physostigmine	Leguminosae	*Physostigma venenosum* Balf.	Calabar bean	LD₅₀ 3 mg/kg orally mice	
	Ergonovine, Ergotamine	Fungi (Pyrenomycetes)	*Claviceps purpurea* L.	Ergot	LD₅₀ 62 mg/kg i.v. rats	Convulsions, madness and death

Table 1 (continued)
ALKALOIDS IN PLANTS TOXIC TO ANIMALS

Alkaloid type	Name	Occurrence Family[18]	Species	Common name	Toxicity[a]	Symptoms
True	Strychnine	Convolvulaceae	Ipomoea sp.	Morning glories		
	Brucine	Strychnaceae (Apocynaceae)	Strychnos nos-vomica	Strychnine	MLD 5 mg/kg orally rats	
	Yohimbine	Rubiaceae	Corynathe yohimba Welv.			
	Ibogaine	Apocyanaceae	Tabernanthe iboga Baill			
	Gelsemine	Loganiaceae	Gelsemium sempervirens (L.) Aitif	Yellow jessamine		Double visions, muscular weakness, respiratory arrest
	Vinoblastine, vincristine	Apocynaceae	Catharanthus roseus G. Don	Periwinkle, Vinca		
	Reserpine	Apocynaceae	Rauvolfia serpentina L.			
Imidazole	Pilocarpine	Rutaceae	Pilocarpus alvaradoi Vahl.			
Steroidal	Solanine	Solanaceae	Solanum sp.	Potato	LD_{50} 42 mg/kg i.p. mice	Nausea and vomiting
			Solandra sp.	Trumpet flower		
	Tomatine	Solanaceae	Lycopersicon esculentum L.	Tomato	LD_{50} 900—1000 mg/kg orally rats	Respiratory depression, unconsciousness and death
	Veratridine	Liliaceae	Veratrum viride Ait	American hellebore		
Diterpenoids	Aconitine	Ranunculaceae	Aconitum napellus L.	Monkshood	LD_{50} 1 mg/kg orally mice	Numbness, weak pulse, respiratory paralysis, convulsions and death
	Delphinine	Ranunculaceae	Delphinium sp.	Larkspur		
	Cyclobuxine taxine	Buxaceae	Buxus semper-virens L.			
		Taxaceae	Taxus baccata L.	Yew	LD_{50} 500 mg/kg s.c. mice	
Biological amines	Mescaline	Cactaceae	Lophophora williamsii L.	Peyote	LD_{50} 132 mg/kg mice	Teratogen, hallucinogenic

	Bufotenine		*Bufa* sp.		
	Psilocybin	Leguminosae	*Piptadenia peregrina* L.		
		Fungi (Agaricaceae)	*Psilocybe mexicana*		
Peptides	Amanitin	Fungi (Agaricaceae)	*Amanita phalloides* (Fr) Secr	Agarics LD_{50} 275 mg/kg mice	Hypoglycemia and death
Miscellaneous	Colchicine	Liliaceae	*Colchicum autumnale* L.	Crocus LD_{50} 0.4 mg/kg mice	Vomiting, kidney and respiratory failure

tures (e.g., strychnine). Most exhibit marked physiological activity, are usually bitter to taste, and as a group are the most toxic in nature. Hegnauer[14] has classified the alkaloids into three sub-classes: the *true* alkaloids which are formed biosynthetically from the five amino-acids — ornithine, lysine, phenylalanine, tyrosine, and tryptophan; the *proto* alkaloids (biological amines) which do not contain heterocyclic nitrogen other than the indole ring from tryptophan, but which are formed from similar precursors to the true alkaloids; and the *pseudo* alkaloids, which include compounds in which the nitrogen is introduced at a late stage in biosynthesis (diterpenoid and steroidal alkaloids) and the unusual peptides which exhibit alkaloid-like toxicity.

By and large the toxicity of alkaloids is generally correlated with the complexity of their structures, the simpler compounds being the least toxic presumably because they are closely related to normal metabolites (e.g., proline, nicotinic acid, tryptophan, etc.) which are rapidly degraded or detoxified in the liver. Exceptions are the steroidal alkaloids (which are among the most toxic known) and the peptide alkaloids of the fungi. It may be assumed that these two latter groups owe their toxicity to their "mimicking" normal hormonal or other controlling metabolites at target cells.[9]

Alkaloids are present in about 25% of all plant species.[15] They are most commonly distributed in the flowering plants among the Apocynaceae, Berberidaceae, Leguminosae (Fabaceae), Papaveraceae, Ranunculaceae, Rubiaceae, and Solanaceae, often occurring in concentrations of up to 10% in some organs. Generally their concentration is much less, and their bitterness usually warns animals about eating plants which contain them. They are mainly confined to certain orders of families and it is of evolutionary significance that the full flowering of alkaloid complexity is not found until the angiosperms. Lower plants contain few such compounds and none derived from the aromatic amino-acids.[16]

The *true* alkaloids from ornithine all contain a five-membered heterocyclic ring akin to that found in proline. Chemically, the most important are classed as pyrrolidine (e.g., nicotine, Figure 1A) and tropane (e.g., atropine, Figure 1B) alkaloids in which a single ornithine moiety is utilized, and the pyrrolizidine (or necine) alkaloids (e.g., retrorsine, Figure 1C) where two ornithines are involved in their biosynthesis. The latter are, as expected, the more toxic to man and other animals, as they contain not only a complex bicyclic *N*-containing ring system, but are acylated by a series of unusual dicarboxylic acids which have no counterpart in normal metabolism.

The lysine alkaloids are similar to the ornithine derivatives, but have one extra carbon atom forming simple six-membered rings — piperidine alkaloids (e.g., coiine, Figure 1D) or those like the tropanes (e.g., pseudopelletierine, Figure 1E) and more complex structures involving two or three lysines in their biosynthesis, the quinolizidines or lupine alkaloids (e.g., lupinine and sparteine, Figures 1F and 1G). Again the latter are the most toxic of their class.

The aromatic amino acids, phenylalanine and tyrosine, give rise to a series of isoquinoline alkaloids — simple isoquinolines or benzylisoquinolines which involve *two* molecules of the aromatic acids in their synthesis (e.g., papaverine, Figure 1H). The latter compounds can rearrange in several ways to give compounds like morphine (Figure 1I) or the apomorphine (Figure 1) alkaloids. Further addition of an extra carbon on the heterocyclic nitrogen gives rise to berberine (Figure 1K) and similar types. Again, by and large, the more complex the resulting alkaloid structure, the more toxic it is.

Tryptophan gives rise to a similar series of simple alkaloids which include the harmalines and the eserine types (e.g., physostigmine, Figure 1L). However, the most toxic alkaloids of this group are the complex indole alkaloids in which a monoterpene moiety is combined to give a multi-ring structure. These include the ergolines (e.g., ergotamine Figure 1M), strychnine, yohimbine, and ibogaine, which are among the most poisonous natural products known.

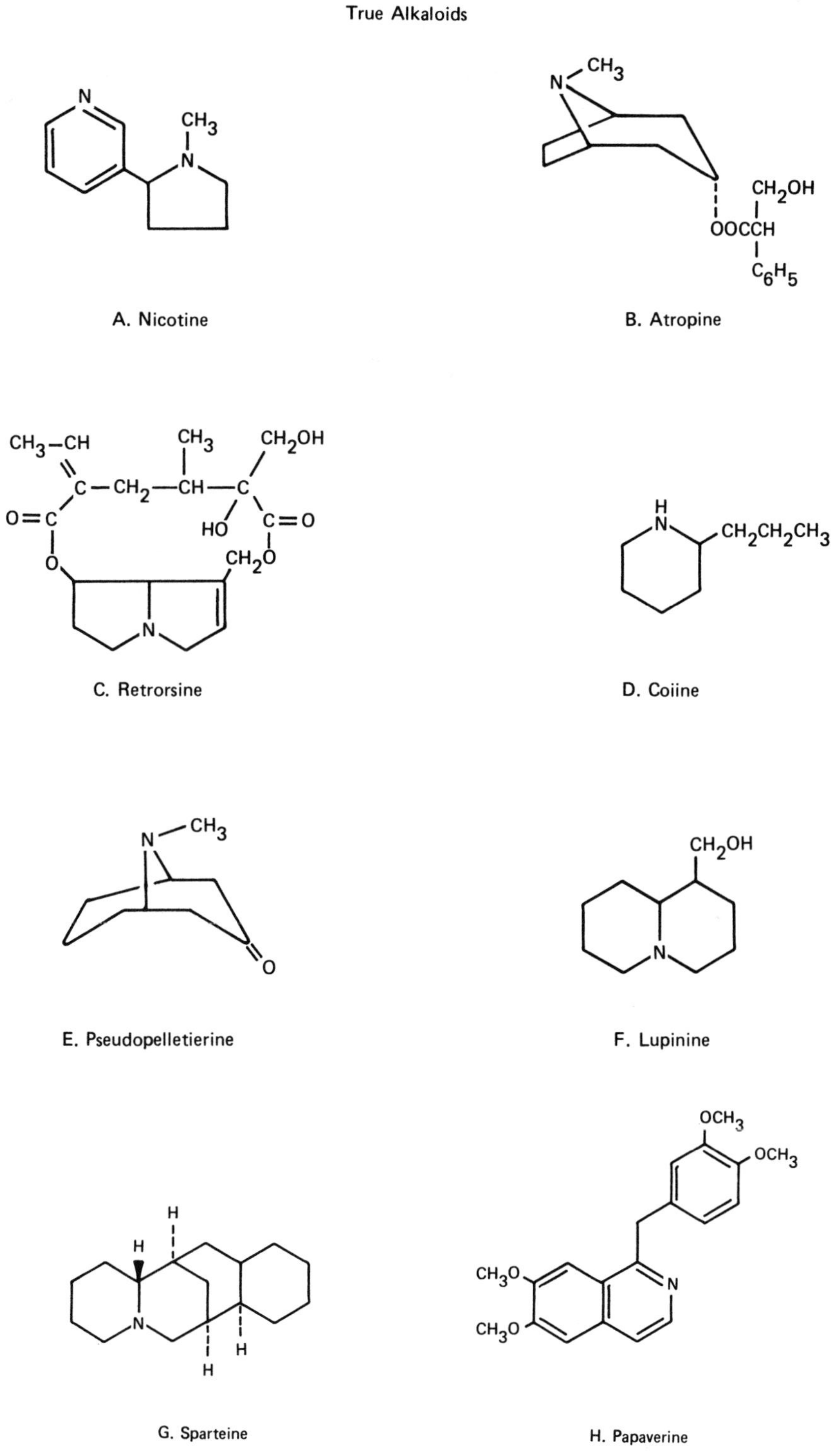

True Alkaloids

A. Nicotine

B. Atropine

C. Retrorsine

D. Coiine

E. Pseudopelletierine

F. Lupinine

G. Sparteine

H. Papaverine

FIGURE 1. Some toxic alkaloids present in plants.

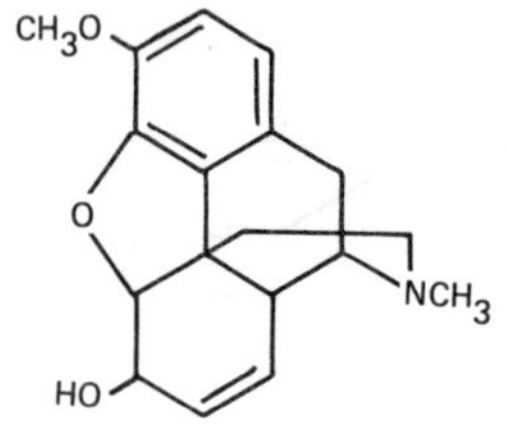

I. Morphine

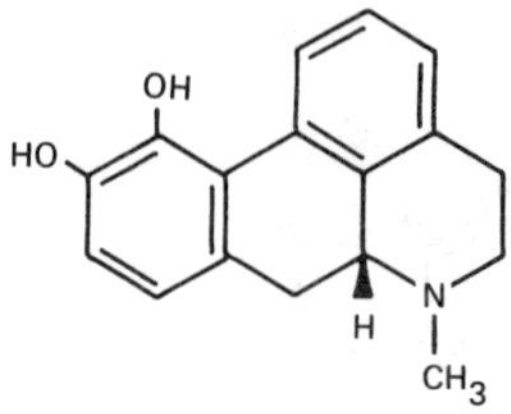

J. Apomorphine

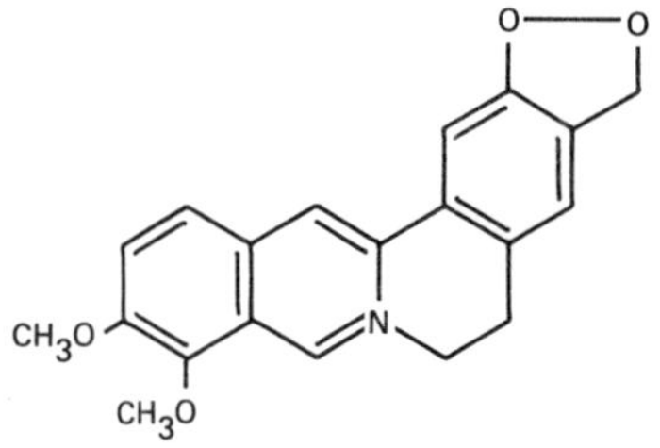

K. Berberine

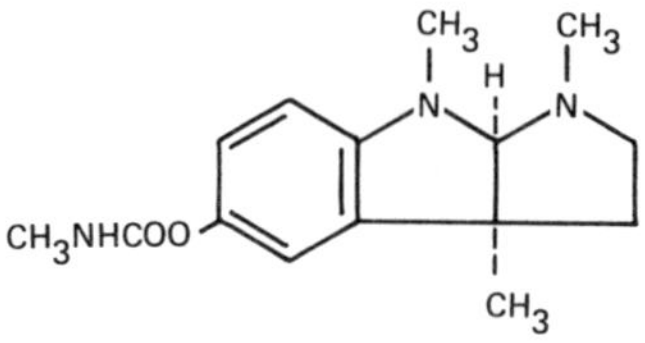

L. Physostigmine

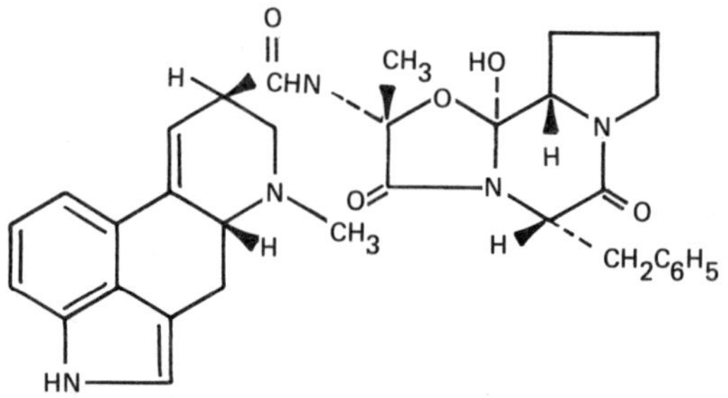

M. Ergotamine

Protoalkaloids

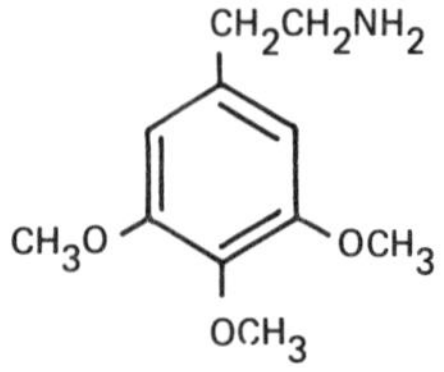

N. Mescaline

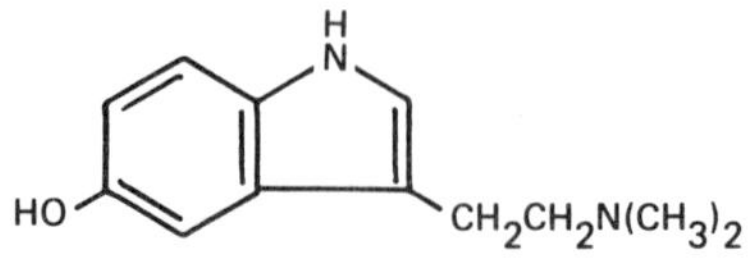

O. Bufotenine

FIGURE 1. Continued.

The majority of the *proto*-alkaloids or biological amines are directly derived from protein amino acids by decarboxylation, the most important being those obtained from the aromatic amino acids phenylalanine, tyrosine, and tryptophan (e.g., mescaline, Figure 1N). The naturally occurring compounds are usually further modified by *N*-methylation and by further hydroxylations of the aromatic ring (e.g., bufotenine, Figure 1O). Although the biological amines are hardly toxic in the generally accepted sense, most produce serious psychological disturbances and hallucinations in extremely small doses. Their use and abuse in modern society has been well documented.[2,17]

Pseudoalkaloids

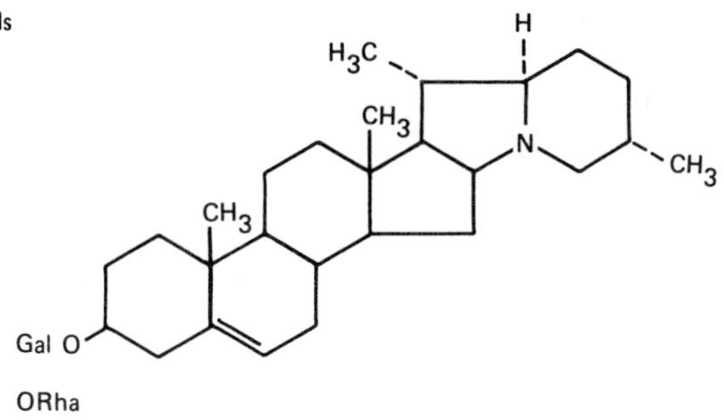

P. Solanine

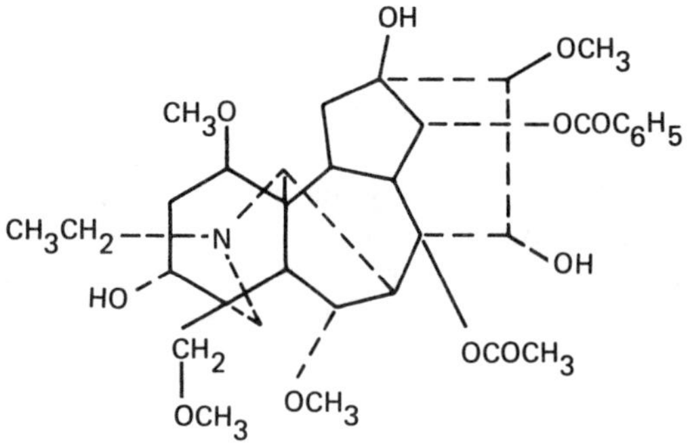

Q. Aconitine

Peptides

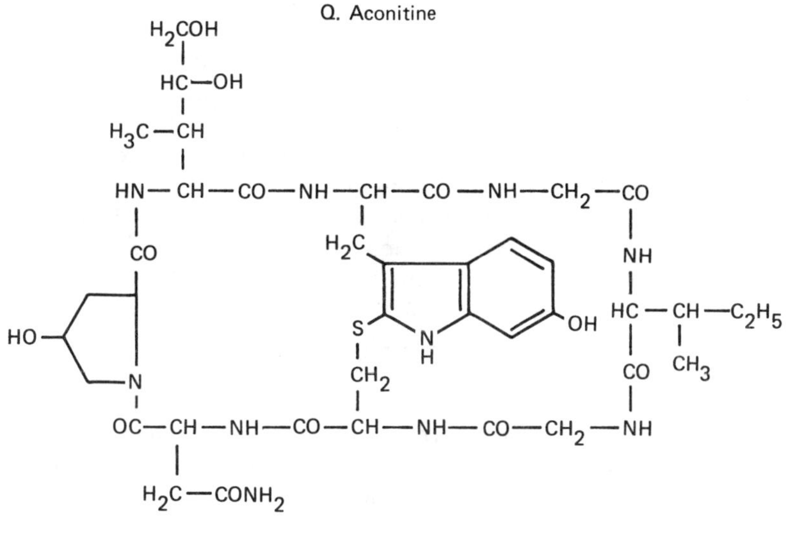

R. α-Amanitin

FIGURE 1. Continued.

Steroidal *pseudo* alkaloids can be as toxic as the complex indole alkaloids. The steroidal group is formed from triterpenoid precursors and the alkaloids formed by the introduction of nitrogen after the formation of this steroidal system. Usually these alkaloids contain complex oligosaccharides attached to the 3-hydroxyl of the triterpenoid nucleus. They include such substances as tomatine and solanine (Figure 1P). Equally toxic are the diterpenoid alkaloids such as taxine from the yew, aconitine (Figure 1Q), and delphine.

Miscellaneous

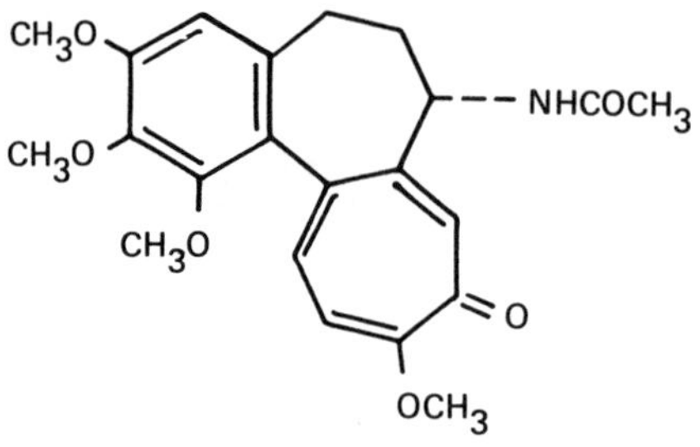

S. Colchicine

FIGURE 1. Continued.

The most important of the peptides toxic to man are those synthesized by the fungi. These are usually cyclic and often contain unusual amino acids or D-forms of normal ones (e.g., amanitin, Figure 1R). By and large, natural peptides are nontoxic, but some may exert toxic properties against other plants.

Other poisonous alkaloids which do not fall readily into any of the above categories include colchicine (Figure 1S) isolated from seeds and corms of *Colchicum autumnale*, a compound which is used in medicine,[9] but can cause kidney and respiratory failure commonly resulting in death if taken in excess.[7,9]

PROTEINS (TABLE 2)

Although proteins are normally regarded as being nutritious, a number are highly toxic if ingested. Perhaps the best known from higher plants is the glycoprotein from precatory bean *Abrus precatorius*, whose attractive bright scarlet seeds contain the highly toxic glycoprotein, abrin.[7,19] Other proteins, though less toxic, may still be fatal if ingested in large amounts. Most appear to be glycoproteins which are akin to the lectins (e.g., Concanavalin A from *Concanavalia ensiformis*, Jack Bean), but others show no hemoglutinating activity, for example ricin from the castor bean.[7,19]

Probably the most troublesome of the toxic proteins in Western countries is the enterotoxin of *Staphylococcus aureus* but although gastrointestinal upsets are common in summer, deaths are rare. However the toxin from *Clostridium botulinum* is one of the most highly toxic proteins known, death occurring in up to two thirds of persons affected.[20]

Proteins on the surface of pollens are undoubtedly responsible for the various allergies known as hay fever and asthma which cause countless lost work and school days during the summer. The proteins induce an immune response in their victim, which results in hypersensitivity reactions when further exposure occurs.[2]

Another toxic protein in plants which has been shown to be fatal in horses and other monogastric animals is the enzyme thiaminase from bracken, *Pteridium aquilinum*.[21] Here, the symptoms are due to thiamine deficiency and death can be averted by administration of the vitamin B_1.[7]

AMINO ACIDS (TABLE 2)

Besides the normal 20-odd protein amino acids, plants produce nearly 400 nonprotein analogues, some of which are extremely toxic.[22] The most important are those causing the disease of lathyrism in man and his domestic animals, which has been

Table 2
PROTEINS AND AMINO ACIDS IN PLANTS TOXIC TO ANIMALS

	Name	Family	Species	Common name	Toxicity	Symptoms
Proteins	Abrin	Leguminosae (Fabaceae)	*Abrus precatorius* L. (seeds)	Jequirity	LD_{50} 0.02 mg/kg i.p. mice humans 0.05 mg	Nausea, diarrhea, circulatory collapse, death
	Ricin	Euphorbiaceae	*Ricinus sanguineus* L. *Ricinus communis* L. (seeds)	Castor oil	LD_{50} 0.4 mg/kg mice	Uremia, convulsions and death
	Thiaminase	Filicinae	*Pteridium aquilinum* (L.) Kuhn *Dryopteris felix-mas* (L.) Schott	Bracken Male fern		Thiamine deficiency
		Sphenopsida	*Equisetum* sp.	Horsetail		
Amino acids	Albizzine	Leguminosae	*Albizzia* sp.			
	Azetidine-2-carboxylic acid	Liliaceae	*Convallaria majalis* L.	Lily of the valley		
	Canavanine	Leguminosae	*Canavalia ensiformis* (L.) D.C.	Jack bean		Mitogenic
	γ-glutamyl-aminopropionitrile	Leguminosae	*Lathyrus* sp.	Indian sweet pea		
	Hypoglycine A	Sapindaceae	*Blighia sapida* Koenig	Akee		

$$\begin{array}{l}\text{CO}-(\text{CH}_2)_2-\text{CH}-\text{COOH}\\|\qquad\qquad\qquad\;\;|\\\text{NH}\qquad\qquad\quad\;\text{NH}_2\\|\\\text{CH}_2-\text{CH}_2-\text{CN}\end{array}$$

A. γ-Glutamylamino propionitrile

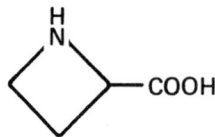

B. Azetidine-2-carboxylic acid

$$\text{NH}_2\text{C} = \text{NH NHO}(\text{CH}_2)_2\text{CHNH}_2\text{CO}_2\text{H}$$

C. Canavanine

FIGURE 2. Some toxic amino acids present in plants.

known since ancient times.[2,7] Ingestion of large amounts of various species of *Lathyrus*, especially *L. sativus* (Indian pea), often eaten in times of famine, produces a paralytic syndrome usually confined to the legs, which can rapidly lead to death. The toxic principle is the γ-glutamyl derivative of amino propionitrile (Figure 2A).

The effect of other nonprotein amino acids undoubtedly could be equally deleterious, but, fortunately, the plants which contain them are rarely eaten by man. Many of these compounds exert their effects by being incorporated into proteins instead of the normal congeners (e.g., azetidine-2-carboxylic acid [Figure 2B] substitutes for proline; canavanine [Figure 2C] for arginine) and thus inhibit many growth processes and result in death if consumed in too large amounts.

TERPENOIDS (TABLE 3)

Many oxygenated sesqui- and diterpenes[23] are as toxic as the steroidal alkaloids.[1,2] Fortunately these compounds appear to be rather rarely found in plants in sufficient quantity to cause dire effects on man or livestock. However, the recent demonstration of the anti-tumor effect of certain of these compounds from the Asteraceae shows their importance, and many of the compounds being screened for anti-tumor cancer activity fall into this group (e.g., vernolepin).[1]

Probably the most troublesome of the diterpenoid derivatives are the grayanotoxins

Table 3
TERPENOIDS IN PLANTS TOXIC TO ANIMALS

Name	Family	Species	Common name	Toxicity	Symptoms
Diterpenoids					
Grayanotoxins	Ericaceae	*Rhododendron* sp.	Rhododendron, azalea		Slow pulse, low blood pressure, convulsions, progressive paralysis, death
	Ericaceae	*Kalmia* sp.	Laurel		
	Ericaceae	*Leucothoe* sp.			
	Ericaceae Thymeliaceae	*Daphne mezereum* L.	Mezereum		Internal bleeding, weakness, coma, death
Phorbol	Euphorbiaceae	*Croton* sp. (seeds)	Hogwort		Purgatives, gastroenteritis
Sesquiterpenes					
Picrotoxin	Menispermaceae	*Amamirta cocculus*, L.		MLD 4 mg/kg i.v. mice	
Illudins	Fungi (Basidiomycete)	*Clitocybe illudens*		LD_{50} 5 mg/kg i.p. mice	
Tremetone	Compositae	*Eupatorium rugosum* Houtt	White snakeroot		Milk sickness, nausea, prostration, trembles

(Figure 3A) of the Ericaceae (*Rhododendron, Kalmia,* and *Leucothoe)* which are extremely important in causing livestock poisoning in the U.S. Other toxic plants containing active diterpenes are *Daphne mezereum* (Thymeliaceae), one of the oldest recorded toxic plants (Dioscorides), and many members of the Euphorbiaceae including *Croton* spp. which contain the active compound phorbol (Figure 3B).[2,7]

Among the toxic sesquiterpenes are picrotoxinin (Figure 3C) from *Anamirta cocculus* and the illudins (Figure 3D) from the mushroom *Clitocybe illudens*. Tremetone (Figure 3E), a toxin from *Eupatorium rugosum* (Compositae), is sequestered in the milk of cattle and thus causes poisoning (milk-sickness) in humans, with a 10 to 25% mortality. It is rumored that Abraham Lincoln's mother died in this way. The plant also affects the animals themselves.[7]

GLYCOSIDES

Most of the compounds which contain one or more hydroxyl groups as part of their structure exist in plants in combined form with various sugars forming what are termed glycosides. In many cases the sugars are the well-known glucose, galactose, and other aldohexoses, but a number of unusual sugars are found, for example, in the cardiac glycosides.

Glycosides are readily hydrolysed by enzymes or by hot mineral acids to yield the sugar(s) and the parent aglycone, which may be a variety of compounds including cyanohydrins, sapogenins, coumarins, and so on. The glycosides therefore are not a *class* of compounds like the amino acids. However, the presence of the sugar moiety often alters substantially the toxicity of the compound to ourselves and other animals, probably by changing the rates of detoxification, excretion, and transport of the functional aglycone to the site of action.

CYANOGENIC GLYCOSIDES (TABLE 4)

Cyanogenic glycosides are themselves nontoxic but on acid or enzymatic hydrolysis yield a sugar (usually glucose and a cyanhydrin or similar compound) which breaks down spontaneously to yield an aldehyde or ketone and hydrogen cyanide (HCN) (Figure 4A).[24,25] Hydrogen cyanide is a potent toxin with LD_{50} in man of about 0.2 to 0.3 mg/kg. Although the poison is not cumulative since man and other animals detoxify the compound to the nontoxic thiocyanate by the action of the liver enzyme rhodanese, nevertheless, plants which contain sufficient amounts of cyanogenic glycosides to yield more than 20 mg HCN per 100 g are dangerous if eaten in relatively small amounts (¼ lb or so). Many of the reports of livestock poisoning are due to their ingestion (e.g., *Lotus corniculatus, Sorghum* spp., etc.). The edible roots of the tropical staple, cassava *(Manihot esculenta),* contain large amounts of linamarin which has to be removed by washing the grated root prior to use.[7,25]

Cyanogenesis was first detected in plants in 1801 in *Prunus amygdalus*. The compound isolated from bitter almonds, amygdalin (mandelonitrile-β-gentiobioside), has recently achieved notoriety as a cancer cure (laetrile). At present over 2000 species are known which produce hydrogen cyanide: most are angiosperms but a few ferns *(Pteridium),* gymnosperms *(Taxus),* and fungi are also known. The majority of cyanogenic flowering plants occur in the super order Rosidae (e.g., in the families Rosaceae, Leguminosae), but examples are also found in other families.

According to the amino acids involved, five main biosynthetic groups of cyanogenic compounds have been found in plants.[25,26] The glycosides, prunasin and amygdalin (Figure 4B), are synthesized from phenylalanine; sambrunigrin and dhurrin (Figure 4C) and taxiphyllin from tyrosine; whereas linamarin (Figure 4D) and lotaustralin (Fig-

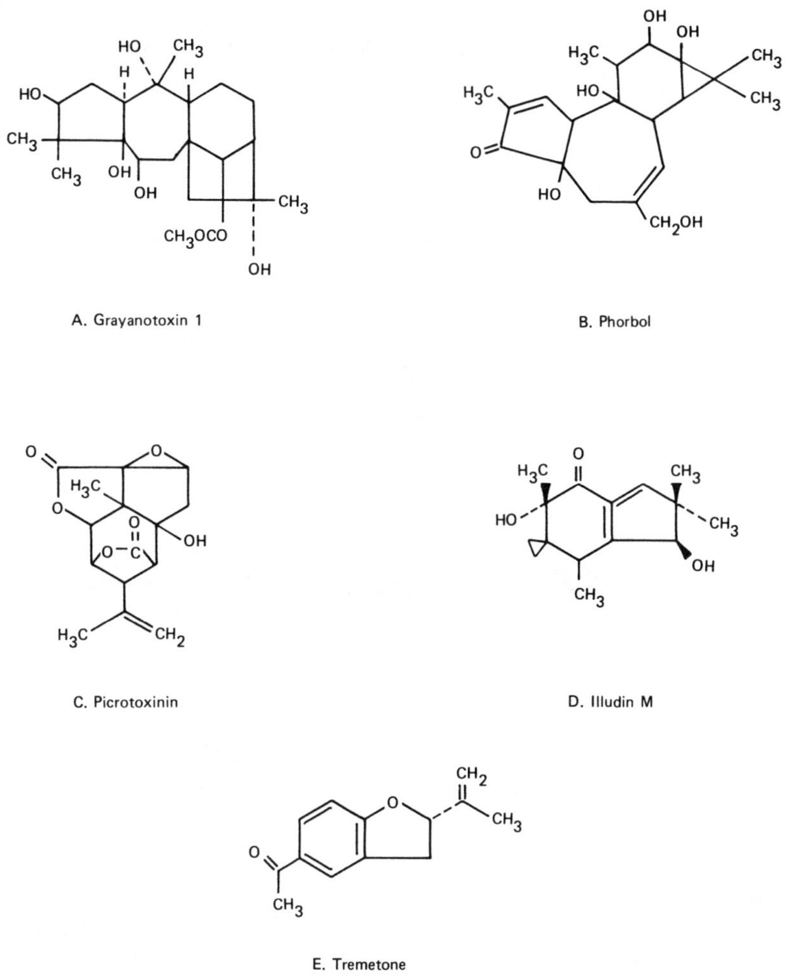

A. Grayanotoxin 1

B. Phorbol

C. Picrotoxinin

D. Illudin M

E. Tremetone

FIGURE 3. Some toxic terpenoids present in plants.

ure 4E) are synthesized from the nonaromatic amino acids valine and isoleucine. Compounds like acacipetalin (Figure 4F) and several cyanolipids (Figure 4G) are leucine-derived cyanogenic plant constituents.

Often cyanogenesis is genetically polymorphic within populations of a given species, i.e., although some individuals will yield HCN on injury, others will not because they lack either the necessary hydrolytic enzyme (most unusual), the glycoside, or both. This fact may have given rise to divergent reports on the toxicity of certain plants.[24]

GLUCOSINOLATES (TABLE 5)

The glucosinolates are a group of sulfur-containing glycosides which also yield toxic constituents on hydrolysis.[27] These are the mustard oils or isothiocyanates, which if ingested in quantity, are toxic to animals. The two most common are allyl isothiocyanate and 3-butenyl isothiocyanate. Fortunately, these mustard oils are so pungent that no fatalities have been reported, but gasteroenteritis may be produced in livestock who ingest large amounts of *Brassica* and related species in the Cruciferae, Resedaceae, and other families in the Capparales. The compounds also occur sporadically in six other families of dicotyledons, but not in any other taxa of plants or in the fungi.

Table 4
PLANTS CONTAINING CYANOGENIC GLYCOSIDES

Name	Family	Species	Common name
Prunasin	Rosaceae	*Prunus* sp.	Cherries
Amygdalin	Rosaceae	*Prunus* sp.	Bitter almonds, apricots, plums, peaches
Dhurrin	Graminae	*Sorghum* sp.	Sorghum
Taxiphyllin	Taxaceae	*Taxus* sp.	Yew
Sambunigrin	Caprifoliaceae	*Sambucus nigra* L.	
Linamarin	Euphorbiaceae	*Manihot esculentum* Crantz	Cassava
	Linaceae	*Linum usitatissimum* L.	Flax
	Leguminosae	*Lotus corniculatus* L.	Bird's foot trefoil
		Trifolium repens L.	White clover
Lotaustralin	Leguminosae	*Lotus australis* L.	Clover
Acacipetalin	Leguminosae	*Acacia* sp.	Acacias
Cyanolipids	Sapindaceae	Many species	
	Boraginaceae (Ehretiaceae)	*Cordia verbenacea* L.	

The type compound is sinigrin from *Sinapis alba* (white mustard), which on hydrolysis (Figure 5A), yields an unstable intermediate which rearranges by loss of sulfate to give the corresponding allyl isothiocyanate. This same reaction is undergone by the other 80-odd compounds in the series, and in a few cases the corresponding nitrile may also be formed.[27]

PROTOANEMONIN GLUCOSIDES (TABLE 6)

Many species of the Ranunculaceae including buttercups and crowfoots (*Ranunculus* spp.), marsh marigolds *(Caltha palustris)*, and anemones *(Anemone nemerosa)* contain a glycoside, ranunculin, which on hydrolysis yields a toxic vesicant volatile oil, protoanemonin.[7,28] This compound slowly dimerizes to the less toxic anemonin (Figure 6A). Again, however, poisoning by buttercups and their allies is rare because the compounds are so distasteful, having an acrid burning taste, that most animals avoid eating ranunculus plants except by accident or through hunger.

CARDIAC GLYCOSIDES AND SAPONINS (TABLE 7)

The cardiac glycosides are the most useful medicinal products obtained directly from higher plants known to man.[7,9] Although the palliative nature of foxglove (*Digitalis purpurea*) has been known for centuries, it was not until the 18th century that its efficiency in dropsy was clearly established by William Withering. Today, in spite of the rapid advances in the production of synthetic medicinals, digitalis (the essential principle and its congeners) is still the drug of choice for cases of congestive heart failure. But the margin between therapeutic and toxic doses is very small, hence cardiac glycosides are used as arrow poison in many parts of the world.

The cardiac glycosides are closely related to the steroids. All possess a 14-hydroxyl group and either a furan (cardenolides) or pyran (bufodienolides) ring at C_{17}. About 500 are known, many containing various unusual sugars at C3 (e.g., lanatoside, Figure 7A).[29] The majority are found in species of the Scrophulariaceae (e.g., digitonin, Figure 7B), Liliaceae (e.g., convallatoxin, Figure 7C), and Apocyanaceae (e.g., oleandrin, Figure 7D).

The saponins are bitter to the taste and form a nonalkaline soapy froth or foam when shaken in water. They are divided into two groups. The noncardioactive steroidal saponins are chemically closely related to the cardiac glycosides and are often found

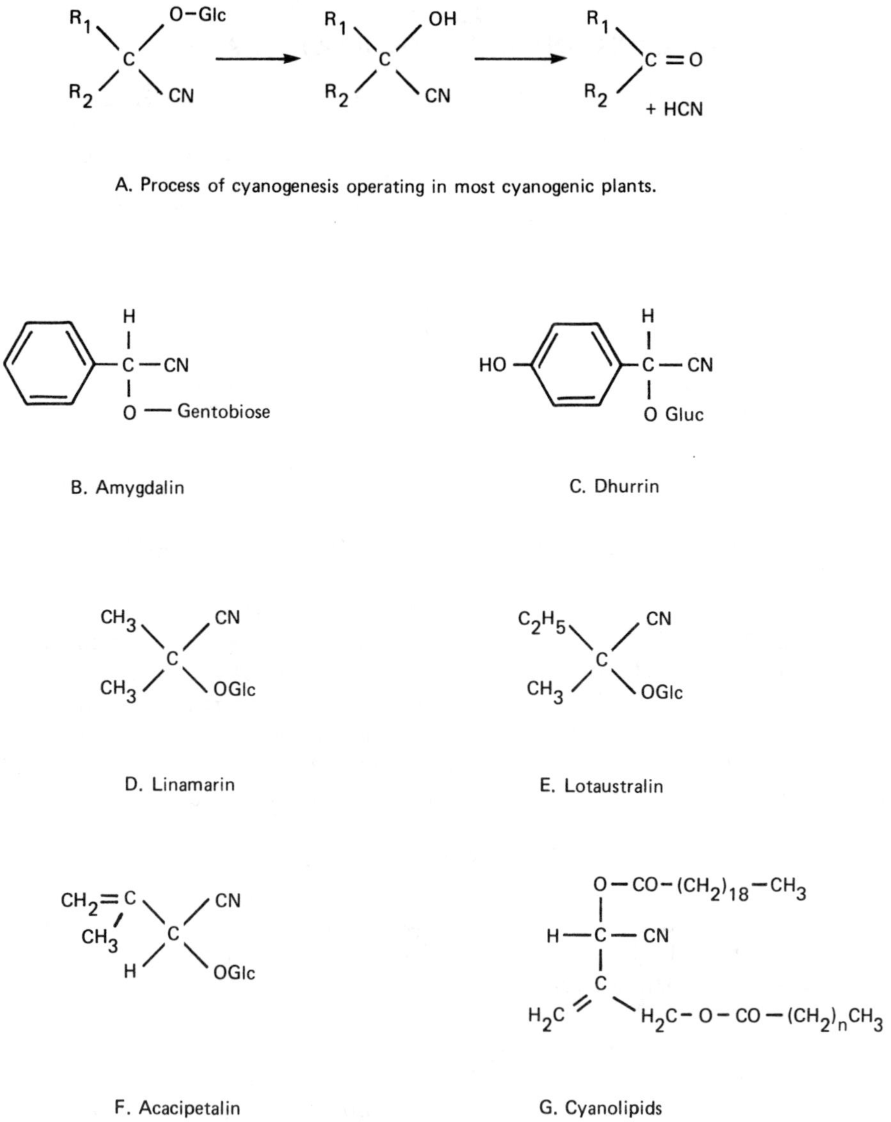

A. Process of cyanogenesis operating in most cyanogenic plants.

B. Amygdalin

C. Dhurrin

D. Linamarin

E. Lotaustralin

F. Acacipetalin

G. Cyanolipids

FIGURE 4. Some cyanogenic glycosides present in plants.

in the same plant. The aglycones of these compounds, e.g., diosgenin (Figure 7E), are used for the preparation of corticosteroids and sex hormones.[2,9,29] The other group of saponins are based on pentacyclic triterpenes, e.g., glycyrrhetic acid (Figure 7F). Both groups have complex sugar derivatives at C_3 and possess a potent hemolytic activity. They are not readily adsorbed into the bloodstream through an uninjured digestive tract and hence are usually nontoxic, but they can cause gastrointestinal upsets in animals if ingested in large quantities. Two plants which are particularly troublesome to livestock because of their saponin content are pokeweed *(Phytolacca americana)* and corn cackle *(Agrostemma githago)*.

POLYKETIDES

The polyketides, par excellence, are the products of fungal metabolism.[30] These compounds formed by head-to-tail condensation of acetic or malonic acid units occur

Table 5
PLANTS CONTAINING GLUCOSINOLATES

Name	Family	Species	Common name
Sinigrin	Cruciferae	Brassica nigra (L.) Koch	Black mustard
		Brassica juncea Cosson	Indian mustard
		Sinapis alba L.	White mustard
Gluconasturtiin	Cruciferae	Nasturtium officinale R. Br	Water cress
Glucoibervin	Cruciferae	Iberis sempervirens L.	
Glucobrassicin	Cruciferae	Brassica oleracea L.	Cabbage
Gluconapin	Cruciferae	Brassica napus L.	Rape
Glucobrassicanapin	Cruciferae	Brassica napus L.	Rape
Gluconringiin	Cruciferae	Conringia orientalis (L.) Dumart	
Glucobarbarin	Resedaceae	Reseda luteola L.	
Glucotropaeolin	Tropaeolaceae	Tropaeolum majus L.	Nasturtium

in all higher plants and some bacteria, but the diversity of structure in this class of compounds is symptomatic of the kingdom Fungi. Many of the compounds of this type are toxic to lower organisms, e.g., patulin, grisofulvin, tetracyclines, and the various lichen acids, but the most important toxic compounds to man are the nonaketides, the aflatoxins which are formed on peanut meal infected by *Aspergillus flavus* and *A. versicolor* used in animal feeds (aflatoxin B_1 LD_{50} orally duckling 0.36 mg/kg).[31]

MISCELLANEOUS (TABLE 8)

There are many other classes of compounds which have been shown to be toxic to man and other animals. Because of their diversity of structure it is useful to group them in terms of the deleterious effects they cause.

Compounds Affecting the Skin[2,32]

By far the most dreaded of plants in the northern U.S. are the poison oak, ivy, and sumac, all of which belong to the genus *Toxicodendron* (Anarcardiaceae). These plants contain lipophenolics (e.g., urishiols, Figure 8A) which induce an immune response resulting in itchy skin in mild cases to death from respiratory failure when the response is severe. There is no real cure, although cortisone or its analogues may relieve the symptoms.

Many other compounds can cause dermititis, especially the mono- and sesquiterpenes, and, of course, acetylcholine and histamine which are found in the stinging hairs of the Urticaceae (nettles) and many other plants.[2,9]

Many compounds affect the skin by inducing a sensitivity to sunlight. When so affected, the animal may show gross erythema and pruritis followed by edematous suffusions and skin necrosis. This photodynamic effect is usually not lethal in itself, but deaths are frequent from secondary infection or liver damage.[2] The major cause of photodermatitis in animals is from ingestion of St. John's Wort (*Hypericum perforatum*, Guttiferae) which contains the dianthrone, hypericin (Figure 8B). Incomplete catabolism of chlorophyll may result in the accumulation of fluorescent phylloerythrin, responsible for photosensitization by many of the grasses and fodder plants, which under normal conditions are harmless.

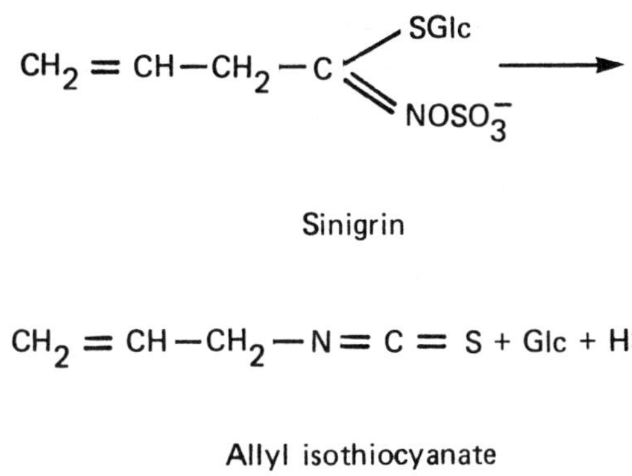

$$CH_2 = CH-CH_2-C \begin{matrix} \diagup SGlc \\ \diagdown NOSO_3^- \end{matrix} \longrightarrow$$

Sinigrin

$$CH_2 = CH-CH_2-N = C = S + Glc + HSO_4^-$$

Allyl isothiocyanate

FIGURE 5. Formation of mustard oils from glucosinolates.

Compounds Affecting Reproduction[2,33]

Substances in plants which cause reduced fertility in domestic animals are the isoflavones (e.g., formononetin, Figure 8C and genistein), found in *Trifolium subterraneum* Leguminosae, which are responsible for the undesirable increase in spontaneous abortion in sheep in Australia. Certain steroidal saponins, alkaloids, and cardiac glycosides may have similar effects.

Hallucinogens[17]

The majority of natural hallucinogenic plants which are used today contain simple biological amines based on β-phenylethylamine (mescaline, Figure 8D from *Lophophora williamsii)*, tryptamine (psilocybin from *Conocybe* spp.), or their derivatives the β-carbolines (harmine, etc. in *Banisteropsis coapi)* and more complex indoles from lysergic acid (from *Claviceps purpurea* and *Ipomoea violacea).*

Nevertheless, a number of other classes of "mind-bending" drugs exist such as Δ^6-tetrahydra cannabinol (Figure 8E), the main active compound in marijuana (pot), *Cannabis sativa*, and a number of common alkaloids (cytosine) and the phenylpropenes (myristicin from *Myristica fragrans).* None of these compounds are toxic taken in "normal" amounts, but can lead to death if ingested in excess.

Inorganic Compounds[7]

Many plants sequester from the soil high concentrations of poisonous inorganic elements (e.g., selenium, copper, lead, molybdenum). *Astragalus* species (Leguminosae) are examples of selenium concentrators and many species are toxic because of this.

Oxalates[2]

The simple organic acid oxalate (LD_{50} dogs 1 g/kg) accumulates in many plants, especially in the Polygonaceae *(Rheum, Rumex)*, Chenopodiaceae *(Beta, Halogeton, Salsola)*, and Oxalidaceae *(Oxalis).* It occurs in plants in the form of soluble (sodium and potassium) and insoluble (calcium) oxalates or acid oxalates. This compound affects calcium metabolism and possible blocking of the renal function by precipitation of insoluble oxalates, and deaths have been reported.

Polyacetylenes[34]

These compounds are mainly found in the Umbelliferae and Compositae. Two toxic acetylenes from the Umbelliferae are oenanthetoxin (Figure 8F) from *Oenantha crocata* and cicutoxin from *Circuta virosa*. These are convulsant poisons isolated from the roots.

Table 6
PLANTS WHICH CONTAIN PROTOANEMONIN GLUCOSIDES

Ranunculaceae	*Caltha palustris* L.	Marsh marigold
	Anenome sp.	Windflower
	Ranunculus sp.	Buttercups, crowfoots
	Clematis vitalba L.	Travellers' joy

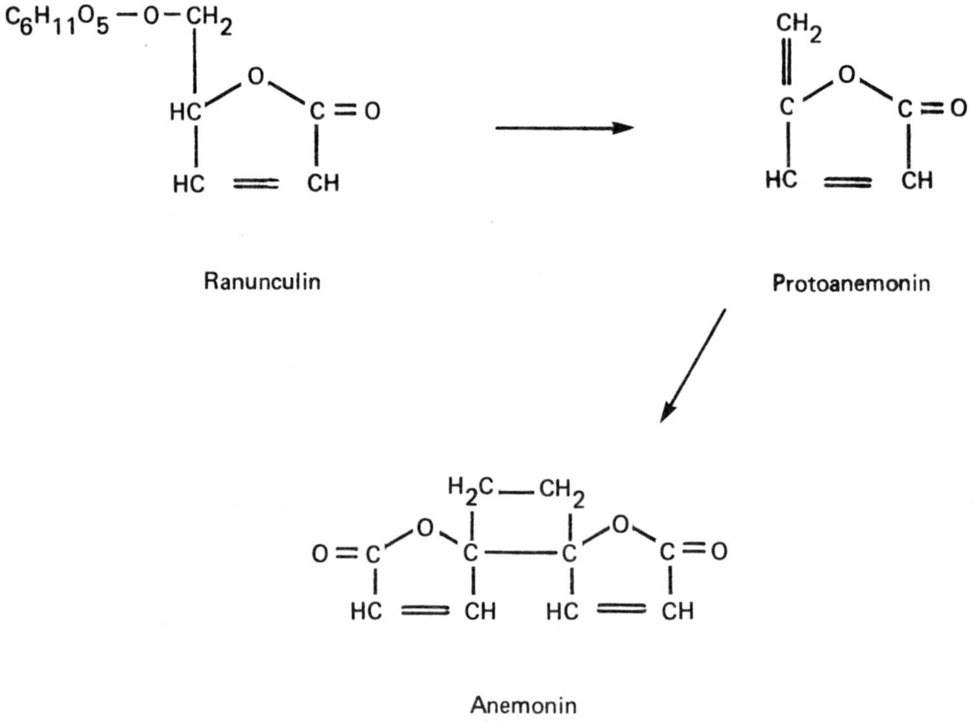

FIGURE 6. Formation of protoanemonin and anemonin from a protoanemonin glycoside.

Others[2,7]

Two other unrelated compounds should be mentioned: gossypol (Figure 8G) from *Gossypium* species, toxic to nonruminants by affecting the oxygen binding capacity of hemoglobin; and dicoumarol (Figure 8H), an artifact produced in spoiled hay from plants containing coumarin (e.g., *Melilotus officinalis*), which reduces blood clotting when ingested.

Many other compounds are only marginally toxic, but can affect young animals if fed in large amounts. For example, tannins, which are present in ferns, gymnosperms, and most woody angiosperms can cause serious protein deficiency and plants containing them (e.g., *Quercus*) are reported to be associated with various cancerous conditions of the esophagus.[35] Many of the Dichopetalaceae accumulate fluoroacetic acid (LD_{50} 2.5 mg/kg), which is highly toxic to livestock as it may be incorporated into lipids and interfere with normal metabolism.

Table 7
CARDIAC GLYCOSIDES AND SAPONINS IN PLANTS TOXIC TO ANIMALS

Name	Occurrence Family	Species	Common name	Toxicity	Symptoms
Cardiac glycosides					
Calotropin	Asclepiadaceae	*Asclepias curassavica* L.	Milkweed	LD cats 0.12 mg/kg	Act directly on heart musculature; nausea, dizziness, blurred vision, and diarrhea
Convallatoxins	Liliaceae	*Convallaria majalis* L.	Lily of the Valley	MLD frogs 0.3 mg/kg	
Scillaren A	Liliaceae	*Urginea maritima* (L.) Baker	Squill		Act directly on heart musculature; nausea, dizziness, blurred vision, and diarrhea
Digitoxins	Scrophulariaceae	*Scrophularia aquatica* L.	Water figwort	LD_{50} rats 0.9 mg/kg	Act directly on heart musculature; nausea, dizziness, blurred vision, and diarrhea
	Scrophulariaceae	*Digitalis purpurea* L.	Foxglove		Act directly on heart musculature; nausea, dizziness, blurred vision, and diarrhea
Lanatoside A	Scrophulariaceae	*Digitalis lanata* Erh.			Act directly on heart musculature; nausea, dizziness, blurred vision, and diarrhea
Oleandrin	Apocynaceae	*Nerium oleander* L.	Oleander	LD_{50} cats 0.32 mg/kg	Act directly on heart musculature; nausea, dizziness, blurred vision, and diarrhea
Saponins					
Diosgenin	Dioscoreaceae	*Dioscorea tokoro* Makino			Severe gastroenteritis; gastro-intestinal irritation
Glycyrrhetic acid	Leguminosae	*Glycyrrhiza glabra* L.			
Hederagenin	Araliaceae	*Hedera helix* L.	English ivy		
Medicagenic acid	Papilonaceae	*Medicago sativa* L.	Lucerne alfalfa		
Saponarin	Caryophyllaceae	*Saponaria officinalis* L.	Soapwort		
	Caryophyllaceae	*Agrostemma githago* L.	Corn cockle		
Phytolaccic acid	Phytolaccaceae	*Phytolacca sp.* L.	Pokeweed		

Cardiac glycosides

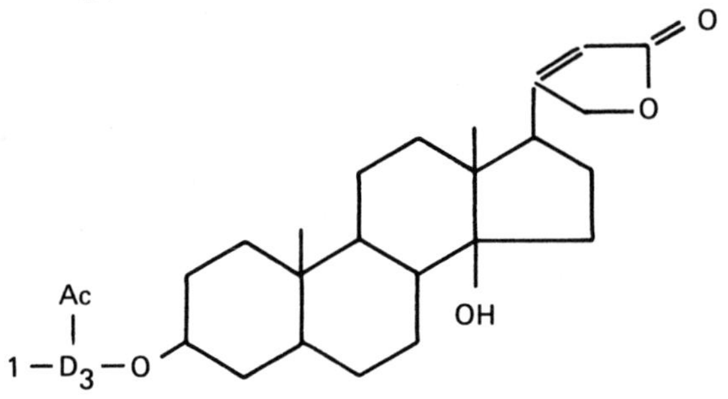

A. Lanatoside A (D = digitoxose)
(G = glucose)

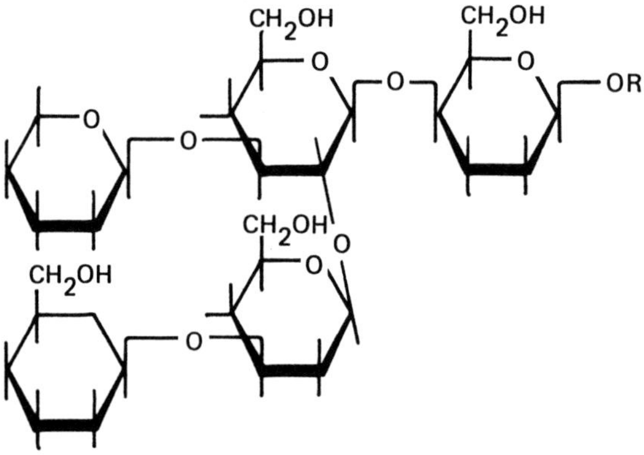

B. Digitonin

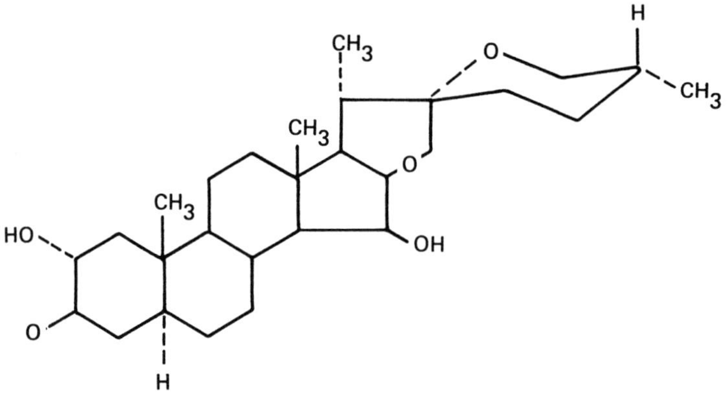

R = digitogenin

FIGURE 7. Some cardiac glycosides and saponins in plants toxic to animals.

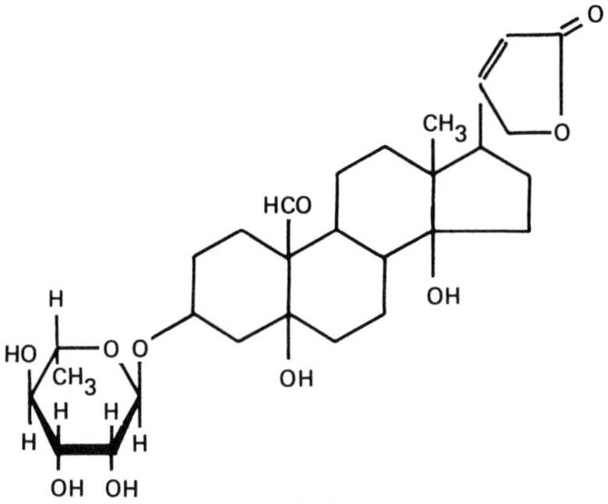

C. Convallatoxin

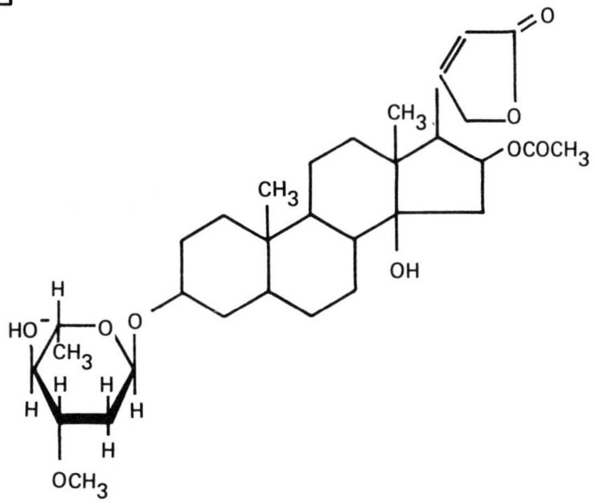

D. Oleandrin

Saponins

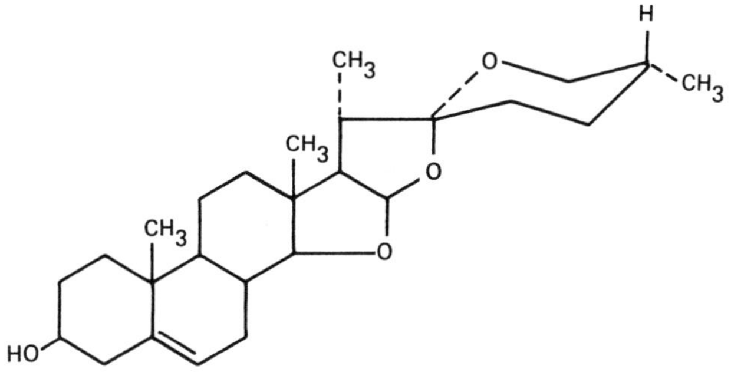

E. Diosgenin

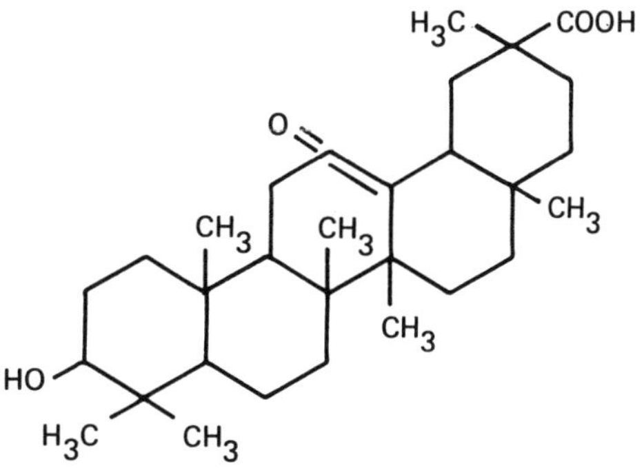

F. Glycyrrhetic acid

FIGURE 7. Continued.

Table 8
MISCELLANEOUS COMPOUNDS IN PLANTS TOXIC TO ANIMALS

Type name	Family	Species	Common name	Toxicity	Symptoms
Skin					
Urushiol	Anarcardiaceae	*Toxicodendron radicans* (L.) Kuntze	Poison ivy		Dermatitis; mucous and alimentary canal membranes may be affected
Photosensitizers					
Fagopyrin	Liliaceae	*Narthecium ossifragum* (L.) Huds	Bog asphodel		Induces sensitivity to sunlight
Fagopyrin	Polygonaceae	*Fagopyrum sagittatum* Gilib	Buckwheat		Induces sensitivity to sunlight
Hypericin	Guttiferae	*Hypericum perforatum* L.	St. John's Wort		Induces sensitivity to sunlight
Psoralen	Umbelliferae	*Cymopterus watsonii* Rafin	Spring parsley		Induces sensitivity to sunlight
Reproduction					
Formononetin	Leguminosae	*Trifolium subterranean* L.	Clover		Increases the rate of spontaneous abortion
Genistein	Leguminosae	*Trifolium subterranean* L.	Clover		Increases the rate of spontaneous abortion
Hallucinogens					
Cannabinol	Cannabidaceae	*Cannabis sativa* L.	Marijuana or hemp		Hallucinogentic dreamlike state
Harmine	Malpighiaceae	*Banisteropsis coapi* C. B. Rob and Small			
Lysergic acid	Fungi (Ascomycete)	*Claviceps purpurea* (Fr.) Tul	Ergot		Madness, delirium, convulsions
Lysergic acid	Convolvulaceae	*Ipomoea violacea* L.	Morning glory		
Mescaline	Cactaceae	*Lophophora williamsii* Coult	Peyote		
Myristicin	Myristicaceae	*Myristica fragrans* R. Br	Nutmeg		

Psilocybin	Fungi (Basidiomycete)	*Coenocybe* sp.		
Inorganics				
Selenium	Leguminosae	*Astragalus* sp.	Vetches	Anorexia, depression; death through respiratory and myocardial failure
Organics				
Oxalates	Araceae	*Arisaema triphyllum* (L.) Schott	Jack-in-the pulpit	Dullness, colic, depression, prostration, and coma
Oxalates	Araceae	*Symplocarpus foetidus* (L.) Salisl.	Skunk cabbage	Dullness, colic, depresssion, prostration, and coma
Oxalates	Chenopodiaceae	*Beta* sp.	Sugar beet	Dullness, colic, depression, prostration, and coma
Oxalates	Chenopodiaceae	*Halogeton* sp.	Mangolds	Dullness, colic, depression, prostration, and coma
Oxalates	Chenopodiaceae	*Salsola* sp.	Dumb cane	Dullness, colic, depression, prostration, and coma
Oxalates	Oxalidaceae	*Oxalis* sp.	Sorrels	Dullness, colic, depression, prostration, and coma
Oxalates	Polygonaceae	*Rheum* sp.	Rhubarb	Dullness, colic, depression, prostration, and coma
Acetylenes				
Cicrutoxin	Umbelliferae	*Circuta virosa* L.	Water hemlock	Violent convulsions
Oenanthotoxin	Umbelliferae	*Oenantha crocata* L.	Water dropwort	Violent convulsions
Others				
Dicoumarol	Leguminosae	*Melilotus officinalis* Lam.	Sweet clover	LD_{50} rats 5.0 g/kg orally Hemorrhagic diseases; bleed to death both internally or externally
Gossypol	Malvaceae	*Gossypium* sp.	Cotton	LD_{50} rats 2.57 g/kg orally Widespread congestion and edema; progressive heart failure
Fluoroacetic acid	Dichapetalaceae	*Dichapetalum* sp.		
Tannins	Fagaceae	*Quercus robur* L.	Oak	Cancer of the esophagous, protein deficiency

238 CRC Handbook of Naturally Occurring Food Toxicants

Skin

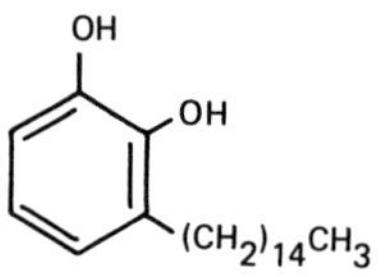

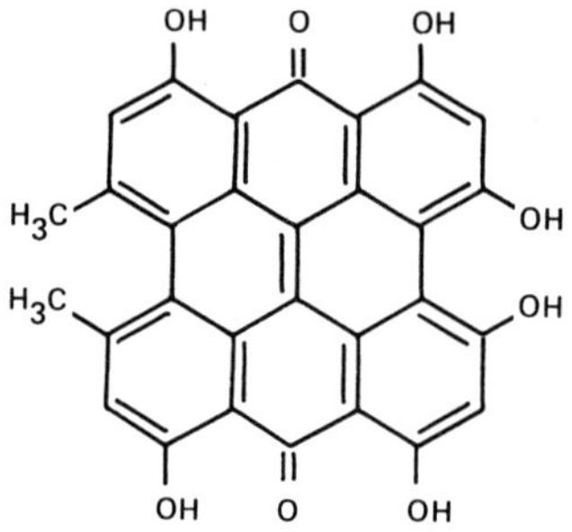

B. Hypericin

Reproduction

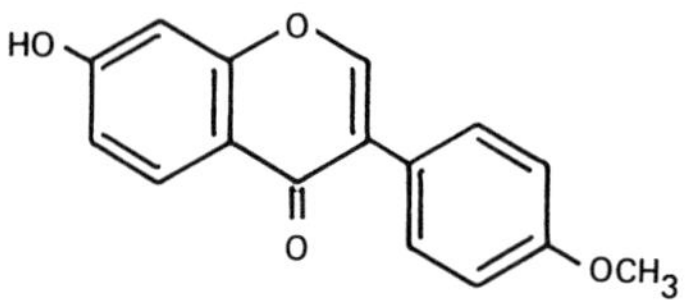

C. Formononetin

Hallucinogenic

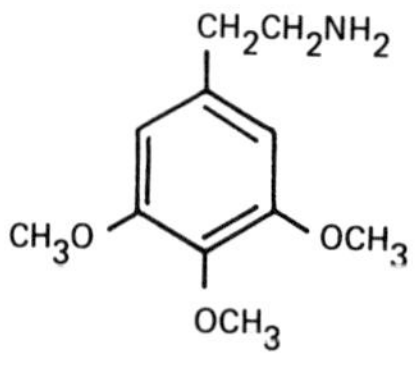

D. Mescaline

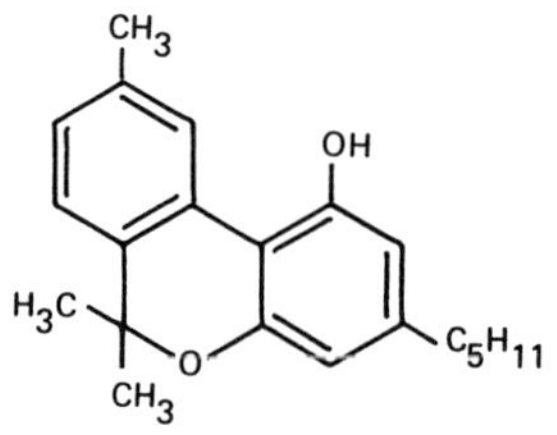

E. Cannabinol

FIGURE 8. Some miscellaneous compounds in plants toxic to animals.

Polyacetylenes

$$HOCH_2CH = CH(C \equiv C)_2 (CH=CH_2) (CH_2)_2 CHOH (CH_2)_2 CH_3$$

F. Oenanthetoxin

Others

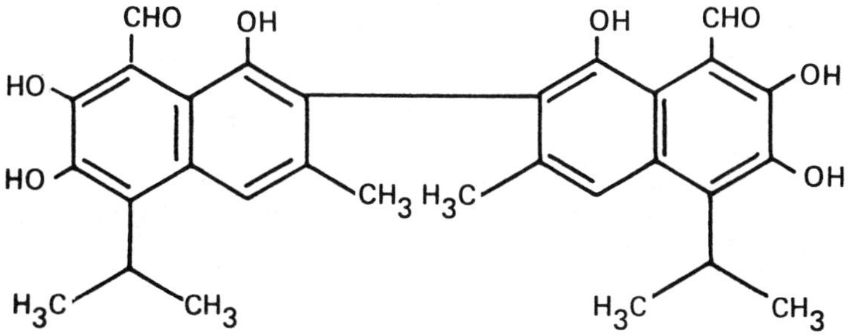

G. Gossypol

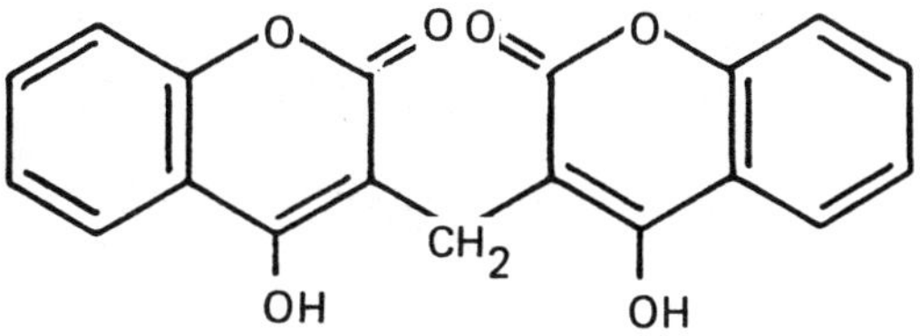

H. Dicoumarol

FIGURE 8. Continued.

REFERENCES

1. **Swain, T.**, *Plants in the Development of Modern Medicine,* Harvard University Press, Cambridge, 1972.
2. **Lewis, W. H. and Elvin-Lewis, M. P. F.**, *Medical Botany — Plant's Affecting Man's Health,* Wiley-Interscience, New York, 1977, 11—63.
3. **Geissman, T. A. and Crout, D. H. G.**, *Organic Chemistry of Secondary Metabolism,* W. H. Freeman, San Francisco, 1969.
4. **Luckner, M.**, *Secondary Metabolism in Plants and Animals,* Chapman and Hall, London, 1972, 259—336.

5. Levin, D. A., The chemical defenses of plants to pathogens and herbivores, *Ann. Rev. Ecol. Syst.*, 7, 121—159, 1976.
6. Swain, T., Secondary plant compounds as protective agents, *Ann. Rev. Plant Physiol.*, 28, 479—501, 1977.
7. Kingsbury, J. M., *Poisonous plants of the United States and Canada*, Prentice-Hall, Englewood Cliffs, New Jersey, 1964, 70—503.
8. *Merck Index*, 9th ed., Merck, Rahway, New Jersey, 1976.
9. Meyers, F. M., Jawetz, E., and Goldfein, A., *Medical Pharmacology*, Lange, Los Altos, Calif., 1974.
10. Hughes, D. W. and Genest, K., Alkaloids, in *Phytochemistry*, Vol. 2, Miller, L. P., Ed., Van Nostrand Rheinhold, New York, 1973, 118—170.
11. Manske, R. H. F., *The Alkaloids*, Vols. I and XII, Academic Press, New York, 1950 and 1970.
12. Pelletier, S. W., *Chemistry of the Alkaloids*, Van Nostrand Rheinhold, New York, 1970.
13. Raffauf, R. F., *A Handbook of Alkaloids and Alkaloid Containing Plants*, Wiley-Interscience, New York, 1970.
14. Hegnauer, R., Comparative phytochemistry of alkaloids, in *Comparative Phytochemistry*, Swain, T., Ed., Academic Press, New York, 1966, 211—230.
15. Levin, D. A. and York, B. M., Jr., The toxicity of plant alkaloids: an ecogeographic perspective, *Biochem. Syst. Ecol.*, 6, 1978, 61—76.
16. Swain, T., *Comprehensive Biochemistry*, Vol. 29A, Elsevier, Amsterdam, 1974, 279.
17. Schultes, R. E. and Hofmann, A., *The Botany and Chemistry of Hallucinogens*, Charles C Thomas, Springfield, Ill., 1973.
18. Airy-Shaw, M. K., *A Dictionary of the Flowering Plants and Ferns*, 8th ed., J. C. Willis, Ed., Cambridge University Press, London, 1973.
19. Harborne, J. B., *Introduction to Ecological Biochemistry*, Academic Press, London, 1977, 58—82.
20. Schuhardt, V. T., *Pathogenic Microbiology*, Lippincott, New York, 1978.
21. Evans, W. C., Bracken thiaminase-mediated neurotoxic syndromes, *Bot. J. Linn. Soc.*, 73, 113—132, 1976.
22. Fowden, L. B., The non-protein amino acids of plants, in *Progress in Phytochemistry*, Vol. 11, Reinhold, L. and Liwschitz, T., Eds., Interscience, London, 1970, 203—266.
23. Runeckles, V. C. and Mabry, T. J., Terpenoids: structure, biogenesis and distribution, in *Recent Advances in Phytochemistry*, Academic Press, New York, 1973.
24. Jones, D. A., Cyanogenic glucosides and their function, in *Phytochemical Ecology*, Harborne, J. B., Ed., Academic Press, London, 1972, 103—124.
25. Siegler, D. S., Isolation and characterization of naturally occurring cyanogenic compounds, *Phytochemistry*, 14, 9—29, 1975.
26. Hegnauer, R., Cyanogenic compounds as systematic markers in the Tracheophyta, *Plant Syst. Evol.*, Suppl. 1, 191—209, 1977.
27. Kjaer, A., Glucosinolates in the Cruciferae, in *The Biology and Chemistry of the Cruciferae*, Vaughan, J. G., Macleod, A. G., and Jones, B. M. G., Eds., Academic Press, London, 1976, 207—220.
28. Ruijgrok, H. W. L., The distribution of ranunculin, in *Comparative Phytochemistry*, Swain, T., Ed., Acacemic Press, London, 1966, 175—186.
29. Newman, A. A., *Chemistry of Terpenes and Terpenoids*, Academic Press, London, 1972.
30. Turner, W. B., *Fungal Metabolites*, Academic Press, New York, 1971.
31. Moss, M. O., Aflatoxins and related mycotoxins, *Phytochemical Ecology*, Harborne, J. B., Ed., Academic Press, London, 1972, 125—144.
32. Mitchell, J. C., Contact allergies from plants, *Rec. Adv. Phytochem.*, 9, 119—138, 1975.
33. Shutt, D. A., The effects of plant oestrogens on animal reproduction, *Endeavour*, 35, 110—113, 1976.
34. Sørensen, N. A., Polyacetylenes in the Compositae, in *The Biology and Chemistry of the Compositae*, Heywood, V. H., Harborne, J. B., and Turner, B. L., Eds., Academic Press, London, 1977.
35. Swain, T., Tannins and lignins, in *Herbivores: Their Interrelationships with Plant Secondary Constituents*, Rosenthal, G. A. and Janzen, D. H., Eds., Academic Press, New York, 1979.

ALKALOIDS IN TALL FESCUE AND REED CANARYGRASS: A REVIEW*

A. W. Hovin and R. C. Buckner

ALKALOIDS AND LIVESTOCK PROBLEMS

Livestock disorders and low productivity may result when animals graze certain pasture grasses. Fescue toxicity or "fescue foot", poor animal performance or "summer syndrome", and fat necrosis are some physiological disorders observed in cattle grazing tall fescue, *Festuca arundinacea* Schreb.[1,2] Poor animal performance associated with the symptoms of loss of weight and/or milk production during summer, generally referred to as summer syndrome, is the most important response of animals grazing tall fescue.[3] Alkaloids in the plant, mycotoxins, and other secondary metabolites from systemic fungi, and organic acids have been implicated.[4-10] Alkaloids have also been implicated in the etiology of "ryegrass staggers" in the closely related genus *Lolium*.[11] Usually alkaloids produced by a plant are closely related structurally; however, tall fescue produces two types of alkaloids. One type (N-acetyl and N-formyl loline) contains a pyrrolizidine nucleus; the other type contains a diazaphenanthrene nucleus (perloline and perlolidine).[3] In late summer, perloline levels of 2000 to 3000 µg/g dried forage have been observed frequently in tall fescue pastures.[12,13] Perlolidine levels of 800 to 1300 µg/g and levels of loline derivatives of 1000 to 2000 µg/g have also been observed in tall fescue pastures during summer.[3] In tall fescue, leaf blades had 44% as much perloline and 61% as much total alkaloids as the stems when sampled at the dough stage in June.[12] The concentration of total alkaloids in mature shoots was 89% of that found in shoots of pasture plants sampled in June. Several quantitative procedures have been developed for determination of total alkaloid concentration.[2,14,18]

Mycotoxins may be involved in the occasional outbreak of a gangrenous-type poisoning resulting when cattle graze tall fescue.[6,7] Rumen content of fistulated steers that subsequently developed fescue toxicosis showed a high fungal population count, particularly of *Aspergillus terreus* Thom.[7] The systemic, claviceptaceous fungus *Balansia epichloe* (Weese), was isolated from smutgrass (*Sporobolus poiretii* [Roehm. & Schult.] Hitchc.) grown in 'Kentucky 31' tall fescue pastures.[9] The fungus produces ergot-type indole alkaloids but has not been causally associated with fescue toxicity.[19] The fungus is parasitic on several economically important forage grasses grown in Southeastern U.S.[20] If fungi are not responsible for fescue toxicity or fescue foot, then the causative agent is produced in the plant. Research at the University of Missouri demonstrated that the ethanol-extracted anion fraction of tall fescue hay infused into cattle caused fescue foot symptoms.[10,21]

The endophytic and seed-transmitted fungus *Sphacelia typhina* (Pers.) Socc., the imperfect stage of *Epichloe typhina* (Fr.) Tul., has been isolated from several tall fescue cultivars, including a low-perloline experimental strain.[22] This fungus has been isolated from repeated sampling of tall fescue in Kentucky and Georgia and from tall fescue and orchardgrass (*Dactylis glomerata* L.) pastures in Maryland and Missouri but not from Minnesota. Observations of poor performance of cattle grazing tall fescue and incidence of *E. typhina* in the grass suggested that the phytopathogen might be involved in the summer syndrome malady of cattle.[23]

Evidence of low cattle productivity caused by tall fescue has come from feeding studies and from direct observations at grazing trials.[24] The grass has several good

---

* Contribution from Minnesota Agricultural Experiment Station, Scientific Series 10, 413. Contribution from Kentucky Agricultural Experiment Station; 78-3-126.

nutritional characteristics.[13,25] Feeding trials with sheep resulted in lower voluntary intake but higher digestibility when animals were offered low-, as compared to high-perloline strains.[26] Contrary to expectation, steers assigned to the low-perloline strain had poor average daily gains and showed signs of emaciation, rough haircoat, elevated respiration rate, and less tolerance to heat stress than steers grazing a high-perloline strain.[27] In a 2-year study with lactating dairy cows fed soilage of Kentucky 31, high and low perloline strains, cows consuming the low perloline strain had the lowest intake and milk production.[28] These studies indicated that in the selection for low perloline, compound(s) more toxic and detrimental to animal performance were increased in the low perloline strain. Recent research showed a direct positive association of *E. typhina* with N-acetyl and N-formyl loline production in tall fescue.[29,30] When tall fescue seeds and forage containing different levels of the loline alkaloids were fed to young cattle under high ambient temperature stress, a direct positive association was found for the alkaloid levels and the summer syndrome symptoms of the cattle.[31,32] Thus, N-acetyl and N-formyl loline concentrations are related to *E. typhina* infestation, and toxic effects to the animal are potentiated by elevated environmental temperature.[31]

In tall fescue, concentration of perloline is negatively associated with *in vitro* cellulose disappearance by inhibiting rumen fermentation.[33,34] Perloline added to the diet of sheep reduced apparent crude protein and cellulose disappearance and increased body temperature.[35] The derivative perlolidine was inhibitory to cellulose digestion and rumen bacterial protein production only at high concentration.[36] Rumen bacteria have been shown to detoxify the pyrrolizidine alkaloids in tall fescue.[37] It is evident, therefore, that no single factor in tall fescue can account for the physiological disorders observed when cattle graze this species.

Of the 11 reported alkaloids in the genus *Phalaris*, 10 belong to the indole group which includes gramine, tryptamines, and β-carboline derivatives; the other is an unrelated phenol, hordenine.[38-41] Alkaloids in the former group are biosynthetic derivatives of the amino acid tryptophan, whereas hordenine is synthesized from tyrosine.[42,43]

The tryptamine alkaloids in *Phalaris* species have been implicated as the cause of "phalaris staggers" and may also be associated with bovine emphysema.[44,45] Sheep showing the phalaris staggers syndrome have been observed when grazing Hardinggrass, *Phalaris aquatica* L. (*P. tuberosa* var. *stenoptera* [Hack.] Hitchc.), in California. The disorder occurs only in certain areas and is much more severe in some seasons. Both soil nutrients such as cobalt and climatic factors have been investigated, but the cause of the etiology has not been clarified as yet.[46] The incidence of phalaris staggers has not been reported in North America for animals grazing reed canarygrass, *Phalaris arundinacea* L. Over long time periods, ruminants may consume large quantities of reed canarygrass without showing symptoms of these diseases, but with incidence of severe diarrhea and weight loss.[47,48]

The strong negative correlation in reed canarygrass between palatability to livestock and total indole alkaloid concentration has had biological significance in that animals forced to consume unpalatable genotypes have had either reduced intake, reduced daily liveweight gains, or both.[48-50] Total alkaloid concentration was highly negatively correlated with average daily gains by lambs and steers ($r = -0.90$ or above for each of 3 grazing seasons).[47] In a similar study with lambs, the relationship was $r = -0.97$ (year 1) and $r = -0.66$ (year 2).[48] Furthermore, animals in these trials had more diarrhea when grazing plants containing tryptamine-carboline as compared to gramine-containing plants. The indole alkaloid concentration threshold is about 0.20% dry weight or above, at which lambs will show reduced gain when grazing reed canarygrass.[48]

The forage quality of reed canarygrass is comparable to that of other forage grasses.[25,50] The alkaloids do not usually affect *in vitro* fermentation of cellulose or forage dry matter.[41,51] The concentrations of indole alkaloids in the forage are highest in the leaf blade and lowest in the stem.[52] Concentration of hordenine, on the other hand, is highest in the sheath fraction of first-growth forage.[53,54] Concentration of hordenine and gramine may be two times and ten times higher, respectively, in regrowth forage as compared to first growth of the season.[54]

EFFECT OF PLANT GENOTYPE

Comparisons of cultivars and genetic studies of alkaloid types and concentration levels have been reported for *Festuca, Lolium,* and *Phalaris.* Perloline concentration in tall fescue was shown to differ among and within cultivars.[12,13] Perloline levels of 6700 µg/g of dry weight (0.67%) was observed in commercial cultivars and as high as 11,900 µg/g in breeding material.[13]

Heritability in the broad sense for concentration of perloline has been in the 0.57 to 0.98 range.[55] Genes controlling low concentration of perloline expressed dominance over high concentration in annual ryegrass-tall fescue hybrid derivatives, but no plants were completely free of perloline.[56] General and specific combining ability were significant sources of variation for perloline concentration in tall fescue.[57] A significant genotype × environment interaction suggested that selections be evaluated over years and locations.[55,57]

In *Phalaris* species, a wide range exists for total indole alkaloid concentration, but no plants have been reported free of alkaloids.[41,58-60] The total alkaloid concentration in available cultivars may reach 5000 µg/g and varies slightly among cultivars in comparative trials.[61] Individual plants may range from 20,000 µg/g to less than 10 µg/g.[41] Somewhat lower maximum concentration levels have been recorded in Australia for *Phalaris aquatica* L. (*P. tuberosa* L.).[58]

Heritability estimates for total indole alkaloids in reed canarygrass indicated high additive genetic variance.[59] Narrow sense heritability estimates for concentration of gramine (0.72) and hordenine (0.53) were relatively high when determined in a greenhouse environment.[53] Slightly higher estimates were reported for field-grown material.[54] High narrow sense heritability (0.82) was also reported for alkaloid concentration in *Phalaris aquatica*.[58] In reed canarygrass, gramine is recessive to tryptamines and their carboline derivatives.[60,62] The genetic evidence supports the hypothesis of an inverse biosynthetic relationship between gramine and the tryptamine and β-carboline alkaloids, in that *Phalaris* plants containing gramine are usually free of tryptamine alkaloids.[40] Hordenine is apparently inherited independently of the indole alkaloids.[53,54]

EFFECTS OF CULTURAL PRACTICES AND ENVIRONMENT

Epichloe typhina and, consequently, N-acetyl and N-formyl loline alkaloids were absent in tall fescue plants established from seeds 2 years old or older.[63] These data suggest that *E. typhina* does not survive in seed that is a minimum of 2 years old. Therefore, the fungus and N-acetyl and N-formyl lolines may be eliminated from tall fescue by planting seed that is at least 2 years old.

Nitrogen fertilization and moisture stress are among the crop management and climatic factors that influence alkaloid concentration most. In tall fescue, the highest alkaloid concentration occurs following high rates of N, particularly during July and August.[12,13] Good management practices to improve yield may not necessarily result in better animal performance when grazing either tall fescue or reed canarygrass. In reed canarygrass, high rates of nitrogen in the form of ammonium nitrate caused greatest increase in total alkaloid concentration.[64] Ammonium-N seems to be incorporated directly into the indole alkaloid, thereby making this source more effective than nitrate-N.[40,44,64] Furthermore, alkaloid concentration in reed canarygrass can be more than doubled when plants are subjected to moisture stress.[65] Other factors such as day length, temperature, and simulated cloud cover have only slight to moderate effects on alkaloid concentration levels.[40,65] Use of forage preservative (86% formic acid) affects alkaloid concentration of reed canarygrass silage. The silage was shown to retain about 78% and the effluent about 14% of the concentration before ensiling. The concentration of effluent dry weight was nearly six times higher than that of the silage.[66]

SUMMARY

Alkaloids in tall fescue and reed canarygrass have been shown to contribute to nonthrifty appearance of animals grazing these forage grasses. The low liveweight gains by animals consuming these grasses at times when alkaloid concentrations are high document the biological and agricultural significance of alkaloids. Several other secondary metabolites may cause problems in feeding these grasses, although the direct cause of some reported animal disorders has not been demonstrated. Mycotoxins, systemic fungi, and anionic fractions of ethanolic extract of tall fescue may be associated with some of the tall fescue-induced disorders. Perloline and the pyrrolizidine alkaloids occur in highest concentration in midsummer. The concentrations of indole alkaloids of reed canarygrass are highest in the leaf blades, particularly those of regrowth forage. Genetic studies demonstrated that alkaloid concentration is highly inherited and has been altered by plant breeding procedures. The highly positive association of the endophytic fungus, *Ephichloe typhina,* with accumulation of N-acetyl and N-formyl lolines in the plant suggests that control of the fungus either through breeding or cultural practices perhaps will overcome the summer syndrome malady of cattle grazing tall fescue during periods of high temperatures. Among cultural practices, high rates of ammonium-nitrogen as fertilizer result in increased alkaloid synthesis in reed canarygrass, particularly when plants have been subjected to a period of moisture stress.

REFERENCES

1. Cunningham, I. J., A note on the cause of tall fescue lameness in cattle, *Aust. Vet. J.,* 25, 27—28, 1948.
2. Bush, L. P. and Buckner, R. C., Tall fescue toxicity, in *Antiquality Components of Forages,* Matches, A. G., Ed., Crop Sci. Soc. Am. Spec. Publ. No. 4, Madison, Wisc., 1973, 99—112.
3. Bush, L. P., Boling, J. A., and Yates, S. G., Animal disorders, in *Tall Fescue Monograph (20),* Buckner, R. C. and Bush, L. P., Eds., Am. Soc. Agron., Madison, Wisc., 1979, 147—292.
4. Bush, L. P. and Jeffreys, J. A. D., Isolation and separation of tall fescue and ryegrass alkaloids, *J. Chromatogr.,* 111, 165—170, 1975.
5. Robbins, J. D., Sweeny, J. G., Wilkinson, S. R., and Burdick, D., Volatile alkaloids of Kentucky 31 tall fescue seed (*Festuca arundinacea* Schreb.), *J. Agric. Food Chem.,* 20, 1040—1043, 1972.
6. Yates, S. G., Tookey, H. L., Ellis, J. J., Tallent, W. H., and Wolff, I. A., Microtoxins as a possible cause of fescue toxicity, *J. Agric. Food Chem.,* 17, 437—442, 1969.
7. Futrell, M. C., Farnell, D. R., Poe, W. E., Watson, V. H., and Coates, R. E., Fungal populations in the rumen associated with fescue toxicosis, *J. Environ. Qual.,* 3, 140—143, 1974.
8. Porter, J. K., Bacon, C. W., Robbins, J. D., and Higman, H. C., A field indicator in plants associated with ergot-type toxicities in cattle, *J. Agric. Food Chem.,* 23, 771—775, 1975.
9. Bacon, C. W., Porter, J. K., and Robbins, J. D., Toxicity and occurrence of *Balansia* on grasses from toxic fescue pastures, *Appl. Microbiol.,* 29, 553—556, 1975.

10. Williams, M., Shaffer, S. R., Garner, G. B., Yates, S. G., Tookey, H. L., Kintner, L. D., Nelson, S. L., and McGinity, J. T., Induction of fescue foot syndrome in cattle by fractionated extracts of toxic fescue hay, *Am. J. Vet. Res.*, 36, 1355—1357, 1975.
11. Cunningham, I. J. and Clare, E. M., A fluorescent alkaloid in ryegrass (*Lolium perenne* L.). V. Toxicity, photodynamic action, and metabolism of perloline, *N.Z. J. Sci. Technol.*, 24, 167B—178B, 1943.
12. Gentry, G., Chapman, R. A., Henson, L., and Buckner, R. C., Factors affecting the alkaloid content of tall fescue (*Festuca arundinacea* Schreb.), *Agron. J.*, 61, 313—316, 1969.
13. Bush, L. and Buckner, R. C., Tall fescue toxicity, in *Antiquality Components of Forages*, Matches, A. G., Ed., Crop Sci. Soc. Am. Spec. Pub. No. 4, Madison, Wisc., 1973, 99—112.
14. Aasen, A. J. and Culvenor, C. C., Abnormally low vicinal coupling constants for O-CH-CH in a highly strained five-membered ring ether; the identity of loline and festucine, *Aust. J. Chem.*, 22, 2021—2027, 1969.
15. Jeffreys, J. A.D., The alkaloids of perennial rye-grass (*Lolium perenne* L.). I. Perloline, *J. Chem. Soc. London*, 4505—4512, 1964.
16. Grimmet, R. E. R. and Waters, D. F., A fluorescent alkaloid in ryegrass (*Lolium perenne* L.). II. Extraction from fresh ryegrass and separation from other bases, *N.Z. J. Sci. Technol.*, Sect. B. 24, 151B, 1943.
17. Yates, S. G., Paper chromatography of alkaloids of tall fescue hay, *J. Chromatogr.*, 12, 423—426, 1963.
18. Kennedy, C. W., Accumulation and Metabolism of Alkaloids in Ryegrass × Tall Fescue Hybrids, Ph.D. thesis, University of Kentucky, Lexington, 1980.
19. Porter, J. K., Bacon, C. W., Robbings, J. D., and Higman, H. C., A field indicator in plants associated with ergot-type toxicities in cattle, *J. Agric. Food Chem.*, 23, 771—775, 1975.
20. Dichl, W. W., *Balansia* and Balansiae in America, Agriculture Monograph No. 4, U.S. Department of Agriculture, Washington, D.C., 1950, 1—82.
21. Garner, G. B., Williams, M., Gates, S. G., and Tookey, H. L., "Fescue-foot" induction from experimental pastures, *J. Anim. Sci.*, 35, 228—229, 1972.
22. Bacon, C. W., Robbins, J. D., and Porter, J. K., The systemic infection of toxic fescue grasses by *Epichloe typhina*, *J. Anim. Sci.*, 45 (Suppl. 1), 397, 1977.
23. Bacon, C. W., Porter, J. K., Robbins, J. D., and Luttrell, E. S., *Epichloe typhina* from toxic tall fescue grasses, *Appl. Environ. Microbiol.*, 34(5), 576—581, 1977.
24. Jacobson, D. R., Carr, S. B., Hatton, R. C., Buckner, R. C., Graden, A. P., Dowden, D. R., and Miller, A. W., Growth, physiological responses and evidence of toxicity in yearling dairy cattle grazing different grasses, *J. Dairy Sci.*, 53, 575—583, 1969.
25. Bryan, W. B., Wedin, W. F., and Vetter, R. L., Evaluation of reed canarygrass and tall fescue as spring-summer and fall-saved pasture, *Agron. J.*, 62, 75—80, 1970.
26. Bull, L. S., Kane, E. P., Boling, J. A., Hemken, R. W., Bush, L. P., and Buckner, R. C., Intake and digestion of improved varieties of fescue, *J. Anim. Sci.*, 45 (Suppl. 1), 290, 1977.
27. Steen, W. W., Gay, N., Boling, J. A., McCormick, J. W., Pendlum, L. C., Buckner, R. C., and Bush, L. P., Response of growing steers grazing four varieties of fescue, *J. Anim. Sci.*, 45 (Suppl. 1), 396, 1977.
28. Hemken, R. W., Bull, L. S., Boling, J. A., Kane, E., Bush, L. P., and Buckner, R. C., Summer fescue toxicosis in lactating dairy cows and sheep fed experimental strains of ryegrass-tall fescue hybrids, *J. Anim. Sci.*, 49(3), 641—646, 1979.
29. Jones, T. A., Buckner, R. C., Bush, L. P., Chapman, R. A., Burrus, P. B., II, and Varney, D. R., Association of the endophytic fungus, *Epichloe typhina*, with loline alkaloid content of tall fescue, *Agron. Abstr.*, 1980.
30. Buckner, R. C., Bush, L. P., Burrus, P. B., II, Boling, J. A., Chapman, R. A., Hemken, R. W., and Jackson, J. A., Jr., Improvement of forage quality of tall fescue through *Lolium-Festuca* hybridization, Proc. 14th Intl. Grassl. Congr., Lexington, Ky., 1981 (in press).
31. Boling, J. A., Hemken, R. W., Bush, L. P., Buckner, R. C., Jackson, J. A., Jr., and Yates, S. G., Role of alkaloids and toxic compound(s) in the utilization of tall fescue by ruminants, Proc. 14th Intl. Grassl. Congr., Lexington, Ky., 1981 (in press).
32. Jackson, J. A., Jr., Hemken, R. W., Boling, J. A., Bull, L. S., Bush, L. P., and Buckner, R. C., Summer fescue toxicosis as a result of feeding tall fescue seed, *J. Dairy Sci.*, 63 (Suppl. 1), 133, 1980.
33. Bush, L. P., Streeter, C., and Buckner, R. C., Perloline inhibition of *in vitro* ruminal cellulose digestion, *Crop Sci.*, 10, 108—109, 1970.
34. Bush, L. P., Boling, J. A., Allen, G., and Buckner, R. C., Inhibitory effects of perloline to rumen fermentation *in vitro*, *Crop Sci.*, 12, 277—279, 1972.
35. Boling, J. A., Bush, L. P., Buckner, R. C., Pendlum, L. C., Burrus, P. B., Yates, S. G., Rogovin, S. P., and Tookey, H. L., Nutrient digestibility and metabolism in lambs fed added perloline, *J. Anim. Sci.*, 40, 972—976, 1975.

36. Bush, L. P., Burton, H., and Boling, J. A., Activity of tall fescue alkaloids and analogues in in vitro rumen fermentation, *J. Agric. Food Chem.*, 30, 869—872, 1976.
37. Lanigan, G. W., Metabolism of pyrrolizidine alkaloids in the ovine rumen. III. The competitive relationship between heliotrine metabolism and methanogenesis in rumen fluid in vitro, *Aust. J. Agric. Res.*, 22, 123—130, 1971.
38. Culvenor, C. C. J., Bon, R. Dal, and Smith, L. W., The occurrence of indole-alkylamine alkaloids in *Phalaris tuberosa* L. and *P. arundinacea* L., *Aust. J. Chem.*, 17, 1301—1304, 1964.
39. Frahn, J. L. and O'Keefe, D. F., The occurrence of tetrahydro-β-carboline alkaloids in *Phalaris tuberosa* (Graminaea), *Aust. J. Chem.*, 24, 2189—2192, 1971.
40. Gander, J. E., Marum, P., Marten, G. C., and Hovin, A. W., The occurrence of 2-methyl-1,2,3,4-tetrahydro-β-carboline and variation in alkaloids in *Phalaris arundinacea*, *Phytochemistry*, 15, 737—738, 1976.
41. Marten, G. C., Alkaloids in reed canarygrass, in *Antiquality Components of Forages*, Matches, A. G., Ed., Crop Sci. Soc. Am. Spec. Publ. No. 4, Madison, Wisc., 1973, 15—31.
42. Snieckus, V., The distribution of idole alkaloids in plants, in *The Alkaloids*, Vol. 11, Manske, R. H. F., Ed., Academic Press, New York, 1968, 1—149.
43. Robinson, Trevor, The biochemistry of alkaloids, in *Molecular Biology, Biochemistry and Biophysics*, Vol. 3, Kleinzeller, A., Springer, G. F., and Whittman, H. G., Eds., Springer-Verlag, New York, 1968, 1—149.
44. Gallagher, C. H., Kock, J. H., and Hoffman, H., Deaths of ruminants grazing *Phalaris tuberosa* L. in Australia, *Aust. Vet. J.*, 43, 495—500, 1967.
45. Parmar, S. S. and Brink, V. C., Tryptamine levels in pasturage implicated in bovine pulmonary emphysema, *Can. J. Plant Sci.*, 56, 175—184, 1976.
46. Rendig, V. V., Cooper, D. V., Dunbar, J. R., Lawrence, C. M., Clawson, W. J., Bushnell, R. B., and McComb, E. A., Phalaris "staggers" in California, *Calif. Agric.*, June 8, 1976.
47. Marten, G. C., Jordan, R. M., and Hovin, A. W., Biological significance of reed canarygrass alkaloids and associated palatability variation to grazing sheep and cattle, *Agron. J.*, 68, 909—914, 1976.
48. Marten, G. C., Jordan, R. M., and Hovin, A. W., Improved lamb performance associated with breeding for alkaloid reduction in reed canarygrass, *Crop Sci.*, 21, 295—298, 1981.
49. Simons, A. V. and Marten, G. C., Relationship of indole alkaloids to palatability of *Phalaris arundinacea* L., *Agron. J.*, 63, 915—919, 1971.
50. Marten, G. C. and Donker, J. D., Determinants of pasture value of *Phalaris arundinacea* L. vs. *Bromus inermis* Lyss., *Agron. J.*, 60, 703—705, 1968.
51. Coulman, B. E., Clark, K. W., and Woods, D. L., Effects of selected reed canarygrass alkaloids on in vitro digestibility, *Can. J. Plant Sci.*, 57, 779—785, 1977.
52. Hagman, J. L., Marten, G. C., and Hovin, A. W., Alkaloid concentration in plant parts of reed canarygrass of varying maturity, *Crop Sci.*, 15, 41—43, 1975.
53. Coulman, B. E., Woods, D. L., and Clark, K. W., Distribution within the plant, variation with maturity and heritability of gramine and hordenine in reed canarygrass, *Can. J. Plant Sci.*, 57, 771—777, 1977.
54. Woods, D. L., Hovin, A. W., and Marten, G. C., Seasonal variation of hordenine and gramine concentrations and their heritabilities in reed canarygrass, *Crop Sci.*, 19, 853—857, 1979.
55. Buckner, R. C., Bush, L. P., and Burrus, P. B., II, Variability and heritability of perloline in *Festuca* sp., *Lolium* sp., and *Lolium-Festuca* hybrids, *Crop Sci.*, 13, 666—669, 1973.
56. Cornelius, P. L., Buckner, R. C., Bush, L. P., Burrus, P. B., II, and Byars, J., Inheritance of perloline content in annual ryegrass × tall fescue hybrids, *Crop Sci.*, 14, 896—898, 1974.
57. Watson, C. E., Jr., Frakes, R. V., Chilcote, D. O., Sleper, D. A., and Matches, A. G., Genetic variation for perloline, N, and digestibility in tall fescue, *Crop Sci.*, 18, 458—460, 1978.
58. Oram, R. N., Genetic and environmental control of the amount and composition of toxins in *Phalaris tuberosa* L., Proc. 11th Intl. Grassl. Congr., Surfers Paradise, Queensland, 1970, 785—788.
59. Barker, R. E. and Hovin, A. W., Inheritance of indole alkaloids in reed canarygrass (*Phalaris arundinacea* L.). I. Heritability estimates for alkaloid concentration, *Crop Sci.*, 14, 50—53, 1974.
60. Woods, D. L. and Clark, K. W., Genetic control and seasonal variation of some alkaloids in reed canarygrass, *Can. J. Plant Sci.*, 51, 323—329, 1971.
61. Hovin, A. W. and Marten, G. C., Distribution of specific alkaloids in reed canarygrass cultivars, *Crop Sci.*, 15, 705—707, 1975.
62. Marum, P., Hovin, A. W., and Marten, G. C., Inheritance of three groups of indole alkaloids in reed canarygrass, *Crop. Sci.*, 19, 539—544, 1979.
63. Buckner, R. C., unpublished data.
64. Marten, G. C., Simons, A. B., and Frelich, J. R., Alkaloids of reed canarygrass as influenced by nutrient supply, *Agron. J.*, 66, 363—368, 1974.

65. **Marten, G. C.** and **Frelich, J. R.,** Alkaloid concentration in *Phalaris arundinacea* L. as influenced by temperature, photoperiod, and water supply, Proc. 13th Intl. Grassl. Congr., Leipzig, German Democratic Republic, 1977, 1497—1499.
66. **Hovin, A. W., Solberg, Y.,** and **Myhr, K.,** Alkaloids in reed canarygrass grown in Norway and the U.S.A., *Acta Agric. Scand.,* 30, 211—215, 1980.

TALL FESCUE TOXINS*

S. G. Yates

INTRODUCTION

Tall fescue (*Festuca arundinacea* Schreb.), a grass used widely as a permanent pasture and a source of hay, is normally an excellent provider of economical feed for beef cattle. However, under certain management conditions which are not entirely understood, tall fescue can become toxic.

Cattle may be allowed to graze tall fescue throughout the year, or it may be utilized as a cool season pasture. Much of the time, tall fescue compares favorably with other pasture grasses, with respect to daily weight gain of cattle on pasture. However, occasionally problems arise, and cattle exhibit clinical signs of fescue toxicosis.

At least three distinct toxicoses are recognized: fescue foot, summer syndrome, and fat necrosis. Each of these is associated with stress to the plant or animal. Perhaps much more important economically are subclinical forms of these toxicoses which result in failure to make expected gains or in loss of weight.

In the course of our studies concerning one of these problems, fescue foot, we have associated toxic tall fescue with alkaloids, mycotoxin-producing fungi, and other unidentified chemicals. Herein is a compilation of toxicants that could be present in a tall fescue pasture.

MYCOTOXINS

Numerous mycotoxins and metabolites have been isolated from in vitro cultures of fungi that were found on tall fescue. Few of these compounds have been isolated from natural sources,[1] and none have so far been isolated from tall fescue pastures. However, since the general climatic and biological conditions and the associated micronutrient content of a tall fescue pasture are ever changing, one cannot assume that one or more of these or other compounds do not occur naturally at any given time.

Aspergillus terreus Toxins

The genus *Aspergillus* is widely distributed in nature; because of the large number of enzymes it produces, it is capable of utilizing many substrates. In fact, if enough moisture is available, it grows on almost any organic matter such as debris and food.[2] *Aspergillus terreus* Thom. is commonly found on decaying vegetation and is particularly abundant in soils of southern and southwestern U.S.[3] This organism produces many oxygenated, aromatic metabolites, some of which are toxic (Table 1).

Futrell et al.[15] implicated *Aspergillus terreus* Thom. as well as *Fusarium tricinctum* (Cda.) Cacc. in the fescue foot syndrome. Fungal counts of rumen fluid from cattle on tall fescue were made by taking 25 g of rumen contents, homogenizing it in a sterilized microblender with 100 mℓ of pH 7 phosphate buffer, and then inoculating warm nonsolidified Czapek's agar (10 mℓ) with 1 mℓ of the buffer solution. After 10 days at room temperature, the colonies of fungi were classified and counted. Fungal counts of pasture samples were made in a similar manner after grinding of surface-sterilized grass samples in pH 7 phosphate buffer. *A. terreus* has been isolated from tall fescue pastures and from the rumina of cattle on pasture when grazing cattle exhibited clinical

---

* The mention of firm names or trade products does not imply that they are endorsed or recommended by the U.S. Department of Agriculture over other firms or similar products not mentioned.

Table 1
PARTIAL LIST OF METABOLITES PRODUCED BY *ASPERGILLUS TERREUS* THOM.

Name	Structure	Ref.
FLAVIPIN		3
TERREIN		3
CITRININ		3
d-GEODIN		3
d,1-ERDIN		3
GEODOXIN		3
PHENOLIC COMPOUND	NOT IDENTIFIED	3
TERRECIN	NOT IDENTIFIED	3
PATULIN		3
TERREIC ACID		3

Table 1 (continued)
PARTIAL LIST OF METABOLITES PRODUCED BY *ASPERGILLUS TERREUS* THOM.

Name	Structure	Ref.
"BIFIDUS FACTOR"		3
ASTERRIC ACID		3
"ETHEREAL SULPHATES"	NOT IDENTIFIED	3
METABOLITE		4
3,6-DIHYDROXYTOLUQUINONE		4
EMODIN		4
QUESTIN		4
SULOCHRIN		4
DIHYDROERDIN		4
ASPULVINONE D	NOT IDENTIFIED	4
COMPOUND C_1	NOT IDENTIFIED	5

Table 1 (continued)
PARTIAL LIST OF METABOLITES PRODUCED BY *ASPERGILLUS TERREUS* THOM.

Name	Structure	Ref.
COMPOUND C_2	NOT IDENTIFIED	5
COMPOUND C_3	NOT IDENTIFIED	5
COMPOUND C_4	NOT IDENTIFIED	5
DIHYDROXY PULVINONE, AND 6 PULVINONE DERIVATIVES		6, 7
3-METHYLORSELLINIC ACID		8
4-0-DEMETHYLBARBATIC ACID		8
ASTERRIQUINONE		8
GLIOTOXIN		9
3, 5-DIHYDROXY-1, 2-DIMETHYLBENZENE		10
QUADRONE		11

Table 1 (continued)
PARTIAL LIST OF METABOLITES PRODUCED BY *ASPERGILLUS TERREUS* THOM.

Name	Structure	Ref.
ASPERGILLIDE B1 AND OTHER ASPERGILLIDES		12
ASPTERRIC ACID		13
TERRETONIN		14

signs of fescue foot, but the organism was not present on the same pastures when the grass was nontoxic. *Fusarium tricinctum* was always present, whether pastures were toxic or not.

Steers dosed intraruminally with 20 petri cultures of *A. terreus* 3 times weekly developed clinical signs of fescue foot. Furthermore, cows treated with thiabendazole (an antifungal compound) at a rate of 5 g/100 lb body weight did not develop clinical signs of fescue foot on a toxic pasture; untreated cows on the same pasture developed clinical signs of fescue foot.[15,16] However, these studies did not determine which, if any, of the metabolites listed in Table 1 produced the toxicosis.

Cladosporium cladosporioides Toxins

The genus *Cladosporium* is found world-wide, in all climates, growing on most organic materials. It can be isolated from soil as well as air. Some *Cladosporium* species cause a great deal of damage to plants, food products, and clothing.[17] *Cladosporium cladosporioides* (Fres.) nov. comb. is commonly found on dead organic matter, but it will infect living plant material that is damaged or weak from poor growing conditions. It may also be a secondary parasite on rust-infected plants.[17] Scott et al.[18] report that this organism produces cladosporin (Table 2) which possesses both bacteriostatic and fungistatic activity.

Keyl et al.[19] implicated *C. cladosporioides* in the fescue foot syndrome. Samples of toxic tall fescue hay were extracted with ether, and the residue from the extract was suspended in olive oil. Some olive oil suspensions produced a hemorrhagic response when applied to the depilated skin of a rabbit's back. Twenty-four molds, isolated from hay samples causing such a rabbit response, were cultured on Sabouraud Maltose Agar at 3°C. Extracts of one of these, *Cladosporium cladosporioides,* produced erythema and edema in the rabbit skin test. A mixture of surface cultures (90-day growth

Table 2
PARTIAL LIST OF METABOLITES PRODUCED BY *CLADOSPORIUM CLADOSPORIOIDES* (FRES) NOV COMB.

Name	Structure	Ref.
CLADOSPORIN	(structure)	18

at 3°C) of *C. cladosporioides* and *Fusarium nivale* (later correctly identified as *F. tricinctum*) were toxic to a sheep when administered via rumen fistula. The resultant ruminal atony was followed by failure to eat or drink. The ensuing dehydration produced fever and increased hematocrit and respiration rate. Other pathology included lipidosis, central necrosis of lobules in the liver, enlargement of bile ducts, uterine stroma with cellular muscle tissue, and atelectasis of the lung.[19]

Nontoxic tall fescue hay was inoculated with aqueous spore suspensions of *C. cladosporioides* and fermented in a glass carboy for 22 days at 7°C (occasional warming to 25°C). An 80% ethanol extract produced no clinical signs when given to 2 cows at an equivalent of 1 to 2 lb of hay per day.[20]

Epicoccum nigrum Toxins

Epicoccum nigrum Link., one of two species in the *Epicoccum* genus, is a common, early secondary invader of plants. It is not uncommon to isolate it from leaf spots, along with other molds, from the air, from animals, and from foodstuffs. It sporulates readily under UV light.[21] This organism produces numerous carotenoid pigments, humic acids, and oxygenated aromatic metabolites (Table 3). Keyl et al.[19] implicated *E. nigrum* in the fescue foot syndrome in the same series of experiments in which they implicated *Cladosporium cladosporioides*. Extracts of each of two isolates of *E. nigrum* cultured on Sabouraud Maltose Agar at 3°C produced erythema and edema in the rabbit skin test. Filtrates of cultures caused death in mice when injected intraperitoneally. Visceral hemorrhage was the most striking pathology.[19] *E. nigrum* inoculum on a nontoxic tall fescue hay failed to grow properly. This hay was not extracted and tested in cattle as was *Cladosporium cladosporioides* and *Fusarium tricinctum*.

Fusarium tricinctum Toxins

The genus *Fusarium*, like other field fungi, is distributed throughout the world, being especially abundant in cultivated soils. These organisms live on numerous organic substrates and are frequently associated with diseases of plants, animals, and man. As plant pathogens, they cause wilt and root rot. On organic substrates, they produce mycotoxins that get into the animal or human food chain.[28] Their ability to adapt rapidly to new environments gives them a tremendous capacity for survival. This ability also contributes to the confusion of classifying *Fusarium* species. Determining which species are synonymous depends on which classification system is followed.[28,29] *F. tricinctum* (also known as *F. sporotrichioides*, *F. poae*, and others) is widely distributed throughout the world, and it produces several mycotoxins (Table 4), including trichothecenes. This latter group of mycotoxins has been associated both with moldy corn toxicosis in livestock and with alimentary toxic aleukia in humans.[29]

F. tricinctum (Corda) Snyd. et Hans. was implicated in the fescue foot syndrome by Keyl et al.[19] when they isolated this organism from toxic tall fescue hay samples and showed that extractives from cultures gave a dermal response in the rabbit and produced visceral hemorrhage and death in mice. Yates et al.[20,35] showed that this

Table 3
PARTIAL LIST OF METABOLITES PRODUCED BY *EPICOCCUM NIGRUM* LINK

Name	Structure	Ref.
ORSELLINIC ACID		22
CRESORSELLINIC ACID		22
PHENOLS, QUINONES, HUMIC ACIDS	NOT IDENTIFIED	22
AUXINS	NOT IDENTIFIED	23
FLAVIPIN		24
PIGMENTS A & B	NOT IDENTIFIED	24
3, 6-DIBENZYL-2, 5-DIOXOPIPERAZINE		25
EPICORAZINE A		26
EPIRODINS	NOT IDENTIFIED	27

isolate plus other *Fusarium* isolates from tall fescue and orchard grass are capable of producing 4-acetamido-4-hydroxy-2-butenoic acid γ-lactone, T-2 toxin, or both (Table 4). However, in a series of experiments over a period of years, neither of these mycotoxins nor *F. tricinctum* cultures produced lameness or gangrene of the feet, which are characteristic of fescue foot in cattle.[20,36-39]

Epichlöe typhina Toxins

Epichlöe typhina (Fries) Tulasne belongs to the family Clavicipitaceae, and is closely related to the genus *Claviceps*. The best-known species of this genus, *Claviceps pur-*

Table 4
PARTIAL LIST OF METABOLITES PRODUCED BY *FUSARIUM TRICINCTUM* (CORDA) SNYD. ET HANS

Name	Structure	Ref.
DIACETOXYSCIRPENOL		30
T–2 TOXIN		31, 32
HT–2 TOXIN		30
NEOSOLANIOL MONOACETATE		33
4-ACETAMIDO-4-HYDROXY-2 BUTENOIC ACID- γ -LACTONE		31, 32
SPOROFUSARIOGENIN		34

purea, is the cause of gangrenous ergotism in livestock and humans.[40] *E. typhina*, a systemic endophyte of numerous grasses, causes "choke disease," so named because of the structural character of stroma, formed around the sheath of the leaf that covers the inflorescence; the white stroma, which later turns orange, encloses the inflorescence.[41] *E. typhina* can infect healthy grasses by inoculation with conidia and ascospores carried by a parasitic fly *(Phorbia phrenione)*.[41] The seed of plants infected with *E. typhina* may carry hyphae and transmit the disease to new plants.[41] Bacon et al.[42] isolated *E. typhina* from hybrids and varieties of toxic tall fescue, and postulated that this fungus is the cause of fescue foot in cattle.

In tall fescue, the fungus goes unnoticed because it does not produce the characteristic stroma. The fungus is detected microscopically by placing pith scrapings removed from longitudinally split culms of fertile tillers on a microscope slide, adding a dye (50 mℓ lactic acid-100 mℓ of 0.1% aqueous aniline blue), and warming the slide in a flame.[42] Tall fescue that produced clinical signs of summer syndrome or fescue foot in cattle always contained hyphae of *E. typhina.* The frequency of *E. typhina* infection of tall fescue that did not produce clinical signs in cattle was 0 to 50%.

Isolates of *E. typhina* from different varieties of tall fescue had different growth characteristics, as did *E. typhina* from other grasses. Because of sparse growth, the first toxicity studies were carried out with *E. typhina* from bent grass, *Agrostis perennans* (Walter) Tuckermann, which produced an uncharacterized metabolite(s) toxic to chicken embryos. All isolates produce a nontoxic steroid (ergosta-4,6,8(14), 22-tetraen-3-one) (Table 5), which is described as a field indicator for toxicity of tall fescue pastures.[43] Cultural conditions necessary to maintain *E. typhina* and other clavicipitaceous fungi were eventually defined, and a two-stage fermentation process was discovered that allowed production of several milligrams of ergot-type alkaloids.[44] Colorimetric determination of alkaloids calculated as ergonovine maleate was 5.5 mg of alkaloid per liter from a 28-day old culture. Ten mℓ of culture filtrate made basic with 0.2 mℓ of 10 N NaOH was extracted with 25 mℓ of chloroform and the chloroform layer was evaporated to dryness at 40°C. The residue was triturated with 2% tartaric acid and the absorbance at 590 nm was calculated as ergonovine maleate.[44] Cultures were maintained at 24 to 28° C on corn meal-maltose agar.[42] For production of alkaloids, cultures were first incubated in 50 mℓ of sporulation medium, M 102[42], in 125 mℓ triple-baffled shake flasks, at 24°C, for 10 days. In the second stage, 2 mℓ of spores from medium 102 were inoculated into 100 mℓ of medium SM[44], in 500 mℓ triple baffled, cotton-stoppered flasks, at 24°C for 10 days on a gyratory shaker, then incubated as stationary cultures until harvested. All cultures were incubated in the dark. Large-scale cultures in 19 ℓ carboys provided enough alkaloid for chemical characterization.

Under these conditions, *E. typhina* was reported to produce ergosine, ergosinine, and chanoclavine 1 (Table 5).[45] Ergosine, a peptide derivative of lysergic acid, produces clinical signs in laboratory animals similar to those observed in cattle on toxic fescue. However, with the aid of isobutane chemical-ionization mass spectra, the major alkaloids were shown to be ergovaline and ergovalinine (Table 5).[46,47] This investigation did not eliminate the possibility that traces of ergosine and ergosinine were present along with the more abundant alkaloids ergovaline and ergovalinine. The potency of ergovaline (as its methane sulfonate derivative) with respect to interruption of early pregnancy in the rat was half that of ergosine methane-sulfonate.[48] Ergovalinine and other isolysergic acid derivatives ending in "inine" are weakly active;[49] likewise, the chanoclavines are weakly active. Other clavine alkaloids represented by agroclavine, penniclavine, and festuclavine (Table 5) possess central nervous system activity, moderate anti-serotonin activity, and weak smooth muscle activity.[49,50]

Balansia epichlöe, B. henningsiana, B. Strangulans, B. Claviceps, Toxins

Balansia belongs in the Clavicipitaceae family, and like *Epichlöe typhina* is closely related to the genus *Claviceps*.[51] *Claviceps purpurea* and *C. paspali,* also in the Clavicipitaceae family, are producers of indole alkaloids.[40] *Balansia epichlöe* (Weese) Diehl, *B. henningsiana* (Moller) Diehl, *B. strangulans* (Mont.) Diehl, and *B. claviceps* Spegazzini are systemic endophytes of grasses;[44] the genus *Balansia* parasitizes 10 tribes of the American Gramineae.[52] These fungi on warm-season grasses, such as smut grass and panicum, are detected by heavy sporulation on the leaf surface. Bacon et al.[51] suggest that in cooler climes, these fungi may not sporulate and may, therefore, go undetected. *B. epichlöe* produces two steroids, ergosta-4,6,8(14),22-tetraen-3-one and ergosta-4,6,8(14),-trien-3-one (Table 6), which are described as field indicators of the presence of this fungus.[43]

Studies with *Balansia* sp. paralleled those of *Epichlöe typhina;* the problem of culture

Table 5
PARTIAL LIST OF METABOLITES PRODUCED BY *EPICHLOE TYPHINA* (FRIES) TULASNE

Name	Structure	Ref.
ERGOSTA—4, 6, 8(14), 22—TETRAEN—3—ONE	SEE TABLE 6	43
TOXIN(S) OF UNKNOWN STRUCTURE		42
ERGOSINE	$R=CH_3$, $R=CH_2CH(CH_3)_2$ ACIDIC FUNCTION AT C_8 EXTENDS FORWARD FROM PLANE	45
ERGOSININE	ACIDIC FUNCTION AT C_8 EXTENDS BEHIND PLANE $R=CH_3$ $R'=CH_2CH(CH_3)_2$	45
CHANOCLAVINE 1		45
ERGOVALINE	SEE ERGOSINE $R' = CH(CH_3)_2$	46
ERGOVALININE	SEE ERGOSININE $R' = CH(CH_3)_2$	46
AGROCLAVINE	$R = CH_3$	46
ELYMOCLAVINE	SEE AGROCLAVINE $R—CH_2OH$	46

Table 5 (continued)
PARTIAL LIST OF METABOLITES PRODUCED BY *EPICHLOE TYPHINA* (FRIES) TULASNE

Name	Structure	Ref.
PENNICLAVINE		46

R_1 = CH$_2$OH EXTENDS BEHIND PLANE.
R_2 = OH EXTENDS FORWARD FROM PLANE.

SECOAGROCLAVINE		46
FESTUCLAVINE		46

maintenance and growth plaguing both. Early studies with *B. epichlöe* from fescue and other grasses present in a toxic tall fescue pasture showed that cultures produced compounds toxic to chicken embryos.[51] Later, in vitro *B. epichlöe* cultures produced three indole alkaloids (Table 6) toxic to the chick embryo.[53] Eventually, a two-stage fermentation was developed (see *Epichlöe typhina* toxins). Under these conditions, *B. epichlöe, B. henningsiana, B. strangulans,* and/or *B. claviceps* isolated from parasitized grasses (not including tall fescue) produced several ergot alkaloids (Table 6).[44] *Balansia epichloe* produced the greatest abundance of alkaloids (390 mg/ℓ), and also the greatest variety of alkaloids (chanoclavine I, ergonovine, ergonovinine, agroclavine, elymoclavine, and penniclavine). Ergonovine, a simple amide of lysergic acid possesses strong uterotonic activity.[49] Additional studies revealed *B. epichlöe* produced other clavine-type ergot alkaloids. *B. claviceps* produced chanoclavine I, ergonovine, and ergonovinine.[54]

Smut grass parasitized with *B. epichlöe* was shown to contain ergot alkaloids (chanoclavine I 16 mg/kg, ergonovine 0.5 mg/kg, unidentified alkaloids 0.5 mg/kg) thereby

Table 6
PARTIAL LIST OF METABOLITES PRODUCED BY THE FUNGUS *BALANSA EPICHLOE*, WEESE

Name	Structure	Ref.
ERGOSTA-4, 6, 8(14), 22-TETRAEN-3-ONE		43
ERGOSTA-4, 6, 8(14), TRIEN-3-ONE		43
4-(3-INDOLYL) BUTANE-1, 2, 3-TRIOL		53
3-(3, 3-DIINDOLYL) PROPANE-1, 2-DIOL		53
3(3-INDOLYL) PROPANE-1, 2, 3-TRIOL		53
CHANOCLAVINE I	SEE TABLE 5	44
AGROCLAVINE	SEE TABLE 5	44
PENNICLAVINE	SEE TABLE 5	44
ELYMOCLAVINE	SEE TABLE 5	44

indicating that *B. epichlöe* produces ergot alkaloids in vivo as well as in vitro.[44] Infected smut grass leaves (15 g) were lyophilized and then defatted with petroleum ether. The defatted plant material was then extracted 1 × 75 mℓ, 3 × 45 mℓ, with 70% aqueous

Table 6 (continued)
PARTIAL LIST OF METABOLITES PRODUCED BY THE FUNGUS *BALANSA EPICHLOE*, WEESE

Name	Structure	Ref.
ERGONOVINE	(structure with COR at C8, N–CH$_3$, indole nucleus; R=NH–CH(CH$_3$)–CH$_2$OH) ACIDIC FUNCTION AT C$_8$ EXTENDS FORWARD FROM PLANE	44
ERGONOVININE	ACIDIC FUNCTION AT C$_8$ EXTENDS BEHIND PLANE	44

acetone containing 2% tartaric acid. After concentrating to remove acetone, the aqueous concentrate was extracted 2 × 60 mℓ with ether to remove nonalkaloidal material. The alkaloids were extracted into ether 1 × 75 mℓ, 3 × 45 mℓ, after making the aqueous concentrate basic with Na$_2$CO$_3$. The ether layer was evaporated to dryness to give total alkaloids.

Additional evidence needed to prove that Clavicipitaceous fungi cause fescue toxicosis is as follows: (a) production of lysergic acid peptide alkaloids by Clavicipitaceous fungi grown on media containing a water extract of tall fescue, (b) isolation of lysergic acid peptide alkaloids from fields of tall fescue that cause fescue toxicosis, (c) production of the clinical signs of fescue toxicosis by feeding pure lysergic acid peptid alkaloids isolated from a toxic tall fescue pasture.

ALKALOIDS

Tall fescue and ryegrass are closely related botanically and can be genetically crossed to yield hybrids. Both grasses produce two types of alkaloids: one type contains a dizaphenanthrene nucleus; the other type contains a pyrrolizidine nucleus. Though published data indicate these bases are only mildly toxic compared to strychnine; if ingested continuously in relatively large dosages, either or both types might produce or potentiate toxicoses associated with tall fescue.

Perloline

Variation in the perloline (Table 7) content of tall fescue results from a complex relationship between soil fertility, availability of moisture, season of the year, disease, stage of maturity, and variety. Perloline content can also be influenced by crossing tall fescue plants of specified perloline concentration.[67-70] Gentry et al.[71] did not find perloline in the dormant seed of Ky-31, Kenwell, Alta, and NK-36 tall fescue; it appeared after germination during formation of primary roots. Perloline was the principal alkloid formed in the seedlings of these varieties. Older plants (grown in green-

Table 7
ALKALOIDS OF TALL FESCUE

Name	Formula	Structure	Physiological activity	Ref.
PERLOLINE	$C_{20}H_{18}N_2O_4$	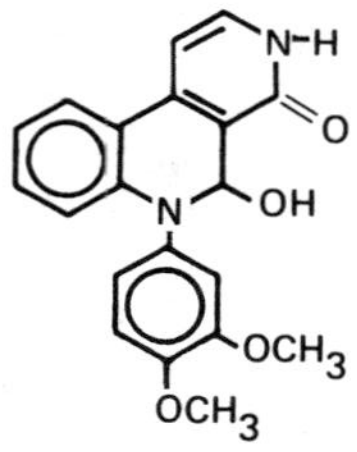 (structure shown)	Mild photosensitization in mice	55
			Mild photosensitization in paramecia, rat blood cells, mice, and sheep	56
			Mild toxicity in paramecia, mice, rabbits, sheep	56
			Did not cause facial eczema in sheep	56
			Effects cellulose digestion	57, 60
			Inhibits root growth of plants	61, 62
LOLINE (FESTUCINE)	$C_8H_{14}N_2O$	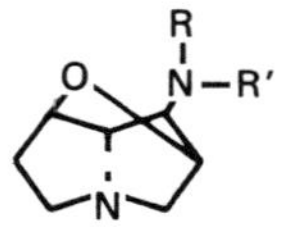 (structure shown) $R=CH_3$, $R'=H$	Mild toxicity mice	63

N–ACETYL LOLINE	R=CH$_3$, R'=OCCH$_3$	Mild toxicity rats	64
		Potentiates action of acetylcholine	65
N–FORMYL LOLINE	R=CH$_3$, R'=OCH		64
DESMETHYL–N–ACETYL LOLINE (N–ACETYL NORLOLINE)	R=H, R'=OCCH$_3$		64
PERLOLIDINE			66

house) contained several alkaloids; three were present in relatively high concentrations, namely perloline, "alkaloid 44," and loline. Perloline was present in all parts of the plant, except the seed head, at the dough stage of maturity. It was present in highest concentration (0.2% of dry matter) in the stems. Perloline decreased in concentration as the plants approached maturity. In vegetative regrowth, the highest concentration of peroline was in the roots. The perloline content of field-cured hay was greatly reduced; only traces were found in 2-year-old hay.[71] Fertilization affected the concentration of perloline in the plant. Applications of nitrogen, phosphorus, and potassium increased perloline concentrations by 50% during summer months when perloline content peaked and by 100% during winter months when perloline content was lowest. Applications of phosphorus and potassium alone decreased perloline concentration.[71]

Gentry[72] found a correlation between peroline and disease resistance in tall fescue. Higher perloline concentrations correlated with resistance to infection by *Rhizoctonia solani* Kuhn or *Helminthosporium vagans* Drech. The perloline content of leaf lesions caused by these organisms was less than that of leaf tissue surrounding the lesions; likewise, leaf tissue surrounding the lesions had less perloline than leaf tissue from healthy plants. This phenomenon appears to be an overall degradation of perloline throughout the entire plant, because there was no increase in perloline in other plant parts, and no other newly formed alkaloids were detected.

The structure of perloline mercurichloride was determined by single crystal X-ray diffraction,[73,74] thus establishing the structure of the pseudobase (Table 7). The hydroxyl moiety of the carbinol amine group is readily replaced

by a methoxyl group in methanol solutions or an ethoxyl group in ethanol solutions, or it is eliminated in chloroform to form the anhydronium base.[75]

Jeffreys[75] reports that the presence of this latter form is the cause of double melting points of perloline and perloline ethyl ether. One of the decomposition products of perloline is perlolidine which has been synthesized by two groups.[76-78] This alkaloid has been detected in tall fescue (Table 7).[66]

Perloline can be analyzed quantitatively by several methods. One early method employed acidic extraction, purification by extraction into chloroform or acidic aqueous solutions at the appropriate pH, then measurement of its color in choloroform.[79] Gentry[72] and Gentry et al.[71] extracted total alkaloids into chloroform-methanol (95:5) after grinding plant material with sand and sodium bicarbonate. The alkaloids were separated by thin-layer chromatography; zones were located and eluted with dilute HCl. Perloline was measured spectrophotometrically at 258 nm (low concentrations), or 393 nm (high concentrations). A later adaptation of this method employed thin-layer densitometry (tld).[80] Jeffreys[75] cautioned that such methods might give high results due to a basic, yellow, nonperloline compound which is extracted along with perloline. Yates et al.[80] observed decomposition of perloline in chloroform solution (cf.[71]) and found that only the absorption at 480 nm paralleled the decreasing concentration of perloline as determined by tld, and that other absorption bands (243, 288 nm) increased.

Shaffer et al.[81] extracted perloline with 50% ethanol, purified the extract by cation exchange chromatography, and measured peroline by fluorometry (excitation at 450 nm, scanning fluorescence from 509 to 515 nm; F max = 512 nm). Tall fescue contained interfering compounds which were removed by cation exchange chromatography; unfortunately, perloline recoveries were affected unless flow rates were controlled carefully. Recoveries of 92% were obtained.

Yates et al.[80] described a simple procedure for isolating perloline from plant material; the procedure can be scaled up to yield large quantities. They isolated about 338 g as perloline monohydrochloride (approximately 42 g isolated from each of 8 batches, 136 kg each).

Perloline has been shown to have a variety of physiological activities, but it is only mildly toxic compared to strychnine, when ingested orally (Table 7). Cunningham and Clare[56] did a series of experiments demonstrating that, in mice and sheep, there was a rapid degradation of perloline, especially if it were administered orally. Only trace amounts of perloline were detected in the blood, feces, or urine of the animals. Mixtures of perloline with organ tissues showed that perloline was destroyed both by the kidney and liver; however, the destruction by the liver was about 20-fold faster than that of the kidney.

Reduced performance of cattle grazing tall fescue pastures during summer months may be related to the effect of perloline on cellulose digestion in the rumen and the effects of perloline on other body functions. Bush et al.[57] showed that perloline inhibits in vitro digestion of cellulose by rumen microorganisms. In a later study, perloline was shown to inhibit the growth of certain rumen bacteria.[58]

Bowling et al.[60] fed sheep approximately 4 g of perloline monohydrochloride per day, along with a control diet. Cellulose digestion of these sheep was compared to sheep fed the control diet alone. Adding perloline resulted in a reduction of cellulose digestion, especially on days 10 and 11.[60] In addition, sheep given perloline showed a lower crude protein digestibility, a decreased

	Cellulose digested (%)	
	Day 10	Day 11
Control sheep	72.6	71.4
Perloline-fed group	67.8	67.4

amount of volatile fatty acids produced in the rumen, and a slight elevation of temperature on days 10 and 11.

Loline

The concentration of loline-type alkaloids (Table 7) in tall fescue may be affected by a variety of factors similar to those that affect the concentration of perloline. Loline was present in the seed of Ky-31 and Kenwell, but was not detected in seed from Alta,

Goar, nor NK-36.[71] During germination, loline content decreased in the seed of Ky-31 and Kenwell tall fescue; it then began to appear in the growing plants. Ten-day-old seedlings contained loline plus five other alkaloids; Alta, Goar, and NK-36 contained loline plus two other alkaloids. The "other alkaloids" are probably the amide forms of loline and norloline (desmethylloline). Older plants produced a greater number of alkaloids, but loline, perloline, and another alkaloid designated as "alkaloid 44" were the principal ones.[71] Mature tall fescue plants from a heavily fertilized field were found to contain 0.2 to 0.5% loline-type alkaloids.[64] Loline, unlike perloline, does not appear in the root of tall fescue.[72]

Although there are no in-depth studies, there is a hint that loline, like perloline, is related to disease resistance in tall fescue. Loline was detected in both healthy and diseased plant tissue, but its concentration was decreased in plant tissue infected with *Rhizoctonia solani*.[72] Boling, et al.[82] showed that the loline-type alkaloid concentration of Gl-307 fescue was related to infestation of *Epichloë typhina*, a systemic fungus. Gl-307 seed treated with a systematic fungicide, Benomyl, produced plants with 44% *E. typhina* infection that contained 115 µg/g of N-acetyl loline plus N-formyl loline. Untreated seed produced plants with 95% *E. typhina* infection that contained 895 µg/g of N-acetyl loline plus N-formyl loline. Steen et al.[83] mention that Gl-307 tall fescue, selected for its low perloline content, has much higher concentrations of loline-type alkaloids than does Gl-306, selected for its high perloline content, or Ky-31, a variety found on most farms.

Loline-type alkaloids and perloline can easily be analyzed qualitatively by paper chromatography.[84] The earliest quantitative method was developed by Gentry[72] who employed thin-layer chromatography. Each alkaloid zone was located, scraped from the plate, and eluted. UV absorption at 264 nm for loline and 307 nm for "alkaloid 44" was related to concentration. Robbins et al.[64] were the first to separate and measure loline-type alkaloids by gas chromatography. Aside from the difficulty of obtaining a known quantity of pure standards, this method affords a sensitive, efficient measurement of loline-type alkaloids. A greater understanding of the metabolic and physiological role of this group of alkaloids should be forthcoming now that a better analytical tool is available.

Though scant information is available concerning what controls loline-type alkaloid content in plants, a greater amount of information has been published concerning the chemistry of these alkaloids. This interest is in part due to the fact that loline-type alkaloids also occur in other plants (*Lolium* sp. and *Adenocarpus decorticans* Boiss.).[85-92] Another point of interest is that loline-type alkaloids are pyrrolizidine bases, the unsaturated alkaloids of which are involved in numerous animal toxicoses.[93-95] The toxicity of this group of alkaloids is related to an allylic ester function (a good alkylating agent)

and/or to a toxic pyrrole derivative, which is formed in the liver from Δ-1,2-unsaturated pyrrolizidines.[96-98] Some saturated pyrrolizidines are

known to be metabolized by the liver into nontoxic pyrroles.[99]

Table 8
EFFECT OF INTRAVENOUS (FEMORIAL) DOSES OF LOLINE DERIVATIVES ON DOGS AND CATS[100]

System	Lolinedihydrochloride	N-Benzoyl-loline methiodide
Narcotic and sedative action of barbamy/or chloral hydrate	Intensifies and prolongs action	—
Blood pressure	1—60 mg/kg, decrease, 2—15 min duration; after atropine sulfate, no effect	1—50 mg/kg decrease, 5—30 min duration; after atropine sulfate, same effect as above
Respiration	Immediate deepening; after vagotomy, same effect as above	Temporary decrease in rate; deeping; after vagotomy, same effect as above
Coronary blood flow	Decrease; weak accelerated systolic beat	Decrease; weak accelerated systolic beat
Parasympathetic ganglia (fibers of vagus nerve)	No effect	Interruption of the impulse transmission
Sympathetic ganglia (nictitating membrane contraction)	No effect	Inhibition of transmission of excitation
Synaptic transmission	No effect	Impaired transmission of impulses

Loline was shown to be mildly toxic to rats[64] and mice.[63] Bruce et al.[65] found that it potentiated the action of acetylcholine to contract smooth muscle if administered before, but not after, acetylcholine. Karimov and Kamilov[100] studied the effects of the amine and amide form of loline (Table 8) and showed that the amide form was the more toxic. Studies on related pyrrolizidine alkaloids suggest that derivatives of loline-type alkaloids may have a wide range of physiological activities. Sadrildinov et al.[101] and Shakhidoyator et al.[102] have shown that bisquaternary pyrrolizidines possess neuromuscular blocking activity similar to that of curare.

UNKNOWN TOXIN(S)

Tall fescue (*Festuca arundinacea* Schreb.) is associated with several cattle diseases, the etiologies of which have not been determined (fescue foot,[103] summer syndrome,[103] and fat necrosis[104]). Aside from grazing tall fescue, a common contributory factor present in all three of these diseases is stress either to animal or pasture. Such stresses are cold weather in the case of fescue foot, hot weather in the case of summer syndrome, and high nitrogen fertilization in the case of fat necrosis. High nitrogen fertilization also appears to be involved in fescue foot.[105]

Fescue Foot Toxin(s)
Early clinical signs of fescue foot generally include a rough hair coat, scouring, lameness, arched back, loss of weight, increased body temperature, increased respiration rate, and other signs that are less obvious to the untrained observer. More advanced clinical signs include formation of gangrenous tissue at the extremities (feet, tail, and occasionally ears). Frequently, cattle showing clinical signs of fescue foot will lose the switch of the tail, and in extreme cases, one or more hoofs may be sloughed.[103]

Several etiological agents have been investigated as the cause of fescue foot. Tall fescue alkaloids (perloline and loline-type) were among the first compounds suspected as the cause of fescue foot. Alkaloidal subfractions prepared from toxic tall fescue hay have been given to cattle; these subfractions did not produce fescue foot.[106,107] However, in the preparation of these subfractions, the alkaloids were in contact with strong mineral acids, which can hydrolyze the amide forms of loline-type alkaloids to yield the less toxic amine forms (cf. alkaloids, loline-type).[64]

Mycotoxins were also suspected as causing fescue foot in cattle. Though 4-acetamido-4-hydroxy-2-butenoic acid γ-lactone, T-2 toxin, molded hay, and molded hay extracts were found toxic to cattle, they did not produce fescue foot (cf. Mycotoxins). The plant, in response to fungal infection and other forms of stress, might produce substances (phytoalexins) that are toxic to cattle. Research on this phytoalexin concept has not been reported.

One group investigating the cause of fescue foot in cattle is fractionating toxic tall fescue hay extracts. A bioassay, production of fescue foot in calves, will be used to determine which fractions contain the toxin(s). Thus far, reported evidence indicates that the anions present in tall fescue, rather than the cationic alkaloids, are responsible for fescue foot.[106-110] Once the specific toxin(s) are characterized, their origin and pharmacodynamic action(s) will be determined.

Summer Syndrome Toxin(s)

Summer syndrome, described by Bush et al.[103] as lack of weight gain and/or poor milk production in cattle, usually occurs during summer months, especially August and September. Also reported as clinical signs of summer syndrome are intolerance of cattle to heat, elevated body temperature, and high respiration rate.[112] Gl-307 tall fescue (a hybrid variety containing a low concentration of perloline [255 to 281 µg/g] and high concentrations of N-acetyl plus N-formyl loline [895 µg/g]) regularly produces severe clinical signs of summer syndrome.[82,83,112] The toxicants are found throughout the growing season, but their effect is observed only at high temperatures (34 to 35°C).[113] The toxicants lower serum prolactin concentration at low, medium, and high temperatures (10 to 13°C, 21 to 23°C, 34 to 35°C), but the effect is magnified at 34 to 35°C. Because ergocryptine, an ergot alkaloid, produces a similar effect, Hurley et al.[114] suggest the toxin(s) are related to ergot alkaloids, thus affecting prolactin secretion at the pituitary level. Clinical signs of summer syndrome are produced by feeding 700 g of Gl-307 seed daily, or feeding Ky-31 or Gl-307 seed at 70% of the ration.[115] Therefore, if ergot-type alkaloids are responsible for summer syndrome, they must be present in the seed as well as the forage. The appearance of the syndrome coincides with the seasonal increase in the concentration of tall fescue alkaloids. The data presented by Bush et al.,[103] indicates that a 250-kg calf could receive as much as 29 ± 7 g total alkaloid (perloline, 14 g; perlolidine, 6 g; loline type, 9 g) per day from grazing tall fescue at this time of year. A concentration of 1 mM of alkaloid per liter of rumen fluid could possibly be surpassed. Bush and Buckner[111] have hypothesized that tall fescue alkaloids inhibit rumen microflora activity. As a result, the rate of digestion decreases, passage of forage through the animal decreases, and forage intake is reduced.

Fat Necrosis Toxins

Fat necrosis, formation of hard fat deposits, is encountered when animals graze tall fescue pastures that are fertilized with large amounts of nitrogen.[116-118] These deposits, distinguished from normal depot fat by their darker yellow color and their texture,[118] are found in the mesentary immediately surrounding the intestines.[116] Gross clinical signs—loss of weight, scanty feces, bloating, etc.—are nonspecific and death of one or more animals of a herd may result due to intestinal strangulation before this disease is diagnosed. Lesions can be detected by rectal palpation or postmortem examination. Stuedemann et al.[117] reported that the incidence of fat necrosis in cows grazing a tall fescue pasture fertilized with broiler litter at 22 ± 2 metric tons/acre/year, increased from 10% the 1st year to 66% the 3rd year. Cattle on a pasture fertilized with ammonium nitrate (79 ± 5 kg/ha/yr) had a low incidence of fat necrosis; one cow had one small lesion. On a pasture receiving an intermediate rate of nitrogen as ammonium nitrate (224 kg/ha/year), the incidence of fat necrosis was 4% the 1st year, 25% the 2nd year, and 20% the 3rd year. Nothing has been reported relating to the specific compounds present in tall fescue pastures that cause this disease. One cow that had a hard fat lesion encircling the intestinal wall was placed on a bermuda grass pasture; after 1 year, no evidence of fat necrosis could be detected.[118]

The following preventive measures are recommended by Stuedemann et al.:[117]

1. Limit broiler litter applications to 4 t/acre/year.
2. Limit nitrogen applications to 200 lb/acre/year.
3. Allow cattle to have access to mineral mixture blocks.
4. Stock pastures with enough cattle to prevent accumulation of forage.
5. Introduce legumes or other forages, or use other pastures.

REFERENCES

1. Hesseltine, C. W., Natural occurrence of mycotoxins in cereals, *Mycopathol. Mycol. Appl.*, 53, 141, 1974.
2. Alexopoulos, C. J., *Introductory Mycology,* 2nd ed., John & Wiley Sons, New York, 1966, 271.
3. Raper, K. B. and Fennell, D. I., The *Aspergillus terreus* group, in *The Genus Aspergillus,* Williams & Wilkins, Baltimore, 1965, 567.
4. Kiriyama, N., Nitta, K., Sakaguchi, Y., Taguchi, Y., and Yamamoto, Y., Studies on the metabolic products of *Aspergillus terreus*. III. Metabolites of the strain IFO 8835, *Chem. Pharm. Bull.*, 25(10), 2593, 1977; *Chem. Abstr.*, 88, 47259Y.
5. Ling, K., Study on mycotoxins. Contamination of food in Taiwan. 2. Tremor-inducing compounds from *Aspergillus terreus*, *Proc. Natl. Sci. Counc.,* Part 2 (Taiwan), 9, 121, 1976; *(Chem. Abstr.* 86, 51316r.)
6. Ojima, N., Takenaka, S., and Seto, S., Structures of pulvinone derivatives from *Aspergillus terreus*, *Phytochemistry,* 14(2), 573, 1975.
7. Ojima, N., Takahashi, I., Ogura, K., and Seto, S., New metabolites from *Aspergillis terreus* related to the biosynthesis of aspulvinones, *Tetrahedron Lett.,* 13, 1013, 1976.
8. Yamamoto, Y., Nishimura, K., and Kiriyama, N., Studies on the metabolic products of *Aspergillus terreus*. I. Metabolites of the strain IFO 6123, *Chem. Pharm. Bull.,* 24(8), 1853, 1976.
9. Cole, R. J., *Aspergillus* toxins other than aflatoxin, *Adv. Chem. Ser.:* No. 149, Mycotoxins and Other Fungal Related Food Problems, Rodericks, J. V., Ed., Am. Chem. Soc., Washington, D.C., 1976, 68.
10. Shinsuke, N., Kaneko, Y., and Doi, S., A new phenolic compound of *Aspergillus terreus, Agric. Biol. Chem. (Tokyo),* 32(6), 781, 1968; *Chem. Abstr.,* 69, 57531c.
11. Ranieri, R. L. and Calton, G. J., Quadrone, a new antitumor agent from *Aspergillus terreus, Tetrahedron Lett.,* (6) 499, 1978.
12. Golding, B. T., Rickards, R. W., and Vanek, Z., New metabolites of *Aspergillus terreus:* 3-Hydroxy-2,5-bis-(p-hydroxyphenyl) penta-2,4-dien-4-olide and derivatives, *J. Chem. Soc., Perkin Trans.,* 1, 1961, 1975.
13. Tsuda, Y., Kaneda, M., Tada, A., Nitta, K., Yamamoto, Y., and Iitaka, Y., Asperterric acid, a new sesquiterpenoid of the carotane group, a metabolite from *Aspergillus terreus* IFO-6123. X-ray crystal and molecular structure of its p-bromobenzoate, *J. Chem. Soc. Chem. Comm.,* 160, 1978.
14. Springer, J. P., Dorner, J. W., Cole, R. J., and Cox, R. H., Terretonin, a toxic compound from *Aspergillus terreus, J. Org. Chem.,* 44(26), 4852, 1979.
15. Futrell, M. C., Farnell, D. R., Poe, W. E., Watson, V. H., and Coats, R. E., Fungal populations in the rumen associated with fescue toxicosis, *J. Environ. Qual.,* 3(2), 140, 1974.
16. Farnell, D. R., Futrell, M. C., Watson, V. H., Poe, W. E., and Coats, R. E., Field studies on etiology and control of fescue toxicosis, *Proceedings of Fescue Toxicity Conference,* Extension Publ., University of Missouri, Columbia, 1973, 24.
17. De Vries, G. A., Contribution to the Knowledge of the Genus *Cladosporium* Link Ex Fr., Doctoral Thesis, Univ. Utrecht, Baarn, Uitgeverij and Drukkerij Holland, 1952, 4, 57.

18. Scott, P. M., Vanwalbeek, W., and MacLean, W. M., Cladosporin, a new antifungal metabolite from *Cladosporium cladosporioides, J. Antibiot., Tokyo,* 24(11), 747, 1971.
19. Keyl, A. C., Lewis, J. C., Ellis, J. J., Yates, S. G., and Tookey, H. L., Toxic fungi isolated from tall fescue, *Mycopathol. Mycol. Appl.,* 31(3 and 4), 327, 1967.
20. Yates, S. G., Tookey, H. L., Ellis, J. J., Tallent, W. T., and Wolff, I. J., Mycotoxins as a possible cause of fescue toxicity, *Agric. Food Chem.,* 17(3), 437, 1969.
21. Ellis, M. B., *Dematiaceous Hyphomycetes,* Commonwealth Mycological Institute, Kew, Surrey, England, 1971, 72.
22. Haider, K. and Martin, J. P., Synthesis and transformation of phenolic compounds by *Epicoccum nigrum* in relation to humic acid formation, *Soil Sci. Soc. Am. Proc.,* 31(6), 766, 1967; *Chem. Abstr.,* 68, 76001a.
23. Buckley, N. G. and Pugh, G. J. F., Auxin production by phylloplane fungi, *Nature (London),* 231(5301), 332, 1971; *Chem. Abstr.,* 75, 45647.
24. Burge, W. R., Buckley, L. J., Sullivan, J. D., Jr., McGrattan, C. J., and Ikawa, M., Isolation and biological activity of the pigments of the mold *Epicoccum nigrum, J. Agric. Food Chem.,* 24(3), 555, 1976; *Chem. Abstr.,* 85, 744a.
25. Baute, M. A., Baute, R., Bourgeous, G., and Deffieux, G., Isolation of 3,6-dibenzyl-2,5-dioxopiperazine from cultures of a strain of mushroom, *Epicoccum nigrum, Bull. Soc. Pharm.,* Bordeaux, 112(4), 169, 1973; *Chem. Abstr.,* 81, 60867v.
26. Deffieux, G., Gadret, M., Leger, J. M., and Carpy, A., Crystal structure of an original fungic metabolite of 3,6-3epidithio-2,5-dioxopiperazines epicorazine A ($C_{18} O_6 N_2 S_2 H_{16} H_2O$), *Acta Crystallogr.,* Sect. B., B33(5), 1474, 1977; *Chem. Abstr.,* 87, 46857j.
27. McGrattan, C. J., The chemistry and biological activity of epirodin, a heptaene antibiotic from *epicoccum nigrum,* Ph.D. thesis, University of New Hampshire, Durham, Order No. 76-23, 129, Diss. Abstr. Int. B, 37(4), 1669, 1976; *Chem. Abstr.,* 86, 1416c.
28. Booth, C., *The Genus Fusarium,* Commonwealth Mycological Institute, Kew, Surrey, England, 1971, 11—13.
29. Ueno, Y., Trichothecenes: overview address, in *Mycotoxins in Human and Animal Health,* Pathotox Publishers, Park Forest South, Ill., 1977, 189—207.
30. Smalley, E. G., Marasas, W. F. O., Strong, F. M., Bamburg, J. R., Nichols, R. E., and Kosuri, N. R., Mycotoxicosis associated with moldy corn, in Proc., 1st U.S.-Japan Conf. Toxic Micro-Organisms, Herzberg, M., Ed., UJNR Joint Panels on Toxic Micro-Organisms and the U.S. Department of the Interior, Washington, D.C., 1968, 163—173.
31. Yates, S. G., Tookey, H. L., Ellis, J. J., and Burkhardt, H. J., Mycotoxins produced by *Fusarium nivale* isolated from tall fescue (*Festuca arundinacea* Schreb.), *Phytochemistry,* 7, 139, 1968.
32. Burmeister, H. R. and Hesseltine, C. W., Biological assays for two mycotoxins produced by *Fusarium tricinctum, Appl. Microbiol.,* 20(3), 437, 1970.
33. Lansden, J. A., Cole, R. J., Dorner, J. W., Cox, R. H., Cutler, H. G., and Clark, J. D., A new trichothecene mycotoxin isolated from *Fusarium tricinctum, J. Agric. Food Chem.,* 26(1), 246, 1978.
34. Bamburg, J. R., Strong, F. M., and Smalley, E. B., Toxins from moldy cereals, *J. Agric. Food Chem.,* 17(3), 443, 1969; See also Olifson, L. E., Mechanism of the reaction of alkali on some toxic substances of cereal plants, *Khim. Nauka i Prom,* 4, 808, 1959; *Chem Abstr.,* 54, 11155b.
35. Yates, S. G., Tookey, H. L., and Ellis, J. J., Survey of tall fescue pasture: Correlation of toxicity of *Fusarium* isolates to known toxins, *Appl. Microbiol.,* 19(1), 103, 1970.
36. Grove, M. D., Yates, S. G., Tallent, W. H., Ellis, J. J., Wolff, I. A., Kosuri, N. R., and Nichols, R. E., Mycotoxins produced by *Fusarium tricinctum* as possible causes of cattle disease, *Agric. Food Chem.,* 18(4), 734, 1970.
37. Kosuri, N. R., Grove, M. D., Yates, S. G., Tallent, W. H., Ellis, J. J., Wolff, I. A., and Nichols, R. E., Response of cattle to mycotoxins of *Fusarium tricinctum* isolated from corn and fescue, *J. Am. Vet. Med. Assoc.,* 157(7), 938, 1970.
38. Tookey, H. L., Yates, S. G., Ellis, J. J., Grove, M. D., and Nichols, R. E., Toxic effects of a butenolide mycotoxin and of *Fusarium tricinctum* cultures in cattle, *J. Am. Vet. Med. Assoc.,* 160(11), 1522, 1972.
39. Grove, M. D., Tookey, H. L., and Yates, S. G., Relation of mycotoxins to fescue toxicity, in *Proceedings of Fescue Toxicity Conference,* Extension Publication, Univ. Missouri, Columbia, 1973, 124—130.
40. Gröger, D., Ergot, in *Microbial Toxins,* Vol. VIII, Kadis, S., Ciegler, A., and Ajl, S., Eds., Academic Press, New York, 1972, 321.
41. Kohlmeyer, J. and Kohlmeyer, E., Distribution of *Epichloë typhina* (Ascomycetes) and its parasitic fly, *Mycologia,* 66(1), 77, 1974.
42. Bacon, C. W., Porter, J. K., Robbins, J. D., and Luttrell, E. S., *Epichloë typhina* from toxic tall fescue grasses, *Appl. Environ. Microbiol.,* 34(5), 576, 1977.

43. Porter, J. K., Bacon, C. W., Robbins, J. D., and Higman, H. C., A field indicator in plants associated with ergot-type toxicities in cattle, *J. Agric. Food Chem.*, 23(4), 771, 1975.
44. Bacon, C. W., Porter, J. K., and Robbins, J. D., Laboratory production of ergot alkaloids by species of *Balansia*, *J. Gen. Microbiol.*, 113(1), 119, 1979.
45. Porter, J. K., Bacon, C. W., and Robbins, J. D., Ergosine, ergosinine, and chanoclavine 1 from *Epichlöe typhina*, *J. Agric. Food Chem.*, 27(3), 595, 1979.
46. Porter, J. K., Bacon, C. W., Robbins, J. D., and Betowski, D., Ergot alkaloid identification in clavicipitaceae systemic fungi of pasture grasses, *J. Agric. Food Chem.*, 29(3), 653, 1981.
47. Porter, J. K. and Betowski, D., Chemical ionization mass spectrometry of ergot cyclol alkaloids, *J. Agric. Food Chem.*, 29(3), 650, 1979.
48. Kraicer, P. F. and Shelesnyak, M. C., Mechanism of nidation. XIII. Relation between chemical structure and biodynamic activity of certain ergot alkaloids, *J. Reprod. Fertil.*, 10(2), 221, 1965; *Chem. Abstr.*, 64; 2627g.
49. Stoll, A. and Hofmann, A., The ergot alkaloids, in *The Alkaloids*, Vol. VIII, Manske, R. H. F., Ed., Academic Press, N.Y., 1965, 725.
50. Floss, H. G., Cassady, J. M., and Robbers, J. E., Influence of ergot alkaloids on pituitary prolactin and prolactin-dependent processes, *J. Pharm. Sci.*, 62(5), 699, 1973.
51. Bacon, C. W., Porter, J. K., and Robbins, J. D., Toxicity and occurrence of *Balansia* on grasses from toxic fescue pastures, *Appl. Microbiol.*, 29(4), 553, 1975.
52. Diehl, W. W., Balansia *and* Balansiae *in America*, in *Agric. Monograph No. 4*, U.S. Department of Agriculture, Washington, D.C., 1950, 1.
53. Porter, J. K., Bacon, C. W., Robbins, J. D., Himmelsbach, D. S., and Higman, H. C., Indole alkaloids from *Balansia epichlöe*(Weese) *J. Agric. Food Chem.*, 25(1), 88, 1977.
54. Porter, J. K., Bacon, C. W., and Robbins, J. D., Lysergic acid amide derivative from *Balansia epichlöe* and *Balansia claviceps*(Clavicipitaceae), *J. Nat. Prod.*, 42(3), 309, 1979.
55. Reifer, I. and Bathurst, N. O., A flourescent alkaloid in rye-grass (*Lolium perenne* L.). III. Extraction and properties, *N.Z. J. Sci. Technol.*, 24B, 155, 1943.
56. Cunningham, I. J. and Clare, E. M., A fluorescent alkaloid in rye-grass (*Lolium perenne* L.). V. Toxicity, photodynamic action, and metabolism of perloline, *N.Z. J. Sci. Technol.*, 24B, 167, 1943.
57. Bush, L. P., Streeter, C., and Buckner, R. C., Perloline inhibition of *in vitro* ruminal cellulose digestion, *Crop Sci.*, 10(1), 108, 1970.
58. Bush, L. P., Boling, J. A., Allen, G. and Buckner, R. C., Inhibitory effects of perloline to rumen fermentation *in vitro, Crop Sci.*, 12(3), 277, 1972.
59. Grenz, G. K., Perloline concentration in tall fescue (*Festuca arundinacea* Schreb.) and its effects on the *in vitro* digestion of cell wall constituents by rumen microorganisms, Ph.D. thesis, Purdue University, Lafayette, Ind., Diss. Abstr. Int. B, 36(7), 3156, 1976.
60. Bowling, J. A., Bush, L. P., Buckner, R. C., Pendlum, L. C., Burrus, P. B., Yates, S. G., Rogovin, S. P., and Tookey, H. L., Nutrient digestibility and metabolism in lambs fed added perloline, *J. Anim. Sci.*, 40(5), 972, 1975.
61. Fejer, S. O., Effects of gibberellic acid, indolylacetic acid IAA, coumarin, and peroline on perennial-rye grass (*Lolium perenne* L.), *N.Z. J. Agric. Res.*, 3, 734, 1960; *Chem. Abstr.*, 55, 11743e.
62. Fejer, S. O., The activity of perloline and of root exudates and shoot extracts of *Lolium* spp. in the cress test, *Naturwissenschaften*, 49(15), 354B, 1962.
63. Yates, S. G. and Tookey, H. L., Festucine, an alkaloid from tall fescue (*Festuca arundinacea* Schreb.): chemistry of the functional groups, *Aust. J. Chem.*, 18(1), 53, 1965.
64. Robbins, J. D., Sweeny, J. G., Wilkinson, S. R., and Burdick, D., Volatile alkaloids of Kentucky-31 tall fescue seed (*Festuca arundinacea* Schreb.), *J. Agric. Food Chem.*, 20(5), 1040, 1972.
65. Bruce, L. A., Robbins, J. D., and Huber, T. L., Smooth muscle response to fescue alkaloids, *J. Anim. Sci.*, 32(2), 373, 1971, Abstr. No. 18.
66. Bush, L. P. and Jeffreys, J. A. D., Isolation and separation of tall fescue and ryegrass alkaloids, *J. Chromatogr.*, 111(1), 165, 1975.
67. Buckner, R. C., Bush, L. P., Burrus, P. B., II, Variability and heritability of perloline in *Festuca* species, *Lolium* species, and *Lolium-Festuca-* hybrids, *Crop Sci.*, 13(6), 666, 1973; *Chem. Abstr.*, 80, 68470k.
68. Cornelius, P. L., Buckner, R. C., Bush, L. P., Burrus, P. B., II, and Byars, J., Inheritance of perloline content in annual ryegrass × tall fescue hybrids, *Crop Sci.*, 14(6), 896, 1974; *Chem. Abstr.*, 82, 108956y.
69. Watson, C. E., Jr., Heritability for perloline, nitrogen and digestibility charactestistics in tall fescue (*Festuca arundinacea* Schreb.) single-crosses grown in two locations, Doctoral Thesis, Oregon State Univ., Corvallis, *Diss. Abstr. Int. B*, 37(7), 3199, 1977.
70. Watson, C. E., Jr., Frakes, R. V., Chilote, D. O., Sleper, D. A., and Matches, A. G., Genetic variation for perloline, nitrogen, and digestibility in tall fescue, *Crop Sci.*, 18(3), 458, 1978; *Chem. Abstr.*, 89, 104067f.

71. Gentry, C. E., Chapman, R. A., Henson, L., and Buckner, R. C., Factors affecting the alkaloid content of tall fescue *(Festuca arundinacea), Agron. J.*, 61(2), 313, 1969; *Chem. Abstr.,* 70: 103672v.
72. Gentry, C. E., Interrelationship of *Rhizoctonia solani* Kühn, environment, and genotype on the alkaloid content of tall fescue, *Festuca arundinacea* Schreb., Doctoral Thesis, Univ. Ky., Lexington, *Diss. Abstr. Int. B*, 30(4), 1446, 1969.
73. Jeffreys, J. A. D., Sim, G. A., Burnell, R. H., Taylor, W. I., Corbett, R. E., Murray, J., and Sweetman, B. J., Perloline, *Proc. Chem. Soc.*, 1963, 171.
74. Ferguson, G., Jeffreys, J. A. D., and Sim, G. A., The alkaloids of perennial rye-grass (*Lolium perenne* L.). II. The crystal structure of the red form of perloline mercurichloride, *J. Chem. Soc., B*, 1966, 454.
75. Jeffreys, J. A. D., The alkaloids of perennial rye-grass (*Lolium perenne* L.). I. Perloline, *J. Chem. Soc.*, 4504, 1964.
76. Powers, J. C. and Ponticello, I., Total synthesis of the diazaphenanthrene alkaloid perlolidine, *J. Am. Chem. Soc.*, 90(25), 7102, 1968. *Chem. Abstr.*, 70, 29147J.
77. Akhtar, M. A., Brouwer, W. G., and Jeffreys, J. A. D., The alkaloids of perennial rye-grass (*Lolium perenne* L.). III. The synthesis of perlolidine, *J. Chem. Soc., C*, 1967, 859.
78. Seelye, R. N. and Stanton, D. W., Synthesis of perlolidine, *Tetrahedron Lett.*, 23, 2633, 1966.
79. Bathurst, N. O., Reifer, I., and Clare, E. M., A fluorescent alkaloid in rye-grass (*Lolium perenne* L.), IV. Methods of estimation, *N.Z. J. Sci. Technol.*, 24B, 161, 1943.
80. Yates, S. G., Rogovin, S. P., Bush, L. P., Buckner, R. C., and Boling, J. A., Isolation of perloline, the yellow alkaloid of tall fescue, *Ind. Eng. Chem., Prod. Res. Dev.*, 14, 315, 1975.
81. Shaffer, S. R., Williams, M., Harmon, B. J., Pickett, E. E., and Garner, G. B., Determination of perloline by a fluorometric method, *J. Agric. Food Chem.*, 23(2), 346, 1975.
82. Boling, J. A., Hemken, R. W., Bush, L. P., Buckner, R. C., Jackson, J. A., Jr., and Yates, S. G., Role of alkaloids and toxic compounds in the utilization of tall fescues by ruminants, 14th Int. Grassland Cong., Lexington, Ky., Agric. Sci. Center, University of Kentucky, Lexington, 1981.
83. Steen, W. W., Gay, N., Boling, J. A., Buckner, R. C., Bush, L. P., and Lacefield, G., Evaluation of Ky-31, G1-306, G1-307 and Kenhy tall fescue as pasture for yearling steers. II. Growth, physiological response, and plasma constituents of yearling steers, *J. Anim. Sci.*, 48(3), 618, 1979.
84. Yates, S. G., Paper chromatography of alkaloids of tall fescue hay, *J. Chromatogr.*, 12(3), 423, 1963.
85. Tookey, H. L. and Yates, S. G., The alkaloids of tall fescue: loline (festucine) and perloline, *An. Quim.*, 68(5,6), 921, 1972.
86. Aasen, A. J. and Culvenor, C. C. J., Abnormally low vicinal coupling constants for O-CH-CH in a highly strained five-membered-ring ether; the identity of loline and festucine, *Aust. J. Chem.*, 22(9), 2021, 1969.
87. Ribas, M., Landa, A., and Ribas, I., Identification of festucine with methyl-*N*-depropionyldecorticasine, *An. Quim.*, 64(5), 515, 1968; *(Chem Abstr.*, 69, 109764c.)
88. Ribas, M. and Ribas, I., Identity of the alkaloid norloline with depropionyldecorticasine, *An. Quim.*, 64(6), 637, 1968; *Chem. Abstr.*, 69, 87265m.
89. Landa-Velon, A. and Ribas-Marques, I., Alkaloids of Papilonaceae. LV. Identification on N-depropionyldecorticasine and higher amides of decorticasine in *Adenocarpus decorticans* Boiss, *An. Quim.*, 70(4), 360, 1974; *Chem. Abstr.*, 81, 60849r.
90. Batirov, E. K., Malikov, V. M., and Yunusov, S. Y., Lolidine, a new chlorine-containing alkaloid from *Lolium cuneatum* seeds, *Khim, Prir. Soedin.*, 1, 63, 1976; *Chem. Abstr.*, 85, 74883s.
91. Batirov, E. K., Khamidkhodzhaev, S. A., Malikov, V. M., and Yunusov, S. Y., Study of alkaloids from *Lolium cuneatum, Khim. Prir. Soedin*, 1, 60, 1976; *Chem. Abstr.*, 85, 59556u.
92. Batirov, E. K., Malikov, V. M., and Yunusov, S. Y., Alkaloids from *Lolium cuneatum* seeds, *Khim. Prir. Soedin.*, 1, 120, 1976; *Chem. Abstr.*, 86, 13792k.
93. Warren, F. L., Senecio alkaloids, in *The Alkaloids*, Vol. 12, Manske, R. F., Ed., Academic Press, New York, 1970, 246.
94. McLean, E. K., Toxic actions of pyrrolizidine (Senecio) alkaloids, *Pharm. Rev.*, 22(4), 429, 1970; *Chem. Abstr.*, 74, 74403h.
95. McLean, E. K., Toxic actions of pyrrolizidine (Senecio) alkaloids, *Pharm. Rev.*, 22(3), 389, 1970; *Chem. Abstr.*, 73, 118613n.
96. Culvenor, C. C. J., Tumor-inhibitory activity of pyrrolizidine alkaloids, *J. Pharm. Sci.*, 57(7), 1112, 1968.
97. Culvenor, C. C. J., Dann, A. T., and Dick, A. T., Alkylation as the mechanism by which the hepatotoxic pyrrolizidine alkaloids act on cell nuclei, *Nature (London)*, 195, 570, 1962.
98. Mattocks, A. R., Toxicity of pyrrolizidine alkaloids, *Nature (London)*, 217, 723, 1968.
99. Mattocks, A. R. and White, I. N. H., Pyrrolic metabolites from non-toxic pyrrolizidine alkaloids, *Nature (London) New Biol.*, 231, 114, 1971.

100. Karimov, V. A. and Kamilov, I. K., Pharmacology of the new loline alkaloid and of its derivative, *Dokl. Akad. Nauk, Uzb. SSR*, 12, 43, 1961. Available from U.S. Dept. Comm., Clearinghouse for Fed. Sci. Tech. Info., Springfield, Va., 22151.
101. Sadritdinov, F. S., Khamdamov, I., and Rustamov, B., Curare-like properties of bisquaternary ammonium derivatives of pyrrolizidine, *Dokl. Akad, Nauk, Uzb. SSR*, 31(12), 22, 1974; *Chem. Abstr.*, 84, 115661t.
102. Shakhidoyatov, K. M., Abdullaev, N. P., Rustamov, B., and Kadyrov C. S., Synthesis and pharmacological properties of bisquaternary salts of the pyrrolizidine series, *Khim-Farm Zh*, 11(2), 44, 1977; *Chem. Abstr.*, 87, 68512v.
103. Bush, L., Boling, J., and Yates, S., Animal disorders, in *Tall Fescue Monograph*, Bush, L. and Buckner, R., Eds., Am. Agron. Soc., 1979, 247.
104. Stuedemann, J. A., Wilkinson, S. R., Williams, D. J., Ciordia, H., Ernst, J. V., Jackson, W. A., and Jones, J. B., Jr., Long-term broiler litter fertilization of tall fescue pastures and health and performance of beef cows, in *Managing Livestock Wastes*, Proc. 3rd Int. Symp. Livestock Wastes, Am. Soc. Agric. Eng., St. Joseph, Mich., 1975, 264.
105. Garner, G. B. and Harmon, B. W., Experimental pastures and field case data, in *Proceedings of Fescue Toxicity Conference*, Ext. Publ., University of Missouri, Columbia, 1973, 42.
106. Jacobson, D. R., Miller, W. M., Seath, D. M., Yates, S. G., Tookey, H. L., and Wolff, I. A., Nature of fescue toxicity and progress toward identification of the toxic entity, *J. Dairy Sci.*, 46(5), 416, 1963.
107. Williams, M., Shaffer, S. R., Garner, G. B., Yates, S. G., Tookey, H. L., Kintner, L. D., Nelson, S. L., and McGinity, J. T., Induction of fescue foot syndrome in cattle by fractionated extracts of toxic fescue hay, *Am. J. Vet. Res.*, 36(9), 1353, 1975.
108. Yates, S. G., Rothfus, J. A., Garner, G. B., and Cornell, C. N., Videothermometry for assay of fescue foot in cattle, *Am. J. Vet. Res.*, 40(8), 1192, 1979.
109. Cornell, C. N., Garner, G. B., Yates, S. G., and Bell, S., Comparative fescue foot potential of fescue varieties, *J. Anim. Sci.*, 55(1), 180, 1982.
110. Garner, G. B., Cornell, C. N., Yates, S. G., Plattner, R. D., Rothfus, J. A., and Kwolek, W. F., Fescue foot: assay of extracts and compounds identified in extracts of toxic tall fescue herbage, *J. Anim. Sci.*, 55(1), 185, 1982.
111. Bush, L. and Buckner, R. C., Tall fescue toxicity, in *Antiquality Components of Forages*, Matches, A. G., Ed., Crop Sci. Soc. Am. Inc., Madison, Wisc., 1973, 99.
112. Hemken, R. W., Bull, L. S., Boling, J. A., Kane, E., Bush, L. P., and Buckner, R. C., Summer fescue toxicosis in lactating dairy cows and sheep fed experimental strains of ryegrass-tall fescue hybrids, *J. Anim. Sci.*, 49(3), 641, 1979.
113. Hemken, R. W., Boling, J. A., Bull, L. S., Hatton, R. H., Buckner, R. C., and Bush, L. P., Interaction of environmental temperature and anti-quality factors on the severity of summer fescue toxicosis, *J. Anim. Sci.*, 52(4), 710, 1981.
114. Hurley, W. L., Convey, E. M., Leung, K., Edgerton, L. A., and Hemken, R. W., Bovine prolactin, TSH, T_4, and T_3 concentrations as affected by tall fescue summer toxicosis and temperature, *J. Anim. Sci.*, 51(2), 374, 1981.
115. Jackson, J. A., Jr., Hemken, R. W., Boling, J. A., Bull, L. S., Bush, L. P., and Buckner, R. C., Summer fescue toxicosis as a result of feeding tall fescue seed, *J. Dairy Sci.*, 63 (Suppl. 1), 185, 1980.
116. Wilkinson, S. R. and Stuedemann, J. A., Fertilizer: animal health and pasture fertilization with poultry litter, in *Yearbook Sci. Technol.*, McGraw-Hill, New York, 1974, 180.
117. Stuedemann, J. A., Williams, D. J., and Wilkinson, S. R., Fat necrosis in beef cattle grazing heavily fertilized fescue pastures, in *Proc. 1974 Beef Cattle Short Course: Water Management Problems of the Cow and Calf Producer*, Coop. Ext. Serv., College of Agric., University of Georgia, Athens, 1974, 6.
118. Williams, D. J., Tyler, D. E., and Papp, E., Abdominal fat necrosis as a herd problem in Georgia Cattle, *J. Am. Vet. Med. Assoc.*, 154(9), 1017, 1969.

Toxic Animal Constituents

FOOD CONTAMINANTS: ANIMAL GROWTH PROMOTORS (ANTIBIOTIC RESIDUES)

Irtaza H. Siddique

INTRODUCTION

The use of antibiotics for about 30 years has made it possible to successfully treat and alleviate the effects of many diseases in both men and animals. In addition, antibiotics have been widely used to promote growth of livestock. An estimated 80% of U.S. livestock and poultry receive some animal drug during their lifespan. Low levels of penicillin, several tetracyclines, and combination products containing these antibiotics are estimated to be used in feed for all turkeys, 30% of chickens, 80% of swine and veal calves, and 60% of cattle raised for food in the U.S.[1] Needless to say, the use of antibiotics in feed has resulted in increased supplies of meat and eggs for the consumers.[2,3] A report by the Council for Agricultural Science and Technology (CAST) indicates that in absence of the antibiotic use, the efficiency of gain will be reduced, and methods of raising animals would become less efficient.

Under the Food, Drug, and Cosmetic Act, foods are considered adulterated when they are contaminated with unapproved residues of drugs. Hence the antibiotic residues which may be found in foods that come from animals in which antibiotics are used may be a source of health hazard in man and are, therefore, undesirable.

An ideal antibiotic should conform to the following criteria for a modern veterinary antibacterial agent;[4]

1. Safe in use
2. Active against a wide range of organisms.
3. Minimal residue problems
4. Will not endanger the efficacy of antibiotics used in the human field
5. Moves rapidly to the site of action in the animal body and the bacterial cell

ANTIBIOTICS IN MILK

The antibiotic residues in milk and dairy products have resulted in problems of concern to the dairy industry. The recurring problem of antibiotics in raw milk supply is a great liability to the dairy industry. Accordingly, in addition to economic loss to the offending dairymen, antibiotic residues in milk increase the cost of milk marketing and create potential health problems for the consumer.[54] Antibiotic residues bring about retardation and complete absence of acid production by bacterial starter cultures employed in many of the manufactured products, including cheese.[57] Antibiotics that are used in the treatment of mastitis are penicillin, streptomycin, neomycin, polymyxin, and others, and are used singly or in combination. It is desirable that the antibiotic levels are adequate in order to be effective.[58]

However, in cases where the drug is not properly used, there is a possibility that the antibiotics are either excreted in milk or are retained in the animal tissues and thus pass on to consumers. The antibiotic residues may result in a number of hazards.

Antibiotic Residues Causing Toxic, Allergic, or Hypersensitive Reactions[5-13]

It is estimated that 17 to 20 million people in the U.S. are sensitive to antibiotics and other chemotherapeutic drugs. Antibiotic contaminated milk or food creates a potential for a harmful allergic reaction which may range from mild sensitizing responses to fatal or near-fatal anaphylactic shock in people who cannot tolerate even very small quantities of these drugs.[54]

Antibacterial Agents Enhancing Pathogenicity of Gram-Negative Bacilli

Many such antibiotic-resistant organisms may cause diseases both in humans and animals. This resistance can then be transferred to bacteria in people and as a consequence antibiotics may be less effective in therapy because the bacteria have increased immunity to these antibacterial agents. Bacteria harboring R-factors both pathogenic and "nonpathogenic" are considered to be particularly hazardous because of their ability to transfer multiple drug resistance. Transferrable drug resistance indicates that the original bacterium is capable of passing the resistance characteristic to other bacteria through special finger-like appendages called "pili". Resistance to a single drug or multiple drugs may be transferred if the donor cell possesses the determinants for these drugs.[14-35]

Antibiotics Changing Florae

The use of antibiotics may change florae and contribute to a build-up of antibiotic resistant bacteria in the intestinal tracts of man and animals. The theoretical possibility that drug-resistant pathogens can be produced by antibiotic selection has become a real threat with the emergence of human diseases (typhoid and childhood meningitis) caused by ampicillin and chloramphenicol-resistant *Salmonella* and *Haemophilus*. The point is that *known routes of transfer exist by which antibiotic use in animals can contribute to such threats.*[36-48]

Orally Administered Antibiotics

Some orally administered antibiotics, e.g., tetracyclines, are incompletely absorbed and large proportions are excreted intact. The effect of such residues on soil microorganisms is largely unknown, but includes the possible development of drug-resistant bacteria.[49]

CONDITIONS RELATED TO ANTIBIOTIC RESIDUES

Because of these possible hazards due to antibiotic residues, the Commissioner of the Food and Drug Administration established a task force of scientists in April 1970, to undertake a comprehensive review of the use of antibiotics in animal feeds. This task force identified, among others, the conditions which were related to its study.

1. The use of antibiotics, especially in subtherapeutic amounts, favors the selection and development of single- and multiple-antibiotic resistance and R-factor bearing bacteria.
2. Animals which are exposed to antibiotics may serve as reservoirs of antibiotic-resistant bacteria which can produce human infections; *Salmonella* and *Escherichia coli* organisms being the most prominent bacteria in this category.
3. The antibiotic-resistant bacteria have been found on meat and meat products and there has been an increase in the prevalence of such organisms in man.

RECOMMENDATIONS

The Task Force on the use of antibiotics in animal feeds in 1972 recommended:

1. The Food and Drug Administration (FDA) review the effectiveness of low and intermediate levels of antibiotics used alone or in combination in feed and discontinue any ineffective uses
2. The FDA prohibit the low-level use in feeds of antibiotics that are also used in human therapy if they fail to meet criteria developed from the Task Force's guidelines, and that such antibiotics be permitted in animals only by a veterinarian's prescription for treatment of disease

3. That antibiotics most critically needed for treatment of disease in man not be used at all in animal feeds. The specific antibiotics named: chloramphenicol, semisynthetic penicillins, gentamycin, and kanamycin. The FDA has never approved any of these drugs for use in animal feeds.
4. The FDA undertake additional research on the safety and efficacy of antibiotics used in animals and on the diseases for which antibiotics are used as the principal treatment
5. That industry begin immediately to develop other drugs that can be used in feeds to increase growth rate and efficiency

In an effort to maintain vigilance for nonpermitted biological residues in food animals, the Meat and Poultry Residue Program is carried out by the U.S. Department of Agriculture (USDA).[50-53]

The USDA regularly monitors tissue samples from slaughtered animals for between 30 and 40 individual agricultural and environmental chemical compounds. Classes of compounds and examples of compounds presently monitored include:

Antimicrobials—Sulfonamides, penicillins, streptomycin, tetracyclines, erythromycin, and neomycin.

Other drugs—Coccidiostats, growth promotants, and other special purpose drugs.

Pesticides—Chlorinated hydrocarbon pesticides, various industrial chemicals, hexachlorobezene, and polychlorinated benzene.

Trace elements—Lead, cadmium, mercury, and arsenic.

DETECTION AND REGULATION

The USDA drug detection program consists of two parts: the monitoring phase and the surveillance phase. Uniform procedures and guidelines have been established to assure compliance with the regulations when residues are suspected or found in edible tissues of animals slaughtered for human food. To monitor the residues, tissue samples are randomly selected from carcasses of normal-appearing animals for residue analysis. Results thus obtained are employed to predict trends, incidence, and provide information for compliance and control. Analytical results of antibiotics and sulfonamides (in ppm) in animal tissues taken as part of National Residue Monitoring Program — USDA 1973 are shown in Table 1.

Table 2 shows the incidence of antibiotic violations in randomly selected animals, and Table 3 shows the incidence of antibiotic violations in different types of cattle.

The USDA announced recently that the percentage of illegal chemical residues in meat and poultry remained constant during the July-September quarter 1977. Among the 7080 samples analyzed, 640 residue violations were found.[54]

Officials of the USDA Food Safety and Quality Service said that the major violation continued to be sulfonamaide residues in swine—614 violations out of 4426 samples — a violation rate of 13.8% as compared with April-June rate of 13.41%.

Other samples analyzed during the 3rd quarter indicated 25 red meat violations out of 1820 samples — a violation rate of 1.37%, as compared with the same rate the previous quarter; 1 poultry residue violation out of 753 samples — a violation rate of 0.13%, as compared with 0.21% the second quarter.

A breakdown of other types of violations for the 3rd quarter of 1977 showed 21 antibiotic, 2 diethylstilbestrol, and 3 halocarbon residue violations.

In the January 20, 1978, *Federal Register,* of the Food and Drug Administration published its proposed regulations which would permit use of penicillin and the tetracyclines in animal feed "only upon the written order of a licensed veterinarian". The restrictions would prohibit livestock and poultry producers from purchasing and using

Table 1
ANALYTICAL RESULTS FOR ANTIBIOTICS AND SULFONAMIDES (IN PPM) IN ANIMAL TISSUES[a] TAKEN AS PART OF THE NATIONAL RESIDUE MONITORING PROGRAM (USDA, 1973)

	Sample	ND[b]	0.01—0.3	0.31—1.0	1.01—1.5	1.51—2.0	2.01—3	Over 3.0
Penicillin	5301	5284	8	2	1	0	0	0
Streptomycin	5299	5206	1	1	3	3	18	67
Tetracycline	5299	5271	0	23	2	1	0	2
Erythromycin	5299	5297	0	1	0	0	0	1
Neomycin	5299	5167	1	5	3	3	2	18
Oxytetracycline	5299	5290	0	5	2	0	0	2
Chlortetracycline	5299	5274	10	11	2	0	1	1
Nonspecific	5301	5147	154	0	0	0	0	0
Sulfas	728	716	0	0	0	0	2	10

[a] All livestock. Does not include poultry. During 1973, 840 poultry tissues were analyzed; no antibiotics or sulfas were detected.[3]
[b] Nondetectable.

Reprinted from *Federation Proceedings* 34:197—201, 1975. With permission.

Table 2
INCIDENCE OF ANTIBIOTIC VIOLATIONS IN RANDOMLY SELECTED ANIMALS, NATIONAL RESIDUE MONITORING PROGRAM 1973—77[53]

	1973	1974	1975	1976	1977[a]
Species	Violation/Sample (%)	Violation/Sample (%)	Violation/Sample (%)	Violation/Sample (%)	Violation/Sample (%)
Cattle	46/1592 (2.9)	18/1336 (1.3)	6/458 (1.3)	8/545 (1.5)	8/389 (2.1)
Calves	147/1882 (7.8)	94/2849 (3.3)	155/2131 (7.3)	81/1378 (5.9)	17/293 (5.8)
Swine	15/838 (1.8)	7/292 (2.4)	4/150 (2.7)	2/247 (0.8)	2/105 (1.9)
Chicken	4/665 (0.6)	2/296 (0.7)	5/177 (2.8)	1/155 (0.6)	0/92 (0.0)
Turkey	0/175 (0.0)	2/218 (0.9)	17/491 (3.5)	0/258 (0.0)	1/101 (1.0)

[a] Data from January to March 1977.

Table 3
INCIDENCE OF ANTIBIOTIC VIOLATIONS IN DIFFERENT TYPES OF CATTLE USDA-FSQS NATIONAL RESIDUE MONITORING PROGRAM 1973—1977[53]

	Samples analyzed	Total No. violations (%)	Penicillin/ Streptomycin	Neomycin	Tetracycline	Chlortetracycline	Erythromycin	UMI
1973								
Steer/Heifer								
Cows	1592	42 (2.6)	31	7		1		3
Bulls								
1974								
Steer/Heifer	35	0 (0.0)						
Cows	1298	17 (1.3)	13	1		1		2
Bulls	3	1 (33.3)	1					
1975								
Steer/Heifer	222	0 (0.0)						
Cows	225	6 (2.7)	2	1		1		1
Bulls	11	0 (0.0)						
1976								
Steer/Heifer	187	0 (0.0)						
Cows	345	7 (2.0)	7					
Bulls	13	1 (7.7)	1					
1977								
Steer/Heifer	75	0 (0.0)						
Cows	285	7 (2.5)	4	2	1			
Bulls	29	1 (3.4)	1					

Table 4
PRESLAUGHTER WITHDRAWAL TIMES FOR SWINES[53]

Swine Drug List

Active ingredients	Withdrawal days	Brand name examples
	Injectable use	
Dihydrostreptomycin	30	Numerous brand names
Lincomycin	2	Lincococin
Oxytetracycline	22	Terramycin®
Procaine Penicillin G	5	Crysticillin, Pro-Pen G, Combiotic, Distrycillin® A.S.
Procaine Penicillin G & dihydrostreptomycin	30	Pennstrep
Tylosin	4	Tylan® 50, Tylan® 200
	Oral use	
Arsanilic acid	5	Pro-Gen-Plus
Carbocox	70	Mecadox
Chlortetracycline	1	Aureomycin®, Vi-Mycin
Chlortetracyclin	2	Klortet, Vita-Treet
Chlortetracycline, sulfamethazine, and procaine penicillin (feed)	7	Chlorachel-250® Aureo SP-250®
Chlortetracycline, sulfathiazole, and procaine penicillin (feed)	7	CSP-250 and 500
Furazolidone	5	Furox®, Furoxone,® NF-180
Hygromycin B	2	Hygromix
Levamisole (feed or water)	3	Ripercol® L, Tramisol
Roxarsone	5	3-Nitro-10
Sodium arsanilate	5	Numerous brand names
Sodium sulfathiazole	10	Duatok
Sulfaquinoxline	10	S. Q. Solution, Tetrachel®
Tetracycline (HCl) (water)	4	Tetracycline HCL, Tetramycin, Tetra-sol,® Vetquamycin®
Tylosin (with vitamins)	2	Tylan® Plus Vitamins
Tylosin and sulamethazine	5	Tylan® Plus Sulfamethazine Tylan-Sulfa

medicated feeds containing these antibiotics without an order from a licensed veterinarian. Similar restrictions on the manufacture of animal feeds containing these antibiotics have been proposed. However, no final decision is expected on these issues until 1979 or later.[55] In addition, because of high incidence of illegal sulfa residues in swine, FDA has taken several steps to reduce the incidence of these residues, including extending the withdrawal time to 15 days for all sulfamethazine-containing products used in swine feed and water. Preslaughter withdrawal times for swine and cattle are given in the number of days between the last treatment and the day the animal is shipped. Times are given in Tables 4 and 5.

The problem of antibiotic residues in milk can be eliminated by withholding the milk of cows treated with antibiotics from the market for enough time to allow clearing of antibiotic residue from the udder. Milk discard time may vary from 36 to 96 hr depending on the antibiotic preparation used.[58] It has been shown that antibiotic from a treated quarter may be carried in the bloodstream and may be found in milk from all quarters; all milk from such a cow may be withheld until it is free from antibiotic residues. The key to the solution of the problem is to reduce incidence of mastitis, thus reducing need for mastitis treatment.[56]

Table 5
PRESLAUGHTER WITHDRAWAL TIME FOR CATTLE[53]

Beef Cattle Drug List

Active ingredients	Withdrawal Days	Brand name examples
	Injectable use	
Erythromycin	14	Enthro-200, Gallimycin®
Levamisole phosphate	7	Ripercol® L, Tramisol®
Oxytetracycline	15	Terramycin® 100
Oxytetracycline	18	Oxy-Tet 50, Oxy-Tet 100
Oxytetracycline	19	Aquachel, Oxyvet
Oxytetracycline	20	Oxyject
Oxytetracycline	22	Liquamycin, Oxytetracycline HCL Terramycin®
Procaine penicillin G and Dihydrostreptomycin sulfate	30	Combiotic, Distrycillin A. S. Mycillin V, Penstrep®, Pro-Mycin, Pro-Pen G in Dyhydrostreptomycin sulfate
Tylosin	8	Tylan® 50, Tylan® 100
	Oral use	
Chlortetracycline	2 (350 mg/head)	Klortet
Chlortetracyline	3	Aureomycin®, Vita-Treet
Chlortetracycline	10 (5 mg/lb)	Klortet
Chlortetracycline, Sulfamethazine	7	Aureomix® S-700
Levamisole	2	Levasole®, Ripercol® L Tramisol®
Melengestrol acetete	2	MGA®
Ronnel	10	Moorman's Rid Ezy, Trolene®
Thiabendazole	3	Mintrate, Moorman's E-Z Ex-Wormer, Omnizole,® Thibenzole
Tetracycline hydrochloride	5	Tetrachel®, Tetracycline HCL, Tetramycin, Tetra-Sol®, Vetquamycin, Panmycin
Tetracycline hydrochloride	12	T-500® Bolus
	Topicals	
Famphur and Xylene	35	Anchor Famphor, Bo-Ana®, Pour On Purina, Grub Kill, Warbex Famphur
Fenthion	35 (Add 45 days if retreated)	Tiguvon Pour On, Tiguvon Spray
Progesterone and estrodiol benzoate	60	Spotton®
Progesterone and estrodiol benzoate	60	Synovex®-Steers
Estrodiol benzoate and testrosterone propionate	60	Synovix-Heifers
Zeranol	65	Ralgro®

Beef Calf Drug List

	Oral Use	
Chlortetracycline and neomycin	1	Calf Scour Oblets
Streptomycin	2	Biolec 25%, Vetstrep® 25%

Note: These withdrawal times may not apply if other drugs or pesticides requiring preslaughter times have been used in the animal.

REFERENCES

1. U.S. Department of Health, Education and Welfare, Food and Drug Administration, HEW News, April 15, 1977.
2. Edwards, S. J., Effects of antibiotics on the growth rate and intestinal Flora *(Escherichia coli)* of calves, *J. Comp. Pathol.*, 72, 420—432, 1962.
3. Mussman, Harry C., Drug and Chemical residues in domestic animals, *Fed. Proc., Fed. Am. Soc. Exp. Biol.*, 34, 197—201, 1975.
4. Brander, G. C., History of semisynthetic penicillins, *Vet. Med. Small Anim. Clin.*, 72, 804, 1977.
5. Vickers, H. R., Dermatological hazards of the presence of penicillin in milk, *Proc. R. Soc Med.*, 57, 1091—1092, 1964.
6. Zimmerman, M. C., Chronic penicillin urticaria from dairy products, proved by penicillinase cures, *Am. Med. Assoc. Arch. Dermatol.*, 79, 1—6, 1959.
7. Caldwell, J. R. and Cluff, L. E., Adverse reactions to antimicrobial agents, *J. Am. Med. Assoc.*, 230, 77—80, 1974.
8. Martin, R. R., Warr, G. A., Couch, R. B., Yeager, H., and Knight, V., Effects of tetracycline on leukotaxis, *J. Infect. Dis.*, 129, 110—116, 1974.
9. Forsgren, A. and Schmeling, D., Effects of antibiotics on chemotaxis of human leukocytes, *Antimicrob. Agents Chemother.*, 11, 580—584, 1977.
10. Appel, G. B. and Neu, H. C., The nephrotoxicity of antimicrobial agents — medical progress, *N. Engl. J. Med.*, 296, 722—728, 1977.
11. Nickas, G. M., Antibiotics and the Kidney. II. Antibiotic induced nephrotoxicity, *Ariz. Med.*, 33, 577—578, 1978.
12. Alexander, J. W., Antibiotic agents and the immune mechanisms of defence, *Bull. N. Y. Acad. Med.*, 51, 1039-1045, 1975.
13. Smith, D. H. Antibiotics in agriculture and the health of man, U.S. Food and Drug Administration Papers, September 10, 1968.
14. Huber, W. G., The impact of antibiotic drugs and their residues., *Adv. Vet. Sci. Comp. Med.*, 15, 101—132, 1971.
15. Bernard, H. R., Dangers of indiscriminate antibiotic therapy, *Surg. Clin. N. Am.*, 55, 1303—1308, 1975.
16. Loken, K. I., Wagner, L. W., and Henke, C. L., Transmissible drug resistance in enterobacteriaceae isolated from calves given antibiotics, *Am. J. Vet. Res.*, 32, 1207—1212, 1971.
17. Smith, H. W., The effect of the use of antibacterial drugs on the emergence of drug resistant bacteria in animals, *Adv. Vet. Sci. Comp. Med.*, 15, 67—100, 1971.
18. Porcurull, D. W., Gaines, S. A., and Mercer, H. D., Surveys on infectious multiple drug resistance among Salmonella isolated from animals in the United States, *Appl. Microbiol.*, 21, 358—362, 1971.
19. Gill, F. A. and Hook, E. W., Salmonella with transferable antimicrobial resistance, *JAMA*, 198, 1267—1269, 1966.
20. Bissett, M. I., Abbot, S. L., and Wood, R. M., Antimicrobial resistance and R-factors in Salmonella isolated in California (1971-1972), *Antimicrob. Agents Chemother.*, 5, 161—168, 1974.
21. Williams-Smith, H. The incidence of transmissible antibiotic resistance amongst Salmonellae isolated from poultry in England and Wales, *J. Med. Microbiol.*, 3, 181, 1970.
22. Cooksey, R. C., Thorne, G. M., and Farrer, W. Ed., Jr., R Factor-medicated antibiotic resistance in *Serratia marcescens*, *Antimicrob. Agents Chemother.*, 10, 123—127, 1976.
23. Burt, S. J. and Woods, D. R., Solution of transferable antibiotic resistance in coliform bacteria from remote environments, *Antimicrob. Agents Chemother.*, 10, 567—568, 1976.
24. Neu, H. C., Cherubin, C. E., Longo, E. D., Flouton, B., and Winter, J., Antimicrobial resistance and R-factor transfer among isolates of Salmonella in Northeastern United States: a comparison of human and animal isolates, *J. Infect Dis.*, 132, 617—622, 1975.
25. Rennie, R. P. and Duncan, I. B. R., Emergence of gentamycin-resistant Klebsiella in a general hospital, *Antimicrob. Agents Chemother.*, 11, 179—184, 1977.
26. Dorn, C. R., Tsutakawa, R. K., Fein, D., Burton, G. C., and Blenden, C. D., Antibiotic resistance patterns of *Escherichia coli* isolated from farm families consuming home-raised meat, *Am. J. Epidemiol.*, 102, 319—326, 1975.
27. Fein, D., Blenna, B., Tsutakawa, R., and Blenden, D., Matching of antibiotic resistance patterns of *Escherichia coli* of farm families and their animals, *J. Infect. Dis.*, 140, 274—279, 1974.
28. Levy, S. B., Fitzgerald, G. B., and Macone, B. S., Change in intestinal flora of farm personnel after introduction of tetracycline-supplemented feed on a farm, *N. Engl. J. Med.*, 295, 583—588, 1976.
29. Wells, D. M. and James, O. B., Transmission of infectious drug resistance from animals to man, *J. Hyg.*, 71, 209—215, 1973.

30. Neu, H. C., Cherubin, C. E., Longo, E. D., Flouton, B., and Winter, J., Antimicrobial resistance and R-factor transfer among isolates of Salmonella in the Northeastern United States: comparison of Human and Animal Isolates, *J. Infect. Dis.*, 132, 617—622, 1975.
31. Smith, H. W., The incidence of infective drug resistance in strains of *Escherichia coli* isolated from diseased human beings and domestic animals, *J. Hyg.*, 64, 465—474, 1966.
32. Smith, H. W., The transfer of antibiotic resistance between strains of enterobacteria in chicken, calves and pigs, *J. Med. Microbiol.*, 3, 165—180, 1970.
33. Harry, E. G., The ability of low concentrations of chemotherapeutic substances to induce resistance in *E. coli, Poultry Sci.*, 3, 85—93, 1964.
34. Corey, R. and Byrnes, J. M., Oxytetracycline, coliforms in commercial Poultry Products, *Appl. Microbiol.*, II 481—484, 1963.
35. Girard, A. E., English, A. R., Evangelisti, D. G., Lynch, J. E., and Solmons, I. A., Influence of subtherapeutic levels of a combination of neomycin and oxytetracycline on *Salmonella typhimurium* in swine, calves and chickens, *Antimicrob. Agents Chemother.*, 10, 89—95, 1966.
36. Evangelisti, D. B., English, A. R., Girard, A. E., Lynch, J. E., and Solomons, I. A., Influence of subtherapeutic levels of oxytetracycline on *Salmonella typhimurium* in swine, calves and chickens, *Antimicrob. Agents Chemother.*, 8, 664—672, 1975.
37. Walton, J. R., Indirect consequences of low-level use of antimicrobial agents in animal feeds. Food sources of incidental drug exposure, *Fed. Proc., Fed. Am. Soc. Exp. Biol.*, 34, 205—208, 1975.
38. Seigel, D., Huber, W. G., and Enloe, F., Continuous nontherapeutic use of antibacterial drugs in feed and drug resistance of the gram-negative enteric flora of food producing animals, *Antimicrob. Agents Chemother.*, 6, 697—701, 1974.
39. Smith, H. W. and Crabb, W. E., The effect of the continuous administration of diets containing low levels of tetracyclines on the incidence of drug-resistant *Bacterium coli* in the faeces of pigs and chickens: the sensitivity of *Bact. coli* to other chemotherapeutic agents, *Vet. Rec.*, 69, 24—30, 1957.
40. Mercer, H. D., Pocurull, D., Gaines, S., Wilson, S., and Bennett, J. V., Characteristics of Antimicrobial resistance of *Escherichia coli* from animals: relationship to veterinary and management uses of antimicrobial agents, *Appl. Microbiol.*, 22, 700—705, 1971.
41. Linton, A. H., Hadley, B., Osborne, A. D., Whaw, B. G., Roberts, T. A., and Hudson, W. R., Contamination of pig carcasses at two abattoirs by *Escherichia coli* with special reference to 0-serotypes and antibiotic resistance, *J. Appl. Bacteriol.*, 42, 89—111, 1977.
42. Katz, S. E., Fassbender, C. A., Dinnerstein, P. S., and Dowlin, J. J., Jr., Effects of Feeding Penicillin to Chickens, *J. Assoc. Off. Anal. Chem.*, 57, 522—526, 1974.
43. Schroeder, S. A., Terry, P. M., and Bennett, J. V., Antibiotic resistance and transfer factor in Salmonella, United States 1967, *JAMA*, 205, 903—906, 1968.
44. Babcock, G. F., Berry-ill, D. L., and Marsch, D. H., R-factors of *Escherichia coli* from dressed beef and humans, *Appl. Microbiol.*, 25, 21—23, 1973.
45. Anderson, J. W., Gillespie, W. A., and Richmond, M. H., Chemotherapy and antibiotic-resistance transfer between enterobacteria in the human gastro-intestinal tract, *J. Microbiol.*, 6, 461—473, 1973.
46. Lundback, A. and Nordstrom, K., Effect of R-factor mediated drug metabolizing enzymes on survival of *Escherichia coli* K-12 in presence of ampicillin, chloram phenicol or streptomycin, *Antimicrob. Agents Chemother.*, 5, 492—499, 1974.
47. U.S. Department of Health Education and Welfare, Food and Drug Administration, Bureau of Veterinary Medicine, Animal Drug Memo, May 16—31, 1977.
48. U.S. Department of Health Education and Welfare, Food and Drug Department of Health, Education and Welfare, Public Health Service, Food and Drug Administration, Bureau of Veterinary Medicine, Rockville, Md., Publication No. (FDA) 76-7011.
49. Anon., Residue violations in meat and poultry remain constant, *J. Am. Vet. Med. Assoc.*, 172, 133, 1978.
50. Freeman, A., Veterinarians order of antibiotics in feed, *J. Am. Vet. Med. Assoc.*, 172, 658, 1978.
51. U.S. Department of Agriculture, Animal and Plant Health Inspection Service, Meat and Poultry Inspection Program, Washington, D.C., MPI Directive 917.1, 1976.
52. Cazier, P. D. and Arnold, J. S., Monitoring drug use in food animals, FDA Consumer September 1975, DHEW Publ. No. (FDA) 76—3006.
53. Leese, W. F., United States Department of Agriculture, Food Safety and Quality Service, Washington, D.C., 1977, (personal communications).
54. Anon., Dairy men must solve problem of antibiotics in milk, *Hoard's Dairyman*, Feb. 10, 1978.
55. Siddique, I. H., Antibiotic residues in foods, in *The Safety of Foods,* AVI Publ. Westport, Conn. 1968, 358—360.
56. Siddique, I. H., Loken, K. I., and Hoyt, H. H., Antibiotic residues in milk transferred from treated to untreated quarters in dairy cattle, *J. Am. Vet. Med. Assoc.*, 146, 589—593, 1965.
57. Albright, J. L., Tuckey, S. L., and Woods, G. T., Antibiotics in milk — review, *J. Dairy Sci.*, 34, 779—807, 1961.

58. Siddique, I. H., Loken, K. I., and Hoyt, H. H., Concentrations of neomycin, dihydrostreptomycin and polymyxin in milk after intramuscular or intramammary administration, *J. Am. Vet. Med. Assoc.*, 146, 594—599, 1965.

NATURALLY OCCURRING HORMONES IN ANIMAL FOODS: TESTOSTERONE

Bernd Hoffmann

INTRODUCTION

Testosterone is a steroid hormone with 19 carbon atoms, thus belonging to the group of androgens, having a β-OH-group in the C-17 position, a 3-keto group at C-3, and a double bond in ring A from C-4 to C-5 (Figure 1); the systematic name is 17β-Hydroxy-4-androsten-3-one.[1] It is the principal hormone produced by the male gonad, the testis,[2] and was first identified by David et al.[3] in 1935. Testicular androgen production has been demonstrated to occur during all developmental stages, including fetal life.[4-9] The female gonads as well as the adrenals also possess the basic capacity to produce testosterone.[4,10-12] Another way for formation of testosterone is from peripheral metabolism of certain precursors like androstenedione (4-androstene-3, 17-dione).[4] Apart from these endogenous sources, testosterone can enter the body due to certain treatments, for example when given as a replacement therapy, or, like in animal production, as a constituent of certain anabolic preparations.[13,14] Regardless of its origin, but with some species-specific differences, testosterone is predominantly metabolized to biologically less active forms (catabolism of steroids) which are primarily excreted after conjugation to glucuronic acid with the urine or appear as free steroids in the feces.[4,13,15,16] The route of elimination via the feces is of particular interest, since the steroids are originally secreted as conjugates with the bile into the gut, where a majority are hydrolyzed due to the presence of hydrolytic enzymes, mostly of bacterial origin. The free steroid can then be reabsorbed and enter the enterohepatic circulation. However, it should be kept in mind that, in the case of endogenous steroids like testosterone, usually only biologically deactivated metabolites will undergo enterohepatic circulation.[13,17,18] As was shown for the human, the male liver exhibits a bigger capacity to metabolize testosterone then the female liver.[19]

The primary activity of testosterone in the male is to allow and stimulate development of the genital tract and to maintain its function thereafter. Similarly, testosterone is responsible for the expression of the secondary sex characteristics.[2] In the female, testosterone seems to be involved in the processes of follicular maturation and ovulation, either directly or as a precursor for estrogen production.[10,20]

Apart from its sex hormone activities, testosterone also exerts some extragonadal, anabolic activities which, however, seem to be related, but not uniquely, to the androgenic activity in general.[13,21-24] Thus, testosterone and other biologically active androgens, usually in combination with an estrogen, are applied as constituents of anabolic preparations in animals, particularly in beef, veal, and lamb production[13,14] (for example 200 mg testosterone in combination with 20 mg estradiol-17β are suggested to be used as a subcutaneous (s.c.) implant at the base of the ear in female veal calves, at least 70 days before slaughter).

OCCURRENCE OF TESTOSTERONE IN FOOD ANIMALS

The definition of a food animal may vary between countries, depending on the eating habits. However, in this chapter reference will be made only to those animals which are generally accepted throughout the world as food animals. In general the availability of data on tissue levels of hormones, not to mention concentrations in processed food, is rather limited, while the occurrence of testosterone in peripheral plasma has been

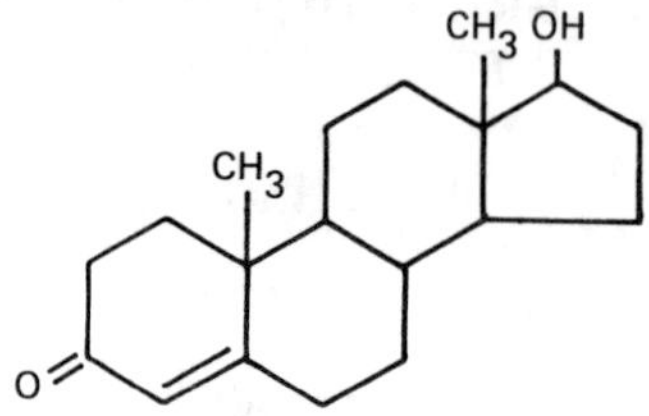

FIGURE 1.

studied to a greater extent. Therefore, until more data on the actual tissue levels of hormones have been compiled, the peripheral plasma data have in part to be accepted as an indicator for the presence of hormones in food of animal origin.

Blood Levels
Male Animals

Table 1 shows the values seen in male animals. Obviously they show a wide range of concentrations but can be quite high (up to 28 ng/mℓ in the ram), which is also reflected in the production rate which, for example, was calculated to be between 40 to 50 mg testosterone per 24 hr in the bull.[42] For some species like cattle and sheep, diurnal rhythms for the concentrations of testosterone in peripheral plasma have been established.[25,28,31] Similarly, seasonal changes in the testosterone production have been observed in the sheep, goat, and stallion.[31,43]

Among the species listed in Table 1, only males from cattle and domestic fowl enter the food chain in substantial numbers. Particularly in the pig for reasons of meat hygiene, people object to the marketing of the intact, sexually mature male animal due to the occurrence of a specific "boar taint steroid" with the approach of puberty. This highly odorous compound (androstenon, 5α-androst-16-en-3-one), related in its biosynthesis to that of testosterone, can be measured in concentrations between 2 and 30 ng/mℓ peripheral plasma,[47,48] and can reach levels of more than 7 µg/g adipose tissue.[33,44-46]

Female Animals

From the data available it is evident that levels are generally 10 to 100 times lower in females than those determined in male animals (Table 2). Similarly the testosterone production in the ewe from an autotransplanted ovary was calculated to stay in the low microgram range (up to 2 µg/24 hr).[54] In the mare, the concentrations of androstenedione, which can act as a precursor for testosterone, were between 0.18 and 0.38 ng/mℓ plasma.[55]

Castrate and Prepubertal Animals

As for the female animal, only limited data are available on testosterone levels in male-castrated animals. As far as determined, levels are in the same range or even lower than those in intact female animals (Table 3).

Concerning the prepubertal animal, probably only the calf can be considered as a regular food animal (veal calf). The testosterone levels determined in peripheral plasma of male calves are higher than those in normal female and testosterone-treated female calves. Still slightly higher levels were determined in male piglets (Table 4).

Tissue Levels and Concentrations in Milk

In respect to the occurrence of tissue levels of testosterone, only cattle have been studied in any detail.[57] Table 5 gives the values for free testosterone determined in muscle, liver, kidney, and fat of mature slaughter bulls, heifers, and untreated and

Table 1
TESTOSTERONE CONCENTRATIONS IN PERIPHERAL PLASMA OF MALE FOOD ANIMALS

Species	Testosterone, ng/ml (range)	Ref.
Cattle	1—18	25
	2—20	26
	2—10	27—29
Sheep	1.3—8.9	30
	0.5—28	31
Goat	3.1—7.7	32
Pig	2—23	15
	1.2—16	33, 34
	4—7	35
Horse	1.5—3.2	36
	0.08—1.6	37
Rabbit	1.1	38
Domestic fowl	7—11.3	39
	0.35—2.4	40
Fish	6—13	41

Table 2
TESTOSTERONE CONCENTRATIONS IN PERIPHERAL PLASMA OF FEMALE FOOD ANIMALS

Species	Testosterone, ng/ml (range)	Ref.
Cattle	0.010—0.047	49
Sheep	0.3	50
Goat	0.04—0.2	32
Pig	0.4—1.9	33
Rabbit	0.05	51
Domestic fowl	0.00—0.26	52
	0.15—0.62	53
	0.36—0.96	40

Table 3
TESTOSTERONE CONCENTRATIONS IN PERIPHERAL PLASMA OF MALE-CASTRATED FOOD ANIMALS

Species	Testosterone, ng/ml (range)	Ref.
Cattle	0.09	56
Sheep	<0.05	50
Pig	1.5—2.4	33
Horse	0.015	37

treated veal calves. It is evident that beyond the age- and sex-dependent relationship a certain tissue-dependent relationship also exists within each animal. Testosterone is highest (possibly due to the occurrence of receptor sites) in the kidney of animals with a low production rate (calf, heifer) and highest in fat of animals with a high testosterone production rate (bull). Probably the equilibrium achieved in the bull between production and metabolic clearance rate of testosterone allows its simple partitioning into fat based on physical and chemical properties (testosterone is rather lipophilic). It is

Table 4
TESTOSTERONE CONCENTRATIONS IN
PERIPHERAL PLASMA OF
PREPUBERTAL FOOD ANIMALS

Species	Testosterone, ng/ml (range)	Ref.
Calf (male)	0.5—0.6	13
Calf (female)	0.060—0.064	13
Calf (female-treated)[a]	0.26—0.51	13
Piglet (male)	1.5	35

[a] Concentrations determined 35—71 days after s.c. implantation of 20 mg extradiol-17β and 200 mg testosterone.

Table 5
CONCENTRATIONS OF UNCONJUGATED
(FREE) TESTOSTERONE (ng/g) IN VARIOUS
BOVINE TISSUE SAMPLES: MEAN VALUES OF
3—5 ANIMALS

Tissue	Veal calf Untreated	Veal calf Treated[a]	Feedlot heifer	Slaughter bull
Muscle	0.016	0.070	0.092	0.535
Liver	0.039	0.047	0.183	0.749
Kidney	0.256	0.685	0.595	2.783
Fat	0.178	0.340	0.250	10.950

[a] 20 mg estradiol-17β plus 200 mg testosterone as a s.c. implant 77 days before slaughter.

From Hoffmann, B. and Rattenberger, E., *J. Anim. Sci.*, 45, 342 1977. With permission.

interesting to note that the testosterone levels seen in treated calves are only slightly higher (not significantly) than those in untreated animals and very similar to those measured in heifers. Apart from free testosterone, Hoffmann and Rattenberger[57] have also determined the presence of conjugated testosterone which exceeded the concentrations of free testosterone only in liver (Table 6) and was not detectable in fat. As for tissues, no sex or age differences in the ratios of free to conjugated testosterone were seen. To allow some comparison, the total testosterone content in bull testes increases from less than 100 μg in animals 39 to 90 days old to a content of more than 3000 μg in fully mature animals;[58,59] calf ovaries contained between 20 and 100 ng testosterone.[12]

Finally, the testosterone levels determined in cows' milk varied between <0.05 and 0.122 ng/ml, depending on the stage of the cycle.[57]

Other than for cattle, only some isolated data are available for the boar where testosterone reached concentrations between 8 and 24 ng/g in the fat while those of androsterone could be above 7 μg/g.[48,68]

CONCLUSIONS

Though the information is still limited, it can be said with confidence that practically all food of animal origin contains endogenous hormones, one of them being testoster-

Table 6
CONJUGATED TESTOSTERONE IN PERCENT OF TOTAL TESTOSTERONE (FREE AND CONJUGATE) IN BOVINE MUSCLE, LIVER AND KIDNEY TISSUE

Tissue	Conjugate testosterone (%)
Muscle	8.6
Liver	76.8
Kidney	37.5

From Hoffmann, B. and Rattenberger, E., *J. Anim. Sci.*, 45, 342, 1977. With permission.

one. It is highly unlikely that the steroid testosterone, which is also quite stable under rather extreme conditions like gas chromatography (temperature up to about 280°C), will be destroyed during the common food-processing procedures. However, under certain conditions, some microbial or special chemical degradation (reduction) would have to be anticipated. From the studies performed in cattle,[57] it can be concluded that the testosterone concentrations in muscular tissue never exceed those determined in plasma; on the contrary, they can be expected to be lower. Apart from the site of production, accumulation of testosterone only seems to occur in tissues with receptor sites (kidney among the edible tissues) and in the liver (conjugated testosterone), which is the center regulating the metabolism of testosterone. Apparently only in male animals with a high testosterone production rate can the hormone concentrations accumulate in fat, reaching or exceeding the levels seen in peripheral plasma. Thus, testosterone can be considered a natural constituent of our food and the species probably contributing most to the human intake are poultry and cattle, especially if it is taken into account that in some countries, like Germany, the intact mature bull is the major beef-producing animal. It has further been demonstrated that the use of testosterone with anabolic implants in calves seems to increase the testosterone tissue concentrations seen at slaughter. However, the values are still well within the physiological range seen in heifers, and well below the levels observed in tissues from bulls (Table 5) or in testes, which occasionally are eaten as a local delicacy. Lastly it should be said that, based on normal eating habits and the low oral activity of testosterone, it cannot be expected that the rather minute amounts of testosterone consumed with food will significantly or measurably add to the endogenous testosterone already present in any human (testosterone production per 24 hr: 4.4 to 6.6 mg in men, 0.35 mg in women).[4]

REFERENCES

1. Schulster, D., Burstein, S., and Cooke, B. A., *Molecular Endocrinology of the Steroid Hormones*, John Wiley & Sons, New York, 1976, chap. 1.
2. Paulsen, C. A., The testes, in *Textbook of Endocrinology*, 5th Ed., Williams, R. H., Ed., W. B. Saunders, Philadelphia, 1974, chap. 6.

3. David, K., Dingemanse, E., Freud, J., and Laqueur, E., Über kristallinisches männliches Hormon aus Hoden (Testosteron), Wirksamer als aus Harn oder aus Cholesterin bereitetes Androsteron, *Zeitschr. Physiol. Chem.*, 233, 281, 1935.
4. Vermeulen, A., Plasma levels and secretion rate of steroids with anabolic activity in man, in *Environmental Quality and Safety, Suppl., Vol. V, Anabolic Agents in Animal Production*, Lu, F. C. and Rendel, J., Eds., Georg Thieme Verlag, Stuttgart, 1976, 171.
5. Struck, H. J. and Karg, H., Extraktion und dünnschichtchromatographische Bestimmung von Testosteron und Androstendion aus Testesgewebe von Rinderfoeten, *J. Chromatography*, 36, 74, 1968.
6. Attal, J., Levels of testosterone, androstenedione, estrone and estradiol-17β in the testes of fetal sheep, *Endocrinology*, 85, 280, 1969.
7. Meusy-Desolle, N., Evolution du taux de testostérone plasmatique an cours de la vie foetale chez le porc domestique, *C. R. Acad. Sci.*, 278, 1257, 1974.
8. Mongkonpunya, K., Oxender, W. D., and Hafs, H. D., Serum and testicular androgens in bovine fetuses, *J. Anim. Sci.*, 37, 321, 1973.
9. Elsaesser, F., König, A., and Smidt, D., Der Testosterone-und Androstendiongehalt in Eberhoden in Abhängigkeit vom Alter, *Acta Endocrinol. (Kbh)*, 69, 553, 1972.
10. Ross, T. G. and Van de Wiele, R., The ovaries, in *Textbook of Endocrinology*, 5th ed., William, R. H., Ed., W. B. Saunders, Philadelphia, 1974, chap. 7.
11. Turner, C. D. and Baguara, J. T., *General Endocrinology*, 5th ed., W. B. Saunders, Philadelphia, 1971, 361.
12. Rattenberger, E., Rückstandsanalytik von Testosteron im Gewebe vom Rind mit Hilfe des Radioimmunotest, Diss. Agric. Techn. Univ. München, 1976.
13. Hoffmann, B. and Karg, H., Metabolic fat of anabolic agents in treated animals and residue levels in their meat, in *Environmental Quality and Safety, Suppl., Vol. V, Anabolic Agents in Animals Production*, Lu, F. C. and Rendel, J., Eds., Georg Thieme Verlag, Stuttgart, 1976, 181.
14. Hoffmann, B., Karg, H., Vogt, K. and Kyrein, H. J. Aspekte zur Anwendung, Rückstandsbildung und Analytik von Sexualhormonen bei Masttieren, in *Forschungsbericht Deutsche Forschungsgemeinschaft, Rückstände in Fleisch und Fleischerzeugnissen*, Harold Boldt Verlag K. G., Boppard 1975, 32.
15. Velle, W., Endogenous anabolic agents in farm animals, in *Environmental Quality and Safety, Suppl., Vol. V., Anabolic Agent in Animals Production*, Lu, F. C. and Rendel, J., Eds., Georg Thieme Verlag, Stuttgart, 1976, 159.
16. Martin, R. P., Fecal metabolism of testosterone-4-^{14}C in the bovine male castrate, *Endocrinology*, 78, 907, 1966.
17. Gassner, F. X., Martin, R. P., Shimoda, W., and Algeo, J. W., Metabolism of radioactive steroid esters in the bovine male and female, *Fertil., Steril.*, 11, 49, 1960.
18. Martin, R. P., Loriaux, D. L., and Farnham, G. S., Enterohepatic cycling of metabolized testosterone in the male dog, *Steroids*, Suppl. 2, 149, 1965.
19. Nieschlag, E. and Cüppers, H., Plasma androgens in normal subjects and patients with liver diseases after oral administration of testosterone, *Acta Endocrinol. (Kbh)*, Suppl. 193, 56, 1975.
20. Lindner, H. R., Amsterdam, A., Salomon, Y., Tsafriri, A., Nimrod, A., Lamprecht, S. A., Zor, U., and Koch, Y., Intraovarian factors in ovulation: determination of follicular response to gonadotrophins, *J. Reprod. Fertil.*, 51, 215, 1977.
21. Martin, C. R., *Textbook of Endocrine Physiology*, Williams & Wilkins, Baltimore, 1976, 254.
22. Heitzman, R. J., The effectiveness of anabolic agents in increasing rate of growth in farm animals: report on experiments in cattle, in *Environmental Quality and Safety, Suppl., Vol. V., Anabolic Agents in Animal Production*, Lu, F. C. and Rendel, J., Eds., Georg Thieme Verlag, Stuttgart, 1976, 89.
23. Van Weerden, E. J. and Grandadam, J. A., The effect of an anabolic agent on N deposition, growth, and slaughter quality in growing castrated male pigs, in *Environmental Quality and Safety*, Suppl., Vol. V., Lu, F. C. and Rendel, J., Eds., Georg Thieme Verlag, Stuttgart, 1976, 115.
24. Gassner, F. X., Martin, R. P., and Algeo, J. W., Hormone in der Tiermast: 6. Symposium, Deutsche, Gesellschaft f. Endocrin, Springer-Verlag, Berlin, Göttingen, Heidelberg, 1959, 151.
25. Karg, H., Giménez, T., Hartl, M., Hoffmann, B., Schallenberger, E., and Schams, D., Testosterone, luteinizing hormone (LH) and follicle stimulating hormone (FSH) in peripheral plasma of bulls: levels from birth through puberty and short term variations, *Zentralbl. Veterinaermed. Reihe A.*, 23, 793, 1976.
26. Katangole, C. B., Naftolin, F., and Short, R. V., Relationships between blood levels of luteinizing hormone and testosterone in bulls, and the effect of sexual stimulation, *J. Endocrinol.*, 50, 457, 1971.
27. Smith, O. W., Mongkonpunya, K., Hafs, H. D., Convey, E. M., and Oxender, W. D., Blood serum testosterone after sexual preparation or ejaculation, or after injection of LH or prolactin in bulls, *J. Anim. Sci.*, 37, 979, 1973.

28. Sanval, P. C., Sundby, A., and Edqvist, L. E., Diurnal variation of peripheral plasma levels of testosterone in bulls measured by a rapid radioimmunoassay procedure, *Acta Vet. Scand.*, 15, 90, 1974.
29. Thibier, M. and Rolland, O., Levels of testosterone and luteinizing hormone in the plasma of young post-pubertal bulls after injection of human chorionic gonadotrophin or dexamethasone and human chorionic gonadotrophin, *J. Endocrinol.*, 75, 451, 1977.
30. Galloway, D. B., Cotta, J., Pelletier, J., and Terqui, M., Circulating luteinizing hormone and testosterone response in rams after luteinizing hormone releasing hormone treatment, *Acta Endocrinol. (Kbh)*, 77, 1, 1974.
31. Katangole, C. B., Naftolin, F., and Short, R. V., Seasonal variations in blood luteinizing hormone and testosterone levels in rams, *J. Endocrinol.*, 60, 101, 1974.
32. Zlotnik, G., Testosterone levels in intersex goats, *J. Reprod. Fertil.*, 32, 287, 1973.
33. Hoffmann, B., Claus, R., and Karg, H., Bestimmung von Testosterone im peripheren Blut von Schwein und Rind mit einer Doppelisotopen-Derivat-Verdünnungsmethode, *Acta Endocrinol. (Kbh)*, 64, 377, 1970.
34. Claus, R. and Alsing, W., Einfluб von Choriongonadtropin, Haltungsänderung und sexueller Stimulierung auf die Konzentrationen von Testosterone in Plasma sowie des Ebergeruchsstoffes in Plasma und Fett eines Ebers, *Berl. Munch. Tierarztl. Wschr.*, 89, 354, 1976.
35. Elasesser, F., Pomerantz, D. K., Ellendorff, F., Kreikenbaum, K., and König, A., Plasma LH, testosterone and DHT in the pig from birth to sexual maturity, *Acta Endocrinol. (Kbh)*, 72 (Suppl. 173), 148, 1973.
36. Berndtson, W. E., Picket, B. W., and Nett, T-M., Reproductive physiology of the stallion. IV. Seasonal changes in the testosterone concentrations in peripheral plasma, *J. Reprod. Fertil.*, 39, 115, 1974.
37. Cox, J. E., Williams, J. H., Rowe, P. H., and Smith, J. A., Testosterone in normal, cryptorchid and castrated male horses, *Equine Vet., J.*, 5, 85, 1973.
38. Falvo, R. E. and Nalbandov, A. V., Radioimmunoassay of peripheral plasma testosterone in males from eight species using a specific antibody without chromatography, *Endocrinology*, 95, 1466, 1974.
39. Schanbacher, B. D., Gomes, W. R., and Van Demark, N. L., Diurnal rhythm in serum testosterone levels and thymidine uptake by testes in the domestic fowl, *J. Anim. Sci.*, 38, 1245, 1974.
40. Schröcksnadel, H., Bator, A., and Frick, J., Plasma testosterone levels in cocks and hens, *Steroids*, 18, 359, 1971.
41. Idler, D. R., Horne, D. A., and Sangalang, G. B., Identification and quantification of the major androgens in testicular and peripheral plasma of atlantic salmon *(Salmo salar)* during sexual maturation, *Gen. Comp. Endocrinol.*, 16, 257, 1971.
42. Rhynes, W. E. and Ewing, L. L., Testicular endocrine function in Hereford bulls exposed to high ambient temperature, *Endocrinology*, 92, 509, 1973.
43. Leidl, W., Hoffmann, B., and Karg, H., Endokrine Regulation und jahreszeitlicher Rhythmus der Fortpflanzung beim Ziengenbock, *Zentralbl. Veterinaermed. Reihe A.*, 17, 623, 1970.
44. Claus, R., Hoffmann, B., and Karg, H., Determination of 5α-androst-16-en-3-one, a boar taint steroid in pigs, with reference to relationships to testosterone, *J. Anim. Sci.*, 33, 1293, 1971.
45. Claus, R. Dosage Radioimmunologique du 5α-androst-16-en-3-one, steroide reponsable de l'odeur de verrat, dans le tissue adipeux des porcs, *C. R. Acad. Sci.*, 278, 299, 1974.
46. Andresen, O., 5α-Androstenone in peripheral plasma of pigs, diurnal variation in boars, effects of intravenous HCG administration and castration, *Acta Endocrinol. (Kbh)*, 78, 385, 1975.
47. Andresen, O., A radioimmunoassay for 5α-androst-16-en-3-one in procine adipose tissue, *Acta Endocrinol. (Kbh)*, 79, 619, 1975.
48. Claus, R., Messung des Ebergeruchstoffes im Feff von Schweinen mittels eines Radioimmunotests. I. Mitteilung: Geruchsdepotbildung in Abhängigkeit vom Alter, *Z. Tierzuchtg. Zuchtungsbiol.*, 92, 118, 1975.
49. Shemesh, M. and Hansel, W., Measurement of bovine plasma testosterone by radioimmunoassay (RIA) and by a rapid competitive protein binding (CPB) assay, *J. Anim. Sci.*, 39, 720, 1974.
50. Purvis, K., Illius, A. W., and Haynes, N. B., Plasma testosterone concentrations in the ram, *J. Endocrinol.*, 61, 241, 1974.
51. Bahr, J., personal communication, 1978.
52. Shahabi, N. A., Norton, H. W., and Nalbandov, A. V., Steroid levels in follicles and plasma of hens during the ovulatory cycle, *Endocrinology*, 96, 962, 1975.
53. Laverne, R., Development and Validation of a Bioassay for Chicken LH and Application to Chicken Serum, Ph.D. thesis, University of Illinois, Urbana, 1978.
54. Baird, D. T., Goding, J. R., Ichikawa, J., and McCracken, J. A., The secretion of steroids from the autotransplanted ovary in the ewe spontaneously and in response to systemic gonadotropin, *J. Endocrinol.*, 42, 283, 1968.

55. **Noden, P. A., Oxender, W. D., and Hafs, H. D.**, The cycle of oestrus, ovulation and plasma levels of hormones in the mare, *J. Reprod. Fert.*, Suppl. 23, 189, 1975.
56. **Sitarz, N. E., Erb, R. E., Martin, T. G., and Singleton, W. L.**, Relationships between blood plasma testosterone, weaning treatment, daily gains and certain physical traits of young angus bulls, *J. Anim. Sci.*, 45, 342, 1977.
57. **Hoffmann, B. and Rattenberger, E.**, Testosterone concentrations in tissue from veal calves, bulls and heifers and in milk samples, *J. Anim. Sci.*, 45, 342, 1977.
58. **Lindner, L. R.**, Androgens in bovine testis and spermatic vein blood, *Nature (London)*, 183, 1605, 1959.
59. **Lindner, H. R. and Mann, T.**, Relationship between the content of androgenic steroids in the testis and the secretory activity of seminal vesicles in the bull, *J. Endocrinol.*, 21, 341, 1960.
60. **Claus, R.**, Pheromone bei Säugetieren unter besonderer Berücksichtigung des Ebergeruchsstoffes und seiner Beziehung zu anderen Hodensteroiden. Habilitationsschrift, Fachbereich für Ladwirtschaft und Gartenbau, Techn. Univ. München/Weihenstephan, 1977.

NATURALLY OCCURRING HORMONES IN ANIMAL FOODS: GLUCOCORTICOIDS

H. Allen Tucker

INTRODUCTION

The principle glucocorticoid hormones secreted from the adrenal cortex into the blood of animals are cortisol and corticosterone. These hormones produce a diversity of effects. In some cells glucocorticoids are catabolic, whereas in others they are anabolic. More specifically, glucocorticoids suppress tissue utilization of carbohydrates, promote formation of glucose from tissue protein, increase deposition of glycogen in liver, cause breakdown of protein in some tissues but increase synthesis of protein in other tissues, decrease fat synthesis from carbohydrate, and diminish numbers of eosinophils and lymphocytes in blood.

Glucocorticoids are bound to corticoid binding globulin in blood. To accomplish their biological function, the glucocorticoids dissociate from corticoid binding globulin, cross the plasma membrane of the target cells and combine with a protein-binding site in the cytoplasm of the cell. The hormone-binding site complex becomes activated, and translocates to the nucleus where it binds to chromatin and increases the transcription rates of specific genes.[1] Subsequently, the glucocorticoids dissociate from their binding sites and exit from the cells. Thus, binding of glucocorticoids to intracellular receptors probably represents the first step in a series which culminates in the physiological response characteristic of the target tissue-glucocorticoid interaction. Since glucocorticoids affect most animal tissues and intracellular binding sites for glucocorticoids have been detected in a wide variety of tissues,[2,3] it seems likely that many, if not all, animal tissues used for food will contain these hormones. However, to this author's knowledge, with the exception of mammary tissue and milk, there are no reports of direct measurements of the glucocorticoids in tissues used for food consumption. Therefore, this review will emphasize factors which affect the concentration of glucocorticoids in milk.

FACTORS AFFECTING MILK GLUCOCORTICOIDS

Simultaneous measurements of concentrations of total glucocorticoids in a mammary artery and vein suggest that the mammary glands of goats and cows remove glucocorticoids from blood,[4,5] especially at milking.[6] Indeed, in pregnant and in lactating cows, corticosterone averaged 2.3 and 3.2 ng/g of mammary tissue, respectively; cortisol averaged 15.6 and 6.8 ng/g, respectively.[7] Consequently glucocorticoids might be expected to be excreted into milk.

Normal Physiological Concentrations

Total glucocorticoids in pathogen-free milk from cows of unspecified reproductive status ranged from 0.7 to 1.4 ng/mℓ.[8] During the estrous cycle of lactating cows, total glucocorticoids ranged from 6.8 to 13.4 ng/mℓ in serum, and from 0.19 to 0.62 ng/mℓ in milk (Table 1).[9] However, changes in concentrations of glucocorticoids in either milk or serum were not associated with various stages of the estrous cycle.[9]

In another experiment, serum and milk were sampled from approximately 3 weeks before parturition through 1 week after parturition.[9] Although total glucocorticoids in sera did not change significantly during the periparturient period, concentrations in milk were increased ($p < 0.01$) on the day of parturition (3.08 ng/mℓ) relative to con-

Table 1
CONCENTRATIONS OF TOTAL GLUCOCORTICOIDS IN SERUM AND MILK DURING THE ESTROUS CYCLE OF SIX HOLSTEIN COWS

Day of estrous cycle	Glucocorticoid			
	Serum		Milk	
	$\bar{X}$	SE	$\bar{X}$	SE
0 (estrus)	7.8	1.9	0.46	0.21
2	8.5	1.2	0.22	0.08
5	13.4	7.5	0.23	0.10
8	9.1	3.0	0.19	0.04
11	7.7	1.1	0.35	0.11
15	9.7	4.2	0.51	0.15
18	6.8	1.6	0.62	0.42
20	12.6	8.6	0.23	0.06

From Schwalm, J. W. and Tucker, H. A., *J. Dairy Sci.*, 61, 550—560, 1978. With permission.

Table 2
CONCENTRATIONS OF TOTAL GLUCOCORTICOIDS IN SERUM AND MILK DURING TEN PERIPARTURIENT PERIODS OF EIGHT HOLSTEIN COWS

Source of glucocorticoid	Days from parturition									
	−24 to −18	−17 to −11	−10 to −4	−3 to −1	0	0.5	1	2	3	7
(ng/mℓ) Serum $\bar{X}$	10.6	6.4	4.9	7.7	8.5	4.8	4.6	5.7	4.2	3.0
SE	2.7	1.1	0.6	2.3	1.3	0.4	0.4	1.0	1.0	0.7
(ng/mℓ) Milk $\bar{X}$	0.38	0.33	0.50	0.65	3.08	1.30	1.32	1.49	2.92	0.47
SE	0.08	0.05	0.06	0.24	1.07	0.46	0.32	0.54	1.36	0.10

From Schwalm, J. W. and Tucker, H. A., *J. Dairy Sci.*, 61, 550—560, 1978. With permission.

centrations 3 weeks before (0.38 ng/mℓ or 1 weeks after (0.47 ng/mℓ) parturition (Table 2). The increase on the day of parturition is probably associated with stress of delivery of the calf.

When viewed over an entire lactation, total glucocorticoids in sera did not change, whereas in milk, there was a slight decrease ($p < 0.01$) as lactation progressed (Table 3). The results of partitioning total glucocorticoids into cortisol and corticosterone by column chromatography are in Table 3. Although cortisol appeared to decline in milk while corticosterone increased with advancing lactation, these trends were not significant. Thus, the sum of cortisol and corticosterone (assayed following chromatography) remained reasonably constant while the ratio of cortisol to corticosterone declined. The sum of cortisol and corticosterone greatly exceeded the total glucocorticoid concentration obtained by direct assay (Table 3). Possible reasons for this discrepancy

Table 3
CONCENTRATIONS OF TOTAL
GLUCOCORTICOIDS IN SERUM AND MILK
DURING THREE STAGES OF LACTATION
AND CONCURRENT PREGNANCY

	Months of lactation		
	0 to 2 (0)[a]	5 to 7 (3 to 5)[a]	9 to 11 (7 to 9)[a]
	ng/ml		
Serum			
Total	8.2 ± 0.5	9.8 ± 0.6	8.5 ± 0.5
Cortisol	7.6 ± 0.7	9.2 ± 0.9	7.3 ± 0.7
Corticosterone	3.1 ± 0.3	4.0 ± 0.3	4.8 ± 0.5
Milk			
Total	0.59 ± 0.11	0.28 ± 0.04	0.25 ± 0.02
Cortisol	1.75 ± 0.38	0.97 ± 0.16	0.91 ± 0.11
Corticosterone	2.58 ± 0.39	2.84 ± 0.43	3.46 ± 0.54

[a] Months pregnant.

From Schwalm, J. W. and Tucker, H. A., *J. Dairy Sci.*, 61, 550—560, 1978. With permission.

have been described.[9] The ratio of cortisol to corticosterone in sera was approximately 2:1, whereas in milk the ratio averaged less than 1:1. In other words, cortisol was the predominant glucocorticoid in serum while in milk corticosterone concentrations were greater than those of cortisol. These data may suggest that corticosterone is preferentially taken up by the mammary gland, that catabolism of cortisol occurs in the mammary gland, or that substantial conversion of cortisol to corticosterone occurs in the mammary gland.

In all physiological states studied, concentrations of total glucocorticoids in sera greatly exceed concentrations in milk. This is in marked contrast to the ovarian steroids which are generally at least as great in milk as in sera.[10] Furthermore, there is no positive correlation between percentage of milk fat and concentrations of glucocorticoids in milk.[8,9] Studies of distribution of glucocorticoids suggest that cortisol and corticosterone are associated primarily with aqueous phases of milk, whereas ovarian steroids are located primarily in milk fat.[9] Corticoid binding globulin has been reported in whey of colostrum and milk of several species and may be associated with the mechanism whereby glucocorticoids are seqestered in the nonlipid phase of milk.[11-13] Indeed, corticoid binding protein in milk is only 7 to 15% of that in serum although both proteins appear to be identical.[13,14] This reduced corticoid binding globulin in milk coincides with the reduced concentrations of glucocorticoids in milk as compared with serum.

Effects of Milk Processing

None of the commonly used methods of pasteurization, homogenization, or separation of milk alter total glucocorticoid concentrations (Table 4).[15]

Injection of Cortisol or Adrenocorticotropin (ACTH)

Intramuscular injection of 1.6 g of cortisol or 100 to 250 IU of repository form ACTH markedly increased concentrations of total glucocorticoids in whole and skim

Table 4
EFFECTS OF VARIOUS COMBINATIONS OF MILK PROCESSING METHODS ON CONCENTRATIONS OF GLUCOCORTICOIDS IN MILK

Processing method	Total glucocorticoids (ng/mℓ)
Raw whole milk	0.53 ± 0.02
HTST[a] pasteurized, whole milk	0.61 ± 0.02
HTST pasteurized, homogenized, whole milk	0.50 ± 0.02
Bulk pasteurized,[b] whole milk	0.56 ± 0.02
Bulk pasteurized, homogenized, whole milk	0.65 ± 0.02
HTST pasteurized skim milk[c]	0.55 ± 0.02
HTST pasteurized, homogenized, skim milk	0.58 ± 0.03
Bulk pasteurized, skim milk	0.46 ± 0.02
Bulk pasteurized, homogenized, skim milk	0.60 ± 0.02

[a] HTST = pasteurization at 71°C for 15 sec.
[b] Bulk pasteurized = pasteurization at 63°C for 30 min.
[c] Whole milk was separated by centrifugation to cream (milk fat) and skim milk. Cream was discarded.

From Schwalm, J. W., Kirk, J., Secrest, S., and Tucker, H. A., *J. Dairy Sci.*, 61, 1517—1518, 1978. With permission.

Table 5
CONCENTRATIONS OF TOTAL GLUCOCORTICOIDS IN WHOLE AND SKIM MILK BEFORE AND AFTER INJECTION OF CORTISOL OR ACTH

	Whole milk		Skim milk	
Treatment	Before injection	After injection	Before injection	After injection
Cortisol, 1.6 g	0.7 ± 0.2	5.6 ± 1.2	0.7 ± 0.2	3.5 ± 0.6
ACTH, 250 IU	1.0 ± 0.3	23.4 ± 5.7	0.9 ± 0.3	24.6 ± 7.6
ACTH, 100 IU	1.4 ± 0.2	11.5 ± 1.4	1.3 ± 0.2	14.3 ± 3.8

From Gwazdauskas, F. C., Paape, M. J., and McGillard, M. L., *Proc. Soc. Exp. Biol. Med.*, 154, 543—545, 1977. With permission.

milk (Table 5).[8] Furthermore, intramuscular injection of 200 IU ACTH increased cortisol from 2.5 to 8.7 ng/mℓ in whole milk collected 12 hr later.[16] Cortisol in milk remained above preinjection concentrations for approximately 48 hr. The concentrations of cortisol in plasma were parallel, though greater than concentrations in milk.

A single intramuscular injection of 40 IU ACTH did not affect milk cortisol concentrations, whereas 4 injections of 40 IU ACTH at 2-hr intervals increased cortisol approximately 5-fold in milk collected at the subsequent milking.[17] Cortisol in milk was highly correlated with cortisol measured in multiple blood plasma samples collected between milkings.[16,17] Thus, cortisol in milk is an integrated measure of plasma cortisol.

Stress of Movement of Cattle

Shipment of dairy cows by truck about 6 hr before the afternoon milking increased cortisol in milk approximately 30%.[16] Whether other stressful conditions will increase glucocorticoids in milk remains to be determined, although preliminary data suggest that placing cattle in unfamiliar housing facilities increased milk cortisol 0.6 to 1 ng/mℓ with 10 of 12 cows responding.[18] It may be concluded that effects of various management practices on cortisol secretion may be monitored in milk.

Mastitis

Infusion of 300 to 700 colony-forming units of strain 305 *Staphylococcus aureus* (courtesy of F.H.S. Newbould, University of Guelph, Ontario) into the right front teat cistern of lactating cows did not affect concentrations of cortisol in milk, whereas concentrations of corticosterone decreased 25% within 12 hr.[19] But within 24 hr concentrations of corticosterone had returned to normal.

Season

Subjection of cattle or hogs to increasing ambient temperatures above their thermoneutral zone leads to increased followed by reduced concentrations of glucocorticoids in serum;[20-22] thus, one might expect to observe seasonal changes in concentrations of these hormones in milk. However, total glucocorticoids, cortisol and corticosterone, did not change significantly among milk samples collected in cold (December, February) or warm (May, August) seasons in East Lansing, Mich.[19] For example, cortisol in milk averaged 0.39 and 0.48 ng/mℓ, and corticosterone averaged 0.67 and 0.56 ng/mℓ during the cold and warm months, respectively.

SUMMARY

A small portion of the glucocorticoids in blood sera are excreted into milk. Estimates of total glucocorticoids in normal milk range from approximately 0.2 to 1 ng/mℓ. Glucocorticoids in milk decrease slightly as lactation advances. Intramuscular injection of cortisol or ACTH, and movement of cattle to unfamiliar surroundings (stress?) increase concentrations of cortisol in milk. Inflammation of the mammary gland (mastitis) decreases the concentrations of corticosterone by 25% without altering the concentrations of cortisol. Glucocorticoids are associated primarily with the aqueous phase of milk and are not affected by milk fat percentage, commonly used milk processing methods, or by seasonal changes. Milk glucocorticoids represent an integrated measure of the plasma concentrations. Thus, it is likely that subjection of animals to managemental protocols which markedly alter blood plasma concentrations of glucocorticoids will produce corresponding changes in milk concentrations of these hormones.

REFERENCES

1. Cake, M. H. and Litwack, G., The glucocorticoid receptor, in *Biochemical Actions of Hormones*, Vol. 3, Litwack, G., Ed., Academic Press, New York, 1975, 317—390.
2. King. R. J. B. and Mainwaring, W. I. P., *Steroid-Cell Interactions*, University Park Press, Baltimore, 1974, 102—161.
3. Ballard, P. L., Baxter, J. D., Higgins, S. J., Rousseau, G. G., and Tomkins, G. M., General presence of glucocorticoid receptors in mammalian tissues, *Endocrinology*, 94, 998—1008, 1974.
4. Paterson, J. Y. F. and Linzell, J. L., The secretion of cortisol and its mammary uptake in the goat, *J. Endocrinol.*, 50, 493—499, 1971.
5. Paterson, J. Y. F. and Linzell, J. L., Cortisol secretion rate, glucose entry rate and the mammary uptake of cortisol and glucose during pregnancy and lactation in dairy cows, *J. Endocrinol.*, 62, 371—383, 1974.
6. Gorewit, R. C. and Tucker, H. A., Lactational events related to glucocorticoid binding in bovine mammary tissue, *J. Dairy Sci.*, 60, 889—895, 1977.
7. Shirley, J. E., Emery, R. S., Convey, E. M., and Oxender, W. D., Enzymic changes in bovine adipose and mammary tissue, serum and mammary tissue hormonal changes with initiation of lactation, *J. Dairy Sci.*, 56, 569—574, 1973.
8. Gwazdauskas, F. C., Paape, M. J., and McGilliard, M. L., Milk and plasma glucocorticoid alterations after injections of hydrocortisone and adrenocorticotropin, *Proc. Soc. Exp. Biol. Med.*, 154, 543—545, 1977.
9. Schwalm, J. W. and Tucker, H. A., Glucocorticoids in mammary secretions and serum during reproduction and lactation and distributions of glucocorticoids, progesterone and estrogens in fractions of milk, *J. Dairy Sci.*, 61, 550—560, 1978.
10. Erb, R. E., Chew, B. P., and Keller, H. F., Relative concentrations of estrogen and progesterone in milk and blood excretion of estrogen in urine, *J. Anim. Sci.*, 45, 617—626, 1977.
11. Payne, D. W., Peng, L. H., Pearlman, W. H., and Talbert, L. M., Corticosteroid-binding proteins in human colostrum and milk and rat milk, *J. Biol. Chem.*, 251, 5272—5279, 1976.
12. Rosner, W., Beers, P. C., Awan, T., and Khan, M. S., Identification of corticosteroid-binding globulin in human milk: measurement with a filter disk assay, *J. Clin. Endocrinol. Metab.*, 42, 1064—1073, 1976.
13. Raymoure, W. J. and Kuhn, R. W., Steroid-binding proteins in guinea pig milk and plasma, *Endocrinology*, 106, 1747—1754, 1980.
14. Pearlman, W. H., Skrzynia, C., Hampel, M. R., Peng, L. H., and Berko, R. M., The levels of corticosterone-binding proteins in rat milk and coincidental serum, and the dissociation rates of the corticosterone protein complexes, *Endocrinology*, 108, 741—746, 1981.
15. Schwalm, J. W., Kirk, J., Secrest, S., and Tucker, H. A., Effects of processing milk on concentrations of glucocorticoids in milk, *J. Dairy Sci.*, 61, 1517—1518, 1978.
16. Bremel, R. D. and Gangwer, M. I., Effect of adrenocorticotropin injection and stress on milk cortisol content, *J. Dairy Sci.*, 61, 1103—1108, 1978.
17. Natzke, R. P. and Fox, L., personal communication, 1978.
18. Abilay, T. A., Johnson, H. D., and Madan, M., Influence of environmental heat on peripheral plasma progesterone and cortisol during the bovine estrous cycle, *J. Dairy Sci.*, 68, 1836—1840, 1975.
19. Schwalm, J. W. and Tucker, H. A., unpublished data, 1981.
20. Christison, G. I. and Johnson, H. D., Cortisol turnover in heat-stressed cows, *J. Anim. Sci.*, 34, 1005—1010, 1972.
21. Lee, J. A., Roussel, J. D., and Beatty, J. F., Effect of temperature-season on bovine adrenal cortical function, blood cell profile, and milk production, *J. Dairy Sci.*, 59, 104—108, 1976.
22. Marple, D. N., Aberle, E. D., Forrest, J. C., Blake, W. H., and Judge, M. D., Effects of humidity and temperature on porcine plasma adrenal corticoids, ACTH and growth hormone levels, *J. Anim. Sci.*, 34, 809—812, 1972.

TOXIC CONSTITUENTS OF ANIMAL FOODSTUFFS: EGGS OF FISHES AND AMPHIBIANS

Frederick A. Fuhrman

INTRODUCTION

The classification of poisonous fish according to the tissue that is the predominant source of the toxin, as suggested by Halstead,[1] has been convenient during a time when most of the toxins were unknown or poorly characterized. With the identification of the chemical nature of these toxins, it now seems more logical to classify poisonous fishes on the basis of the chemistry of the toxin. Thus, the most important example of ichthyosarcotoxism, ciguatera (for review cf. Banner),[2] is caused by a chemically well-characterized toxin (ciguatoxin) produced by a dinoflagellate.[3] This article shall discuss those toxins that are found principally or exclusively in the eggs and ovaries (roe) of marine and fresh-water fishes and amphibians (ichthyootoxins). Two of these have now been identified chemically: tetrodotoxin and dinogunellin. It is to be hoped that the chemical nature of the other toxins will soon be known. For a more detailed account of some of this material an earlier review[4] should be consulted.

The old literature on fish poisoning is replete with lucid descriptions of symptoms following ingestion of the roe of various fishes that are now commonly eaten without harm. It must be assumed that many such instances of poisoning are attributable to bacterial spoilage of the eggs rather than to a toxin inherent in them. Such food poisoning may result from toxins produced by bacteria that have grown on the eggs (e.g., staphylococci), or from infection with bacteria transmitted with the eggs (e.g., salmonella). Other sections of this handbook may be consulted for further information on food spoilage. One disease resulting from spoilage of fish eggs and other fish products is fish-borne botulism. The older European literature contains a number of accounts of paralytic ichthyism or *Fischvergiftung* following ingestion of various fish products including the eggs. The symptoms included muscular weakness, headache, difficulty in swallowing, diplopia, muscular paralysis and respiratory failure. These differ markedly from the gastrointestinal symptoms of the usual bacterial poisoning, and early in this century it gradually became clear that they were attributable to fish-borne botulism.[5,6] The paralysis produced should not be confused with that of paralytic shellfish poisoning (caused by the dinoflagellate toxin saxitoxin) or that of tetrodotoxin, both of which occur within a few minutes after ingestion of the fish rather than 12 to 36 hr later. In North America, fish-borne botulism is usually caused by the rather uncommon Type E *Clostridium botulinum*. The methods of preserving fish eggs used by the Indians of the Pacific Northwest provide excellent culture conditions for *Cl. botulinum*, and a number of instances of fish-borne botulism have been attributed to fish eggs.[6,7]

EGGS CONTAINING TETRODOTOXIN

Occurrence of Tetrodotoxin and Related Toxins

It has been known for at least 2000 years that the eggs, ovaries, and liver of the puffer fish (blowfish, globe fish, fugu) are poisonous. The history of the puffer fish poison has been recounted elsewhere[8-10] and will not be repeated here. Even though the viscera of these fish are well known to be poisonous, and the Japanese try to clean the fish thoroughly in the fish markets and to license restaurants to serve them, puffer fish poisoning is still a public health problem in the Orient. It is clear that the toxicity of the roe and liver of puffer fish is caused by tetrodotoxin.

Table 1
FISHES AND AMPHIBIANS CONTAINING TETRODOTOXIN OR PHYSIOLOGICALLY RELATED SUBSTANCES IN THE EGGS AND OVARIES

Pisces
  Class: Osteichthyes
    Order: Plectognathi (Tetraodontiformes)

      Family: Canthigasteridae (sharp-nosed puffers)
        Canthigaster rivulatus Temminck and Schlegel

      Family: Diodontidae (porcupine fish)
        Chilomycterus sp.
        Diodon hystrix Linnaeus

      Family: Tetraodontidae (puffers, swellfish, fugu)
        Arothron hispidus Linnaeus
        Arothron meleagris Lacepede
        Arothron setosus Smith
        Fugu basilevskianus Basilewsky
        Fugu chrysops Hilgendorf
        Fugu niphobles Jordan and Snyder
        Fugu ocellatus ocellatus Linnaeus
        Fugu paradalis Temminck and Schlegel
        Fugu poecilonotus Temminck and Schlegel
        Fuge pseudommus Chu
        Fugu rubripes rubripes Temminck and Schlegel
        Fugu strictonotus Temminck and Schlegel
        Fugu vermicularis porphyreus Temminck and Schlegel
        Fugu vermicularis radiatus Abe
        Fugu vermiculars vermicularis Temminck and Schlegel
        Fugu xanthopterus Temminck and Schlegel
        Lagocephalus sceleratus Forster
        Sphaeroides annulatus Jenyns

        Sphaeroides maculatus Bloch and Schneider

        Sphaeroides testudineus Linnaeus

    Order: Gobiesociformes
      Family: Gobiidae
        Acanthogobius flavimanus Temminck and Schlegel
        Gillichthys mirabilis Cooper

Amphibia
  Order: Caudata
    Family: Salamandridae
      Taricha torosa
      Taricha rivularis
  Order: Salientia
    Family: Atelopidae
      Atelopus chiriquiensis

Note: Tetrodotoxin has been isolated chemically from those designated by *. In other instances the toxin has been established by bioassay. For other species (not included in the table) tetrodotoxin or related substances may occur in other organs as discussed in text.

Tetrodotoxin has been isolated from the ovaries of three species of puffer fish: *Fugu rubripes*,[11,12] *F. vermicularis*,[13] and *F. sticnotus*.[14] The ovaries of a total of 23 species of fish belonging to the order Tetraodontiformes (Table 1) have been shown to be toxic when extracts are injected into experimental animals. Although the symptoms of

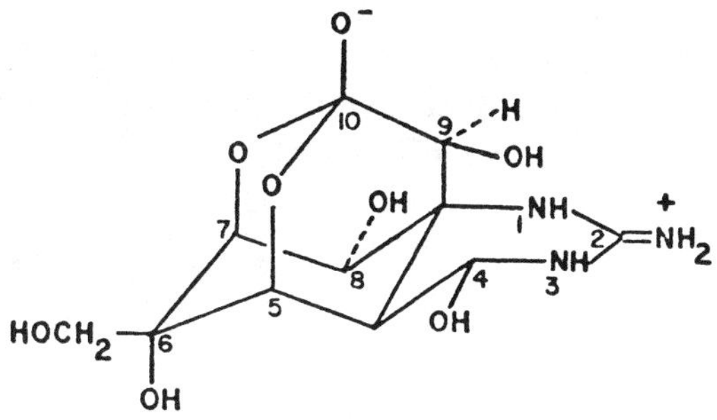

FIGURE 1. Tetrodotoxin.

toxicity resemble those of tetrodotoxin, there is at present no proof that the toxin is in fact tetrodotoxin. It is now becoming evident that tetrodotoxin and related substances are considerably more widely distributed among marine animals and amphibians than was originally supposed. This was first shown by demonstration that the crystalline toxin[15] isolated from the eggs of the California newt, *Taricha torosa,* is actually tetrodotoxin.[16] The eggs of another newt, *Taricha rivularis,* also contain tetrodotoxin, and a total of ten species of newt belonging to the family Salamandridae contain substances that produced symptoms resembling those of tetrodotoxin in mice.[17]

Tetrodotoxin was also isolated in crystalline form from the ovaries and liver of the goby, *Gobius criniger,* from the western Pacific.[18] Three species of goby from California contain toxins that resemble tetrodotoxin pharmacologically.[19] We reported[20] that three closely related species or subspecies of Central American frog of the genus *Atelopus* contain tetrodotoxin and that one of them, *A. chiriquiensis,* also contains a related toxin that differs chemically by a substitution at C-6. Both toxins are present in the eggs of this species.[21] Finally, and more surprising, the toxin occurring in the salivary glands of the Australian blue-ringed octopus *(Octopus [Hapalochlaena] maculosa)* has now been identified as tetrodotoxin.[22]

The animals listed in Table 1 are only those for which there is good experimental evidence that the eggs or ovaries contain tetrodotoxin or physiologically related substances determined by bioassay. Longer lists of fishes suspected of containing tetrodotoxin are available elsewhere.[1,10,23] Tetrodotoxin was isolated from whole *Gobius criniger,* but it is not known whether it is present in the ovaries.[18] Several other species of newts[17] and frogs[20] were found to contain tetrodotoxin or a related toxin, but again the ovaries or eggs were not separately analyzed. Most of the fish containing tetrodotoxin are found in the Western Pacific and Indian oceans. Several studies have been made of toxicity of the Atlantic puffers that occur along the eastern coast of the U.S. The gonads of the Northern puffer, *Sphaeroides maculatus* (possibly actually *S. nephelus),*[24] and the checkered puffer, *S. testudineus,* taken off Florida, were usually, but not invariably, toxic.[25,26] Lynch et al.[27] could detect only about 0.005 µg/g of tetrodotoxin-like activity in the ovaries of *S. maculatus* caught off New Jersey during May to July. We[28] found toxicity equivalent to about 0.05 µg/g of tetrodotoxin in the ovaries of *S. maculatus* caught off Coney Island in September. Robinson and Schwartz[29] reported the ovaries of one group of *S. maculatus* from Chesapeake Bay to be toxic. *S. nephelus* from the Gulf coast of Florida were not toxic.[30] See "Tetrodotoxin Poisoning in Man" of this article.

Chemistry of Tetrodotoxin

Tetrodotoxin was first prepared in crystalline form from the ovaries of the Japanese puffer or blowfish *Fugu rubripes* by Yokoo[11] in 1950. The structure (Figure 1) is unu-

Table 2
DISTRIBUTION OF TETRODOTOXIN-LIKE SUBSTANCES IN TISSUES OF FEMALE FISH AND AMPHIBIANS

	Ovaries		Liver	
	(µg/g)	Total (µg)	(µg/g)	Total (µg)
Tetraodontidae[8]				
Fugu niphobles	400	200	1,000	1,000
F. aloplumbeus	200	4,400	1,000	14,000
F. pardalis	200	5,100	1,000	22,000
F. vermicularis	400	6,400	200	3,200
F. porphyreus	400	10,000	200	65,000
F. ocelatus	100	6,520	40	1,200
F. rubripes	100	24,000	100	20,000
Lagocephalus inermis	0.4	15	1	75
Gobiidae[19]				
Gillichthys mirabilis	10	170	30	200
Salamandridae[17]				
Taricha torosa	25	a	<0.1	—
Atelopidae[21]				
Atelopus chiriquiensis	200	150	—	—

a From eggs collected from ponds.

sual and distinctive and was arrived at independently in 1964 by Mosher et al.,[9] Woodward,[31] Goto et al.,[32] and Tsuda.[33] The cyclic hemilactal structure is unknown in any synthetic compound and occurs in nature only in one toxin, chiriquitoxin,[34] that is closely related to tetrodotoxin. The pure crystalline toxin does not easily dissolve in water, but is readily soluble in weak acids. Aqueous solutions are reasonably stable at pH 7 and are not inactivated by boiling for 1 hr. However, in both acid and alkaline solutions, particularly the latter, inactivation occurs rapidly.[35] Consequently, the toxin in fish eggs may persist after short periods of cooking if the pH is near neutral. In puffer fish canned by the common commercial method in ½ lb tins, some, but not all, of the toxin was inactivated.[36]

Distribution of Tetrodotoxin in Tissues

Tetrodotoxin and related substances occur not only in the eggs and ovaries of fish but also in the liver and to a lesser extent in other tissues. Some of these data, principally from Tani[8] are listed in Table 2. It should be noted that in some cases where the toxin concentration per unit weight is not the highest, the total toxin content of the organ is very large because of the large size of the liver or ovaries.

In amphibia, the skin is the principal toxic organ other than the eggs and ovaries.

In fish there is a marked seasonal variation in toxicity of the ovaries, according to Tani. The concentration of tetrodotoxin in the ovaries of *Fugu rubripes rubripes* is very low (less than 1 µg/g) during October and November when the ovaries are small. As eggs develop during December to April, the concentration ranges from 7 to 19 µg/g and the weight of the ovaries increases enormously so that the total amount of tetrodotoxin at this time may be a thousand times greater than when the ova are immature.

Pharmacology of Tetrodotoxin
Detection

In the absence of adequate chemical methods for detection of tetrodotoxin, it is necessary to rely on bioassay. Horsburgh et al.[37] adapted an assay procedure devised by Sommer and Meyer[38] for paralytic shellfish poison and applied it to crude extracts of newt eggs containing tetrodotoxin; Ogura[39] used the same method for puffer fish extracts. The method depends upon the fact that there is a rough exponential relationship between the rapidity of death and the dose administered to mice. By adjusting the concentration so that a given dose gives a death time between 1 and 15 min, the method is reproducible and much faster than the conventional determination of LD_{50}. It can be made more specific by determining the toxicity of dialysates of acidic (pH 5) suspensions of tissue.[17] The result is usually expressed in mouse units (M.U.): 1 M.U. is the amount of toxin necessary to kill a 20 g mouse in 10 min after injection of 0.2 mℓ. Since 1 mg of crystalline tetrodotoxin is equivalent to about 7000 M.U., 1 M.U. is equal to about 140 ng of tetrodotoxin.

Effects in Experimental Animals

Tetrodotoxin is lethal to all vertebrates so far examined except those that contain it.[40,41] In mice there is an extremely steep dose-response relationship, and the LD_{50} is about 10 μg/kg intraperitoneally.[42,43] Tetrodotoxin is only about 1/20 as toxic orally as intraperitoneally.

In experimental animals lethal doses (>10 μg/kg) of tetrodotoxin produce principally a progressive paralysis of the voluntary muscles, hypotension, and respiratory paralysis. The effect on voluntary muscles results, in rodents, in a peculiar wobbling gait in which the hind limbs appear to be paralyzed.[42,43] This is not, as some had supposed, an ascending spinal paralysis. It is now clear that tetrodotoxin exerts its effect on conduction in nerve axons (see below). Both motor[40] and sensory[44] axons are affected and, usually somewhat later, a direct blocking effect on skeletal muscle fibers can be demonstrated.[45]

In experimental animals, one of the most dramatic effects of tetrodotoxin is the profound hypotension that occurs after intravenous injection of doses as small as 0.5 μg/kg. Both systolic and diastolic pressures may fall by 50% after doses of 2 μg/kg. A marked depression of respiration usually occurs simultaneously and with similar doses. It is now clear, largely through the work of Kao and his associates,[46,47] that these effects are due to peripheral effects of tetrodotoxin rather than to effects on the respective medullary centers. The original publications cited above and the reviews by Kao[10] and Evans[48] should be consulted for details.

Mechanism of Action

The pharmacological effects of tetrodotoxin mentioned above can all be explained by the effect of tetrodotoxin on the generation of action potentials in nerve axons and in skeletal muscle. The nerve axons and muscle fibers of vertebrates are surrounded by selectively permeable membranes that maintain an electrical potential difference of about 70 mV between the inside and outside of these cells. The inside is electrically negative to the outside and contains relatively little Na^+ and Cl^-, but high concentrations of K^+. In the resting state the membranes are permeable to K^+ but not to Na^+. With excitation these membranes become suddenly and briefly permeable to Na^+ and later to K^+. These changes in ionic permeabilities are the origins of the propagated action potentials. It is now clear from the work of Narahashi[49] and others[50] that tetrodotoxin selectively prevents the transient increase in permeability to Na^+ without effect on permeability to K^+, and thus blocks the action potential in both nerve axons and in skeletal muscle cells. Action potentials of nerve[41] and muscle[51] from animals that contain tetrodotoxin are insensitive to the action of the toxin.

Tetrodotoxin Poisoning in Man

Intoxication in many may become evident in 30 to 60 min. The symptoms consist of numbness of the lips, tongue, and often the fingers and arms, muscular paralysis, ataxia, and incoordination. Loss of consciousness and respiratory depression occur before death from respiratory paralysis. There is no effective antidote. Obviously, efforts should be made to remove tetrodotoxin from the gastrointestinal tract. A dose equivalent to 1 to 2 mg of crystalline tetrodotoxin may be fatal in man, and this might be contained in 1 to 10 g of roe or liver.

Poisoning from eating fish roe containing tetrodotoxin occurs principally in Japan, where these fish are used as food. The puffer most prized as food, *Fugu rubripes rubripes* (Tora Fugu), contains rather large amounts of tetrodotoxin in the ovaries and liver (Table 2). It is eaten mainly in the winter, when it is most poisonous, because the flesh loses flavor after spawning.[33] Although efforts are made to control poisoning,[43] deaths from tetrodotoxin still occur. Most instances of poisoning result from confusing puffer roe for edible roe.

The number of deaths from tetrodotoxin poisoning in Japan has remained fairly constant at about 100 per year for 70 years.[52] In 1958 there were 289 cases of poisoning with a mortality of 60.9% and in 1959 there were 211 cases with a mortality of 56%.[33] Elsewhere in the world, only occasional poisonings from puffer fish are known. In Florida two fatalities were reported in 1956.[52] Since then only a single case of poisoning from puffer fish has been reported.[53] It also occurred in Florida, but the species responsible was not identified.

EGGS CONTAINING DINOGUNELLIN

Occurrence

Dinogunellin is a toxic lipoprotein that has so far been identified in the roe of only two species of the order Perciformes. The northern blenny or stickelback, *Stichaeus (Dinogunellus) grigorgjewi* (family Stichaeidae), is widely distributed in the sea surrounding northern Japan and is used as a food fish in Hokkaido. A series of poisonings occurred there in 1952 to 1953, and Takayanagi et al.[54] succeeded in reproducing the symptoms of poisoning in human subjects by feeding them 20 to 30 g of raw fish roe. The toxin does not occur in other organs.[55]

The other species from which dinogunellin has been isolated is the Cabezon or marbeled sculpin, *Scorpaenichthys marmoratus* (family Cottidae), a common fish on the Pacific coast of North America from Canada to Mexico, where it is of some commercial importance and is frequently taken by sport fishermen. The toxicity of cabezon roe was discovered by the ichthyologist Carl Hubbs, who unknowingly poisoned himself and later demonstrated that roe fed to experimental animals is toxic.[56] We confirmed these observations and studied the chemical nature and physiological effects of the toxin.[57,58]

Chemistry

Asano and Itoh[59,60] extracted a toxic lipoprotein from blenny roe that they designated lipostichaerin. Hatano[61] characterized lipostichaerin as containing 22% lipid and 78% protein with a molecular weight of about 4×10^5. The LD_{50} of lipostichaerin (i.p., mice) was 180 mg/kg. Lipostichaerin could be split into a nontoxic protein moiety and a toxic lipid fraction. A similar toxic lipid could be extracted from fresh roe with acetone. Hatano[62] showed that the toxic principle of the acetone extract was a peculiar phospholipid that amounted to about 1.6% of lipostichaerin. The phospholipid was designated dinogunellin (after the former name of the genus) by Hatano and Hashimoto,[63] who found the LD_{50} to be about 25 mg/kg and the degradation products to be adenine, glycerophosphate, and an unknown compound. They[64] later determined the structure to be that shown in Figure 2.

We[57] fractionated the roe of the cabezon by several methods and obtained an unsta-

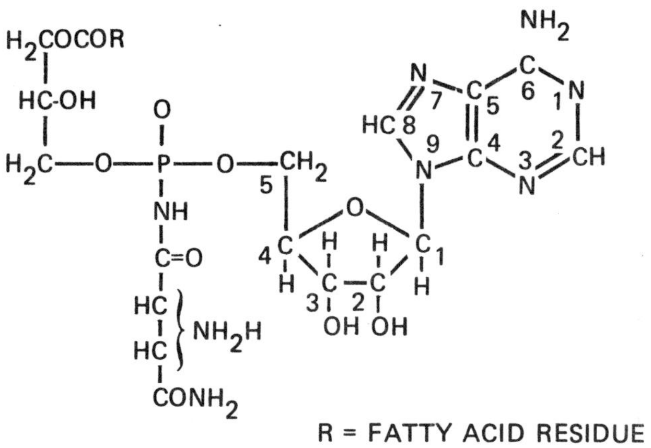

FIGURE 2. Dinogunellin.

ble lipoprotein mixture that was toxic orally in rats and had an LD_{50} (i.p., mice) of about 200 mg/kg. Hashimoto et al.[65] later obtained from cabezon roe a phospholipid that they consider to be dinogunellin, identical to that obtained from *Stichaeus*.

Effects in Man and Animals

Ingestion of fish roe containing dinogunellin produces, within a few hours, diarrhea, nausea, vomiting, and epigastric distress. In severe cases, including one fatal case described by Asano and Itoh,[59] the symptoms also include respiratory distress, chest pain, syncope, and coma.[66] I do not know of any fatalities from eating cabezon roe.

Laboratory rodents given crude dinogunellin orally or intraperitoneally show little effects for about 12 hr. They then exhibit ruffled fur, seek corners of the cage, become inactive, and finally comatose before death in 15 to 24 hr.[57,67] Hatano[61] found that lipostichaerin and dinogunellin from *Stichaeus* decreased the concentration of total lipid, neutral lipid, and cholesterol in the plasma of rats without changing total protein, globulins, glucose, bilirubin, Na, or K. Increased serum glutamic-oxaloacetic transaminase (GOT), serum glutamic-pyruvic transaminase (GPT), serum lactic dehydrogenase, and amylase were found. These studies suggest that dinogunellin produces pathological changes in the liver (GOT and GPT are normally intracellular and are released following damage to parenchymal cells) and possibly in the spleen and pancreas as well. Somewhat earlier, Saunders and Fuhrman[68] found that extracts of cabezon roe, then not known to contain dinogunellin, produced focal necrosis in the liver and depletion of lymphocytes from the red pulp of the spleen. Thus, with the establishment of dinogunellin as the toxic agent in both blenny and cabezon roe, the pathological effects are quite consistent: dinogunellin produces pathological effects in both spleen and liver with focal necrosis of the latter organ. Cabezon roe extracts also inhibited growth of mouse fibroblasts grown in tissue culture.[58]

EGGS OF OTHER FISHES

Gars

The gar family, Lepisosteidae, consists of fewer than ten species found in the fresh and brackish waters of North America. Over a century ago Brooks[69] described a "burning sensation in the pit of the stomach, which was soon succeeded by vomiting, purging, and cramping, in their most aggravated form" in an Illinois family of five who ate the roe of a freshly caught gar for dinner. Similar symptoms were experienced by others[70] and the several reviewers reported gar eggs to be poisonous without citing specific evidence.[71-73]

There is also experimental evidence that gar roe is poisonous. Greene et al.[74] found that fresh gar roe fed to chickens in divided doses over several days produced loss of appetite, diarrhea, muscular weakness, circulatory disturbances in the comb and depression of the central nervous system. In rats, 5 g orally was fatal and death was preceded by weakness and diarrhea. The toxic substance occurred in the globulin fraction of the eggs. Netsch and Witt,[75] apparently unaware of Greene's experiments, fed roe of the longnose gar, *Lepisosteus osseus,* to chickens and mice and found that they became ill. Eggs of the short nose gar, *L. platostomus,* also produced toxic effects in mice. We[57] established that the eggs of the spotted gar, *L. productus,* are toxic when fed to rats and that the toxin is not tetrodotoxin.

Cyprinidae

The family Cyprinidae is a large one including carp and minnows. The roe of several of these fish may produce mild to severe nausea, vomiting, and diarrhea when eaten raw or cooked. Although these symptoms may be confused with those of bacterial food poisoning, their repeated association with eating the roe of certain fishes strongly suggests that specific toxic substances are present in the eggs.

Barbels *(Barbus barbus* and *B. meridionalis)* are European freshwater fish whose eggs have been known for centuries to produce diarrhea ("Barbencholera") after ingestion. In the book *Corona Florida Medicinae* (Venice, 1491), Antonio Gaza records that to test the validity of folk tales that the roe of barbels is poisonous, he ate some and experienced vomiting and diarrhea.[76] Other instances of diarrhea from barbel roe are recorded by Meyer-Ahrens,[77] von Franque,[78] and Münchmeyer.[79] The symptoms reported include nausea, diarrhea, epigastric pain, cold extremities, malaise, and vomiting. No fatalities are reported. McCrudden[80,81] reported chemical and pharmacological experiments on barbel roe, but the experimental design was poor and no results after oral administration are given.

Related fishes whose roe are usually listed as poisonous include the tench *(Tinca tinca),*[77,82-84] the bream *(Abramis brama),*[77,82] and the snow trout *(Schizothorax intermedius).*[82]

Miscellaneous Fishes

The roe of the pike *(Esox lucius)* is reported to produce symptoms similar to those of the barbel.[77,82,85] The effect, however, is not so well documented, and McCrudden[80,81] failed to produce any effects by feeding 324 g of pike roe to a 6-kg dog.

Aqueous extracts of the roe of the creolefish, *Paranthias farcifer* (family Serranidae) were reported by Halstead and Schall[86] to be toxic when injected intraperitoneally into mice.

Evidence for the toxicity of the roe of other fish is poorly documented. The publications of Halstead[1] and Fuhrman[4] may be consulted for references.

POISONOUS EGGS FROM AMPHIBIANS

The California newt, *Taricha torosa,* lays eggs in clusters of some 20 ova each in ponds and streams. These eggs contain tetrodotoxin[9] as described above. I do not know of any evidence of human poisoning from them, but they are toxic to bass. The eggs of the Costa Rican frog, *Atelopus chiriquiensis,* contain both tetrodotoxin and the related toxin chiriquitoxin.[21]

The eggs of *Bufo marinus* are reported to be responsible for the fatal poisoning of a woman and child when they were consumed as soup.[87]

REFERENCES

1. Halstead, B. W., Poisonous and Venomous Marine Animals of the World, Vol. 2, U. S. Government Printing Office, Washington, D.C., 1967.
2. Banner, A. H., Ciguatera: a disease from coral reef fish, in *Biology and Geology of Coral Reefs*, Vol. 3, Jones, O. A. and Endean, R., Eds., Academic Press, New York, 1976, chap. 6.
3. Yasumoto, T., Nakajima, I., Bagnis, R., and Adachi, R., Finding of a dinoflagellate as a likely culprit of ciguatera, *Bull. Jpn. Soc. Sci. Fish,* 43, 1021—1026, 1977.
4. Fuhrman, F. A., Fish eggs, in *Toxic Constituents of Animal Foodstuffs,* Liener, I. E., Ed., Academic Press, New York, 1974, chap. 3.
5. Dolman, C. E., Chang, E., Kerr, D. E., and Shearer, A. R., Fish-borne and type E botulism: two cases due to homepickled herring, *Can. J. Pub. Health,* 41, 215—229, 1950.
6. Dolman, C. E., Type E (Fish-borne) botulism: a review, *Jpn. J. Med. Sci. Biol.,* 10, 383—395, 1957.
7. Sakaguchi, G., Botulims — type E, in *Food-borne Infections and Intoxications,* Rieman, H., Ed., Academic Press, New York, 329—358, 1969.
8. Tani, I., *A Study of the Toxicity of Japanese Fugu,* Teikoku Tosho, Tokyo, 1945, (in Japanese).
9. Mosher, H. S., Fuhrman, F. A., Buchwald, H. D., and Fischer, N. G., Tarichatoxin-tetrodotoxin: a potent neurotoxin, *Science,* 144, 1100—1110, 1964.
10. Kao, C. Y., Tetrodotoxin, saxitoxin, and their significance in the study of excitation phenomena, *Pharmacol. Rev.,* 18, 997—1049, 1966.
11. Yokoo, A., Toxic substance of a globe fish, *Spheroides rubripes:* isolation of spheroidine, *J. Chem. Soc. Jpn.,* 71, 590—592, 1950 (in Japanese).
12. Nagai, J., Isolation of poison of the Fugu fish by use of ion exchange, *Hoppe-Seylers Ztschr. Physiol. Chem.,* 306, 104—106, 1956.
13. Kakisawa, H., Okamura, Y., and Hirata, Y., An extraction and structure of tetrodotoxin, *J. Chem. Soc. Jpn.,* 80, 1483, 1959.
14. Arakawa, H., Chemical studies on fugu poison, *J. Chem. Soc. Jpn.,* 77, 1295—1297, 1956 (in Japanese).
15. Brown, M. S. and Mosher, H. S., Tarichatoxin: isolation and purification, *Science,* 140, 295—296, 1963.
16. Buchwald, H. D., Durham, L., Fischer, H. G., Harada, R., Mosher, H. S., Kao, C. Y., and Fuhrman, F. A., Identity of tarichatoxin and tetrodotoxin, *Science,* 143, 474—475, 1964.
17. Wakely, J. F., Fuhrman, G. J., Fuhrman, F. A., Fischer, H. G., and Mosher, H. S., The occurrence of tetrodotoxin (tarichatoxin) in amphibia and the distribution of the toxin in the organs of newts (Taricha), *Toxicon,* 3, 195—203, 1966.
18. Noguchi, T. and Hashimoto, Y., Isolation of tetrodotoxin from a goby, *Gobius criniger, Toxicon,* 11, 305—307, 1973.
19. Elam, K. S., Fuhrman, F. A., Kim, Y. H., and Mosher, H. S., Neurotoxins from three species of California goby: *Clevelandia ios, Acanthogobius flavimanus,* and *Gillichthys mirabilis, Toxicon,* 14, 45—49, 1977.
20. Kim, Y. H., Brown, G. B., and Mosher, H. S., Tetrodotoxin: occurrence in Atelopid frogs of Costa Rica, *Science,* 189, 151—152, 1975.
21. Pavelka, L. A., Kim, Y. H., and Mosher, H. S., Tetrodotoxin and tetrodotoxin-like compounds from the eggs of the Costa Rican frog *Atelopus chiriquiensis, Toxicon,* 15, 135—139, 1977.
22. Sheumack, D. D., Howden, M. E. H., Spence, I., and Quinn, R. J., Maculotoxin: a neurotoxin from the venom glands of the octopus *Hapalochlaena maculosa* identified as tetrodotoxin, *Science,* 199, 188—189, 1978.
23. Bouder, H., Cavallo, A., and Bouder, M. J., Poissons vénéneux et ichthyosarcotoxisme, *Bull. Int. Oceanogr. (Monaco),* 1240, 1—66, 1962.
24. Shipp, R. L. and Yerger, R. W., Status, characters, and distribution of the northern and southern puffers of the genus *Sphoeroides, Copeia,* 3, 425—433, 1969.
25. Lalone, R. C., DeVillez, E. D., and Larson, E., An assay of the toxicity of the Atlantic puffer fish *Spheroides maculatus, Toxicon,* 1, 159—164, 1963.
26. Larson, E., Lalone, R. C., and Rivas, L. R., Comparative toxicity of the Atlantic puffer fishes of the genera *Spheroides, Lactophrys, Lagocephalus,* and *Chilomycterus, Fed. Proc. Fed. Am. Soc. Exp. Biol.,* 19, 388, 1960.
27. Lynch, P. R., Coblentz, J. M., and Hamer, P., An evaluation of the northern puffer, *Spheroides maculatus,* for possible toxic properties, *Am. J. Med. Sci.,* 254, 173—177, 1967.
28. Fuhrman, F. A. and Fuhrman, G. J., unpublished data, 1966.
29. Robinson, P. F. and Schwartz, F. J., Toxicity of the northern puffer *Sphaeroides maculatus* in the Chesapeake Bay and its environs, *Chesapeake Sci.,* 9, 136—137, 1968.
30. Burklew, M. A. and Morton, R. A., The toxicity of Florida gulf puffers, genus *Sphoeroides, Toxicon,* 9, 205—210, 1971.

31. Woodward, R. B., The structure of tetrodotoxin, *Pure Appl. Chem.*, 9, 49—74, 1964.
32. Goto, T., Kishi, Y., Takahaski, S., and Hirata, Y., Tetrodotoxin, *Tetrahedron Lett.*, 21, 2059—2088, 1965.
33. Tsuda, K., Über tetrodotoxin, Giftstoff der Bowlfische, *Naturwissenschaften*, 53, 171—176, 1966.
34. Fuhrman, F. A., Fuhrman, G. J., Kim, Y., and Mosher, H. S., Pharmacology and chemistry of chiriquitoxin, a new tetrodotoxin-like substance from the Costa Rican frog *Atelopus chiriquiensis*, *Proc. West. Pharmacol. Soc.*, 19, 381—384, 1976.
35. Waterfield, C. J. and Evans, M. H., A method for distinguishing tetrodotoxin from saxitoxin by comparing their relative stabilities when heated in acid solution, *Experientia*, 28, 670—671, 1972.
36. Halstead, B. W. and Bunker, N. C., The effect of the commercial canning process upon puffer poison, *Calif. Fish Game*, 39, 219—228, 1953.
37. Horsburgh, D. B., Tatum, E. L., and Hall, V. E., Chemical properties and physiological actions of *Triturus* embryonic toxin, *J. Pharmacol. Exp. Ther.*, 68, 284—291, 1940.
38. Sommer, H. and Meyer, K. F., Paralytic shellfish poisoning, *Arch. Pathol.*, 24, 537—559, 1937.
39. Ogura, Y., Some recent problems on fugu-toxin, particularly on crystalline tetrodotoxin, *Seitai No Kagaku*, 9, 281—287, 1958, (in Japanese).
40. Ishihara, F., Über die physiologischen Wirkungen des Fugutoxins, *Mitth. Med. Fak. Tokio Univ.*, 20, 375—426, 1918.
41. Kao, C. Y. and Fuhrman, F. A., Differentiation of the actions of tetrodotoxin and saxitoxin, *Toxicon*, 5, 25—34, 1967.
42. Kao, C. Y. and Fuhrman, F. A., Pharmacological studies on tarichatoxin, a potent neurotoxin, *J. Pharmacol. Exp. Ther.*, 140, 31—40, 1963.
43. Ogura, Y., Fugo (puffer-fish) poisoning and the pharmacology of crystalline tetrodotoxin in poisoning, in *Neuropoisons*, Vol. 1, Simpson, L. L., Ed., Plenum Press, New York, 1971, chap. 6.
44. Watanabe, M., The effect of tetrodotoxin on the afferent impulses from sensory nerves, *Igaku Kenkyu*, 28, 876—884, 1958, (in Japanese).
45. Hagiwara, Y., Electromyographic studies of the action of drugs on neuromuscular excitation, *Folia Pharmacol. Jpn.*, 56, 387—403, 1960, (in Japanese).
46. Kao, C. Y., Suzuki, T., Kleinhaus, A. L., and Siegman, M. J., Vasomotor and respiratory depressant actions of tetrodotoxin and saxitoxin, *Arch. Int. Pharmacodyn.*, 165, 438—450, 1967.
47. Kao, C. Y., Nagasawa, J., Spiegelstein, M. Y., and Cha, Y. N., Vasodilatory effects of tetrodotoxin in the cat, *J. Pharmacol. Exp. Ther.*, 178, 110—121, 1971.
48. Evans, M. H., Tetrodotoxin, saxitoxin, and related substances: their applications in neurobiology, *Int. Rev. Neurobiol.*, 15, 83—166, 1972.
49. Narahashi, T., Moore, J. W., and Scott, W., Tetrodotoxin blockage of sodium conductance increase in excitation, *J. Gen. Physiol.*, 47, 965—974, 1964.
50. Takata, M., Moore, J. W., Kao, C. Y., and Fuhrman, F. A., Blockage by tarichatoxin of sodium conductance change in excitation, *J. Gen. Physiol.*, 49, 967—988, 1966.
51. Kidokoro, Y., Grinell, A. D., and Eaton, D. C., Tetrodotoxin sensitivity of muscle action potentials in puffer-fishes and related fishes, *J. Comp. Physiol.*, 89, 59—72, 1974.
52. Ogura, Y., Statistical survey of tetrodotoxin poisoning, *Ann. Rep. Inst. Food Microbiol. Chiba Univ.*, 11, 79—86, 1958, (in Japanese).
52a. Benson, J., Tetraodon (blowfish) poisoning. A report of two fatalities, *J. Forens. Sci.*, 1, 119—125, 1956.
53. Gasteazoro, J., Enriquez, M., Nitzkin, J. L., Saslaw, M. S., Schneider, N. J., and Nayfield, C. L., Puffer fish poisoning — Florida, Morbid. Mortal. Weekly Rep., U.S. Department of Health, Education and Welfare, 75, 68, 1975 (Feb. 15).
54. Takayanagi, F., Kitamura, T., and Satoh, T., Dinogunellus roe poisoning, Soc. Publ. Hlth. Hokkaido, 5th Meeting, 1953 (unpublished), cited from Asano and Itoh Ref. 59.
55. Sakai, M., Kimura, T., Shinano, H., Ezura, Y., Ban, M., and Hayashi, I., A food poisoning caused by the roe of *Stichaeus grigorjewi*. I. Toxicity of the roe of *Stichaeus grigorjewi*, *Shokuhin Eiseigaku Zasshi*, 5, 420—425, 1964, (Japanese).
56. Hubbs, C. L. and Wick, A. N., Toxicity of the roe of the cabezon, *Scorpaenichthys marmoratus*, *Calif. Fish Game*, 37, 195—196, 1951.
57. Fuhrman, F. A., Fuhrman, G. J., Dull, D. L., and Mosher, H. S., Toxins from eggs of fishes and amphibia, *Agric. Food Chems.*, 17, 417—424, 1969.
58. Fuhrman, F. A., Fuhrman, G. J., and Roseen, J. S., Toxic effects produced by extracts of eggs of the cabezon *Scorpaenichthys marmoratus*, *Toxicon*, 8, 55—61, 1970.
59. Asano, M. and Itoh, M., Toxicity of a lipoprotein and lipids from the role of a blenny *Dinogunellus grigorjewi* Herzenstein, *Tohoku J. Agric. Res.*, 13, 151—167, 1962.
60. Asano, M. and Itoh, M., Lipoproteins (Lipostichaerins) in the roe of blenny, *Stichaeus grigorjewi* Herzenstein, *Tohoku J. Agric. Res.*, 16, 299—316, 1966.

61. Hatano, M., Toxic substance of the roe of northern blenny. VI. Comparison of effects on rats administered with lipostichaerin and toxic phospholipid, *Bull. Fac. Fish. Hokkaido Univ.*, 21, 331—335, 1971, (Japanese).
62. Hatano, M., Toxic substance of the roe of northern blenny. VIII. Partial purification and characterization of toxic phospholipid, *Bull. Fac. Fish. Hokkaido Univ.*, 22, 177—186, 1971, (Japanese).
63. Hatano, M. and Hashimoto, Y., Properties of a toxic phospholipid in the nothern blenny roe, *Toxicon*, 12, 231—236, 1974.
64. Hatano, M., Marumoro, R., and Hashimoto, Y., Structure of a toxic phospholipid in the northern blenny roe, *Proc. 4th Int. Symp. Animal, Plant Microbiol. Toxins*, 2, 145—151, 1976.
65. Hashimoto, Y., Kawasaki, M., and Hatano, M., Occurrence of a toxic phospholipid in cabezon roe, *Toxicon*, 14, 141—143, 1976.
66. Russell, F. E., Marine toxins and venemous and poisonous marine animals, *Adv. Marine Biol.*, 3, 255—383, 1965.
67. Hatano, M., Toxic substance of the roe of the northern blenny. IV. Relationship between lipostichaerin and toxic phospholipid, *Bull. Fac. Fish. Hokkaido Univ.*, 21, 315—323, 1971, (Japanese).
68. Saunders, A. M. and Fuhrman, F. A., Pathological effects of cabezon roe toxin, unpublished, 1968.
69. Brooks, W., A family poisoned by eating a gar, *Northw. Med. Surg. J.*, 7, 437—439, 1850.
70. Moore, G. A., Personal communication, 1972.
71. Coker, R. E., Studies of common fishes of the Mississippi river at Keokuk, *Bull. U. S. Bur. Fish.*, 45, 141—219, 1930.
72. Taft, C. H., Poisonous marine animals, *Texas Rep. Biol. Med.*, 3, 339—352, 1945.
73. Colby, M., Poisonous marine animals in the Gulf of Mexico, *Trans. Tex. Acad. Sci.*, 26, 62—69, 1943.
74. Greene, C. W., Nelson, E. E., and Baskett, E. D., Evidence of toxic action of ovaries of gar, *Am. J. Physiol.*, 45, 558—559, 1918.
75. Netsch, N. F. and Witt, A., Jr., Contributions to the life history of the longnose gar *(Lepisosteus osseus)* in Missouri, *Trans. Am. Fish. Soc.*, 91, 251—262, 1962.
76. Gazio, A., *Corona Florida Medicinae sive De Conservatione Sanitatis*, Venice, 1419; cited from Halstead, B. W., Poisonous and Venomous Marine Animals of the World, Vol. 1, U. S. Government Printing Office, Washington, D.C., 1965, 30.
77. Meyer-Ahrens, K. M., Von den giftigen Fische, *Schweiz. Z. Med. Chir. und Geburtshilfe*, 3, 188—230 and 4, 269—332, 1855.
78. von Franque, A., Vergiftungsfälle nach dem Genusse der Eier der Barbe (Cyprinus barbus), *Deutsch. Klin.*, 10, 133, 1858.
79. Münchmeyer, F., Vergiftung durch Rogen von *Cyprinus barbus, Berl. klin. Wochenschr.*, 12, 46—47, 1875.
80. McCrudden, F. H., The toxic action of certain fish ovaries, *J. Chem. Soc. (London)*, 100 (Abstr. II), 421, 1911.
81. McCrudden, F. H., Pharmakologische und chemische Studien über Barben — und Hechtrogen, *Arch. Exp. Pathol. Pharmacol.*, 91, 46—80, 1921.
82. Pawlowsky, E. N., *Gifttiere und ihre Giftigkeit*, G. Fischer, Jena, 1927.
83. Hiyama, Y., Poisonous Fishes of the South Seas, U. S. Department of Interior, Fish and Wildlife Service, Special Sci. Rep., Fisheries No. 25, Washington, D.C., 1950.
84. Phisalix, M., *Animaux Venimeux et Venins*, Masson, Paris, 1922.
85. Romano, S., Animali velenosi della fauna Italiana, *Natura (Milano)*, 31, 137—167, 1940.
86. Halstead, B. W. and Schall, D. S., Poisonous fishes of La Plata island, unpublished data, cited from Ref. 1, p. 911.
87. Light, L. E., Death following possible ingestion of toad eggs, *Toxicon*, 5, 141—142, 1967.

QUAIL POISONING (COTURNISM)

Theodore Ouzounellis

INTRODUCTION

Coturnism is an acute myoglobinuric syndrome which affects only sensitive individuals when they eat *Coturnix coturnix* (quail). This bird, for reasons which remain unknown, sometimes becomes nosogenous.

The term "Coturnism" is derived from the Greek, oτtikiasis, which is from the Greek word, oτtiki, meaning quail. This type of poisoning has a number of common points with two other food poisonings, the myoglobinuria caused by fish (Haff Disease) and the hemoglobinura caused by fava beans (Favism). We will deal with these similarities later. From among all the different types of quails, only the one that lives in the Mediterranean region and migrates every spring to Europe and every fall to North and Central Africa causes poisonings.

HISTORY

The fact that quail could be poisonous has been known since ancient times. The Bible talks about the group poisoning of the Jews during the exodus.[1] Many writers of ancient and Byzantine times, like Didymus of Alexandria,[2] Lucretius, Plinius the elder, Galen, Avicena, Cassianos Vassos, and others inform us that quail often causes illness or even death, because they eat poisonous seeds and especially the seeds of hemlock, elebore, and aconite.[2-6]

More clear is Galen who writes, "In Dorida, in Boetia, in Thessalia (regions in Greece between Thessaloniki and Athens) and in the neighboring areas muscular contractions appeared in some people after eating quails which have been fed on elebore and I know the same occurs in the area of Athens."

In the contemporary literature, the matter has reappeared with Sergent's publication of cases observed in Algeria and Southern France. The publication of Plichet and Brehant referred to the very same cases.[7-10]

Komvos and Giotsas,[11] Karamanos,[12] and Hadjigeorge[13] report poisonings which were observed in Lesbos, a small island in the east Aegean Sea.

In these recent publications, the disease is characterized as in the ancient times; that is, as a usual poisoning from the substances which are engulfed in the poisonous seeds of the hemlock which the quails eat without being poisoned themselves.

Considerable progress has been made in the study of Coturnism since 1968 when it was confirmed by the author that the cases in Lesbos are not poisoning per se, but myoglobinuric syndromes appearing in only sensitive individuals. The causitive factor is innocuous for normal persons.[14-16]

The observations made during the last decade in Lesbos are the most complete that exist. For this reason, the clinical and laboratory findings from these observations are recorded below.

CLINICAL FINDINGS

Symptoms start 1 to 9 hr after eating quails. Muscular exertion before and particularly after the meal accelerates and aggravates the manifestation of the syndrome. Rest after the meal retards or averts it completely, which is why 80% of the incidents have occurred after lunch and only 20% after dinner which is normally followed by sleep.

The first symptoms are extremely intense pains which appear suddenly in the legs, arms, and the trunk, (but never in the head) according to the recent activity of this or that muscular area. For instance, if the individual is walking, the symptoms start from the legs and if he is writing, from his forearm. Pains spread quickly and they are intensified by every movement. Sometimes muscular weakness of varying degree or complete paralysis precedes or coexists with the pains.

In more severe cases, brownish or reddish urine appears soon and in some cases is followed by oliguria or anuria and azothemia.

The duration of the attack is usually short. A feeling of muscular weakness remains for a few days. In more serious cases complicated by anuria and azothemia recovery is prolonged.

Examination of various systems present nothing significant. Muscular masses are soft and painful on palpation.

LABORATORY FINDINGS

Since 1968, when it was established that Coturnism is a myoglobinuric syndrome, a number of laboratory tests have been used to confirm the diagnosis and to follow up the evolution of the disease.

Blood examination shows the presence of large amounts of substances liberated from muscle cells. Thus serum glutamic oxaloacetic transaminase (SGOT) was up to 1700 units (normal up to 40, aldolase up to 17 (normal 3), lactic dehydrogenase up to 1500 (normal 190), creatine phosphokinase up to 18,000 (normal 200). Blood serum is never reddish as it is in the case of hemoglobinuria. The reason being that unlike hemoglobin, myoglobin does not combine with haptoglobin and is excreted directly into the urine. So the presence of haptoglobin in a case with a positive benzidine test in the urine suggests that this positivity was not due to hemoglobinuria but to myoglobinuria. In the cases of Coturnism the haptoglobin is always normal.

Urine examination discloses the presence of myoglobin in various concentrations and the other findings of myoglobinuric nephrosis (albumin custs). If oliguria or anuria exists, then increased values of blood urea and uric acid are noted. The myoglobinuria, which is a constant symptom, lasts for some hours (10 to 15) and the albumin and custs are found in urine and remain for some days (2 to 10). See Table 1.

DIAGNOSIS

The characteristic clinical symptoms and laboratory findings which appear some hours after eating quail make the diagnosis easy.

THERAPY

Absolute bedrest is of utmost importance and analgesics alleviate the pains.

RELATIONS BETWEEN THE POISONINGS APPEARING IN LESBOS AS COMPARED TO THOSE APPEARING IN ALGERIA AND FRANCE

The study conducted so far indicates that all the different types of quail poisonings are of the same form, independent of the geographical origin of quails: Lesbos, Sinai, and Algiers.

The symptoms which Sergent, Plichet, and Brehart have reported for Algerian and French cases are similar to those of Lesbos.[7-10] If one takes into consideration the fact that Sergent used as his primary source of information the symptoms as described by

Table 1
SOME OBSERVATIONS ON COTURNISM IN LESBOS 1950—1977

1. Number of cases: Total: 121 (120 humans, 1 dog) Without laboratory studies: 91 With laboratory studies: 30
2. Age: Younger than 25 years, 16 cases (13.3%)
    Older than 25 years, 104 cases (86.6%)
3. Sex: Male, 85, (71%), Female, 35, (29%)
4. Attacks after lunch: 96 (80%), after dinner 24 (20%)
5. Patients reporting repeated attacks (2, 3 or 4): 9 (7.5%)
6. Patients reporting cramps: 54 (45%)
7. Familial occurrence of the disease: 8
8. Clinical findings: Muscular pains and stiffness 120 cases (100%)
    Severe weakness, 54 cases (45%)
    Red-colored urine which impressed the patients, 24 cases, (28.4%)
    Vomiting, 42 cases, (35%)
    Diarrhea, 3 cases, (2.5%)
    Fever: None
    Anuria (1 to 5 days), 6 cases (5%)
    Usual duration of the disease: 24—48 hr
    Death, 1 case of a 70 year old male diabetic; death
    occurred 32 hr after the onset of the disease with
    symptoms of severe collapse[a]
9. Laboratory findings:
    Blood: Aldolase, GOT, CPK, and LDH at consistently high levels
    which returns to normal in 4 to 6 days
    Lactic acid: slightly increased in the first 24 hr
    Haptoglobin: always normal
    Urine:benzidine test — constantly positive, the first 10—
    15 hr; control for the pigment for hemoglobin, always
    negative; control of the pigment for myoglobin, always
    positive[b]
    Albumin custs: constant finding the first 1 to 3 days
    Urobilin—urobilinogen, always normal

[a] It was my father-in-law.
[b] The pigment has been controlled in all cases by the $(H_4N)_2SO_4$ fractional precipitation method,[21] and in some of them spectroscopically (Prof. Gardikas, Evangelismos Hospital, Athens).

nondoctor inhabitants of this region (because he himself did not want direct contact with the sick persons), one could easily comprehend small differences. The fact that dark-colored urine is not reported should not come as a surprise to us because in many cases from Lesbos, patients are not specifically instructed to watch for this symptom and they often do not observe it.

In his attempt to prove that quail poisoning is a result of hemlock, Sergent succeeded in inducing paralysis in dogs which had eaten quails which had been fed ground hemlock seeds by catheter. Of course, such feeding conditions are not found in nature, nor is there any proof that the poisoning which was induced in the dogs is the same as that which quails induce in humans.

Even the information of previous times is scarce concerning muscular system symptoms similar to those found in Lesbos. Ancient writers report muscular contractions (Galen),[5] tetanus-like spasms (Avicenne),[6] stiffness and dizziness (Cassianus Bassos),[2] and epileptic form or tetanic form reaction (Aldrovadi).[17]

THE GEOGRAPHICAL DISTRIBUTION OF THE DISEASE

Figure 1 indicates the distribution of the quail poisoning cases together with the myoglobinuria from fish[18] and the area (Bordeaux, France) where Prof. Beylot treated

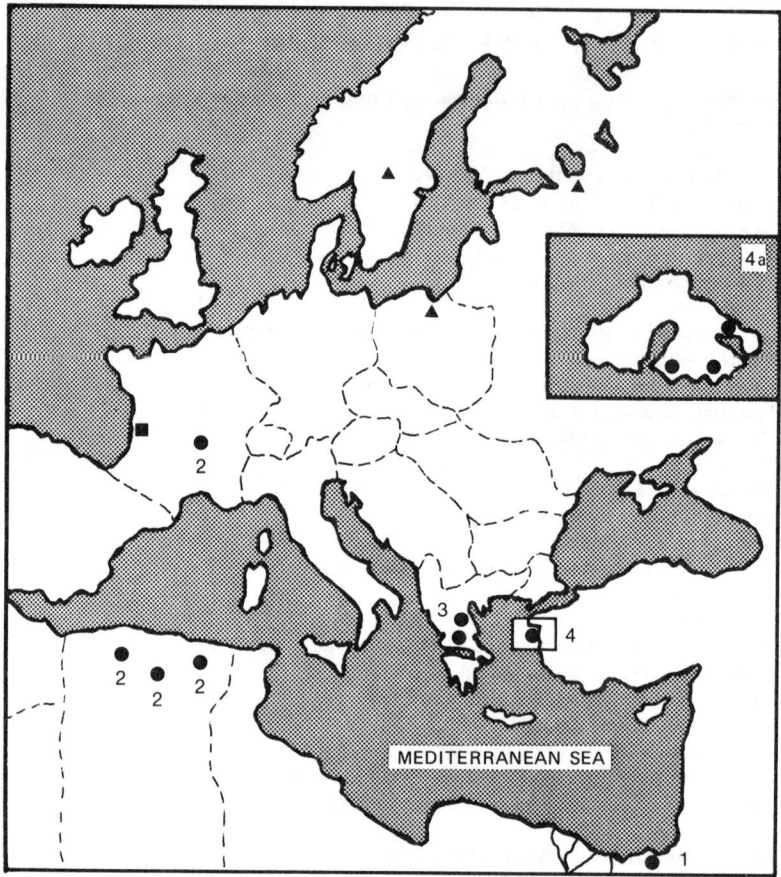

FIGURE 1. Areas where poisoning cases from quails, fishes, and skylarks have been observed. ● — Quail poisoning according to 1. the Bible, 2. Sergent, 3. Galen, 4. Ouzounellis — 4a. island of Lesbos. ▲ — Myoglobinuria after eating fishes. ■ — Myoglobinuria after eating skylarks.

four cases of myoglobinuria caused by eating skylarks.[22] It is noteworthy that while in Lesbos there were 120 cases observed between 1950 and 1977, in the other Aegean islands no such cases had been reported.

THE CAUSATIVE FACTOR

The quail itself cannot be the causative factor since the incidents are few. One could support the view that the poisoning is due to a metabolite which is accumulated in the muscles of the quails during their migratory journey. But in such a case incidents would also have been more frequent because in Lesbos all quails are shot shortly after their arrival on the island and all are exhausted.

The only plausible explanation then is that the causative factor exists in the leaves or seeds of a certain plant which is eaten by certain quails. This could easily explain why certain flocks present many incidents and others none.[16]

Table 2 shows the kind of seeds which were found in the stomachs of quails. Many of them are known to be poisonous. The poisoning, though, caused by them is completely irrelevant to quail poisoning in man.

THE SENSITIVITY FACTOR

According to all indications, the causative factor is harmful only to certain sensitive individuals. This can be concluded by the following observations. In Lesbos, as a means of avoiding severe poisonings, people divide each quail into more individual portions. In this way, should a bird be poisonous, only a small amount of the poisonous flesh will be consumed by any one person. Many attacks have been observed under these circumstances. Usually only one person among those having eaten the same bird is affected, whereas the others did not present any symptoms. In some cases in which two persons affected, those belonged to the same genetic tree.

The same is also indicated by the fact that some persons are attacked by the disease two, three, and even four times.

This sensitivity is transmitted hereditarily. This is clearly shown by the three family trees in Figure 2 which were selected from many others in Lesbos.

It seems that this sensitivity is due to an abnormality of the carbohydrate metabolism in the muscle cells.[14-15] There is not yet proof for this hypothesis.

SIMILARITIES WITH HAFF DISEASE

Fish-Caused Myoglobinuria

This poisoning presents the same clinical picture as quail poisoning. Both are myoglobinuric syndromes. In both, the factor of personal sensitivity is crucial. A difference exists in the time of the clinical manifestation. In quail poisoning it is 1 to 9 hr and in Haff disease about 18 hr.

SIMILARITIES WITH FAVISM

Fava Bean-Caused Hemoglobinuria

It is interesting to note certain similarities existing between Coturnism and Favism. In both, the causative factor is a substance innocuous for normal persons but harmful for those with a hereditarily transmitted sensitivity.

The myoglobin of muscle cells in Coturnism and the hemoglobin of red cells in Favism which are liberated during the poisoning have similar chemical structure and biological role.

In the case of Favism, the hemolysis appears when the three contributing factors mentioned below reach a certain level.[19] That is to say, causative factor (fava beans) and sensitivity factor (lack of defect of Glycine 6-P dehydrogenase) and other predisposing factors (prolonged malnutrition[20] and other unknown factors) hemolysis → hemoglobinuria.

Indications lead to the speculation that the same pathogenetic scheme exists for Coturnism. Causative factor (the substance existing in some quails) and sensitivity factor (the suspected abnormality of muscle cell carbohydrate metabolism) and other predisposing factors (muscular exercise) → myolysis → myoglobinuria.

The clarification of the enzymatic deficiency which produces favism has resulted in the classification in the same group of many seemingly irrelevant hemoglobinurias (from fava beans, antimalaria drugs, sulfamides, naphthalene, chloramphenicol, and others).

It is hoped that similar results concerning different forms of myoglobinuria (from quails, fishes, alcohol, barbiturates, licorice, sea snake bites, and others) may follow if a similar enzymatic deficiency causing quail poisonings is established in the future.

Table 2
SEEDS FOUND IN THE STOMACH OF QUAILS IN LESBOS (FROM 300 QUAILS)

Setaria sp.[a]
Polygonum persicaria L.[a]
Polygonum sp.
Polygonum convulvulus L.
Trifolium sp.[a]
Graminae
Nutlets of Boraginacea or Lubiatae probably
? *Trigonella* sp.[a]
Pods of Vicia sp.
? *Grataegus* sp.
Galium sp.[a]
Onopordun acanthrium L.
Milium sp.
? Boraginaceae
? Stachy of Nutlets
Vicia sp.[a]
Lathyrus sp.[a]
Crotalaria sp.[a]
Amaranthus sp.
Carthamus tinctorius L.
Leguminosae
? Caryophyllaceae
Trifolium arvense L.
Not identified
Some others too damaged for identification

[a] Seeds with poisonous properties, as identified by Dr. Angel of the Royal Botanic Gardens of London. The seeds have been identified upon the request of Dr. J. B. Bateman, Dr. J. P. M. Brenan of the Royal Botanic Gardens of London (Director: Prof. J. Heslop-Harrison).

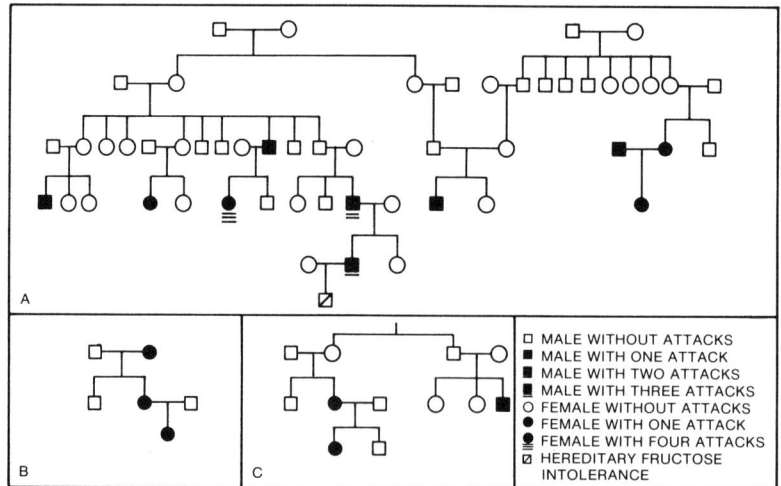

FIGURE 2. Hereditary sensitivity shown by three family trees selected in Lesbos.

REFERENCES

1. The Bible, Number II.
2. Cassianos Bassos, *Geoponica,* Hbeckh, Lipsiae, W. Germany, 1895, XIV, 24.
3. Lucrece, De la nature, trad. A., Ermont, *Les Belles Lettres,* Vol. IV, 2nd ed., Paris, 1924, 640—641.
4. Pline l'ancien. Histoire natur., trad. E., de Saint Denis, *Les Belles Lettres,* Vol. XXIII 33, 69, Paris, 1961.
5. Galeni, in *Hippocratis Epidemiarum Librum. VI. Comentaria,* Wenkebach, E., Ed., Fr. Pfaff. ed., alt. Vol. 34, Acad. Litterarum Berolini, 1956, 306—307.
6. Avicennae, *Arabum medicorum principis,* Canonis lib. II tract 2, cap 153, ex. G. Gremonensis versione Apud luntas Venetiis, 1595 I, p. 298.
7. Sergent, E., Les cailles empoisonneuse dans la Bible et en Algerie de nos jours, *Arch. Inst. Pasteur Alger.,* No. 2, 161—192, 1942.
8. Sergent, E., Les cailles empoisoneuses, *Arch. Inst. Pasteur Alger.,* No. 26, 249—260, 1948.
9. Plichet, A., Les cailles empoisoneuses, *Presse Med.,* 56, 1189, 1952.
10. Brehant, J., A propos d'une intoxication collective par le miel: celles des Hebreux au desert par les cailles, *Presse Med.,* 74, 1157, 1966.
11. Komvos, K. and Giotsas, Z., Illness after eating quail, *Evangelismos Hosp. Rev. (Athens),* 15, 6, 1953.
12. Karamanos, G., Syndrome after eating quails, *Iatriki Proodhos,* 99, 202, 1951.
13. Hadjigeorge, E., Les Cailles Empoisonneuses, *Presse Med.,* 68, 1469, 1952.
14. Ouzounellis, Th., Myoglobinuries par ingestion de cailles, *Presse Med.,* 39, 1863, 1968.
15. Ouzounellis, Th., Myoglobinuria from quail poisoning, *Iatriki,* 14, 213—217, 1968.
16. Ouzounellis, Th., Some notes on quail poisoning, *JAMA,* 211, 1187, 1970.
17. Aldrovandi, Ulyssis, Ornithologiae, II, Apud I. B. Bellagambam., Lib. XIII, Bononiae, 1600, p. 171.
18. Berlin, Ragnar, Haff Disease in Sweden, *Acta Medica Scandinavica,* 139, 560—572, 1947.
19. Katakis, Favism, *Iatriki,* 4, 251, 1963.
20. Hadjigeorge, E. and Ouzounellis, Th., On sixty cases of Favism, *Nosokomeiaka Chronika,* 9, 3, 1950.
21. Blondheim, Sh., Margoliash, E., Shafris, E., A Simple Test for Myoglobinuria, *JAMA,* 167, 453—454, 1958.
22. Beylot, J., personal communication, 1974.

Index

INDEX

A

Abramis brama (bream), 308
Abrin, 222
Abrus precatorius (precatory bean), 222
Acacia sp., 4
Acacipetalin, 227
4-Acetamido-4-hydroxy-2-butenoic acid γ-lactone, 255
Acetate, 103
Acetic acid, 229
Acetylcholine, 230
Acetyl derivatives, 3
N-Acetyl loline, 241, 242, 266, 268
N-Acetyl loline alkaloids, 243
Acetylphenylhydrazine, 64, 73, 74
1-Acetyl-2-phenylhydrazine, 63
Achlorhydria, 135
Acid oxalates, 231
Aconitine, 221
ACTH, see Adrenocorticotropin
Acute hemolysis, 63
Acute toxicity of nitrosamines, 139
Additives to food
    nitrosamines and, 151—152
    PAH and, 161
Adenocarpus decorticans, 266
Adenomas of lung, 51
Adenosine triphosphatase (ATP), 56, 74
Adlupulon, 81
Adrenocorticotropin (ACTH), 297
Affinity chromatography, 31
Aflatoxins, see also specific aflatoxins, 230
Agaricus
    bisporus, 205
    brunnescens, 205
    capestris, 204
Agglutination, 31
Aglucones, 110
    antithyroid effect of, 116—118
    cabbage and, 117
    metabolism of, 111—116
Aglycones, 66—70
Agricultural chemicals nitrosamines, 148—149
Agroclavine, 257, 259
Agrostemma githago (corn cackle), 229
Albizzine, 3
Alcohol sensitivity induced by mushrooms, 198
Aldehyde oximes, 103
Aldehydes, 152, 226
Aldohexoses, 226
Alfalfa, 84, 85, 87
Algae, 172
Ali cyclic compounds, 136
Aliphatic solvent, 163
"Alkali disease", 6
Alkaline phosphatase, 56
Alkaloids, 213—222, 231, 241—244, 259, 261—267

N-acetyl loline, 243
apomorphine, 218
β-carboline, 243
clavine, 257
diterpenoid, 221
eserine, 218
N-formyl loline, 243
indole, 218, 221, 243, 244, 257
isoquinoline, 218
loline-type, 245, 265—267
lupine, 218
lysergic acid peptide, 261
lysine, 218
peptide, 218
piperidine, 218
proto, 218
pseudo, 218
reed canarygrass and, 241—247
separation of, 264—265
steroidal, 218, 224
steroidal psuedo, 221
tall fescue and, 241—247
true, 218
tryptamine, 242
Alkyl compounds, 136
7-Alkyl guanine, 141
Alkylnitrosamides, 136
Alkyl-oxazolidine-2-thiones, 105
Allergies, 222
    to antibiotic residues, 277
    to mushrooms, 205
Alloxan, 67
Allyl-cyanide, 105
Allyl-glucosinolate (sinigrin), 17, 103, 105, 228
Allyl-GS, 24
Allyl-isothiocyanate, 17, 102, 105, 227, 228
    antithyroid effect of, 117
3-Allyl-2-thiohydantoin, 115
Almonds, 107
ALS, see Amyotrophic lateral sclerosis
Amaninamide, 200
Amanita
    bisporigera, 200
    gemmata, 203
    muscaria, 193, 197
    ocreata, 200
    pantherina, 197, 203
    phalloides, 193, 200—202
    sp., 200
    verna, 200
    virosa, 200
Amanitin, 222
Amatoxins, 200
Ames test, 205
Amines, 131, 134
    biological, 218, 220
    primary, 133, 150
    secondary, 139

tertiary, 133, 150
Amino acids, see also specific amino acids, 3—10, 115, 150, 178, 213, 222—224
    aromatic, 218
    nonaromatic, 227
    nonprotein (uncommon), 3, 6, 224
    protein, 3, 220
    sulfur, 6, 7
L-2-Amino-6-amidinohexanic acid (indospicine), 10
Aminoenol, 68
2-Amino-4-(guanidinooxy)butyric acid (canavanine), 10, 224
2-Amino-3-methylaminopropionic acid, 9
3-Aminopropionitrile, 4
Aminopyrine, 135
Ammonium-N, 244
Ammonium quaternary compounds of, 133—134, 150
Amphibian eggs, 301—311
    poisonous, 308
Ampicillin, 278
Amygdalin, 226
Amyotrophic lateral sclerosis (ALS), 43, 44
Anacardiaceae, 230
Anamirta cocculus, 226
Anchovies, 148
Androgens, 81, 287
Anemia
    hemolytic, 8
    kale, 26
Anemone nemerosa, 228
Anemones, 228
Anethole, 81
Angiosperms, 226, 232
Animal growth promotors, 277—286
Anthracene, 171, 172, 179, 180
Anthranthrene, 177, 179
Antibiotics, see also specific antibiotics
    residues of, 277—286
Antithyroid effects, 101, 115—118
Apocyanaceae, 218, 228
Apomorphine alkaloids, 218
Apples, 171
Apricots, 107, 171
Aquarium fishes, 50
Aquatic environment PAH, 173
Araucaria araucana (pinon), 107
Arginine, 3, 10, 134, 224
Armyworm (*Prodenia eridania*), 8
Aromatic amino acids, 218
Aromatic hydrocarbons, see Polycyclic aromatic hydrocarbons
Aromatic isothiocyanates, 102
Aryl compounds, 136
Ascochyta imperfecta, 84
Ascorbate, 134
Ascorbic acid, 68, 72, 105
Aspartic acid, 3, 115
Aspergillus
    flavus, 230
    sp., 249

terreus, 249—253
versicolor, 230
Aspirate, 200
Asteraceae, 224
Asthma, 222
    extrinsic, 204
Astragalus sp., 6, 231
Atelopus
    chiriquiensis (Costa Rican frog), 308
    sp., 303
ATP, see Adenosine triphosphatase
Atropine, 218
Australian blue-ringed octopus (*Octopus maculosa*), 303
Azetidine-2-carboxylic acid, 3, 224
Azomethane, 48
Azoxyglucoside, 44
Azoxyglycoside, see also specific azoxyglycosides, 46—47
Azoxymethane, 48

B

Bacilli, 278
Bacon, 151, 152
    nitrosamines in, 146—147
    smoked, 169
Bacteria
    drug-resistant, 278
    nitrosamine production of, 135
    PAH synthesis by, 171
    water-contaminating goitrogens originating from, 121
Balansia
    claviceps, 257—261
    epichloe, 257—261
    henningsiana, 257—261
    sp., 257
    strangulans, 257—261
Bamboo shoots, 107
Banisteropsis coapi, 231
Barbecued ribs, 178
Barbels, 308
"Barbencholera", 308
Barbus
    barbus, 308
    meridionalis, 308
Barley, 81, 172
    malted, 181
Barnacles, 175
Bass, 177
Beans, 107, 177
    broad (*Vicia faba*), 8, 63, 65—72
    castor, 32, 222
    fava, see Fava beans
    garden (*Phaseolus vulgaris*), 32—35
    jack (*Concanavalia ensiformis*), 222
    lectins in, 32—35
    navy, 35
    precatory (*Abrus precatorius*), 222

Beef
   drippings from, 171
   grilled, 178
Beneficial effects of phytoestrogens, 87
Benomyl, 266
Benz(a)anthracene, 162, 164—167, 170, 177—181
Benz(a)anthracene-chrysene, 165
Benzofluoranthene, 164, 177, 179
Benzo(b)fluoranthene, 162, 163, 165, 181
Benzo(k)fluoranthene, 162, 164, 173
Benzo(k)fluoranthene-benzo(b)fluoranthene, 165
Benzo(g,h,i)perylene, 162, 163, 179, 180
Benzo(a)pyrene, 161—181
   petroleum-linked, 175
Benzo(e)pyrene, 162, 163, 165, 170, 179, 181
Benzthiazuron (N-Methyl-N^1 (2-benzothiozolyl)-urea), 135
Benzylglucosinolate (benzyl-GS), 15, 103
Benzyl-GS, see Benzylglucosinolate
Benzylisoquinolines, 218
Benzypyrenes, 165
Berberidaceae, 218
Berberine, 218
Beverage PAH, 181
BH x BT, see N,N'-bis-(p-Hexyloxybenzylidene)-a,a'-bi-p-toluidine
Binding assays, 200
Biochanin A, 82, 83, 93
Biochemistry
   cycasin, 54—57
   goitrogens, 101—107
Biological amines (proto-alkaloids), 218, 220
Biological effects
   cycasin, 50—58
   glucosinolates, 17—23
Biological fluids, 149—150
Biological properties of nitrosamines, 139—141
Biosynthesis
   goitrogens, 102—104
   PAH by plants, 172, 173
Biphenyls, 121
Biscuits, 177
Black pepper, 148
Black sea bass, 177
Blighia sapida, 7
"Blind-staggers" (chronic selenosis), 6
Blood levels of testosterone, 288
Blowfish (*Fugu rubripes*), 302, 303
Blue-ringed octopus (*Octopus maculosa*), 303
BMBT, see N,N'-*bis*(p-Methoxybenzylidene)-a,a'-bi-p-toluidine
Boletus
   edulis, 204, 205
   luridus, 198
   luteus, 205
Bologna, 169
Bourbon, 181
Bovine emphysema, 242
Bowenia sp., 43, 47
BPhBT, see N,N'-bis(p-Phenylbenzylidene)-a,a'-bi-p-toluidine

Bracydanio reris, 50
Brassica
   campestris (Chinese cabbage)-, 17, 24, 120, 121
   carinata, 24
   hirta (white mustard seed), 15, 120
   juncea, 120
   kale, 15, 26
   napus (rutabagas), 17, 24, 105, 120
   oleracea, see Cabbage
   sp., 25, 26, 105, 118, 227
      fodder of, 23
"Brassica factor" chemical nature, 117
Bream (*Abramis brama*), 308
Broad bean (*Vicia faba*), 8, 63, 65—72
p-Brom-phenylisothiocyanate, 115
Brussels sprouts, 17
B-sitosterol, 82
Bufodienolides, 228
Bufo marinus, 308
Bufotenine, 220
Burley tobaccos, 150
Butenyl-GS, 17
3-Butenyl isothiocyanate, 227
Butter, 171
Buttercups, 228
Butterfish, 177

C

Cabbage, 17, 25, 101, 105, 121
   aglucones in, 117
   Chinese (*Brassica campestris*), 17, 24, 120
Cabbage goiter, 116
Calcium, 231
California newt (*Taricha torosa*), 303, 308
Caltha palustris (marsh marigolds), 228
Camelina sativa, 120
Canavalia ensiformis, 10
Canavanine, see 2-Amino-4-(guanidinooxy)butyric acid
Cancer, see also specific types
   liver, 50
Cannabis sativa, 231
Capparales, 227
Carbazole, 180
Carbohydrase inhibitors, 39—42
Carbohydrates, 178
β-Carboline, 231, 242
β-Carboline alkaloids, 243
Carbon-14-heptadecane, 175
Carbon-14-naphthalene, 175
Carbon-14-zearalenone, 94
Carbonyl-conjugated enediol, 68
Carcinogenicity
   cycads, 44
   cycasin, 50—52, 57
   nitrosamines, 140
   PAH, 162
   phytoestrogens, 93
Carcinomas, see also Cancer, 51

Cardenolides, 228
Cardiac glycosides, 213, 226, 228—229, 231
Carica papaya, 15
Carrots (*Daucas carota*), 81, 171
Cassava, 107
Cassava goiter, 117
Castor beans, 32, 222
Catalytic effects on nitrosation reaction, 133
Cation exchange chromatography, 265
Cattle movement, 299
Cauliflower, 121, 171
Ceratozamia sp., 43
Chanoclavine, 259
Charcoal broiled meats, 161, 178
Cheese, 148
  smoked, 169
Cheirolin, see 3-Methylsulfonylpropyl isothiocyanate
Chemical decomposition of goitrogens, 105—107
Chemical properties
  aglycones, 66—70
  "Brassica factor", 117
  convicine, 66—70
  cycasin, 46—50
  nitroso compounds, 137—138
  vicine, 66—70
Chemical reactions of nitrosamines, 136—139
Chemical structure
  aglycones, 66—70
  convicine, 66—70
  lectins, 31
  vicine, 66—70
  zearalenone, 93
Chemical substances in plants, 213—240
Chemiluminescent detectors, 145
Chenopodiaceae, 231
Cherries, 107
Chinese cabbage, see *Brassica campestris*
Chiriquitoxin, 308
Chloramphenicol, 278
Chromatography
  affinity, 31
  cation exchange, 265
  column, 142, 162, 163
  gas, 110, 144, 162, 166, 175, 179
  gas-liquid, 142—144, 164, 180
  high pressure liquid, 165, 166
  paper, 49, 115, 162, 266
  thin-layer, 49, 142, 143, 162, 163, 200, 265, 266
Chronic selenosis ("blind-staggers"), 6
Chrysanthemum roots, 171
Chrysene, 163—165, 170, 177, 179—181
Chrysene-triphenylene-benz(a)anthracene, 164
Cicutoxin, 231
Circuta virosa, 231
Citrulline, 3
Cladosporium
  cladosporioides, 253—254
  sp., 253
Classical lathyrism (neurolathyrism), 4
Clavaria flava, 205

Claviceps
  paspali, 257
  purpurea, 231, 255—257
  sp., 255, 257
Clavicipitaceae, 255, 257, 261
Clavine alkaloids, 257
Clean-up of nitrosamines, 142
Clitocybe
  clavipes, 198
  illudens, 226
  sp., 194
Clostridium botulinum, 222
Clover
  New Zealand white (*Trifolium repens*), 117
  subterranean, 84
  white, 107
Clover disease (mastitis), 88
Clover goiter, 117
Coconut oil, 170
Cod, 148
Coffee, 177
Coffee substitutes, 177
Coiine, 218
Colchicine, 222
Colchicum autumnale, 222
Colletotricum trifolii, 84
Column chromatography, 142, 162, 163
Colupulon, 81
Coma associated with deliriant mushrooms, 197
Commercial crops, 17
Competition binding assay, 200
Compositae, 226, 231
Concanavalia ensiformis (jack bean), 222
Concanavalin A, 222
Condiments, 15, 24
Conocybe
  filaris, 200
  sp., 196, 231
Contact dermatitis, 205
Convallatoxin, 228
Convicine, 66
  chemical structure and properties of, 66—70
  chemical synthesis of, 70—71
Copelandia sp., 196
Copper, 231
Coprine, 198
Coprinus
  atramentarius, 193, 198
  insignis, 198
  quadrifidus, 198
  variegatus, 198
Corda, 254
Corn, 81, 92, 107, 172
Corn cackle (*Agrostemma githago*), 229
Cornflakes, 93
Cornification, 81
Corn products, 93
Coronene, 162, 177, 179
Corticosteroids, 229
Cortinarius
  gentilis, 203

orellanus, 203
sp., 193, 203
speciosissimus, 203
Cortisol, 297—299
Costa Rican frog (*Atelopus chiriquiensis*), 308
Cottonseed oil, 170
Coturnism, see Quail poisoning
Coturnix coturnix (quail), 313
Coumarin, 226, 232
Coumestans, 82, 87, 88
Coumestrol, 81—85, 93
Crab, 177
Crambe
  abyssinica, 105, 102
  hispanica, 120
Croaker, 148
Crops, see also specific crops
  commercial, 17
  crucifer, 25—26
  oilseed, 15
Crotalaria sp., 4
Croton sp., 226
Crowfoots, 228
Cruciferae, 227
Cruciferous seed meal, 23—24, 120
Crucifer plants, 15, 25—26, 101, 120
Cultural practices, 243—244
Curing of meat, 152
Cyanate donors, 113
Cyanide, 113
3-Cyanoalanine, 5—6
Cyano compounds, 107
Cyanogen, 107
Cyanogenesis, 226
Cyanogenic glucosides, 107, 117
Cyanogenic glycosides, 213, 226—227
Cyanogenic plant constituents, 227
Cyanohydrins, 107, 226
1-Cyano-2-hydroxy-3-butene, 107
1-Cyano-2-(S)-hydroxy-3-butene, 17
1-Cyano-2-hydroxy-3,4-epithiobutane diasteromeric isomers, 107
1-Cyano-2(S)-hydroxy-3-(R)(S)-*epi*thiobutanes, 18
Cyanolipids, 227
1-Dyano-3-methylsulfinylpropane, 25
1-Cyano-3,4-*epi*thiobutane, 17
Cycad, 107
  as food, 43—44
  carcinogenicity of, 44
  distribution of, 43
  flour from, 57
  toxicity of, 44
Cycas
  circinalis, 9, 43, 44, 46, 50, 57
  revoluta, 43, 47, 57
  sp., 9, 43, 47
Cycasin, 43—61
  biochemical actions of, 54—57
  biological effects of, 50—58
  carcinogenicity of, 50—52, 57
  chemical properties of, 46—50

effect of on humans, 57
enzymatic hydrolysis of, 48
hydrolysis of, 48
isolation of, 47
mutagenicity of, 54
neurotoxicity of, 52—54
physical properties of, 49
radiomimetic effects of, 54
Cyclic heptapeptides, 200
Cyclic octapeptides, 200
Cyclic polypeptides, 200
Cyclohexane, 163
Cyclopropanone hydrate, 198
Cylindrocladium scoparium, 84
Cyprinidae, 308
Cystathionase, 10
Cystathionine, 5
Cystathionine synthetase, 10
Cysteine, 10, 103, 115
Cystic glandular hyperplasia of endometrium, 88
Cystine, 7
L-Cystine, 7
Cytidine incorporation, 55
Cytosine, 231
Cytosol, 84

D

Dactylis glomerata (orchardgrass), 241
Daidzein, 82—84, 93
Daphne mezereum, 226
Daucas carota (carrots), 81, 171
DBN, 145
DDT, 81
Decarboxylation, 220
Decomposition
  dialkylnitrosamines, 141
  glucosinolates, 108, 111
  goitrogens, 105—107
Deep frying, 178
Deficiency
  glucose-6-phosphate dehydrogenase, 63—65
  GSSG reductase, 73
  thiamine, 222
Deliriant mushrooms associated with sleep or coma, 197
Delphine, 221
Delta-9-tetrahydrocannabinol, 81
DEN, see Diethylnitrosamine
Deoxynivalenol, 92
Dermatitis, 205, 230
DES, see Diethylstilbestrol
Dhurrin, 226
Diagnosis of systemic mushroom poisoning, 193—194
Dialkylnitrosamines, 139
  decomposition of, 141
Diallylbutylnitrosamine, 140
Dialuric acid, 67
L-2,4-Diaminobutyric acid, 4

Dianthrone, 230
Diasteromeric isomers of 1-cyano-2-hydroxy-3,4-epithiobutane, 107
Diazoalkane, 136
Dibenzanthracene, 179
Dibenz(a,h)anthracene, 178, 180
Dibenz(a,j)anthracene 163
Dibenz(a,h)anthracene-benzo(g,h,i)perylene, 164
Dibenzylbutylnitrosamine, 140
Dibutylnitrosamine, 146
Dichopetalaceae, 232
Dicotyledons, 227
Dicoumarol, 232
Diethylnitrosamine (DEN), 132, 135, 140, 145, 146
Diethylstilbestrol (DES), 83, 84, 92, 93
Diffraction studies, 136
Digitalis, 228
Digitalis purpurea (foxglove), 228
Digitonin, 228
3,4-Dihydroxyphenylalanine, 72—73
L-3,4-Dihydroxyphenylalanine (L-Dopa), 3, 8
Dimethylamine, 134
N,N-Dimethylformamide-water-cyclohexane, 163
1,2-Dimethylhydrazine, 48, 49
Dimethylnitrosamine (DMN), 131, 132, 135, 140, 141, 145—150
Dimethyl-OT, see 5-Dimethyl-oxazolidine-2-thione
5,5-Dimethyloxazolidinethione, 20
5-Dimethyl-oxazolidine-2-thione (dimethyl-OT), 105
Dimethyl sulfoxide, 163
Dinogunellin, 306—307
Dioclea sp., 10
Dioon sp., 43
Dioscorides, 226
Diosgenin, 229
Diphenylbutylnitrosamine, 140
Disulfides, 74, 107
Disulfiram, 135, 198
Diterpenes, 224, 226
Diterpenoid, 218
  alkaloids of, 221
  derivatives of, 224
Divicine, 67, 68, 70—72
  chemical synthesis of, 70—71
DMN, see Dimethylnitrosamine
L-Dopa, see L-3,4-Dihydroxyphenylalanine
Down's syndrome (mongolism), 9
Drippings from beef, 171
Dropsy, 228
Drosophila melongaster, 54
Drugs, see also specific drugs
  bacteria resistant to, 278
  hemolysis induced by, 74
  nitrite interaction with, 135
  sensitivity to, 63

E

Edible mushrooms, 171
Eggs
  amphibian, 301—311
  fish, 301—311
  poisonous, 308
Electron capture detector, 144
Elymoclavine, 259
Emphysema, 242
Encephalartos sp., 43, 47
Endemic goiter, 119—120
Endogenous formation of thiocyanate, 112—113
Endometrial cystic glandular hyperplasia, 88
Enediol, 68
Enterotoxin, 222
Environment
  effects of, 243—244
  nitrosamines in, 145—150
  PAH in, 173
Enzymatic decomposition
  glucosinolates, 108, 111
  goitrogens, 105—107
Enzymatic hydrolysis, 15, 17
  cycasin, 48
Epichloe typhina, 241—243, 255—257, 266
Epicoccum
  nigrum, 254
  sp., 254
Epi-goitrin, 23
Epi-progoitrin, 17, 18, 20, 26, 105
Episulfide, 15
Epithiospecifier protein, 105
Ergolines, 218
Ergonovine, 259
Ergonovinine, 259
Ergosine, 257
Ergosinine, 257
Ergotamine, 218
Ergovaline, 257
Ergovalinine, 257
Ericaceae, 226
Erucic, 120
Erucic acid, 120
Erythorbate, 134
Eserine alkaloids, 218
Esox lucius (pike), 308
Estradiol-17β, 83, 84, 92, 93
Estradiol-17β-cyclo-pentylpropionate, 84
Estradiol dipropionate, 84
Estriol, 81
Estrogenic metabolite, 91
Estrogen receptors, 83
Estrogens, see also specific estrogens, 81—100
  fungal, 91
Estrone, 81, 83, 93
p-Ethyl phenol, 93
Ethyl *tert*-butylnitrosamine, 140
Eupatorium rugosum, 226
Euphorbiaceae, 226
European freshwater fish, 308
Exogenous preformed thiocyanate, 114, 119
Extracellular fluid, 115
Extract incubation with myrosinase, 109—110
Extraction of glucosinolates, 109

Extrinsic asthma, 204

F

Fabaceae, 218
Farm animals, 25—26
Fat necrosis, 241, 249, 267—269
Fats, 169—171
Fatty acids, 178
Fava beans, 63, 313, 317
   fractionation of extracts of, 66
   hemoglobinuria caused by, 317
Favism, 8, 313, 317
   causative agent of, 65—71
   epidemiological aspects of, 63
   etiology of, 63—65, 72—73
   pathogenesis of, 71—74
Favism-producing agents, 63—79
Ferns, 232
Fertilization with nitrogen, 243
Fescue (*Festuca arundinacea*), 241, 267
Fescue foot, 241, 249, 253—255, 267—268
Fescue toxicity, see Fescue foot
Festuca
   arundinacea (tall fescue), 241, 249—273
      alkaloids in, 241—247
   sp., 243
Festuclavine, 257
Fish, see also specific types of fish, 148, 163, 173, 174, 177, 313, 315
   aquarium, 50
   eggs of, 301—311
   European freshwater, 308
   myoglobinuria caused by, 317
   poisonous, 301
   smoked, 161, 167, 169, 179
Fishmeal, 131, 148
Flax, 120
Florae changing by antibiotics, 278
Flounder, 177
Flour from cycad, 57
Flower pigments, 84
Fluoranthene, 164, 170, 171, 179—181
Fluorene, 179
Fluorescence, 164
Fluoroacetic acid, 232
Fluorometry, 265
Fodder, 23
Food additives
   nitrosamines and, 151—152
   PAH and, 161
Food analyses, 162—166
Formononetin, 82—84, 93, 231
N-Formyl loline, 241, 242, 266, 268
N-Formyl loline alkaloids, 243
Foxglove (*Digitalis purpurea*), 228
Fractionation of fava bean extracts, 66
Frankfurters, 134, 147
   smoked, 169
Free radicals, 74

Freeze drying, 152
Freshwater algae, 172
Freshwater fish, 308
Frogs, 303
   Costa Rican (*Atelopus chiriquiensis*), 308
Frying, 178
Fugu
   rubripes (Japanese puffer or blowfish), 302, 303
   sticnotus, 302
   vermicularis, 302
Fungal estrogen, 91
Fungi, see also specific fungi, 222, 226, 230, 241, 243, 257, 261
Furan, 228
Fusarium
   graminearum, 84
   poae, 254
   roseum, 92
   sp., 86, 91, 93, 255
   sporotrichioides, 254
   tricinctum, 249, 253—255

G

Galactopoiesis, 87
Galactose, 226
Galerina
   autumnalis, 200
   marginata, 200
   venenata, 200
Garden beans (*Phaseolus vulgaris*), 32—35
Gars, 307—308
Gas chromatography, 110, 144, 162, 166, 175, 179
Gas-liquid chromatography (GLC), 142—144, 164, 180
Gastric aspirate, 200
Gastroenteric irritants in mushrooms, 194
Genistein, 82—84, 89, 93, 231
Genistin, 82, 88—90
Genotype, 243
Gibberella zeae, 81, 92
Glandular hyperplasia, 88
LGC, see Gas-liquid chromatography
Globulins, 83
Glucobrassicin, 26, 105, 116
Glucobrassicin-1-sulfonate, 105
Glucoconringiin, 105
Glucocorticoids, 295—300
Glucoiberin, 20
Glucono-δ-lactone, 134
S-Glucopyranoside of thiohydroximyl-*O*-sulfate, 101
Glucose, 226
D-Glucose, 105
Glucose-6-phosphatase, 56
Glucose-6-phosphate dehydrogenase (G6PD), 8, 64, 73
   deficiency of, 63—65
   structure of, 64
β-Glucosidase, 45, 51, 52, 107
Glucosides

cyanogenic, 107, 117
mustard oil, see Glucosinolates
protoanemonin, 228
Glucosinolate aglucones, 107
Glucosinolates, 15—30, 101—107, 120, 213, 227—228
   biological effects of, 17—23
   commercial crops and, 17
   decomposition of, 108, 111
   enzymatic decomposition of, 108, 111
   estimation of, 108—111
   extraction of, 109
   hydrolytic products from, 15—17
   identification of, 109
   separation of, 109
   total, 110—111
β-Glucosyl-cycasins, 47
Glucothiohydroximic acid, 103
γ-Glutamyl, 3
3-N-(4-L-Glutamyl)aminopropionitrile, 3—4
4-Glutamylcyanoalanine, 5—6
Glutathione (GSH), 8, 63, 65, 66, 69, 73, 74
   instability of, 64
   level of, 64
   oxidation of, 72, 73
Glutathione disulfide (GSSG), 63, 73
Glutathione disulfide (GSSG) reductase, 64, 73, 74
   deficiency of, 73
Glutathione (GSH) peroxidase, 73, 74
Glycine, 3, 102, 115
Glycine 6-P dehydrogenase, 317
Glycolysis, 74
Glycoprotein, 222
β-Glycoside, 8
Glycosides, 9, 213, 226
   cardiac, 213, 226, 228—229, 231
   cyanogenic, 213, 226—227
   sulfur-containing, 227
Glycyrrhetic acid, 229
Gobius criniger (goby), 303
Goby (*Gobius criniger*), 303
Goiter, 101, 107
   cabbage, 116
   cassava, 117
   endemic, 119—120
   goitrogens and, 116—118
   white clover, 117
Goitrin, 15, 17, 23, 25, 105, 110, 111, 116, 118, 119
   antithyroid effect of, 117
   liberation of, 105—107
   milk and, 26
epi-Goitrin, 23
R-Goitrin, 107
Goitrogens, 101—129
   biochemistry of, 101—107
   biosynthesis of, 102—104
   chemical decomposition of, 105—107
   decomposition of, 105—107
   enzymatic decomposition of, 105—107
   experimental goiter and, 116—118

human thyroid and, 118—121
water-contaminating, 121
Gossypium sp., 232
Gossypol, 232
G6PD, see Glucose-6-phosphate dehydrogenase
Grains, see also specific grains, 86, 172, 173
Gramine, 242, 243
Gram-negative bacilli pathogenicity, 278
Grasses, see specific grasses
Grayanotoxins, 224
Griffonia simplicifolia, 9
Grilling of meat, 178
Grisofulvin, 230
Ground nuts, 107
Growth hormone, 89, 90
Growth promotors, 277—286
GSH, see Glutathione
GSSG, see Glutathione disulfide
Guttiferae, 230
Gymnopilus sp., 193, 196
Gymnosperms, 226, 232
Gyromitra esculenta, 193, 198—199, 205
Gyromitrin, 199

H

Haddock, 148
Haemophilis sp., 278
Haff disease, 313, 317
Hake, 148
   red, 177
Halides, 133
Hallucinogens, 231
Halogeton sp., 231
Ham, 152
Hapten, 31
Harding-grass (*Phalaris aquatica*), 242, 243
Harmalines, 218
Harmine, 231
Hay, 92
Hay fever, 222
HCN, see Hydrogen cyanide
Heinz bodies, 73
Heinz-Ehrlich bodies, 73
Helminthosporium vagans, 264
Hemagglutinating test, 32
Hemagglutination specificity, 35
Hemagglutinins, 31
Hemoglobinura, 313
   from fava beans, 317
Hemolysis
   acute, 63
   drug-induced, 74
Hemolytic anemia, 8
Hemolytic reactions to mushrooms, 205
Hepatocellular carcinomas, 51
Heptadecane, 175
Heptapeptides, 200
Herbage, 15
Herbicides, 135

Herring, 148
Hexanal, 199
Hexokinase, 74
N,N'-bis-(p-Hexyloxybenzylidene)-a,a'-bi-p-toluidine (BH x BT), 164
High-dosage penicillin G therapy, 202
High-dosage vitamin therapy, 202
High pressure liquid chromatography (HPLC), 165, 166
Histamine, 230
Homomethionine, 102
Hops (*Humulus lupulus*), 81
Hordenine, 242, 243
Hormones, see also specific hormones, 287—300
  growth, 89, 90
  luteinizing, 84, 92
  sex, 229, 287
  steroid, 228, 257, 287
  thyroid, 101
Horseradish, 17
HPLC, see High pressure liquid chromatography
5HT, see 5-Hydroxytryptamine
5HTP, see 5-Hydroxy-L-tryptophan
Humulus lupulus (hops), 81
Hydrazine, 139
Hydrazones, 199
Hydrocarbons, polycyclic aromatic, see Polycyclic aromatic hydrocarbons
Hydrocyanic acid, 107
Hydrogen-3-benzo(a)pyrene, 175
Hydrogen cyanide (HCN), 226, 227
Hydrolysis, 136, 227, 228
  enzymatic, see Enzymatic hydrolysis
Hydrolytic products from glucosinolates, 15—17
Hydroxyazoxymethane, 46
p-Hydroxybenzyl-GS (sinalbin), 15, 20
2-Hydroxy-3-butenyl-GS, 20
Hydroxynitrile lyase, 107
Hydroxynitriles, 107
2-Hydroxy-2-phenylethyl-GS, 23
Hydroxyproline, 134, 150
3-Hydroxy-4(1H)-pyridone, 10
3-N-3-Hydroxypyridone-4)-2-aminopropionic acid (mimosine), 9—10
5-Hydroxytryptamine (5HT, serotonin), 9
5-Hydroxy-L-tryptophan (5HTP), 3, 8—9
Hyperestrogenism, 86, 88
Hypericin, 230
Hypericum perforatum (St. John's Wort), 230
Hyperplasia, 88
Hypersensitivity
  to antibiotic residues, 277
  to mushrooms, 204—205
Hypertrophy, 87, 88
  thyroidal, 101
  uterine, 81, 84
Hypholoma fasciculare, 203
Hypoglycin A (3-methylenecyclopropylpropionic acid), 7—8

I

Ibogaine, 218
Ibotenic acid, 197
Illudins, 226
6-Iminodialuric acid, see Isouramil
Immunohemolytic reaction to mushrooms, 205
Impaired glycolysis, 74
Incubation of extracts with myrosinase, 109—110
Indenopyrene, 177
Indeno(1,2,3-cd)pyrene, 163, 179
Indian pea (*Lathyrus sativus*), 3—6, 224
Indigofera spicata, 10
Indole alkaloids, 218, 221, 243, 244, 257
Indolylmethyl-GS, 15, 17
3-Indolylmethyl-GS, 25, 26
Indospicine (L-2-amino-6-amidinohexanic acid), 10
Industrial chemicals, 148—149
Inhibitors
  carbohydrase, 39—42
  invertase, 39
  pectinase, 39
Inocybe sp., 194
Inorganic compounds, 213, 231
Intracellular level of ATP, 74
Invertase inhibitors, 39
Iodine, 107, 115, 121
Ipomoea violacea, 231
Isatis tinctoria, 26
Isoenzymes, 105
Isoflavones, 81, 82, 84, 87, 88, 231
Isolectins, 32
Isoleucine, 227
Isolysergic acid, 257
Isoquinoline alkaloids, 218
Isoquinolines, 218
Isothiocyanates, 15, 17, 25, 26, 105, 110, 111, 115—118, 227
  antithyroid effect of, 115
  aromatic, 102
  liberation of, 105
Isouramil, 67, 70—72
  chemical synthesis of, 70—71

J

Jack bean (*Concanavalia ensiformis*), 222
Japanese blowfish or puffer (*Fugu rubripes*), 302, 303
Japanese shiitake (*Lentinus edoles*), 205
Juglans regis (walnut), 107

K

Kale, 121, 172
  Brassica, 15, 26
Kale anemia, 26

Kalmia sp., 226
Ketone, 226
Kinetics of nitrosation, 132—133

L

Lactarius
  deliciosus, 205
  helvus, 205
  necator, 205
  rufus, 205
  sp., 205
  torminosus, 205
Lactones, 82
Laetrile, 226
Lanatoside, 228
Lateral sclerosis, 43, 44
Lathrogens, 3—6
Lathyrism, 3, 4, 6, 222
  classical (neurolathyrism), 4
Lathyrus
  cicera, 3, 4
  clymenum, 3, 4
  latifolius, 4
  odoratus, 4
  sativus (Indian pea), 3—6, 224
  sp., 3, 5, 6, 107, 224
LD, see Lethal dose
Lead, 231
Lebistes reticulatus, 50
Lectins, 222
  beans and, 32—35
  chemical structure of, 31
  detection of, 32
  foods and, 32
  function of, 31—32
  nutritional significance of, 31—38
  Phaseolus vulgaris and, 32—35
  soybean, 32
Lecythis ollaria, 7
Legumes, see also specific species, 3, 32
Leguminosae, 218, 226, 231
Lentinus edodes (Japanese shiitake), 205
Lepiota
  brunneoincarnata, 200
  helveola, 200
  subincarnata, 200
Lepisosteidae, 307
Leptosphaerulina briosiana, 84
Lethal dose (LD), 213
Lettuce, 173
Leucaena leucocephala, 9
Leucine-derived cyanogenic plant constituents, 227
Leucothoe sp., 226
LH, see Luteinizing hormone
Lichen acids, 230
Licorice roots, 81
Liliaceae, 228
Linamarin, 226
Linseed oil, 170

Lipid peroxidation, 74
α-Lipoic acid (thioctic acid), 202
Lipophenolics, 230
Lipoproteins, 306
Liquid smoke flavors, 180—181
Litchi chinensis (lychee), 8
Liver
  cancer of, 50
  carcinoma of cells of, 51
Loline, 265—267
  N-acetyl, 241—243, 266, 268
  N-formyl, 241—253, 266, 268
Loline-type alkaloids, 265—267
Lolium sp., 241, 243, 266
Lophophora williamsii, 231
Lossen, 105
Lotaustralin, 226
Lotus corniculatus, 226
Lung
  adenomas of, 51
  carcinomas of, 51
  "mushroom worker's", 204
Lupine alkaloids, 218
Lupinine, 218
Lupulon, 81
Luteinizing hormone (LH), 84, 92
Lychee (*Litchi chinensis*), 8
Lysergic acid, 231, 257, 259
Lysergic acid peptide alkaloids, 261
Lysine alkaloids, 218
Lysines, 218
  N-methylated, 3

M

Machaerantha sp., 6
Macrozamia
  communis, 55
  sp., 43, 47
  spiralis, 46
Macrozamin, 46, 55
Maize, see Corn
Malonic acid, 103, 229
Malt-coffee, 177
Malted barley, 181
MAM, see Methylazoxymethanol
MAM-Ac, see Methylazoxymethanol-acetate
Mandelonitrile-β-gentiobioside, 226
Manihot
  esculenta, 226
  utilissima, see Cassava
Manioc, see Cassava
Margarine, 171
Marsh marigolds (*Caltha palustris*), 228
Masitis (clover disease), 88
Mass spectrometry (MS), 144, 164, 166
Mastitis, 299
Meatss, see also specific meats, 151, 163, 179
  charcoal-broiled, 161
  curing of, 152

grilling of, 178
pickled, 152
smoked, 152, 161, 169
Melilotus officinalis, 232
β-Mercaptopyruvate (mercaptopyruvate sulfurtransferase), 113
Mercaptopyruvate sulfurtransferase (β-mercaptopyruvate), 113
Mescaline, 220, 231
Metabolic conversion of thiocyanate, 114—115
Metabolism
    aglucones, 111—116
    nitrosamines, 140—141
    N-nitrosomorpholine, 140
    phytoestrogens, 93—94
Methanol-water-cyclohexane, 163
Methemoglobin, 73
Methionine, 7, 102, 103
N,N'-bis-(p-Methoxybenzylidene)-*a,a'*-bi-*p*-toluidine (BMBT), 164
3-(*N*-Methoxy)indolymethyl-GS, 26
Methylaniline, 134
N-Methylaniline, 134
N-Methylated lysines, 3
N-Methylation, 220
Methylation of nucleic acids, 55
Methylazoxymethanol (MAM), 44—46, 48—52, 54—56
    in milk, 52
Methylazoxymethanol-acetate (MAM-Ac), 48, 49, 53, 54
N-Methyl-*N*¹(2-benzothiozolyl)-urea (benzthiazuron), 135
N-Methylbenzylamine, 134
3-Methylbutanal, 199
4'-*O*-Methylcoumestrol, 82
S-Methylcysteine sulfoxide, 26
2-Methylenecyclopropylglycine, 8
3-Methylenecyclopropylpropionic acid (hypoglycin A), 7—8
N-Methyl-*N*-formylhydrazine, 199
7-Methyl-guanine, 55
3-Methyl-6-methoxy-8-hydroxy-3,4-dihydroisocoumarin, 81
Methylselenocysteine, 6
Methylsulfinylpropyl-GS, 20
3-Methylsulfinylpropyl-GS, 25
3-Methylsulfinylpropyl isothiocyanate, 20
3-Methylsulfonylpropyl isothiocyanate (cheirolin), 20
Microcycas sp., 43
Microencephaly, 52, 53
Milk
    antibiotics in, 277—278, 282
    effects of processing of, 297
    glucocorticoids in, 295—299
    goitrin in, 26
    MAM in, 52
    testosterone in, 288—290
    toxicants from, 25—26
Milk-sickness, 226

Mimosine (3-*N*-3-hydroxypyridone-4)-2-aminopropionic acid), 9—10
Miroestrol, 81
Molds, 86, 91
Molybdenum, 231
Mongolism (Down's syndrome), 9
Monocyclic peptides, 200
Monomethylhydrazine, 199
Monoterpenes, 230
Morphine, 213, 218
Morpholine, 133, 134
MS, see Mass spectrometry
Mucuna sp., 8
Mugicha, 177
Muscimol, 197
Mushrooms, see also specific species, 193, 200—202
    allergic contact dermatitis to, 205
    amatoxin-containing, 200
    deliriant, 197
    edible, 171
    gastroenteric irritant-containing, 194
    hemolytic reactions to, 205
    hypersensitivity to, 204—205
    immunohemolytic reaction to, 205
    mutagenicity of, 205
    poisoning from, 193—194
    psilocybin-containing, 196—197
    sensitivity to alcohol induced by, 198
    sleep or comma-associated, 197
    sweat-inducing, 194
    systemic intoxication from, 194—203
    systemic poisoning from, 193—194
    unclassified toxic, 203—204
"Mushroom worker's lung", 204
Mussels, 176, 177
Mustard, 120
Mustard oil glucosides, see Glucosinolates
Mustard oils, 227
Mustard seed, 15
    white (*Brassica hirta* or *Sinapis alba*), 15, 120, 228
Mutagenicity
    cycasin, 54
    mushrooms, 205
Mycoestrogen, 92
Mycotoxins, see also specific mycotoxins by name, 91, 92, 241, 249—261
    Fusarium, 93
Myoglobinuria, 313, 315
    fish-caused, 317
Myristica fragrans, 231
Myristicin, 231
Myrosinase, 15, 24, 101, 105, 108, 111
    inactivation of, 108
    incubation of extracts with, 109—110

N

NADP, 64

NADPH, 64, 73
Naematoloma fasciculare, 203
Naphthalene, 175
"Natural products", 213
Navy beans, 35
Necrosis of fat, 241, 249, 267—269
Neocycasins, 47
Neoglucobrassicin, 105
Nettles, 230
Neurolathyrism (classical lathyrism), 4
Neurotoxicity of cycasin, 52—54
Newts (*Taricha torosa*), 303, 308
New Zealand white clover (*Trifolium repens*), 117
Nicotine, 218
Nicotinic acid, 218
Nikethamide, 135
Nitrate-N, 244
Nitrates, 131, 134, 152
Nitric dioxide, 150
Nitriles, 15, 25, 26, 228
   liberation of, 105
Nitrites, 131, 134, 151, 152
   drug interaction with, 135
6-Nitro-*m*-cresol, 151
Nitrogen fertilization, 243
Nitrosamines, 131—159
   acute toxicity of, 139
   agricultural chemicals and, 148—149
   bacon and, 146—147
   bacterial production of, 135
   biological properties of, 139—141
   carcinogenicity of, 140
   chemistry of, 132—139
   clean-up of, 142
   concentration of, 142
   determination of, 141—145
   environment and, 145—150
   food preservation and, 151—152
   identification of, 143—145
   industrial chemicals and, 148—149
   isolation of, 141—142
   metabolism of, 140—141
   oxidation of, 139
   physical properties of, 135—136
   reduction of, 139
   structure of, 135—136
   synthesis of, 132—135
   tobacco smoke condensates and, 150
N-Nitrosamines, 132, 135
Nitrosation, 132—133
Nitroso compounds
   chemical proeprties of, 137—138
   nonvolatile, 150—151
   physical properties of, 137—138
C-Nitroso compounds, 131, 151
N-Nitroso compounds, 131, 136
S-Nitroso compounds, 131
N-Nitrosomorpholine metabolism, 140
p-Nitrosophenol, 136
N-Nitrosopiperidine, 134, 146, 148
Nitrosoproline, 134

6-Nitroso-4-propylguaiacol, 151
N-Nitrosoureas, 145
N-Nitrosourethanes, 145
Nitrosyl chloride, 132
Nitrosyl tetrafluoroborate, 132
Nonaketides, 230
Nonaromatic amino acids, 227
Nonprotein (uncommon) amino acids, 3, 6, 224
Nonvolatile nitroso compounds, 150—151
Northern blenny (*Stichaeus grigorgjewi*), 306
Nucleic acid methylation, 55
5-Nucleotidase, 56
Nutritional significance of lectins, 31—38

O

Oats, 81, 172
Octadecylsilane (ODS), 165
Octapeptides, 200
Octopus, Australian blue-ringed (*Octopus maculosa*), 303
Octopus maculosa (Australian blue-ringed octopus), 303
ODAP, see 3-*N*-Oxalyl-L-2,3-diaminopropionic acid
ODS, see Octadecylsilane
Oenantha crocata, 231
Oenanthetoxin, 231
Oils
   coconut, 170
   cottonseed, 170
   linseed, 170
   mustard, 227
   palm, 170
   palm kernel, 170
   peanut, 170
   rapeseed, 170
   safflower, 170
   soybean, 170
   sunflower, 163, 170, 179
   vegetable, 169—171
Oilseed crops, 15
Oilseed meals, 23—24
Oleandrin, 228
Oligosaccharides, 221
Omphalotus
   olearius, 204
   sp., 194
Onion volatiles, 107
Opium poppy, 213
Orally administered antibiotics, 278
Oranges, 172
Orchardgrass (*Dactylis glomerata*), 241
Organic acids, 231, 241
Ornithine, 3, 218
Orotic acid incorporation, 55
Osouramil, 68
Osteolathyrism, 4
Oxalates, 231
Oxalidaceae, 231
Oxalis sp., 231

3-*N*-Oxalyl-L-2,3-diaminopropionic acid (ODAP), 4—6
Oxazolidinethione, see Goitrin
Oxazolidine-3-thione, see Goitrin
Oxidation
  GSH, 72, 73
  nitrosamine, 139
Oxytetracycline, 135
Oysters, 175, 177

P

PAH, see Polycyclic aromatic hydrocarons
Palm (*Phoenix dactylifera*) seeds, 81
Palm kernel oil, 170
Palm oil, 170
Panaeolus sp., 196
Pantherine syndrome, 197
Papain, 15
Papaveraceae, 218
Papaverine, 218
Paper chromatography, 49, 115, 162, 266
Paralytic shellfish poison, 305
Paranthias farcifer, 308
Parkinson's disease, 8
Pathogenicity of gram-negative bacilli, 278
Patulin, 230
Paxillus involutus, 205
Peanut meal, 230
Peanut oil, 170
Peanut products, 171
Peanuts, 178
Peas, see also specific types, 3, 5, 6, 24
  Indian (*Lathyrus sativus*), 3—6, 224
Pectinase inhibitor, 39
Penicillin, 277
Penicillin G therapy, 202
Penniclavin, 257, 259
Pentacyclic triterpenes, 229
Pentanal, 199
Pepper, 148
Peptide alkaloids, 218
  lysergic acid, 261
Peptides, 222
  monocyclic, 200
Perciformes, 306
Perlolidine, 241, 242, 268
Perloline, 241—243, 261—266, 268
Perloline mercurichloride, 264
Peroxidation of lipids, 74
Perylene, 162—165, 170, 179
Pesticides, see also specific pesticides, 135
Petroleum-linked benzo(a)pyrene, 175
Phalaris
  aquatica (Harding-grass), 242, 243
  arundinacea, 242
  sp., 242, 243
  tuberosa, 243
"Phalaris staggers", 242
Phallotoxins, 200

Pharmacology of tetrodotoxin, 304—306
Phaseolus vulgaris (garden beans), 32—35
Phenanthrene, 170, 179, 181
Phenols, 152, 242
Phenylacetaldehyde oxime, 103
Phenylalanine, 102, 103, 218, 220, 226
N,N'-bis(*p*-Phenylbenzylidene)-*a,a'*-bi-*p*-toluidine (BPhBT), 164
β-Phenylethylamine, 231
2-Phenylethyl-GS, 23
2-Phenylethyl isothiocyante, 23
Phenylhydrazine, 74
5-Phenyloxazolidinethione, 23
Phenylpropenes, 231
3-Phenyl-2-thiohydantoin, 115
Phloretin, 84
Phloridzin, 84
Phoenix dactylifera (palm), 81
Phorbol, 226
Photochemistry, 139
Photodermatitis, 230
Photosensitive compounds, 213
Photosensitization, 230
2-Phthalimido-propyltrichlorosilane (PPS), 166
Phylloerythrin, 230
Physical properties
  cycasin, 49
  nitrosamines, 135—136
  nitroso compounds, 137—138
Physiologic effects of phytoestrogens, 87
Physostigmine, 218
Phytoestrogens, 81—84
  beneficial effects of, 87
  carcinogenicity of, 93
  detection of, 93—94
  metabolism of, 93—94
  physiologic effects of, 87
  "toxic" effects of, 87—92
Phytolacca americana (pokeweed), 229
Phytoplankton, 173
Pickled meats, 152
Picrotoxinin, 226
Pigments from flowers, 84
Pike (*Esox lucius*), 308
Pinon (*Araucaria araucana*), 107
Piperazine, 134
Piperidine, 134
Piperidine alkaloids, 218
Plants, see also specific types, specific species
  biosynthesis of PAH by, 172, 173
  chemical substances of, 213—240
  genotypes of, 243
  leucine-derived cyanogenic constituents of, 227
  PAH in, 171—173
  reactions of skin to, 230
  synthesis of PAH by, 171
Pleurotus ostreatus, 204
Pluteus sp., 196
Poison ivy, 230
Poison oak, 230
Poison sumac, 230

Pokeweed (*Phytolacca americana*), 229
Polarography, 49, 143
Polyacetylenes, 231
Polychlorinated biphenyls, 121
Polycyclic aromatic hydrocarbons (PAH), see also specific types, 161—190
  aquatic environment and, 173
  bacterial synthesis of, 171
  beverages and, 181
  biosynthesis of by plants, 172, 173
  carcinogenicity of, 162
  food additives and, 161
  liquid smoke flavors and, 180—181
  plants and, 171—173
  seafoods and, 173—177
  sources of, 161
  synthesis of, 171—173
  vegetable fats and, 169—171
  vegetable oils and, 169—171
  yeasts and, 179—180
Polygonaceae, 231
Polyketides, 213, 229—230
Polypeptides, 200
Polysulfides, 107
Pomegranate (*Punica granatum*) fruit, 81
Poppy, 213
Potassium, 231
Potassium sorbate, 152
Potatoes, 32, 171
Poultry, 163
PPS, see 2-Phthalimido-propyltrichlorosilane
Pratensein, 82
Precatory bean (*Abrus precatorius*), 222
Preformed thiocyanate, 114, 119
Preservatives
  nitrosamines and, 151—152
  PAH and, 161
Primaquine, 73, 74
Primary amines, 133, 150
Primeverose (6-(β-D-Xylopyranoxyl)-D-glucopyranose), 46
Processing of milk, 297
Prodenia eridania (southern armyworm), 8
Progesterone, 81
Progoitrin, 20, 23, 105
epi-Progoitrin, 17, 18, 20, 26, 105
Proline, 134, 150, 218
Propionitrile, 224
n-Propyl-disulfide, 107
Protein amino acids, 3, 220
Proteins, see also specific proteins, 31, 213, 222
  epithiospecifier, 105
  foods rich in, 163
  inhibition of synthesis of, 55
  synthesis of, 55
Proto-alkaloids (biological amines), 218, 220
Protoanemonin, 228
Protoanemonin glucosides, 228
Protoxins, 199
Prunasin, 226
Prunes, 107

Prunus amygdalus, 226
Psalliota
  capestris, 204
  hortensis, 204
Pseudo alkaloids, 218
  steroidal, 221
Pseudopelletierine, 218
Pseudopeziza medicagnis, 84
Psilocin, 196
Psilocybe
  mexicana, 196
  sp., 196
Psilocybin, 196, 231
  mushrooms containing, 196—197
Pteridium
  aquilinum, 222
  sp., 226
Pueraria mirifica, 81
Puffer fish, 302, 303
Punica granatum (pomegranate), 81
PYR, 146, 147, 148
Pyran, 228
Pyrene, 162, 170—172, 179—181
Pyrene-fluoranthene, 164
Pyridoxal, 5
Pyridoxal phosphate, 10
Pyridoxine, 199
Pyrrolidine, 134, 218
Pyrrolizidines, 266, 267

Q

Quail (*Coturnix coturnix*), 313
Quail poisoning (coturnism), 313—319
Quaternary ammonium compounds, 133—134, 150
Quercus sp., 232
Quinolizidines, 218

R

Radioimmunoassay, 200
Radiomimetic effects of cycasin, 54
Radish, 17, 120
Ranunculaceae, 218, 228
Ranunculin, 228
Ranunculus sp., 228
Rape, 120
  Brassica napus, 24
  turnip, 120
Rapeseed, 15, 101, 120
Rapeseed oil, 170
Raphanus sativus, 120
Red blood cells
  G6PD-deficient, 65
  survival of, 74
Red hake, 177
Reductic acid, 68
Reduction of nitrosamines, 139
Reductones, 69

Reed canarygrass alkaloids, 241—247
Reproduction effects, 231
Resedaceae, 227
Resorcyclic acid, 82
Resorcyclic acid lactones, 82
Reticuloendothelial system, 73
Rheum sp., 231
Rhizobium sp., 31
Rhizoctonia solani, 264, 266
Rhodanese, 112, 113, 226
Rhododendron sp., 226
Rice, 81
Ricin, 32, 222
RNA-polymerase competition binding assay, 200
Roasted peanuts, 178
Roasting, 178
Rosaceae, 226
Rosidae, 226
Rubiaceae, 218
Rumex sp., 231
Rutabagas, see *Brassica napus*
Rye, 171, 173, 178
Ryegrass, 261
"Ryegrass staggers", 241

S

Sable, 148
Safflower oil, 170
Salad greens, 171, 172
Salamandriade, 303
Salmon, 148
Salmonella
　sp., 278
　typhimurium, 54
Salmonella/mammallian microsome assay, 93
Salsola sp., 231
Sambrunigrin, 226
Sapogenins, 226
Saponins, 213, 228—229
　steroidal, 231
Sarcosine, 151
Scallops, 175, 177
Schizothorax intermedius (snow trout), 308
Scleroderma aurantium, 204
Sclerosis, 43, 44
SCN, 15, 17, 23, 26
Scotch whisky, 181
Scrophulariaceae, 228
Scup, 177
Sea bass, 177
Seafoods, see also specific seafoods
　PAH in, 173—177
Sea scallops, 175, 177
Secondary amines, 139
"Secondary products", 213
Selenium, 6, 7, 74, 231
Selenoamino acids, 6—7
Selenocystathionine, 6, 7
Selenocystine, 7

Selenomethionine, 7
Selenosis, 6
Sensitivity
　to alcohol induced by mushrooms, 198
　to drugs, 63
Separation of glucosinolates, 109
Serotonin, see 5-Hydroxytryptamine
Serranidae, 308
Sesame meal, 81
Sesquiterpenes, 224, 226, 230
Sex hormones, 229, 287
Shad, 148
Shellfish, 175, 177
　paralytic poisoning from, 305
Simulated food systems, 134—135
Sinalbin (*p*-hydroxybenzyl-GS), 15, 20
Sinapis alba (white mustard seed), 15, 228
Sinigrin, 17, 103, 105, 228
B-Sitosterol, 82
Skin reactions to plants, 230
Sleep associated with deliriant mushrooms, 197
Smoked foods, 152, 161, 167—169, 179
Smoke flavors, 180—181
Smutgrass (*Sporobolus poiretti*), 241
Snow trout (*Schizothorax intermedius*), 308
Sodium, 231
Sodium nitrite, 134, 152
Solanaceae, 218
Solanine, 221
Solvents, 163
Sorghum, 81, 92, 107, 226
Southern armyworm (*Prodenia eridania*), 8
Soybean lectin, 32
Soybean oil, 170
Soybeans, 81, 107, 173
Sparteine, 218
Spectrophotometry, see also Mass spectrometry, 200
　ultraviolet, 164, 166
Sphacelia typhina, 241
Sphaeroides
　maculatus, 303
　testudineus, 303
Spinach, 172
Sporobolus poiretii (smutgrass), 241
Staggers, 241, 242
Staphylococcus aureus, 222
Steaks, 178
Steroidal alkaloids, 218, 224
　pseudo, 221
Steroidal saponins, 231
Steroid-binding globulin, 83
Steroid hormones, 228, 257, 287
Stichaeidae, 306
Stichaeus grigorgjewi (northern blenny or stickelback), 306
Stickelback (*Stichaeus grigorgjewi*), 306
St. John's Wort (*Hypericum perforatum*), 230
Stress of movement of cattle, 299
Stropharia coronilla, 204
Strychnine, 218
N,N-Substituted hydrazine, 139

Subterranean clover, 84
Sugar cane, 107
Sugars, see also specific sugars, 226, 228, 229
Sulfate, 105
N-Sulfate ester, 103
3-(N-Sulfonate)indolylmethyl-GS, 26
Sulfur amino acids, 6, 7
Sulfur-35-p-brom-phenylisothiocyanate, 115
Sulfur-containing glycosides, 227
Sulfur donors, 113
Sulfur-35-methionine, 103
Sulfur-35-thiocyanate, 115
Summer syndrome, 241, 249, 267, 268
Sunflower oil, 163, 170, 179
Sweat-inducing mushrooms, 194
Systemic mushroom intoxications
    with delayed onset, 198—203
    with rapid onset, 194—198
Systemic mushroom poisoning, 193—194

T

Tall fescue (*Festuca arundinacea*), 249—273
    alkaloids in, 241—247
Tannins, 232
Tar, 177
Taricha
    rivularis, 303
    torosa (California newt), 303, 308
Taxine, 221
Taxiphyllin, 226
Taxus sp., 226
T-bone steaks, 178
Temperature effect on nitrosation reaction, 133
Tench (*Tinca tinca*), 308
Terpenoids, 213, 224—226
Tertiary amines, 133, 150
Testosterone, 287—294
    blood levels of, 288
    milk and, 288—290
    tissue and, 288—290
Tetracyclines, 230, 277, 278
Δ^6-Tetrahydra cannabinol, 231
delta-9-Tetrahydra cannabinol, 81
Tetraodontiformes, 302
Tetrodotoxin, 301—306, 308
    chemistry of, 303—304
    detection of, 304—305
    humans and, 305—306
    mechanism of action of, 305
    pharmacology of, 304—306
    tissues and, 304
Thatched barnacles, 175
Therapy, see also specific types
    penicillin G, 202
    vitamin, 202
Thermal energy analyzer, 145
Thiamine deficiency, 222
Thin-layer chromatography (TLC), 49, 142, 143, 162, 163, 200, 265, 266

Thioctic acid (α-lipoic acid), 202
Thiocyanate, 26, 110, 112, 115—118, 133, 226
    antithyroid effect of, 117
    balance of, 115
    distribution of, 114
    endogenous formation of, 112—113
    exogenous preformed, 114, 119
    extracellular fluid and, 115
    ions of, 23
    liberation of, 105
    metabolic conversion of, 114—115
Thioglucose, 103
Thioglucosidase, see Myrosinase
Thioglucosidase glucohydrolase, see Myrosinase
Thioglucoside glucohydrolase, see Myrosinase
Thioglucosides, see Glucosinolates
Thioglycolic acid, 115
2-Thiohydantoins, 115
Thiohydroximide, 103
Thiohydroximyl-*O*-sulfate, 101
Thiosulfatecyanide sulfur transsulfurase, 113
Thymeliaceae, 226
Thyroid
    aglucones and, 118
    goitrogens and, 118—121
    hypertrophy of, 101
Thyroid hormone, 101
Thyroid peroxidase, 118
Thyroxine, 118
Tinca tinca (tench), 308
Tissues, see also specific tissues
    testosterone in, 288—290
    tetrodotoxin in, 304
TLC, see Thin-layer chromatography
Tobacco, 173
    Burley, 150
Tobacco smoke condensate nitrosamines, 150
Tomatine, 221
Tomatoes, 172
Toxicodendron sp., 230
Tremetone, 226
Trichothecenes, 91, 93
Trifolium
    repens (New Zealand white clover), 117
    subterraneum, 231
2,4,5-Trihydroxy-6-aminopyrimidine 5-(β-D-glucopyranoside, 67
Triose reductone, 68
Triphenylene, 164, 180
Triphenylene-crysene-benz(a)anthracene, 165
Triterpenes, 229
Triterpenoid, 221
Tropanes, 218
Trout, snow (*Schizothorax intermedius*), 308
True alkaloids, 218
Tryptamine, 231, 242, 243
Tryptamine alkaloids, 242
Tryptophan, 218, 220, 242
TSH, 218
T-2 toxin, 255
Tumefaction, 84

Turnip rape, 120
Turnips, see also *Brassica campestris*, 121
Tyrosinase, 8
Tyrosine, 115, 218, 220, 226, 242

U

Ultraviolet spectrophotometry, 164, 166
Umbelliferae, 231
Unclassified toxic mushrooms, 203—204
Uncommon (nonprotein) amino acids, 3, 6, 224
Unhydrolyzed allyl-GS, 24
Urethane, 93
Uridine triphosphate (UTP) incorporation, 55
Urishiols, 230
Uromyces striatus, 84
Urticaceae, 230
Uterine cytosol, 84
Uterine hypertrophy, 81, 84
Uterotropic activity, 82
UTP, see Uridine triphosphate

V

Vaginal cornification, 81
Valine, 115, 227
Vegetable fats, 169—171
Vegetable oils, 169—171
Venturia inaequalis, 84
Vernolepin, 224
Verpa bohemica, 198, 204
Vetch (*Vicia sativa*), 5, 6, 66, 67
Vicia
  fava (broad bean), 8, 63, 65—72
  sativa (vetch), 5, 6, 66, 67
Vicine, 66—70
Vinyl-oxazolidine-2-thione, 101, 105
5-Vinyloxazolidinethione, see Goitrin
L-5-Vinyl-2-thiooxazolidone, 105
Vitamin b
  deficiency of, 22
  uptake of, 35
Vitamins, see also specific vitamins
  high-dosage, 202
Volatiles of onion, 107
Vulvar tumefaction, 84
Vulvovaginitis, 91

W

Walnut (*Juglans regia*), 107
Water-contaminating goitrogens of bacterial origin, 121
Wheat, 81, 171—173, 178
Wheat germ, 32
Whiskies, 181
White clover, 107
  New Zealand (*Trifolium repens*), 117

White clover goiter, 117
White herring, 148
White mustard seed, 15, 120, 228

X

X-ray diffraction studies, 136
6-(β-D-Xylopyranosyl)-D-glucopyranose (primeverose), 46

Y

Yams, 107
Yeast, 163
  PAH in, 179—180
Yellow croaker, 148
Yohimbine, 218

Z

Zamia
  floridana, 50
  sp., 9, 43, 47
Zearalenol, 81, 82, 84, 87, 92, 93
Zearalenone, 81—84, 86, 87, 91—94
  carbon-14-labeled, 94
  chemical structure of, 93
  detection of, 93